SPIRITUALITY AND RELIGION WITHIN THE CULTURE OF MEDICINE

The editors express gratitude to the John Templeton Foundation for support in producing this volume. We also thank our colleagues at Harvard University's Initiative on Health, Religion, and Spirituality.

Spirituality and Religion Within the Culture of Medicine

FROM EVIDENCE TO PRACTICE

Edited by

Michael J. Balboni, Ph.D.
INSTRUCTOR, DEPARTMENT OF PSYCHIATRY
HARVARD MEDICAL SCHOOL
INSTRUCTOR, PSYCHOSOCIAL ONCOLOGY AND PALLIATIVE CARE
DANA-FARBER CANCER INSTITUTE
BRIGHAM AND WOMEN'S HOSPITAL

John R. Peteet, M.D.
ASSOCIATE PROFESSOR OF PSYCHIATRY
HARVARD MEDICAL SCHOOL
FELLOWSHIP SITE DIRECTOR, ADULT PSYCHOSOCIAL ONCOLOGY
DEPARTMENT OF PSYCHOSOCIAL ONCOLOGY AND PALLIATIVE CARE
BRIGHAM AND WOMEN'S HOSPITAL

OXFORD
UNIVERSITY PRESS

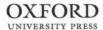
OXFORD
UNIVERSITY PRESS

Oxford University Press is a department of the University of Oxford. It furthers
the University's objective of excellence in research, scholarship, and education
by publishing worldwide. Oxford is a registered trade mark of Oxford University
Press in the UK and certain other countries.

Published in the United States of America by Oxford University Press
198 Madison Avenue, New York, NY 10016, United States of America.

CIP data is on file at the Library of Congress
ISBN 978–0–19–027243–2 (hardcover) | ISBN 978–0–19–755396–1 (paperback)

9 8 7 6 5 4 3 2
Printed in the United States of America

CONTENTS

PART TWO: SCHOLARLY DISCIPLINARY
PERSPECTIVES

PART THREE: SYNTHESIS AND INTEGRATION

CONTRIBUTORS

Alan B. Astrow, M.D.
Chief, Hematology/Medical Oncology
New York-Presbyterian Brooklyn
  Methodist Hospital
Professor of Clinical Medicine, Weill
  Cornell Medical College
Brooklyn, New York

Michael J. Balboni, Ph.D.
Instructor, Department of Psychiatry
Harvard Medical School
Instructor, Psychosocial Oncology
  and Palliative Care
Dana-Farber Cancer Institute
Brigham and Women's Hospital
Boston, Massachusetts

Tracy A. Balboni, M.D., M.P.H.
Associate Professor
Radiation Oncology
Harvard Medical School
Brigham and Women's Hospital
Dana-Farber Cancer Institute
Boston, Massachusetts

Raymond Barfield, M.D., Ph.D.
Associate Professor of Pediatrics
  and Christian Philosophy
Pediatric Oncology and Palliative Care
Director, Medical Humanities
Trent Center for Bioethics, Medical
  Humanities, and History of Medicine
Duke University
Durham, North Carolina

Linda L. Barnes, M.T.S., M.A., Ph.D.
Professor, Department of Family Medicine
Boston University School of Medicine
Graduate Division of Religious Studies
Boston University
Boston, Massachusetts

Sarah Jean Barton, M.T.S., M.S., O.T.R/L.
Department of Physical Therapy and
  Occupational Therapy
Duke University Health System
Duke Divinity School
Duke University
Durham, North Carolina

Dan G. Blazer, M.D., Ph.D.
JP Gibbons Professor of Psychiatry
  and Behavioral Sciences
Duke University School of Medicine
Duke University
Durham, North Carolina

Philip Choi, M.D.
Department of Medicine
Duke University School of Medicine
Durham, North Carolina

Alexandra Cist, M.D.
Pulmonary & Critical Care Medicine
Massachusetts General Hospital
Center for Bioethics
Harvard Medical School
Boston, Massachusetts

Farr A. Curlin, M.D.
Josiah C. Trent Professor of Medical
    Humanities
Co-Director, Theology, Medicine,
    and Culture Initiative
Duke University
Durham, North Carolina

Timothy P. Daaleman, D.O., M.P.H.
Professor and Vice Chair
Department of Family Medicine
University of North Carolina at Chapel Hhill
Chapel Hill, North Carolina

Lydia S. Dugdale, M.D.
Assistant Professor and Associate Director
    for the Program for Biomedical Ethics
Yale School of Medicine
Yale University
New Haven, Connecticut

Gary B. Ferngren, Ph.D.
Professor of History
School of History, Philosophy, and Religion
Oregon State University
Corvallis, Oregon

Professor of the History of Medicine
Department of History of Medicine, Natural
    History, and Culturology
I.M. Sechenov First Moscow State Medical
    University
Moscow, Russia

Marta Herschkopf, M.D., M.St.
Beth Israel Deaconess Medical Center
Center for Bioethics
Harvard Medical School
Boston, Massachusetts

Jonathan B. Imber, Ph.D.
Jean Glasscock Professor of Sociology
Wellesley College
Editor-in-Chief, *Society*
Wellesley, Massachusetts

Najmeh Jafari, M.D.
Post-Doctorate Scientist
George Washington Institute for Spirituality
    and Health
The George Washington University School of
    Medicine and Health Sciences

Warren Kinghorn, M.D., Th.D.
Associate Research Professor of Psychiatry
    and Pastoral and Moral Theology
Duke Divinity School
Duke University
Durham, North Carolina

Harold G. Koenig, M.D.
Professor of Psychiatry & Behavioral Sciences
    Associate Professor of Medicine Director,
    Center for Spirituality, Theology,
    and Health
Duke University Medical Center
Durham, North Carolina, USA
Adjunct Professor, King Abdulaziz University
Jeddah, Saudi Arabia
Adjunct Professor of Public Health, Ningxia
    Medical University
Yinchuan, P.R. China

Lance D. Laird, M.Div., Th.D.
Assistant Professor, Department
    of Family Medicine
Boston University School of Medicine
Graduate Division of Religious Studies
Boston University
Boston, Massachusetts

James A. Marcum, Ph.D.
Department of Philosophy
Baylor University
Waco, Texas

Gary Maslow, M.D., M.P.H.
Assistant Professor of Pediatrics and
  Psychiatry and Behavioral Sciences
Co-Division Director, Division of Child
  and Family Mental Health and
  Developmental Neurosciences
Department of Psychiatry and Behavioral
  Sciences
Duke University School of Medicine
Durham, North Carolina

Brett McCarty, M.Div.
Duke Divinity School
Duke University
Durham, North Carolina

Michael P. Moreland, M.A., Ph.D., J.D.
Professor of Law
Villanova University
Villanova, Pennsylvania

Kenneth Pargament, Ph.D.
Professor of Psychology
Bowling Green University
Bowling Green, Ohio

Rachel Peragallo, M.D., M.S.
Department of Obstetrics and Gynecology
University of North Carolina School
  of Medicine
Chapel Hill, North Carolina

John R. Peteet, M.D.
Department of Psychiatry
Harvard Medical School
Department of Psychosocial Oncology
  and Palliative Care
Brigham and Women's Hospital
Boston, Massachusetts

Christina Puchalski, M.D., M.S.
Director, George Washington Institute
  for Spirituality and Health
Professor, Dept of Medicine and Health
  Services
George Washington University School
  of Medicine
Professor, Health Leadership and
  Management
George Washington University School
  of Public Health
George Washington University
Washington, DC

Lucy Selman, Ph.D.
Research Fellow,
School of Social and Community Medicine,
University of Bristol,
Bristol, UK

O. Carter Snead, J.D.
William P. and Hazel B. White Director
Center for Ethics and Culture
Notre Dame Law School
University of Notre Dame
Notre Dame, Indiana

Daniel P. Sulmasy, M.D., Ph.D.
André Hellengers Professor
  of Biomedical Ethics
Georgetown University
Washington, DC

John Swinton, Ph.D., R.M.N., R.M.N.D.
School of Divinity, History, and Philosophy
King's College
University of Aberdeen
Aberdeen, United Kingdom

John Tarpley, M.D.
Department of Surgery
Vanderbilt University Medical Center
Nashville, Tennessee

Margaret Tarpley
Department of Surgery
Vanderbilt University Medical Center
Nashville, Tennessee

John Thorp, M.D.
Department of Obstetrics and Gynecology
University of North Carolina School
    of Medicine
Chapel Hill, North Carolina

Kelly M. Trevino, Ph.D.
Joan and Sanford I. Weill Department
    of Medicine
Weill Cornell Medical College
New York Presbyterian Hospital
New York, New York

Lynne Vanderpot, Ph.D.
University of Aberdeen
Aberdeen, United Kingdom

Tyler J. VanderWeele, Ph.D.
Departments of Epidemiology
    and Biostatistics
Harvard T.H. Chan School of Public Health
Director, Program on Integrative Knowledge
    and Human Flourishing
Institute of Quantitative Social Science
Harvard University
Boston, Massachusetts

CHAPTER 1

INTRODUCTION

Michael J. Balboni and John R. Peteet

BACKGROUND FOR THE BOOK

There has long been a gap between religion and spirituality on the one hand, and academic medicine on the other. Thirty or forty years ago at elite American universities, a physician could not whisper about these issues without expecting ridicule or worse. Religion was largely understood to belong in the private realm, and medicine was practiced by physician scientists who were objective in their approach toward disease and neutral in their professional stance regarding religion (Imber, 2008). While some still vigorously maintain this perspective (Lawrence, 2002; Sloan, 2006), there has been a noticeable shift taking place both in the wider culture and within the medical profession itself that appears to allow for a new consideration of the relationship between medicine and spirituality. Evidence suggests that while there is still a major gap in professional practices pertaining to engagement with patient spirituality, there are some signs of growing openness within the medical profession to consider the place of patient spirituality within the experience of illness (M. J. Balboni et al., 2013; Curlin et al., 2007).

What are the reasons for this shift? There are several potential causes, of which we highlight three. First, the golden age of medicine that engendered enormous public confidence in science and medical progress may now be in some decline (Burnham, 1982). Despite tremendous advances in public health and medical technologies, suffering, old age, and death remain inevitable. As Western culture begins to come to terms with its denial of suffering and death (Becker, 1973; Hayslip, 2003), patients and medical professionals are forced to realize the limits of medicine and employ a wider lens of meaning that deals with human finitude and mortality, especially within chronic and serious illness (Sulmasy, 2006). This may explain, for example, why palliative care has greatly expanded over the past decade, how it includes spiritual care among its core domains of practice (National Consensus Project, 2009), and how the Joint Commission, a major hospital accrediting agency in the United States, has been increasingly requiring hospitals to address patient spirituality (Joint Commission, 2011). Second, within the American context, the demographics of the medical profession have been shifting to the point where now half of medical students are female, and the numbers of ethnic and racial minorities are growing (Curlin, Lantos, Roach, Sellergren, & Chin, 2005). Females and minorities are historically more religious or spiritual, and such demographic shifts may be slowly altering the religious demographic of the medical profession. Physicians who are more religious or spiritual themselves are likely to be more predisposed to see their patients' spirituality and have greater openness to respond to it (Curlin et al., 2007). These demographic changes ironically cut across secular narratives that suggest that the direction of Western society is increasingly less religious (Martin, 1978). The opposite appears to be happening among physicians in the United States. Finally, there has been a growing body of medical research stretching back into the 1990s that has consistently demonstrated a relationship between spirituality and health (Koenig, King, & Carson, 2012). While this research has been appropriately criticized for its limitations (Sloan, 2006; Sloan, Bagiella, & Powell, 1999), research throughout the field is also becoming increasingly sophisticated in its conceptualization, measurement, and ability to demonstrate relationships with health outcomes. Research has also reported problems and tensions related to religion and health, which demonstrates that this new research field is not merely about advancing a pro-religious hidden agenda but is inclusive of how religion can be problematic. For some of these reasons the medical guild appears more open to considering this intersection than perhaps at any time during the twentieth century.

Reflective of these changes, four of the ten highest ranked universities in the United States now have faculty-led active programs focusing on the intersection of spirituality and health. Elite universities including Duke, the University of Chicago, Yale, and Harvard have established new programs and centers, with an increasing number of faculty and students engaging in research, scholarship, coursework, and advancing national dialogue.[1] Such programs have also been increasingly interdisciplinary, including a wide range of academic disciplines and faculty across medical, public health, and divinity schools. These are joined by a wide range of institutional programs that have been leading the way for years such as the Institute for Spirituality and Health at Texas Medical Center, the George Washington Institute for Spirituality and Health, Emory's Religion and Public Health Collaborative, and Loyola University Chicago's Physician Vocation Program.[2] In addition, the Conference on Medicine and Religion, begun in 2012, is a growing venue that has provided physicians, nurses, health scientists, ethicists, and theologians an opportunity to engage one another through scholarship and research.[3] Many of these are small examples of larger shifts that appear to be taking place at this controversial intersection of medicine and faith.

Our observations of these changes originated during the lecture series sponsored by the Harvard Initiative on Health, Religion, and Spirituality between 2013 and 2016 and funded by the John Templeton Foundation. The lecture series included academic physicians from different specialties who reviewed the evidence for a relationship between religion and spirituality within their medical area of expertise (e.g., surgery, psychiatry, palliative care, etc.) and considered its personal and practical implications in the care of patients.[4] To our surprise, the lecture series attracted nearly 1,500 Harvard faculty and students (and many thousands who have since watched videos of the lectures through our Initiative website) as it sought to create conversation oriented around the question, *What do medicine and spirituality have to do with one another?* One of the most intriguing aspects of the series was the response to their Grand Rounds at leading Harvard teaching hospitals such as Massachusetts General Hospital, Brigham and Women's Hospital, Beth Israel Deaconness Medical Center, and Dana-Farber Cancer Institute. Many of those who attended the Grand Rounds presentations were not predisposed to consider this intersection, yet they consistently provided positive feedback as they were engaged by the empirical work related to their medical subspecialty. Most were not aware of existing research but showed surprising openness to collaborate in hosting the lectures and to consider methodologically rigorous scientific evidence.

Discussion of these issues convinced us both of the broad relevance of religion and spirituality for understanding the culture of medicine, and of the need for establishing evidence based recommendations for clinicians practicing in different contexts. Interest continues to grow in the relationship between religion and health outcomes, varieties of integrative medicine, and ethical challenges arising at the interface between medicine, religion, and spirituality. Yet consensus is frequently lacking about how to understand the place of religion and spirituality within the culture of medicine, or how to implement research findings across widely diverse forms of clinical practice— from assistance at birth to mental health treatment to care at the end of life.

CONCEPTUALIZING RELIGION AND SPIRITUALITY

To begin with, there is a lack of consensus about defining religion and spirituality. Two differing approaches have emerged in considering the relationship of medicine, religion, and spirituality. Some emphasize the concept of "religion and medicine," whereas others highlight the idea of "spirituality and medicine." Proponents of religion resist the concept of spirituality in part because they worry about its connotations of individualism and seeming lack of connection to tradition or theology. There is a legitimate concern that when de-emphasizing the concept of religion, the particular beliefs and practices of a particular religious faith will be co-opted or reduced to something thin and amorphous (Hall, Koenig, & Meador, 2004). Proponents of spirituality, on the other hand, understand religion to be only one of multiple expressions of a larger, broadly conceived category. This view has developed alongside a widening recognition of the diverse cultural and religious practices and beliefs operating in Western society. Proponents of this approach suggest that understanding spirituality this way enables dialogue among different religious groups by emphasizing the common starting point of a shared humanity and softening stark differences responsible for unnecessary conflict. Emphasizing spirituality over religion also includes those who do not easily fit into religious categories or definitions, such as those who describe themselves as "spiritual, not religious." On this view, an inclusive approach facilitates the provision of spiritual care within pluralistic contexts to those who either do not identify with, or are for various reason alienated from, a religious tradition.

The term *religion*, which in its modern usage can be traced to the Enlightenment (Cavanaugh, 2009; Smith, 1998), has been a highly debated construct among religious scholars over the past century. However, as the religious historian Martin Marty has argued, it is generally marked by five characteristics (Marty & Moore, 2000): a focus on "ultimate concern," important roles for myth and symbol, reliance on rite and ceremony, behavioral or ethical obligations, and the presence and role of community (Marty & Moore, 2000). The most critical building block of Marty's definition is the focus on "ultimate concern." He indicates that this refers to an "overarching purpose," what we care about most, or what we are willing to die for (Marty & Moore, 2000). The phrase comes from Harvard theologian Paul Tillich, who taught that religion was about what was of ultimate concern, one's relationship to which would bring ultimate fulfilment

(Tillich, 1958). Tillich argued that "Religion, in the largest and most basic sense of the word, is ultimate concern". In Marty and in Tillich's views, ultimate concern may include not only self-described religious systems such as Christianity or Islam, but also ideologies such as Marxism or New Age astrology, which may not consider themselves religious at all. The object of ultimate concern varies according to religion, but its distinguishing mark is that which is "ultimate" in contrast to what a person identifies as ordinary, mundane, or penultimate ends or concerns. This perception of ultimacy, in Marty's understanding, will eventually become systematized and codified in a social ordering that is categorized as a religion or religious-like phenomenon. Thus, religion is life centered on what is ultimate and therefore brings human fulfilment. The other four characteristics in Marty's definition of religion flow out of and support this primary identifying mark.[5] In other words, every "ultimate concern" will eventually produce its own dogmas, practices, rituals, symbols, relationships, and institutional support structures.

In contrast to the idea of religion, since the 1970s there has been growing use of the term *spirituality* (McGinn, 2005). Spirituality has been both a historically Christian term (McGinn, 2005; Schneiders, 2003) and one favored by those in the New Age movement (McGinn, 2005; Peteet & D'Ambra, 2011). It has been increasingly employed as a construct consciously distinguished from religion (Wuthnow, 1998). A 2009 consensus conference on spirituality for palliative care produced a broad definition for spirituality as the aspect of humanity that refers to the way individuals seek and express meaning and purpose, and the way they experience their connectedness to the moment, to self, to others, to nature, and to the significant or sacred (C. Puchalski et al., 2009; C. M. Puchalski & Ferrell, 2010). Spirituality may include religion and other worldviews but also encompasses far more general ways in which these experiences are expressed, including through the arts, relationships with nature and others—and for some, through the concept of secular humanism, which emphasizes reason, scientific inquiry, individual freedom and responsibility, human values, compassion, and the needs for tolerance and cooperation. This approach understands spirituality to be rooted in the human person prior to the development of religious or theological formulations (Schneiders, 2003; Sulmasy, 2006; Van Ness, 1996). Schneiders says that spirituality "has become a generic term for the actualization in life of the human capacity for self-transcendence, regardless of whether that experience is religious or not" (Schneiders, 2003). She argues that spirituality is a human seeking after self-transcendence cutting across cultural and religious traditions. Peter Van Ness serves as an example of a scholar who has approached spirituality as fundamentally independent and without necessary engagement with a religious tradition. He argues that spirituality itself (1) is derived phenomenologically rather than metaphysically or institutionally, and (2) moves toward a psychological *telos* of human immanence (Van Ness, 1996). Thus, what holds this construct together is that it highlights that there is more to human experience than the material universe. There is an immaterial dimension to being human, experienced by all but especially within a clinical context, which is insufficiently captured by the category of religion. Thus, the concept of spirituality gives expression to many immaterial aspects of being human, and conceptually frees us from the constraints of religion.

A constructive approach through this impasse, suggested by Harold Koenig, is to prefer the concept of religion when the focus of concern is on research, and to prefer the concept of spirituality when the focus of concern is the clinical encounter (Koenig, 2008). Within the research domain it is essential to perform conceptually sound studies that carefully define the phenomenon under investigation. Since the concept of spirituality is intentionally employed as a vague or broader construct, it is problematic for research related purposes. When spirituality is not characterized by what is "ultimate" (as absent in the 2009 Consensus Conference definition), then it becomes impossible to differentiate it from any other dimension of human meaning-making or purpose. If all human meaning—from ethereal to ultimate—is spiritual, then it is not a phenomenon that can be studied empirically. Nebulous objects of study are difficult to describe, rightly intensify objections from the scientific community, and are not conducive to developing future interventions that are replicable or scalable. For this reason we agree with Koenig that employing the construct of religion—as especially defined by Marty and Tillich—is necessary within the context of medical and health research. Religion is particularly identifiable when what is ultimate is present in human experience. We also highlight for those who prefer the concept of spirituality that Tillich and Marty's "ultimate concern" does not presume a theistic object or superhuman beings. "Religion" can refer to a wide array of human phenomena that include the world's great religions but also other objects that humans may deem ultimate. A broader conceptualization of religion that includes non-theistic phenomena—what has been argued for by religious scholars for decades—appears to be functionally equivalent to what is often intended by those who prefer the term spirituality. Thus, it may be that differences between religion and spirituality are less significant within academic perspectives than in how terms are conceived in popular usage.

As Western societies grow increasingly pluralistic, there is a growing consensus that within the patient-clinician relationship, employing the language of spirituality is preferable to the language of religion because it is inclusive of patients from prototypical religions (e.g. Judaism), as well as of those who do not identify with any religion (Koenig, 2008). From this perspective, there is a good deal of practical wisdom to be gained by physicians from invoking the language of spirituality to initiate questions concerning a patient's ultimate meanings and purposes. Most patients who are religious will identify with this language and sense what the doctor is asking about. Patients who identify themselves as "spiritual not religious" will find this language to be inviting rather than off-putting, especially if a particular patient feels some animosity toward religion, such as a faith from his or her upbringing that has been rejected. For patients who are neither religious nor consider themselves spiritual, general questions such as "Is spirituality important to you?" or "What especially gives you meaning during this challenging time?" invite patients to answer in diverse ways with little chance of taking offense. The employment of spirituality rather than religion can be a rhetorical strategy (Cadge, 2012) that is not intended for research or scholarly purposes but as a means to positively communicate with strangers without causing offense or assuming too much.

With this background in mind, this book combines the terms *religion/spirituality*, not to conflate the two concepts as identical but instead to indicate that it is not our current aim to solve this debate. While we recognize that chapter authors in Part One may be employing somewhat different concepts, we specifically instructed them to not use space in their chapter to discuss definitions or argue for their preferred term. Instead, we invited them to review the key literature within their respective fields that covers religion/spirituality and then, within any particular description of a research study, to describe what specifically was being measured. Although this approach has limitations, its strength is that it enables readers to quickly assess the amount and quality of research that currently exists within a subdiscipline of medicine. Combining religion/spirituality also anticipates what we believe will be the future trend of all empirical research in the field—namely, that study tools will increasingly move from fuzzy measurements to assessments with greater resolution and specificity. Specificity will largely bypass normative debates of religion versus spirituality, since research will be able to identify specific variables of religious/spiritual beliefs, practices, and relationships—or more likely some combination of them—that are associated with spiritual health, medical outcomes, and public health (Hall, Meador, & Koenig, 2008). In fact, within a few decades we expect that research in the field will develop spiritual interventions, which will by necessity be based on highly specified information related to religious/spiritual beliefs, practices, and relationships. Earlier measures such as "How religious are you?" or "How spiritual are you?" (Institute, 2003), or single-item questions measuring the frequency of religious service attendance, though demonstrating themselves to have predictive validity, will no longer be viable or descriptively adequate as the field begins to turn to interventions. While generic measures have served an important place in the early phases of the field, and while the field has a way to go in creating meaningful measures pertaining to the multiplicity of "ultimate concerns," the current directions of the field suggest that religion/spirituality will be more readily recognized as only a general construct that includes a variety of religious and spiritual experiences. The implication is that for both research and clinical practice, it will become less important whether we classify something as religion or spirituality, and far more critical to identify the specific beliefs, practices, and relationships that constitute a person's religion/spirituality.

WHOSE ROLE?

There is also a lack of consensus on who should provide spiritual care within the medical context. Differing assumptions about this can sometimes lead to "turf wars" regarding who owns spiritual care as their professional domain (de Vries, Berlinger, & Cadge, 2008). We used our editorial discretion to focus especially in this book on physicians, as the recognized leaders of the patient care team. While certain readers may be surprised that the book has little specific to say about the role of clergy or hospital chaplains, the absence of their voices in this collection should not be taken as a slight against hospital chaplains. We believe it is largely uncontroversial for community clergy and hospital chaplains to be engaging patients in their experience of illness (Rodin et al., 2015). By contrast, there is a great deal of controversy concerning the role of medical professionals, especially physicians, in dealing with patients' spirituality/religion. Thus, as editors of this volume, we encouraged chapter contributors to focus particularly on the role of physicians, engaging questions of what is less known rather than what is already accepted.

Both theoretical presuppositions and practical concerns inform decision making about professional roles. One basic theoretical question is how relevant religion/spirituality is to medical care. Many within Western culture assume that these are what Stephen Jay Gould called "non-overlapping magisteria" (Gould, 1999). From this Cartesian perspective, body and soul are differentiated aspects of human anthropology (McKenny, 1997). If human persons can be deftly divided into distinct material and immaterial domains, then social systems created to care for human persons can also logically be based on a division of labor (M. J. Balboni, Puchalski, & Peteet, 2014). In such systems, physicians focus on the body and clergy on the soul (M. J. Balboni & T. A. Balboni, 2010). While we agree that there can be a great deal of efficiency in this approach, it risks reinforcing rather than overcoming the structural divisions that prevent holistic patient care. Its adherents may acknowledge that patient spirituality is one of several domains of the illness experience, but not the possibility that religion/spirituality is infused within every dimension of illness and caring from the ontological and epistemological to the institutional and professional (M. J. Balboni et al., 2014). In other words, by circumscribing religion/spirituality within a particular domain of the illness experience addressed by a specialized discipline, a division of labor approach does not allow or enable a theological critique of the larger system of medical care or make possible a deeper integration (Bishop, 2011).

Regarding practical matters concerning professional roles, research is beginning to show that a division of labor is difficult to employ in the current medical context because physicians' practice cannot be separated from physicians' spiritual commitments (see Medical Ethics chapter) and that patient medical decision-making is frequently informed by religious/spiritual beliefs (see Palliative Care chapter). The intertwining of medical decision making and religion/spirituality does not easily lend itself to a division of labor approach. Whose role is it to deal with a patient's religious beliefs when his or her medical decision is based on them? As an alternative, we have previously contended for a "clinical relevance" model (Peteet & D'Ambra, 2011), which calls for clinicians to be increasingly engaged in patients' religion/spirituality when it shifts from the background of the patient's experience to the foreground of clinical understanding and decision making. Rather than divided by walls, professional roles are distinguished by semi-permeable membranes (M.J. Balboni & T. A. Balboni, 2010).

Thus, this volume is concerned with medical professionals generally and especially with physicians as leaders of the medical team. We assume clergy and chaplains should be directly involved in spiritual care. How should physicians and nurses think about doing so? We explore here the varied ways these questions arise within major medical specialties by asking chapter authors to provide examples of clinician-patient encounters within each of their areas of practice

OUTLINE OF THE BOOK

In Part One, authors explore the interface between religion/spirituality and medicine from the perspective of differing medical specialties, and in Part Two the relationship of religion/spirituality to the culture of medicine from the perspective of relevant scholarly disciplines. Part Three is an extended concluding chapter that attempts to synthesize and offer perspective on the current data regarding religion/spirituality and health.

Chapter authors in Part One review the relevant scientific evidence in the disciplines of Obstetrics and Gynecology (Rachel Peragallo and John Thorp), Pediatrics (Raymond Barfield and Sarah Jean Barton), Family Medicine (Timothy Daaleman), Psychiatry (Dan G. Blazer), Internal Medicine (Lydia Dugdale and Daniel Sulmasy), Surgery (John and Margaret Tarpley), Gerontology (Harold Koenig), Oncology (Alan B. Astrow), Palliative Medicine (Tracy and Michael Balboni), Intensive Care (Alexandra Cist and Philip Choi), Medical Ethics (Farr Curlin), Medical Education (Marta Herschkopf, Najmeh Jafari, and Christina Puchalski), and Nursing (John Swinton and Lynn Vanderpot). Each discusses the implications of religion/spirituality for the doctor patient encounter within that discipline, engaging the following questions:

1. What is the state of the science of religion/spirituality in your specialty?
2. What are important areas for future research?

3. How does religion/spirituality commonly arise in the patient encounter within your medical specialty?
4. What are the best practices for your specialty as they pertain to religion/spirituality?
5. What is the role of clergy, faith communities, and chaplains in your specialty?
6. Specifically, how should physicians facilitate connections with these resources to provide spiritual care or work to overcome medical-spiritual conflicts?
7. How should clinicians provide spiritual care when there are no clergy or chaplains available?

Given the prominence of existential concerns in specialties such as Psychiatry and Palliative Medicine, readers will not be surprised to find that the evidence base for dealing with religion/spirituality issues is better developed in these than in some other areas. They may, however, be surprised to learn how much literature now exists in all specialties, and how much the ethical and clinical challenges overlap in areas as seemingly divergent as Surgery and Nursing.

Chapter authors in Part Two consider fundamental questions about the relationship between medicine and religion/spirituality from the perspective of a non-medical field. Consideration of spirituality and health has been overwhelmingly performed by isolated scholars and small teams of researchers who have approached their study from within a single disciplinary and methodological framework. While this is a general tension across the academy, it is a particularly vexing concern at the intersection of religion/spirituality, health, and medicine because of the complexity of the subject matter. Not only do traditional academic disciplines—theology, psychology, sociology, historical studies, epidemiology, or medicine—lack methodological resources and explanatory models to understand the multifaceted relationships involved in religion, spirituality, health, and illness, but also each discipline is arguably insufficient to study even its own disciplinary locus apart from considerable collaboration with other disciplines. Consequently, the conceptual, methodological, and ideological problems plaguing the advancement of knowledge in this area may be largely symptoms of current disciplinary barriers characterizing the creation of knowledge. In light of these issues, we opted in this project for an interdisciplinary engagement of issues related to the relationship of religion/spirituality and the practice of medicine. One of our intents for Part Two is to draw in additional scholars from the social sciences, law, and humanities to engage questions related to this relationship and to broaden the horizons of empirical researchers to see beyond measurements and statistical associations.

First, three chapters engage the relationship of medicine and religion/spirituality from the social scientific disciplines, of psychology, sociology, and anthropology.

Psychologists Kelly Trevino and Ken Pargament explore the contributions of psychology to understanding the medicine/religion interface at the levels of coping theory, patient and caregiver experience, as well as the evidence base for spiritual interventions including dignity therapy, mindfulness-based therapies, meaning-centered therapy, dignity therapy, and religiously integrated cognitive behavior therapy.

Jonathan B. Imber reviews sociological analyses of Western medicine before depicting spirituality as resistance to forces such as commodification within medicine, which have threatened to eclipse what it means to be a person.

Linda Barnes and Lance Laird trace the history of medical and religious anthropology to explain the biomedicalization of religion and the need for an anthropology of experience. They advocate a stance of cultural humility based on a synthesis of the strengths of religious studies, medical anthropology, and refined tools of spiritual inquiry that reflect the particularities of different traditions.

In addition to the social-scientific, Orlando Snead and Michael Morehead explore the legal questions in the United States and tensions related to religion/spirituality and the clinician-patient relationship, such as conscientious refusal of treatment by patients and clinicians and reproductive health decision making. To our knowledge, this is the first academic account that explores these issues from a legal perspective, which we believe is an important contribution to the field by identifying critical legal approaches for clinicians, especially in the United States.

Three additional chapters are included in this section exploring the relationship of religion/spirituality and medicine from traditional humanities disciplines, including historical, philosophical, and theological.

Historian Gary Ferngren traces the development of professional medicine and medical philanthropy over more than two millennia in an attempt to provide some understanding of how traditional medical care took shape and how religion came to play an essential supporting role in the healing process before it gave way to cultural shifts and scientific and technological advancements that in the last two centuries have largely eliminated spiritual values from medicine.

Philosopher James Marcum considers metaphysical, definitional, epistemological and ethical issues at the interface between medicine and religion. He then suggests, in contrast to a prevailing assumed reductionistic model, a holistic and emergent model relating the spiritual, social, psychological, and physical dimensions of personhood.

Theologians Brett McCarty and Warren Kinghorn, after briefly considering two common but insufficient ways that theology is used within contemporary religion-and-medicine conversations, argue that in the past theology has informed the contexts within which influential medical institutions and practices, including the hospital itself, have developed. They then suggest that theology continues to inform contexts of health care in the present, most obviously in the case of "faith-based" institutions and programs but also, more subtly, in nonsectarian, "secular" medicine. Finally, turning to prescription and recommendation, they discuss several ways that clinicians, patients, and scholars of medicine and health care might draw more deeply on theological context to inform future moral commitments, practices, and institutions in health care.

Finally, in Part Three, Tyler VanderWeele integrates research findings with philosophical and theological perspectives on subjects such as faith community involvement and forgiveness to address how health and public policy should implement findings about religion/spirituality from epidemiological research. He was able to read drafts from both the clinical/empirical chapters (Part One) and humanities viewpoints (Part Two), and was then tasked to provide a preliminary synthesis on where the field of religion/spirituality and health as a whole currently stands. As a body of knowledge that is inherently interdisciplinary, VanderWeele attempts to bring these chapters in closer alignment by summarizing what is currently known within the field. While others may draw some alternative conclusions, what is especially important is that effort and critical engagement include seeing the bigger picture and putting the various pieces into relationship with one another. From this vantage point, Part Three is a notable step forward in scholarship, as it establishes an example for the field by being interdisciplinary and constructive. Rather than merely pitting disciplines against each other, VanderWeele works toward engagement and unity. He concludes that although we have come a long way as an academic field and in engaging clinical and public health questions, even more empirical research and humanities scholarship should be done in the years ahead.

We hope and expect that readers interested in the changing nature of health care will find in this book a unique resource, both bringing together the perspectives of multiple disciplines on the practical question of what religion/spirituality has to do with medicine, and providing evidence-based ways for clinicians to interface with patients' religion/spirituality from the beginning to the end of life.

NOTES

1. At Duke, see the Center for Spirituality, Theology, and Health located at the medical school (http://www. spiritualityandhealth.duke.edu) and Duke Divinity School's Theology, Medicine, and Culture Program (https://tmc.divinity.duke.edu). At the University of Chicago see their Program on Medicine and Religion (https://pmr.uchicago.edu). At Yale, see their Program for Medicine, Spirituality, & Religion (https://medicine.yale.edu/intmed/genmed/education/medspirel/). At Harvard see the Initiative on Health, Religion, and Spirituality (http://projects.iq.harvard.edu/rshm).
2. For the Institute for Spirituality and Health at Texas Medical Center, see: http://ish-tmc.org. For the George Washington Institute for Spirituality and Health, see https://smhs.gwu.edu/gwish/. For Emory's Religion and Public Health Collaborative, see http://ethics.emory.edu/pillars/health_sciences/Religion_PublicHealth.html. For Loyola University Chicago's Physician Vocation Program, see http://hsd.luc.edu/bioethics/content/physicianvocationprogram/.
3. For the Conference on Medicine and Religion, see http://www.medicineandreligion.com.
4. Many of the lectures are available at the Harvard Initiative's website: http://projects.iq.harvard.edu/rshm/events-videos
5. It may also be clarifying to note that Marty has typically not employed the term *spirituality*. His characteristics of religion include the spiritual dimension and the structures of religion. This is common in how most scholars used the term *religion* throughout the twentieth century in that it was used to apply to a wide-range of phenomena that have more recently been associated with spirituality.

REFERENCES

Balboni, M. J., & Balboni, T. A. (2010). Reintegrating care for the dying, body and soul. *Harvard Theological Review, 103*(3), 351–364.

Balboni, M. J., Puchalski, C. M., & Peteet, J. R. (2014). The relationship between medicine, spirituality and religion: Three models for integration. *J Relig Health.* doi:10.1007/s10943-014-9901-8

Balboni, M. J., Sullivan, A., Amobi, A., Phelps, A. C., Gorman, D. P., Zollfrank, A., . . . Balboni, T. A. (2013). Why is spiritual care infrequent at the end of life? Spiritual care perceptions among patients, nurses, and physicians and the role of training. *J Clin Oncol, 31*(4), 461–467. doi:10.1200/JCO.2012.44.6443

Becker, E. (1973). *The denial of death.* New York, NY: Free Press.

Bishop, J. P. (2011). *The anticipatory corpse: Medicine, power, and the care of the dying.* Notre Dame, IN: University of Notre Dame Press.

Burnham, J. C. (1982). American medicine's golden age: What happened to it? *Science, 215*(4539), 1474–1479. Retrieved from http://www.ncbi.nlm.nih.gov/pubmed/7038876

Cadge, W. (2012). *Paging God: Religion in the halls of medicine*. Chicago, IL; London, England: University of Chicago Press.

Cavanaugh, W. T. (2009). *The myth of religious violence: Secular ideology and the roots of modern conflict*. Oxford, England; New York, NY: Oxford University Press.

Curlin, F. A., Lantos, J. D., Roach, C. J., Sellergren, S. A., & Chin, M. H. (2005). Religious characteristics of U.S. physicians: A national survey. *J Gen Intern Med, 20*(7), 629–634. Retrieved from http://www.ncbi.nlm.nih.gov/entrez/query.fcgi?cmd=Retrieve&db=PubMed&dopt=Citation&list_uids=16050858

Curlin, F. A., Lawrence, R. E., Odell, S., Chin, M. H., Lantos, J. D., Koenig, H. G., & Meador, K. G. (2007). Religion, spirituality, and medicine: psychiatrists' and other physicians' differing observations, interpretations, and clinical approaches. *Am J Psychiatry, 164*(12), 1825–1831. Retrieved from http://www.ncbi.nlm.nih.gov/entrez/query.fcgi?cmd=Retrieve&db=PubMed&dopt=Citation&list_uids=18056237

de Vries, R., Berlinger, N., & Cadge, W. (2008). Lost in translation: The chaplain's role in health care. *Hastings Cent Rep, 38*(6), 23–27. Retrieved from http://www.ncbi.nlm.nih.gov/entrez/query.fcgi?cmd=Retrieve&db=PubMed&dopt=Citation&list_uids=19192712

Fetzer Institute. (2003). Multidimensional measurement of religiousness/spirituality for use in health research: A report of the Fetzer Institute/ National Institute on Aging Working Group. Kalamazoo, MI: Fetzer Institute. Retrieved from https://www.gem-beta.org/public/DownloadMeasure.aspx?mid=1155

Gould, S. J. (1999). *Rocks of ages: Science and religion in the fullness of life* (1st ed.). New York, NY: Ballantine Pub. Group.

Hall, D. E., Koenig, H. G., & Meador, K. G. (2004). Conceptualizing "religion": How language shapes and constrains knowledge in the study of religion and health. *Perspect Biol Med, 47*(3), 386–401. Retrieved from http://www.ncbi.nlm.nih.gov/entrez/query.fcgi?cmd=Retrieve&db=PubMed&dopt=Citation&list_uids=15247504

Hall, D. E., Meador, K. G., & Koenig, H. G. (2008). Measuring religiousness in health research: Review and critique. *J Relig Health, 47*(2), 134–163. Retrieved from http://www.ncbi.nlm.nih.gov/entrez/query.fcgi?cmd=Retrieve&db=PubMed&dopt=Citation&list_uids=19105008

Hayslip, B. (2003). Death denial: Hiding and camouflaging death. In Clifton D. Bryant (ed.), *Handbook of Death & Dying*, chapter 4, 34–42. Thousand Oaks, CA: Sage Publications, Inc.

Imber, J. B. (2008). *Trusting doctors: The decline of moral authority in American medicine*. Princeton, NJ: Princeton University Press.

The Joint Commission. (2011). (3.7.0.0 ed., pp. PC.02.02.13): E-dition. Retrieved from https://www.jointcommission.org.

Koenig, H. G. (2008). *Medicine, religion, and health: Where science and spirituality meet*. West Conshohocken, PA: Templeton Foundation Press.

Koenig, H. G., King, D. E., & Carson, V. B. (2012). *Handbook of religion and health* (2nd ed.). New York, NY: Oxford University Press.

Lawrence, R. J. (2002). The witches' brew of spirituality and medicine. *Ann Behav Med, 24*(1), 74–76. Retrieved from http://www.ncbi.nlm.nih.gov/entrez/query.fcgi?cmd=Retrieve&db=PubMed&dopt=Citation&list_uids=12008797

Martin, D. (1978). *A general theory of secularization*. Oxford, England: Blackwell.

Marty, M. E., & Moore, J. (2000). *Politics, religion, and the common good: Advancing a distinctly American conversation about religion's role in our shared life* (1st ed.). San Francisco, CA: Jossey-Bass Publishers.

McGinn, B. (2005). The letter and the spirit: Spirituality as an academic discipline. In E. Dreyer & M. S. Burrows (Eds.), *Minding the spirit: The study of Christian spirituality* (pp. 25–41). Baltimore, MD: Johns Hopkins University Press.

McKenny, G. P. (1997). *To relieve the human condition: Bioethics, technology, and the body*. Albany, NY: State University of New York Press.

National Consensus Project. (2009). NCP clinical practice guidelines for quality palliative care, 2nd ed. Retrieved from http://ww.nationalconsensusproject.org/guideline.pdf

Peteet, J. R., & D'Ambra, M. N. (2011). *The soul of medicine: Spiritual perspectives and clinical practice*. Baltimore, MD: Johns Hopkins University Press.

Puchalski, C., Ferrell, B., Virani, R., Otis-Green, S., Baird, P., Bull, J., . . . Sulmasy, D. (2009). Improving the quality of spiritual care as a dimension of palliative care: The report of the Consensus Conference. *J Palliat Med, 12*(10), 885–904. Retrieved from http://www.ncbi.nlm.nih.gov/entrez/query.fcgi?cmd=Retrieve& db=PubMed&dopt=Citation&list_uids=19807235

Puchalski, C. M., & Ferrell, B. (2010). *Making health care whole: Integrating spirituality into health care*. West Conshohocken, PA: Templeton Press.

Rodin, D., Balboni, M., Mitchell, C., Smith, P. T., VanderWeele, T. J., & Balboni, T. A. (2015). Whose role? Oncology practitioners' perceptions of their role in providing spiritual care to advanced cancer patients. *Support Care Cancer, 23*(9), 2543–2550. doi:10.1007/s00520-015-2611-2

Schneiders, S. M. (2003). Religion vs. spirituality: A contemporary conundrum. *Spiritus, 3*, 163–185.

Sloan, R. P. (2006). *Blind faith: The unholy alliance of religion and medicine* (1st ed.). New York, NY: St. Martin's Press.

Sloan, R. P., Bagiella, E., & Powell, T. (1999). Religion, spirituality, and medicine. *Lancet, 353*(9153), 664–667. Retrieved from http://www.ncbi.nlm.nih.gov/entrez/query.fcgi?cmd=Retrieve&db=PubMed&dopt=Cit ation&list_uids=10030348

Smith, J. Z. (1998). Religion, religions, religious. In M. C. Taylor (Ed.), *Critical terms for religious studies* (pp. 269–284). Chicago, IL: University of Chicago Press.

Sulmasy, D. P. (2006). *The rebirth of the clinic: An introduction to spirituality in health care*. Washington, DC: Georgetown University Press.

Tillich, P. (1958). *Dynamics of faith*. New York, NY: Harper.

Van Ness, P. H. (1996). *Spirituality and the secular quest*. New York, NY: Crossroad.

Wuthnow, R. (1998). *After heaven: Spirituality in America since the 1950s*. Berkeley, CA: University of California Press.

PART 1

RELIGION, SPIRITUALITY, AND MEDICAL SUBSPECIALITIES

CHAPTER 2

RELIGION AND SPIRITUALITY IN OBGYN

Rachel Peragallo and John M. Thorp

Those of us who provide women's reproductive health care accompany women during human events, which for most, have religious and spiritual implications. Some examples include experiencing sexual awakening/sexuality; making choices about bringing a new human life into the world; grappling with fetal anomalies diagnosed prior to birth; mourning the end of fertility or the inability to conceive. Most humans rely on conscience to inform decision-making around their sexuality and reproductive behavior. Conscience has been defined as "a commitment to morality itself; to acting and choosing morally according to the best of one's ability, and the activity of judging that an act one has done or about which one is deliberating would violate that commitment (Sulmasy, 2008)." Conscience is, in turn, affected by religious and spiritual beliefs and identities (Curlin, 2007). Since obstetrics and gynecology (OBG) is a specialty that diagnoses and treats disorders of sexuality and reproduction in women, conscience and religion and spirituality are a part of almost every patient encounter, even when they are not acknowledged. This is true for both providers and patients.

This chapter explores religious and spiritual aspects of OBG care in two main parts. The first summarizes the relevant scientific literature using real case examples as illustrations. The second offers reflections about best practices for providers of women's health care. In addition to offering reflections about interacting with the religion, spirituality, and the conscience of each patient, the chapter discusses how a provider may grapple with how their own spirituality, religion, and conscience affect patient care.

MAJOR RELIGIONS AND REPRODUCTIVE HEALTH CARE

Reproductive health care is unique compared with other fields of medicine. In addition to the patient and her provider, additional entities, who possess corporate or group consciences, are in operation. These entities, including church, state, family, advocacy groups, and health care purchasers, often possess strongly held beliefs around reproductive health care. It is outside the scope of this chapter to discuss the reproductive health implications of the positions of each of these entities. However, it may be instructive to provide a few examples of the types of positions religious institutions take vis a vis reproductive health care.

Orthodox Judaism permits sexual activity only within the context of marriage, and then primarily for reproduction. Sexual activity must occur only during the time of ovulation, and male masturbation is prohibited (Notzer, Levran, Mashiach, & Soffer). Abortion is not considered equivalent to murder (human life is progressively acquired starting 40 days after conception); however, it is still a serious crime except in the case of threats to the mother's health. Difficult cases must be discussed with a Rabbi (Silber, 1980).

Roman Catholic doctrine teaches that using contraceptive medications or devices and undergoing abortion are grave sins (John Paul, 1995). These positions are so well-defined that Catholic health care institutions in the United States are required to adhere to a written set of *Ethical and Religious Directives for Catholic Health Care Services* (United States Conference of Catholic Bishops [USCCB], 2009). Some medical writers claim such guidance may lead to a delay in treatment for life-threatening pregnancy complications (May, Mukamenzi, & Vekemans, 1990; Raghavan, 2007). The public health implications of such claims are important, since one in six patients in the United States seeks care in a Catholic health care institution (*The Official Catholic Directory*, 2015).

Protestant, Muslim, and Hindu groups have specific moral positions on OBG issues that may impact reproductive health decisions and care for their adherents (Schenker, 2000; Tomkins et al., 2015). Despite institutional policies and position statements, individual women usually have a personal spiritual approach to reproductive health care based on a variety of socioeconomic, cultural, and individual spiritual characteristics and experiences.

RESEARCH RELATED TO REPRODUCTIVE HEALTH AND RELIGION AMONG FEMALE PATIENTS

Over three-quarters of US women are religious: 71% are Christian and 6% have non-Christian faiths (Pew Research Center, 2015). In three surveys of the use of complementary and alternative therapies, over a third of US women stated that they used religion, spirituality, and/or prayer to cope with health issues (Bair et al., 2002; Dessio et al., 2004; Upchurch & Chyu, 2005). One of these studies investigated the effects of race/ethnicity on the use of spirituality to cope with health issues. African American women were the most likely to use spiritual practices to promote health (43%), followed by white (37%) and then Mexican (19%) and Chinese Americans (7%; Dessio et al., 2004).

There are limited data suggesting positive effects of religion and spirituality on women's reproductive health. Spiritual resources were associated with less health risk-taking behavior among pregnant women in the Midwest and in Appalachia (Jesse, Graham, & Swanson, 2006; Jesse & Reed, 2004). About of half of a group of 150 midwestern, mostly African American pregnant women stated that religion or spirituality positively impacted their pregnancy. Women cited specific benefits including guidance and support, protection/blessing and rewards, communication with God, strength and confidence, help making difficult decisions, and generalized positive effect (Jesse, Schoneboom, & Blanchard, 2007). In a study among urban women of low socioeconomic status, women who attended church services at least once a week were 10–15% less likely to have a low birth weight baby(Burdette, Weeks, Hill, & Eberstein, 2012). These effects could not be fully explained by lower rates of mental health problems, less care-seeking, or higher rates of substance abuse. Religious service attendance by peri- and postmenopausal women has been associated with higher rates of breast and cervical cancer screening (Salmoirago-Blotcher et al., 2011).

There are a few studies which investigate the potential adverse effects of religion and spirituality on women's health care. Religious groups with high levels of modesty may be less likely to seek necessary care due to concerns about having intimate exams, especially by male providers (Hasnain, Connell, Menon, & Tranmer, 2011; Vu, 1996). Some OBG providers believe that religious women are more likely to have unprotected intercourse, less likely to use contraception, more likely to seek unsafe abortion, and less likely to receive effective fertility treatments. The actual effects of religion/spirituality on each of these outcomes are complicated and will be addressed in detail in the case examples to follow.

SEXUALITY

CASE: ANITA

Anita is a 21-year-old woman who presents to a new gynecologist for an annual exam. She is quite anxious about the exam. She had never been sexually active due to her religious beliefs. She has a boyfriend who is supportive of her beliefs and shares them. In past exams, providers assumed she was not telling the truth about her virginity and would not be able to sustain her lifestyle of abstinence. She felt she was being pushed to use a birth control method even though she did not need it.

Use of barrier methods at first intercourse is lower among religious youth in some studies (Amoako-Agyeman, 2012; Manlove, Terry-Humen, & Ikramullah, 2006; Zaleski & Schiaffino, 2000), but not in others (Cerqueira-Santos, Koller, & Wilcox, 2008; Gold et al., 2010). The most recent Survey of Family Growth in the United States found that religious individuals have a lower rate of reproductive service use regardless of sexual experience (Hall, Moreau, & Trussell, 2012). However, Christian, Jewish, and Muslim religiosity (e.g. frequent church service attendance) have been consistently associated with later sexual debut and fewer sexual partners (Amoako-Agyeman, 2012; Asubiaro & Fatusi, 2014; Fielder, Walsh, Carey, & Carey, 2013; Gold et al., 2010; Haglund & Fehring, 2010; Imudia et al., 2009; Mabiala Babela, Massamba, Bantsimba, & Senga, 2008; Manlove et al., 2006; Notzer et al., 1984; Rostosky, Regnerus, & Wright, 2003). In a study of over 500 American female adolescents, the risks of sexually transmitted infections and unwanted pregnancies were lower among those with higher levels of religiosity (Gold et al., 2010). Measures of religiosity most strongly associated with lower sexual risk taking seem to be those related to religious practice (e.g. church attendance) versus those related to attitudes and identity (e.g. importance of religious beliefs; Lefkowitz, Gillen, Shearer, & Boone, 2004). The majority of young adults with high religiosity eventually do have intercourse outside of marriage (Finer, 2007); however, they seem to have fewer risky sexual encounters and fewer total partners. A study among religious US college students in the 1990s found that the majority condoned intercourse outside of marriage but still wanted sex to take place "in the context of a meaningful relationship"(Murstein & Mercy, 1994). Still, 3% of Americans do successfully abstain from intercourse until marriage (Finer, 2007), and these rates may be higher among populations with high religiosity.

CONTRACEPTIVES

CASE: BETHANY

Bethany is a 35-year-old woman who has seven children. She presents for an annual exam. She is opposed to the use of contraceptive medications and devices due to the teachings of her religion. She has used a fertility awareness-based method (FABM) of family planning for the past 15 years and has planned all of her pregnancies. She gets the feeling that her gynecologist does not believe her pregnancies are planned and is trying to persuade her to use a more effective family planning method.

Use of many contraceptive drugs and devices is considered immoral by several religions including Orthodox Judaism, Catholicism, and some conservative Protestant and Muslim groups. However, women's stated religious affiliation has not been consistently associated with choices for and against certain contraceptive methods. In the most recent US survey of Family Growth, about 70% of reproductive age women use contraceptive drugs or devices, and there are minimal differences according to religious affiliation (Dreweke, 2011). Similar findings were noted in a large survey of Australian women (Richters, Grulich, de Visser, Smith, & Rissel, 2003). In some developing countries, women who identify as Christian or Muslim are actually more likely to use contraceptives compared with those who identify with traditional religions (Agadjanian, 2013; Doctor, Phillips, & Sakeah, 2009). The negative associations between stated religion and contraceptive use found in many smaller studies (Kamal & Islam, 2010; Kansal, Kandpal, & Mishra, 2006; Raine, Minnis, & Padian, 2003) may be due to unmeasured confounding from differences in education level and other social norms between religious groups (Hennink, Diamond, & Cooper, 1999; Johnson-Hanks, 2006; Pillai & Sunil, 2007). Another explanation for the inconsistent findings is that in cultures with high levels of contraceptive use at baseline, differentials based on social constructs such as religion may be less important because they are small relative to the overall rates of use (Martin, 2005). Like sexuality, use of contraceptive drugs and devices has been more consistently related to measures of religiosity (e.g. religious service attendance) than to stated religious identity (Merchant et al., 2007; Tanfer & Horn, 1985).

FABMs are methods of family planning whereby women track signs of fertility such as cervical mucus and basal body temperature. These include the Standard Days Method, Two Day Method, Billings Ovulation Model, Creighton Model Fertility Care System, Marquette Method, and Sensiplan NFP. Couples are not fertile every day of the month. By tracking their fertile days, couples are able to avoid or plan pregnancy by choosing whether or not to have intercourse on these days. FABMs require daily tracking, interpretation, and decision-making, and the typical pregnancy rates for the first year of use are as high as 25–30% (Grimes, Gallo, Grigorieva, Nanda, & Schulz, 2005; Vaughan, Trussell, Kost, Singh, & Jones, 2008). However, for people who use the method correctly and consistently, these methods can result in rates of unplanned pregnancies of <1% to 5% per year (Manhart, Duane, Lind, Sinai, & Golden-Tevald, 2013). Most of the religiously affiliated FABMs encourage abstinence during the fertile time and are known as "natural family planning" methods. Other FABMs support use of a barrier method during the fertile time and are known as "fertility awareness" methods.

CASE 2: CRISTINA

Cristina is a 21-year old mother of three children under the age of four presenting for contraceptive counseling. She has not used contraceptive medications or devices in the past because her mother told her that they cause abortions and that this is against her religion. She and her partner have tried to use condoms, but they have had three unplanned pregnancies. She has a very low income but was recently able to get into nursing school after finally completing her GED. She strongly desires not to have another pregnancy at this time, but she is also worried about going against her religion and her beliefs. She asks whether or not intrauterine devices cause abortions.

There are two major reasons that religious individuals find contraceptives to be immoral. The first is that contraceptive use separates the possibility of procreation from the act of intercourse. In the Roman Catholic tradition, sex, in the context of contraception, is seen as objectifying or using one's partner. Sex is intended to be an act of complete self-giving that has two dimensions: unitive and procreative. Neither is truly possible when either person is purposely withholding their fertility from the act (John Paul, 1995). While some conservative groups believe that even FABM use is not supportive of both the procreative and unitive dimensions of sex (Harrison, 2005), mainline Catholic teaching does include guidance about "responsible parenthood" and allows for the use of FABMs. In a similar vein, some religious groups only oppose permanent separation of the act of intercourse from the possibility of contraception (e.g. sterilization; Chacko, 2001) but not reversible separation (e.g. contraceptive drugs and devices). The second major reason that some religious groups oppose contraceptive use is that certain contraceptives may cause an early abortion by interfering with implantation of a fertilized embryo (Tomkins et al., 2015). The latter assumption is very difficult to study. Prior to implantation, there are no accurate tests to confirm pregnancy. Given that a significant percentage of women using hormonal medications and devices do ovulate and that these treatments also make the uterine lining less receptive to pregnancies, it is theoretically possible for all methods except barrier methods and sterilization to interfere with the implantation of a fertilized embryo. The proportion of cycles in which this occurs has not been measured. There is evidence to believe that the dominant effects of most methods is the suppression of ovulation, decreasing viability of sperm (Stanford, 2002).

Despite religious prohibitions, women and their partners often decide to use contraceptives. In some cases, they may limit themselves to specific categories of family planning methods such as non-permanent methods (Chacko, 2001), methods that do not work after fertilization or implantation (Lopez-del Burgo, Lopez-de Fez, Osorio, Guzman, & de Irala, 2010), or non-medical methods (Cebeci Save et al., 2004). In other cases, couples either live with ambivalence of acting contrary to religious teaching or creatively interpret their religion's teaching to justify use of contraceptives. Mennonite women using contraceptives prohibited by their church did not discuss this openly among their peers (Kulig, Babcock, Wall, & Hill, 2009). In a study of over 400 Polish Catholic women, more than 70% were using contraception and many of these actually used their own interpretation of their faith to justify their choice (e.g. the immorality of having children one could not care properly for; the immorality of the church to oppose contraceptives without offering tangible assistance to needy people; Mishtal & Dannefer, 2010). After studying contraceptive use in a Mexican Catholic population, one researcher concluded, "Rather than rigidly adhere to or blithely ignore the Catholic Church's opposition to family planning, [women] creatively negotiate their intimate relationships and contest particular facets of Church doctrine, insisting on reinterpreting them in order to create a moral space in their lives where they can fuse their modern bodies with their Catholic souls" (Hirsch, 2008). In a study of an Indian Muslim population, a participant said: "We know that children are given by Allah. But we have so many now. We are poor people, eking out an existence. . .We don't want to go against what the *mullah* says. . .But, can you tell us of a pill or an injection that will stop us from having more babies?" (Chacko, 2001). Not much is known about the repercussions of these ambivalent and complicated decisions. However, in a Kuwaiti study, women who believed contraceptives were immoral were more likely to discontinue their use (Shah, Shah, Chowdhury, & Menon, 2007). In the National Survey of Family Growth, US women those who had made an abstinence pledge were no less likely to have had intercourse outside of marriage; however, pledge-breakers were more likely to have HPV and extramarital pregnancies (Paik, Sanchagrin, & Heimer, 2016).

ABORTION

CASE: DOT

Dot is 25 years old and is 8 weeks pregnant. She is estranged from her family. The father of her baby was a fling and she is no longer in touch with him. She started working a new job and is in a probationary period. She feels she has no way of supporting and taking care of a baby. She will get fired if she takes time off for delivery. Despite abortion being against her religion, she is planning to undergo a pregnancy termination.

CASE: EDIE

Edie is a 35-year-old woman with two children who is 10 weeks pregnant after a failure of her birth control method. She has a large abdominal aortic aneurysm that has been partially repaired. Her vascular surgeon has told her that a full-term pregnancy would likely to lead to her death. Her obstetrician is recommending a pregnancy termination as soon as possible. She feels attached to her baby already. Also, she is religious and believes abortion is a sin.

Although the US abortion rate has declined over the last decade, it is estimated that 30% of women will undergo an elective pregnancy termination by the age of 45 (Jones & Kavanaugh, 2011). In a large survey of over 9000 US women who underwent an elective abortion in 2008–2009, almost 75% had a religious affiliation: 35% Protestant, 28% Catholic, 7% "Other" (Jones, Finer, & Singh, 2010). The individual abortion rates for Protestants in this study were 25% lower than for the entire sample, but the rate for Catholics was equivalent. Women with no religious affiliation had rates that were 60% higher than the entire sample (Jones et al., 2010). Only 13% of the abortion cohort attended services once per week compared with 24% of reproductive age American women, suggesting that women with higher levels of religiosity are less likely to seek abortions (Jones et al., 2010). In a study of religious Israeli Jews, the acceptance of abortion declined as levels of religiosity increased, but still 48% of the most religious group would undergo abortion in the case of an unplanned pregnancy (Notzer et al., 1984). In a qualitative survey, North Carolina pregnant women reported that religious beliefs helped them accept unintended pregnancy (Moos et al., 2008).

Religious women who do undergo abortion may continue to have conflicted feelings about their decision. In a study of over 5000 women undergoing abortion in a large clinic in the United States, 43% reported some spiritual concerns with undergoing abortion, and 18% reported feeling afraid or somewhat afraid that God would not forgive them for their decision (Foster, Gould, Taylor, & Weitz, 2012). In a 1970s study of 300 Indian women undergoing abortion, 78% thought it was a sinful act. Their decisions were primarily based on economic considerations (Roy, Lahiri, & Ghosh, 1978). As with contraception, women undergoing abortion despite spiritual concerns may have a "private set of negotiations with God. . .to rely on the personal forgiveness of God" (Petchesky & Judd, 1998).

In the case of serious fetal disease, decisions about pregnancy termination are even more complicated. Many women who are opposed to elective abortion would undergo fetal testing for chromosome abnormalities and would terminate an affected pregnancy (Kyle, Cummins, & Evans, 1988). However, higher religiosity (e.g. church attendance) is still a predictor of deciding to continue versus terminate affected pregnancies (Bell & Stoneman, 2000; Haghpanah, Nasirabadi, Rahimi, Faramarzi, & Karimi, 2012). The effect of religion on decision-making is dependent on the level of severity of the fetal diseases. Pregnancy termination is more acceptable for lethal anomalies or genetic diseases with serious impacts on quality of life (Bell & Stoneman, 2000).

There is limited data showing that spiritual care may be helpful for women undergoing pregnancy termination. In Sweden, 61% of women undergoing elective abortion reported existential concerns (Stalhandske, Ekstrand, & Tyden, 2011). This finding is despite the fact that only 2% of Swedes report moral objections to abortion and only one-third report a religious affiliation. Researchers concluded that women undergoing abortion in Sweden had spiritual needs that were unmet by the current system (Stalhandske et al., 2011; Stalhandske, Makenzius, Tyden, & Larsson, 2012). Among couples attending a multi-disciplinary fetal anomaly clinic in Germany, 56% desired counseling from a religious representative (Patel, Farley, Impey, & Lakhoo, 2008). We identified only one study which investigated a religious intervention for couples undergoing pregnancy termination. Muslim couples at risk for having a fetus with beta thalassemia (a serious genetic blood disorder) underwent genetic counseling that included a religious component (El-Beshlawy et al., 2012). Genetic counselors explained the Islamic teaching on pregnancy termination in situations of grave fetal disease (a religious fatwa allows termination up until 120 days of gestation). After receiving this intervention, 100% of parents with affected fetuses terminated their pregnancies compared with lower numbers in studies of similar populations (El-Beshlawy et al., 2012).

INFERTILITY

CASE: FRANCES

Frances has been trying to conceive for a year. She is extremely frustrated. She wants to have a baby as soon as possible. Her husband's religion is opposed to the use of artificial reproductive technologies, including in vitro fertilization or intrauterine insemination. She wants to be supportive of his beliefs but she also wants to get pregnant and she is worried that this will not happen using less aggressive methods.

Women struggling with infertility may also have spiritual and religious dilemmas about treatment. These tend to be related to beliefs about the sanctity of the marriage relationship and beliefs about the sanctity of human embryos (Dutney, 2007). There are also spiritual concerns about reducing the man to a semen sample, the woman to an egg and uterus, and a baby to embryos or products (Paul, 1968). Such beliefs may result in opposition to the use of donor gametes; procedures that circumvent intercourse as a means to conception; and procedures that create, manipulate, store, and discard embryos. However, some of these concerns may be balanced by the strong value many religions place on parenthood. Similar numbers of religious versus nonreligious women seek care for infertility (Greil et al., 2010). Among a survey of over 1,200 women intending to undergo in vitro fertilization for infertility, 24% self-identified as Catholic, 29% as Protestant, 18% as other Christian, and 5% as other religions, similar to national proportions (Lyerly et al., 2010).

RESEARCH RELATED TO OBG CARE PROVISION AND THE RELIGION OF THE PROVIDER

Although the religious beliefs and practices of each individual patient impact her reproductive health and decision-making, there is at least one other conscience at play: that of her provider.

CASE: GERDA

Gerda is 30 years old and 10 weeks pregnant. She presents for her first prenatal visit. She has three boys at home. She has no risk factors for genetic diseases. The physician discusses options for fetal genetic testing. She asks how soon she could find out the gender of the fetus because she wants to terminate the pregnancy if it is another boy. Her physician is morally opposed to such a plan for religious reasons.

CASE: DOT (CONTINUED)

Dot discusses her decision to undergo an abortion with her physician but the physician is opposed to elective pregnancy termination . The physician is not sure how to respond at first, but tries to find ways of being supportive to her and making sure her decision is fully informed. The physician provides the phone number of a local clinic where she can obtain a safe abortion. After the visit, Dot tells the nurse that she felt disapproval and judgment from the physician's body language.

A large survey of over 1100 US obstetrician gynecologists was performed in 2008–2009 in order to understand how their religious and spiritual beliefs impacted patient care. Fifty-seven percent believed life begins at conception and were more likely to oppose abortion (Chung, Lawrence, Rasinski, Yoon, & Curlin, 2012). Physicians in this category were more likely to be Catholic, Evangelical Protestant, or Hindu. When physicians were asked about whether they would object to abortions in specific scenarios, the responses ranged from 18% when the fetus had a cardiac or pulmonary anomaly to 82% for gender selection (Harris, Cooper, Rasinski, Curlin, & Lyerly, 2011). Rates of objection were higher for Catholic, Evangelical Protestant, and Muslim providers. Religious physicians were less likely to routinely offer emergency contraception and more likely to offer assisted reproductive technology only to married women (Lawrence, Rasinski, Yoon, & Curlin, 2010). Theological pluralism among physicians was associated with reporting less directive counseling when helping patients through a moral dilemma (Yoon, Rasinski, & Curlin, 2010). Smaller studies in Australia and Denmark have shown similar findings (de Costa, Russell, & Carrette, 2010; de la Fuente Fonnest, Sondergaard, Fonnest, & Vedsted-Jacobsen, 2000; McKelvey, Webb, Baldassar, Robinson, & Riley, 1999). We identified no studies that investigated the effects of a provider's religion or spirituality on the reproductive outcomes or choices of their patients.

FUTURE RESEARCH IN REPRODUCTIVE HEALTH AND RELIGION/SPIRITUALITY

Religion and religiosity have been associated with multiple reproductive decisions and health behaviors. It is unclear whether this association is negative, neutral, or positive. It is also not clear if religion or spirituality are simply confounding markers for other cultural factors in the cross-sectional studies conducted to date. Prospective study designs creatively adjusted for other cultural factors that influence decisions are needed in order to describe the role of religion/spirituality on decisions regarding sexuality, contraception, pregnancy termination, and fertility treatments. Future studies should investigate both beneficial and harmful effects of religion on reproductive outcomes.

Intervention studies to evaluate OBG practices that address spiritual concerns are sorely needed. Although most women are religious (Pew Research Center, 2015), and unmet spiritual needs have been identified in women undergoing reproductive decision making (Stalhandske et al., 2011), only one study evaluated a religious intervention in OBG care (El-Beshlawy et al., 2012). This study simply informed women about Islamic teaching during genetic counseling. Studies investigating ways to improve the cultural competence of health care providers related to religion and spirituality and studies investigating the impact of religious concordance or discordance between providers and patients are also needed.

RECOMMENDED BEST PRACTICES
FOR HEALTH CARE PROVIDERS

There is a lack of data to inform best practices for providing spiritual care in OBG settings. Therefore, this portion of the chapter offers reflections about providing spiritual care based mainly on personal experience. These suggestions should be seen as a starting point for future discussion and research.

REFLECTIONS ABOUT PROVIDING RELIGIOUS/ SPIRITUAL WOMEN'S HEALTH CARE

LISTEN

One of the most important things a provider can do is to listen to his/her patient (Van Berckelaer et al., 2012). On average, doctors interrupt patients about 18 seconds after they begin describing their chief complaints (Beckman & Frankel, 1984). This is especially problematic when trying to understand the effect of religious identity on reproductive decisions. These effects are not predictable. Few assumptions should be made. Women like Cristina and Dot who have previously expressed one point of view may change their minds during a life-changing event. For patients like Anita and Bethany, providers must hear what they are saying about their approach to sexuality and contraception. They must understand that their intentional approach to sexuality and contraception is essential to living out their faith. Trying to persuade them to do otherwise is not respectful and risks alienation and humiliation. For patients like Cristina, Dot, Edie, and Frances, it may be important to understand and hear the ambivalence accompanying their reproductive decision making. Providers who listen to patients demonstrate respect for their patients. This may open an opportunity for dialogue and mutual understanding that would not have happened otherwise.

ASK QUESTIONS

After listening, ask questions. When the impact of religion or spirituality remains unclear, ask questions. In some cases, the prudent clinician must also ask about the ethical voices of other entities (e.g. churches, cultural groups, etc.) in order to help the patient balance her actions in light of their guidance and directives. In our practice, we inquire about the religious identity of every new patient. We then ask if and how the patient's religion or other belief system impacts her decisions about reproductive treatments.

EDUCATE YOURSELF

OBG providers should make an effort to learn about how reproductive health issues are addressed by major religious groups in their geographic region. Reading religious position statements and talking with religious leaders directly may be more beneficial than relying on opinion articles and popular literature. For example, an obstetrician working with a Hmong population met with religious leaders in order to understand religious opposition to obtaining informed consent for cesarean section. Together they were able to implement a new informed consent process that was valued by both providers and the religious community. It is essential to state that such education should never be used as a way to coerce patients to do what one wants them to do.

INCORPORATE FERTILITY AWARENESS-BASED METHODS (FABMS)

In our own obstetrics and gynecology practice,[1] we offer FABMs as part of a treatment plan for reproductive health. The methods can be used effectively to avoid getting pregnant as well as to conceive and to monitor health concerns. By integrating these methods into our practice, we are able to offer care for a variety of problems in a way that is compatible with most major religions. For example, instead of using contraceptive agents to treat abnormal bleeding, women can use their fertility charting to detect underlying hormonal patterns. Providers can then use targeted hormone therapy or lifestyle modification to optimize and support the hormone cycle instead of suppressing it. Although not all practices can operate like ours, it is important for all women's health providers to identify local resources for FABM education. Many of the methods offer online or remote-learning options. Although these methods may not be for everyone, it is important to know that patients like Bethany can use these methods quite effectively if they are properly instructed.

OFFER RELIGIOUS/SPIRITUAL RESOURCES

Physicians should offer chaplain referrals to patients who are struggling with difficult reproductive decisions. Providers may find that involving the patient's personal religious leaders would be helpful in specific cases. Of course this will add another level of complexity. However, it may be especially helpful when the patient may not correctly understand the position of her religious leaders or when the religious leaders may not correctly understand the medical concern. In cases in which making the health care decision requires specialized medical knowledge, such as in Edie's case, consider inviting a colleague to be involved in the discussion who has a religious background similar to that of the patient.

SPIRITUAL REFLECTION

Finally, health care professionals need to be aware of and acknowledge how the professional's own religion/spirituality or lack thereof impacts care of patients. We recommend considering how their care impacts patients who share their beliefs as well as those who do not.

Reflections for religious providers of women's health care

While obstetrics and gynecology (OBG) is not unique among medical specialties, over the last century cultural changes, new knowledge about the biology of human reproduction, and a series of legal decisions have presented daily challenges to the practicing OBG whose religious and spiritual life guides her decision making. These challenges largely come about around the principle of individual conscience, although contemporary ethicists often frame them as issues of autonomy. In our clinical opinions, autonomy is the right to receive or provide care or not, according to one's conscience. Many religious OBG providers rely on their religious and spiritual beliefs to inform their conscience. Most cultures and governments acknowledge individual conscience and the right to live according to such in their constitutions and laws. People who resist "authority" to live according to their own conscience are often seen as heroes. A few examples include Thomas Moore, Mahatma Gandhi, and Martin Luther King Jr.

CASE: HANNAH

Hannah is a fourth year medical student who is planning to match into an obstetrics and gynecology residency. She loves providing prenatal care and delivering babies. Given her religious background, she has thought of herself as "pro-life." She starts a sub-internship in high-risk obstetrics. During the course of her rotation, she witnesses her preceptor counseling a variety of women about pregnancy complications ranging from serious birth defects to serious maternal illness. She feels that most of the counseling is directed toward terminating pregnancies. She feels uneasy having participated in these sessions. However, she is unsure about whether or not she would provide the same counsel if she had the same level of training as her preceptor.

As OBG practitioners within academic health systems, we consistently encounter religious trainees who lack clarity about their own individual convictions. This is not unexpected. Developmentally, they are at the end of the prolonged adolescence medical training requires. The sheer weight of technical information they must master leaves little time for meditation, prayer, or reflection. Trainees are often called on by patients to offer advice on subjects trainees have never considered or experienced. They may have poorly developed moral ideas about sexuality and reproduction informed by family and popular culture, but little practical facility in navigating their own consciences while providing OBG care. They definitely are inadequately prepared to relate their own conscience and actions to those of their patients.

Thus, the first and most important step in mastering the integration of religion and spirituality into medical practice is slowing down for a season of intentional reflection and meditation. The explicit purpose of such a time is to discover one's own conscience and the practical implications of what one's core beliefs. This may best occur after some exposure to medical training. Some of the implications of conscience cannot even be considered by those who have not experienced them. Reflection can be reinforced by reading, discussion, and lectures or sermons. It may also benefit from mentoring with a more experienced provider who has already done this work. In the end, it requires a personal investment of time and the discipline to look inward and, if desired outward, to whatever entity or entities the individual sees as authoritative. Until a clinician has done that hard work, he/she will be of little value, and perhaps even dangerous, when counseling others.

Hannah ultimately spends an elective month during her fourth year of medical school investigating her beliefs. She schedules regular time with a spiritual director and for reflection together with a religious community of health care providers. She is connected by her academic advisor to a geneticist. Together they plan a list of core readings and experiencing. Hannah shadows an OBG provider who shares her religious beliefs. During the month, she creates a written record of her thoughts and conclusions. She spends time on a week-long spiritual retreat before making her final decision to become an obstetrician gynecologist.

Reflections for non-religious providers

Even clinicians who lack or refute religious beliefs and would describe themselves as "secular humanists" or "spiritual, not religious" operate under the umbrella of professionalism. As such, they should be practicing virtues such as sensitivity to other cultures, fair allocation of resources, subordination of self-interest, and respect for the consciences of others (American Congress of Obstetricians and Gynecologists, 2011). Thus, the self-study and reflection we suggest for the religious clinician is equally important and fundamental for the non-religious clinician. We believe that all OBG providers should invest time and reflection to consider what they most deeply believe about reproductive issues. Also, they should consider where their beliefs stand compared to the moral traditions that influence all of our beliefs. The non-religious OBG will often face scenarios involving families with religious beliefs. A failure to have spent time in reflection could hinder those interactions and prevent the development of the respect for other people and cultures that professionalism demands.

Telling young learners in medicine with religious and spiritual inclinations to do more work will not be popular, but we must emphasize a major benefit. Seeing individuals and their consciences as important, being given the opportunity to enter their stories, and even having one's advice sought, and occasionally followed, injects real joy into the routine of day-to-day medical practice. It gives an importance to each encounter and each patient that otherwise is easily overlooked or displaced. We have found that the joy arising from such encounters can keep one going through the long days and nights OBG practice entails.

CAREFULLY NAVIGATE RELIGIOUS DISCORD BETWEEN PATIENT AND PROVIDER.

The process of self-discovery is, in our experience, a life-long journey. Once progress has been made, however, the clinician can safely ponder the consciences of their patients. Clinicians should first acknowledge that they all have some degree of influence or authority over their patients. All but the most fundamental and authoritarian beliefs about individual conscience deplore the use of this authority to coerce or force another to do something. This is true even if our conscience tells us their action would be wrong. We may inform, encourage, and question, but we must take exquisite care to respect the conscience of the individuals we have the privilege to treat.

If our patient ultimately makes an informed decision that would violate our conscience, we must first return to our overarching principle: respect individual conscience. For example, a woman may be informed that her fetus has a serious birth defect. The clinician's conscience may ascribe a moral status to her fetus. This would preclude the clinician from terminating a pregnancy if he or she were in similar circumstances as the patient. However, the clinician should not purposefully neglect to mention the possibility of termination. Neither should they falsely inflate the risks of termination to coerce the behaviors they would see as correct. On the other hand, if their conscience did not ascribe moral status to the fetus, they might believe the woman and the family would benefit from a termination of pregnancy. In this case, the clinician should not purposely neglect to mention the possibility of allowing the pregnancy to progress without termination. He or she should not falsely conflate the risks and benefits of termination. These type of situations require the utmost awareness of our own beliefs and those of the patient. We must respect the inherent power differential between the physician and patient and have sympathy for the suffering and powerlessness of our patients.

At times, albeit rarely, a conflict will arise between patient and clinician that cannot be resolved by dialogue and reflection. Examples may include patients who request cesarean delivery for fetal distress in the setting of serious fetal anomalies that are likely lethal, or patients who opt for a pregnancy termination that the clinician's conscience forbids her to perform. In these cases, there are two options. The first option is to request that the patient transfer her care to another provider. This has also been called an "indirect" versus a "direct" referral (Chervenak & McCullough, 2008). When patients make informed decisions guided by their conscience that conflict with our own, we are not obliged to violate our own conscience to serve theirs. In this case, we are obliged by the principle of respect for autonomy to respect her decision. Some providers who conscientiously object to providing certain OBG services feel that providing any type of "referral" means being complicit in the provision of that service. The nomenclature of "transfer of care" or "indirect referral" versus "direct referral" relating to pregnancy termination is important historically. Prior to the legalization of abortion in the United States, clinicians sympathetic to women's request for pregnancy termination would "refer" her to a clandestine abortion provider for the procedure. Once pregnancy terminations became legal, this underground referral system was no longer necessary. Today, abortion and other OBG providers advertise and publicize their services. No secret access or special knowledge is needed. Sending records, lab work, and images to different providers does not make the transferring physician complicit in an act she deems immoral. We believe it does reflect the respect for individual autonomy that forms the foundation of most religious and spiritual ethical systems.

The second approach to consider when provider and patient disagree is a bioethics consultation. In some cases, this will be necessary because no other provider is available to provide the desired service. Ethics consultations are available at most health care institutions. Their goal is to "improve the quality of health care through the identification, analysis and resolution of ethical questions and concerns" (Tarzian & ASBH Core Competencies Update Task Force, 2013). Sometimes an ethics consultation is staffed by a single expert, but in difficult cases, a team is convened. The team members usually comprise a variety of viewpoints, including, among others, religious leaders, philosophers, clinicians, and patient representatives. Ethics teams use a facilitation approach by eliciting and clarifying the nature of the discrepancy and identifying a range of resolutions that would be morally acceptable to all involved parties (Tarzian & ASBH Core Competencies Update Task Force, 2013). Ethics consultations may allow the parties who differ to clear up miscommunications and to identify and embrace shared values. In studies of families dealing with end-of-life decisions, the majority of providers and patients (87%) felt that the consultation was helpful (Schneiderman et al., 2003). To our knowledge, there are no studies evaluating their effects among families making reproductive decisions.

MAKE CAREFUL DECISIONS ABOUT PRACTICE LOCATION AND PARTNERS

In a few countries (Sweden, Finland, and Iceland), those who would conscientiously object to providing certain reproductive services would have to find work in another field of medicine (Fiala, Gemzell Danielsson, Heikinheimo, Guodmundsson, & Arthur, 2016). However, in most countries, conscientious objection is supported in the context of OBG care. We believe that having providers of a diverse religious background in the field of women's health improves the cultural competence of care. If an OBG provider plans or envisions practicing according to conscience, we believe it critical that she find like-minded partners to work with. This again points to the crucial nature of the prior step we suggested—discerning one own' s conscience. Thereafter, one would want to seek practice situations where conscience is respected and clinicians have invested in similar work. This does not preclude practicing with individuals who disagree on particulars but would indicate the need for conversations on how to practically handle these differences.

CONCLUSION

Women's reproductive health care will be impacted by the religion/spirituality of both the patient and her provider. However, the ways in which it is impacted are not always straightforward or predictable. Keeping an open dialogue with patients about how their religion and spirituality are impacting their health care is of great importance. It is just as important for providers to know how their own conscience and religion/spirituality uses will affect patient the care they offer. We believe that it is a great privilege to know one's conscience, practice accordingly, and interact in a positive way with the consciences of our patients and colleagues.

NOTE

1. See www.replyobgyn.com for details.

REFERENCES

Agadjanian, V. (2013). Religious denomination, religious involvement, and modern contraceptive use in southern Mozambique. *Stud Fam Plann, 44*(3), 259–274. doi:10.1111/j.1728-4465.2013.00357.x

American Congress of Obstetricians and Gynecologists. (2011). *Code of professional ethics of the American College of Obstetricians and Gynecologists.* Washington, DC: ACOG.

Amoako-Agyeman, K. N. (2012). Adolescent religiosity and attitudes to HIV and AIDS in Ghana. *SAHARA J, 9*(4), 227–241. doi:10.1080/17290376.2012.745665

Asubiaro, O. Y., & Fatusi, A. O. (2014). Differential effects of religiosity on sexual initiation among Nigerian in-school adolescents. *Int J Adolesc Med Health, 26*(1), 93–100. doi:10.1515/ijamh-2012-0118

Bair, Y. A., Gold, E. B., Greendale, G. A., Sternfeld, B., Adler, S. R., Azari, R., & Harkey, M. (2002). Ethnic differences in use of complementary and alternative medicine at midlife: Longitudinal results from SWAN participants. *Am J Public Health, 92*(11), 1832–1840.

Beckman, H. B., & Frankel, R. M. (1984). The effect of physician behavior on the collection of data. *Ann Intern Med, 101*(5), 692–696.

Bell, M., & Stoneman, Z. (2000). Reactions to prenatal testing: Reflection of religiosity and attitudes toward abortion and people with disabilities. *Am J Ment Retard, 105*(1), 1–13. doi:10.1352/0895-8017(2000)105<0001:rtptro>2.0.co;2

Burdette, A. M., Weeks, J., Hill, T. D., & Eberstein, I. W. (2012). Maternal religious attendance and low birth weight. *Soc Sci Med, 74*(12), 1961–1967. doi:10.1016/j.socscimed.2012.02.021

Cebeci Save, D., Erbaydar, T., Kalaca, S., Harmanci, H., Cali, S., & Karavus, M. (2004). Resistance against contraception or medical contraceptive methods: A qualitative study on women and men in Istanbul. *Eur J Contracept Reprod Health Care, 9*(2), 94–101.

Cerqueira-Santos, E., Koller, S., & Wilcox, B. (2008). Condom use, contraceptive methods, and religiosity among youths of low socioeconomic level. *Span J Psychol, 11*(1), 94–102.

Chacko, E. (2001). Women's use of contraception in rural India: A village-level study. *Health Place, 7*(3), 197–208.

Chervenak, F. A., & McCullough, L. B. (2008). The ethics of direct and indirect referral for termination of pregnancy. *Am J Obstet Gynecol, 199*(3), 232.e231–233.

Chung, G. S., Lawrence, R. E., Rasinski, K. A., Yoon, J. D., & Curlin, F. A. (2012). Obstetrician-gynecologists' beliefs about when pregnancy begins. *Am J Obstet Gynecol, 206*(2), 132. e131–137. doi:10.1016/j.ajog.2011.10.877

Curlin, F. A., Lawrence, R. E., Chin, M. H., & Lantos, J. D. Religion, Conscience, and Controversial Clinical Practices. *NEJM, 2007, 356*:593-600.

de Costa, C. M., Russell, D. B., & Carrette, M. (2010). Views and practices of induced abortion among Australian Fellows and specialist trainees of the Royal Australian and New Zealand College of Obstetricians and Gynaecologists. *Med J Aust, 193*(1), 13–16.

de la Fuente Fonnest, I., Sondergaard, F., Fonnest, G., & Vedsted-Jacobsen, A. (2000). Attitudes among health care professionals on the ethics of assisted reproductive technologies and legal abortion. *Acta Obstet Gynecol Scand, 79*(1), 49–53.

Dessio, W., Wade, C., Chao, M., Kronenberg, F., Cushman, L. E., & Kalmuss, D. (2004). Religion, spirituality, and healthcare choices of African-American women: Results of a national survey. *Ethn Dis, 14*(2), 189–197.

Doctor, H. V., Phillips, J. F., & Sakeah, E. (2009). The influence of changes in women's religious affiliation on contraceptive use and fertility among the Kassena-Nankana of northern Ghana. *Stud Fam Plann, 40*(2), 113–122.

Dreweke, R. J. J. (2011). *Countering conventional wisdom: New evidence on religion and contraceptive use.* Retrieved from New York:

Dutney, A. (2007). Religion, infertility and assisted reproductive technology. *Best Pract Res Clin Obstet Gynaecol, 21*(1), 169–180. doi:10.1016/j.bpobgyn.2006.09.007

El-Beshlawy, A., El-Shekha, A., Momtaz, M., Said, F., Hamdy, M., Osman, O., . . . Petrou, M. (2012). Prenatal diagnosis for thalassaemia in Egypt: What changed parents' attitude? *Prenat Diagn, 32*(8), 777–782. doi:10.1002/pd.3901

Fiala, C., Gemzell Danielsson, K., Heikinheimo, O., Guodmundsson, J. A., & Arthur, J. (2016). Yes we can! Successful examples of disallowing 'conscientious objection' in reproductive health care. *Eur J Contracept Reprod Health Care, 21*(3), 201–206.

Fielder, R. L., Walsh, J. L., Carey, K. B., & Carey, M. P. (2013). Predictors of sexual hookups: A theory-based, prospective study of first-year college women. *Arch Sex Behav, 42*(8), 1425–1441. doi:10.1007/s10508-013-0106-0

Finer, L. B. (2007). Trends in premarital sex in the United States, 1954–2003. *Public Health Rep, 122*(1), 73–78.

Foster, D. G., Gould, H., Taylor, J., & Weitz, T. A. (2012). Attitudes and decision making among women seeking abortions at one U.S. clinic. *Perspect Sex Reprod Health, 44*(2), 117–124. doi:10.1363/4411712

Gold, M. A., Sheftel, A. V., Chiappetta, L., Young, A. J., Zuckoff, A., DiClemente, C. C., & Primack, B. A. (2010). Associations between religiosity and sexual and contraceptive behaviors. *J Pediatr Adolesc Gynecol, 23*(5), 290–297. doi:10.1016/j.jpag.2010.02.012

Greil, A., McQuillan, J., Benjamins, M., Johnson, D. R., Johnson, K. M., & Heinz, C. R. (2010). Specifying the effects of religion on medical helpseeking: The case of infertility. *Soc Sci Med, 71*(4), 734–742. doi:10.1016/j.socscimed.2010.04.033

Grimes, D. A., Gallo, M. F., Grigorieva, V., Nanda, K., & Schulz, K. F. (2005). Fertility awareness-based methods for contraception: Systematic review of randomized controlled trials. *Contraception, 72*(2), 85–90. doi:10.1016/j.contraception.2005.03.010

Haghpanah, S., Nasirabadi, S., Rahimi, N., Faramarzi, H., & Karimi, M. (2012). Sociocultural challenges of beta-thalassaemia major birth in carriers of beta-thalassaemia in Iran. *J Med Screen, 19*(3), 109–111. doi:10.1258/jms.2012.012038

Haglund, K. A., & Fehring, R. J. (2010). The association of religiosity, sexual education, and parental factors with risky sexual behaviors among adolescents and young adults. *J Relig Health, 49*(4), 460–472. doi:10.1007/s10943-009-9267-5

Hall, K. S., Moreau, C., & Trussell, J. (2012). Lower use of sexual and reproductive health services among women with frequent religious participation, regardless of sexual experience. *J Women's Health (Larchmt), 21*(7), 739–747. doi:10.1089/jwh.2011.3356

Harris, L. H., Cooper, A., Rasinski, K. A., Curlin, F. A., & Lyerly, A. D. (2011). Obstetrician-gynecologists' objections to and willingness to help patients obtain an abortion. *Obstet Gynecol, 118*(4), 905–912. doi:10.1097/AOG.0b013e31822f12b7

Harrison, B. (2005). Is natural family planning a heresy. *This Rock, 16*(2), 12–16.

Hasnain, M., Connell, K. J., Menon, U., & Tranmer, P. A. (2011). Patient-centered care for Muslim women: provider and patient perspectives. *J Women's Health (Larchmt), 20*(1), 73–83. doi:10.1089/jwh.2010.2197

Hennink, M., Diamond, I., & Cooper, P. (1999). Contraceptive use dynamics of Asian women in Britain. *J Biosoc Sci, 31*(4), 537–554.

Hirsch, J. S. (2008). Catholics using contraceptives: Religion, family planning, and interpretive agency in rural Mexico. *Stud Fam Plann, 39*(2), 93–104.

Imudia, A. N., Awonuga, A. O., Dbouk, T., Kumar, S., Cordoba, M., Diamond, M. P., & Bahado-Singh, R. O. (2009). Racial disparity in the clinical determinants and outcomes of cesarean hysterectomy. *J Natl Med Assoc, 101*(6), 565–568.

Jesse, D. E., Graham, M., & Swanson, M. (2006). Psychosocial and spiritual factors associated with smoking and substance use during pregnancy in African American and White low-income women. *J Obstet Gynecol Neonatal Nurs, 35*(1), 68–77. doi:10.1111/j.1552-6909.2006.00010.x

Jesse, D. E., & Reed, P. G. (2004). Effects of spirituality and psychosocial well-being on health risk behaviors in Appalachian pregnant women. *J Obstet Gynecol Neonatal Nurs, 33*(6), 739–747. doi:10.1177/0884217504270669

Jesse, D. E., Schoneboom, C., & Blanchard, A. (2007). The effect of faith or spirituality in pregnancy: A content analysis. *J Holist Nurs, 25*(3), 151–158; discussion 159. doi:10.1177/0898010106293593

John Paul, I. (1995). *Encyclical letter, evangelium vitae: On the value and inviobility of human life*. Washington, DC: United States Catholic Conference.

Johnson-Hanks, J. (2006). On the politics and practice of Muslim fertility: Comparative evidence from West Africa. *Med Anthropol Q, 20*(1), 12–30.

Jones, R. K., Finer, L. B., & Singh, S. (2010). *Characteristics of U.S. abortion patients, 2008*. Guttmacher Institute, New York. Retrieved from https://www.guttmacher.org/sites/default/files/report_pdf/us-abortion-patients.pdf

Jones, R. K., & Kavanaugh, M. L. (2011). Changes in abortion rates between 2000 and 2008 and lifetime incidence of abortion. *Obstet Gynecol, 117*(6), 1358–1366. doi:10.1097/AOG.0b013e31821c405e

Kamal, S. M., & Islam, M. A. (2010). Contraceptive use: Socioeconomic correlates and method choices in rural Bangladesh. *Asia Pac J Public Health, 22*(4), 436–450. doi:10.1177/1010539510370780

Kansal, A., Kandpal, S. D., & Mishra, P. (2006). Reasons for not practicing contraception in a rural population of Dehradun District. *J Commun Dis, 38*(1), 97–101.

Kulig, J. C., Babcock, R., Wall, M., & Hill, S. (2009). Being a woman: Perspectives of low-German-speaking Mennonite women. *Health Care Women Int, 30*(4), 324–338. doi:10.1080/07399330802694989

Kyle, D., Cummins, C., & Evans, S. (1988). Factors affecting the uptake of screening for neural tube defect. *Br J Obstet Gynaecol, 95*(6), 560–564.

Lawrence, R. E., Rasinski, K. A., Yoon, J. D., & Curlin, F. A. (2010). Obstetrician-gynecologist physicians' beliefs about emergency contraception: a national survey. *Contraception, 82*(4), 324–330. doi:10.1016/j.contraception.2010.04.151

Lefkowitz, E. S., Gillen, M. M., Shearer, C. L., & Boone, T. L. (2004). Religiosity, sexual behaviors, and sexual attitudes during emerging adulthood. *J Sex Res, 41*(2), 150–159. doi:10.1080/00224490409552223

Lopez-del Burgo, C., Lopez-de Fez, C. M., Osorio, A., Guzman, J. L., & de Irala, J. (2010). Spanish women's attitudes towards post-fertilization effects of birth control methods. *Eur J Obstet Gynecol Reprod Biol, 151*(1), 56–61. doi:10.1016/j.ejogrb.2010.03.012

Lyerly, A. D., Steinhauser, K., Voils, C., Namey, E., Alexander, C., Bankowski, B., . . . Wallach, E. (2010). Fertility patients' views about frozen embryo disposition: Results of a multi-national institutional U.S. survey. *Fertil Steril, 93*(2), 499–509.

Mabiala Babela, J. R., Massamba, A., Bantsimba, T., & Senga, P. (2008). [Sexual behaviour among adolescents in Brazzaville, Congo]. *J Gynecol Obstet Biol Reprod (Paris), 37*(5), 510–515. doi:10.1016/j.jgyn.2007.11.033

Manhart, M. D., Duane, M., Lind, A., Sinai, I., & Golden-Tevald, J. (2013). Fertility awareness-based methods of family planning: a review of effectiveness for avoiding pregnancy using SORT. *Osteopathic Family Physician, 5*(1), 2–8.

Manlove, J., Terry-Humen, E., & Ikramullah, E. (2006). Young teenagers and older sexual partners: Correlates and consequences for males and females. *Perspect Sex Reprod Health, 38*(4), 197–207. doi:10.1363/psrh.38.197.06

Martin, T. C. (2005). Contraceptive use patterns among Spanish single youth. *Eur J Contracept Reprod Health Care, 10*(4), 219–228. doi:10.1080/13625180500282379

May, J. F., Mukamenzi, M., & Vekemans, M. (1990). Family planning in Rwanda: Status and prospects. *Stud Fam Plann, 21*(1), 20–32.

McKelvey, R. S., Webb, J. A., Baldassar, L. V., Robinson, S. M., & Riley, G. (1999). Sex knowledge and sexual attitudes among medical and nursing students. *Aust N Z J Psychiatry, 33*(2), 260–266.

Merchant, R. C., Casadei, K., Gee, E. M., Bock, B. C., Becker, B. M., & Clark, M. A. (2007). Patients' emergency contraception comprehension, usage, and view of the emergency department role for emergency contraception. *J Emerg Med, 33*(4), 367–375. doi:10.1016/j.jemermed.2007.02.031

Mishtal, J., & Dannefer, R. (2010). Reconciling religious identity and reproductive practices: The Church and contraception in Poland. *Eur J Contracept Reprod Health Care, 15*(4), 232–242. doi:10.3109/13625187.2010.498595

Moos, M. K., Dunlop, A. L., Jack, B. W., Nelson, L., Coonrod, D. V., Long, R., . . . Gardiner, P. M. (2008). Healthier women, healthier reproductive outcomes: Recommendations for the routine care of all women of reproductive age. *Am J Obstet Gynecol, 199*(6 Suppl 2), S280–289. doi:10.1016/j.ajog.2008.08.060

Murstein, B. I., & Mercy, T. (1994). Sex, drugs, relationships, contraception, and fears of disease on a college campus over 17 years. *Adolescence, 29*(114), 303–322.

Notzer, N., Levran, D., Mashiach, S., & Soffer, S. (1984). Effect of religiosity on sex attitudes, experience and contraception among university students. *J Sex Marital Ther, 10*(1), 57–62. doi:10.1080/00926238408405790

Official Catholic directory. (2015). New York: P. J. Kennedy.

Paik, A., Sanchagrin, K. J., & Heimer, K. (2016). Broken promises: Abstinence pledging and sexual and reproductive health. *J Marriage Fam, 78*(2), 546–561.

Patel, P., Farley, J., Impey, L., & Lakhoo, K. (2008). Evaluation of a fetomaternal-surgical clinic for prenatal counselling of surgical anomalies. *Pediatr Surg Int, 24*(4), 391–394. doi:10.1007/s00383-008-2118-8

Paul, V. I. (1968). Encyclical humanae vitae, Vol. 487. AAS 60.

Petchesky, R. P., & Judd, K. (Eds.). (1998). *Negotiating reproductive rights: Women's perspectives across countries and cultures.* Atlantic Highlands, NJ: Zed Books.

Pew Research Center. (2015). *America's changing religious landscape.* Retrieved from http://www.pewforum.org/files/2015/05/RLS-08-26-full-report.pdf

Pillai, V. K., & Sunil, T. S. (2007). Contraceptive use in Yemen: A component analysis. *World Health Popul, 9*(4), 65–78.

Raghavan, R. (2007). A piece of my mind. A question of faith. *JAMA, 297*(13), 1412.

Raine, T., Minnis, A. M., & Padian, N. S. (2003). Determinants of contraceptive method among young women at risk for unintended pregnancy and sexually transmitted infections. *Contraception, 68*(1), 19–25.

Richters, J., Grulich, A. E., de Visser, R. O., Smith, A. M., & Rissel, C. E. (2003). Sex in Australia: Contraceptive practices among a representative sample of women. *Aust N Z J Public Health, 27*(2), 210–216.

Rostosky, S. S., Regnerus, M. D., & Wright, M. L. (2003). Coital debut: The role of religiosity and sex attitudes in the Add Health Survey. *J Sex Res, 40*(4), 358–367. doi:10.1080/00224490209552202

Roy, M., Lahiri, B. C., & Ghosh, B. N. (1978). A KAP study on MTP acceptors and their contraceptive practice. *Indian J Public Health, 22*(2), 189–196.

Salmoirago-Blotcher, E., Fitchett, G., Ockene, J. K., Schnall, E., Crawford, S., Granek, I., . . . Rapp, S. (2011). Religion and healthy lifestyle behaviors among postmenopausal women: The women's health initiative. *J Behav Med, 34*(5), 360–371. doi:10.1007/s10865-011-9322-z

Schenker, J. G. (2000). Women's reproductive health: Monotheistic religious perspectives. *Int J Gynecol Obstect, 70*(1), 77–86.

Schneiderman, L. J., Gilmer, T., Teetzel, H. D., Dugan, D. O., Blustein, J., Cranford, R., . . . Young, E. W. D. (2003). Effect of ethics consultations on nonbeneficial life-sustaining treatments in the intensive care setting: A randomized trial. *JAMA, 290*(9), 1166–1172.

Shah, N. M., Shah, M. A., Chowdhury, R. I., & Menon, I. (2007). Reasons and correlates of contraceptive discontinuation in Kuwait. *Eur J Contracept Reprod Health Care, 12*(3), 260–268. doi:10.1080/13625180701440560

Silber, T. J. (1980). Abortion: A Jewish view. *J Relig Health, 19*(3), 231–239.

Stalhandske, M. L., Ekstrand, M., & Tyden, T. (2011). Women's existential experiences within Swedish abortion care. *J Psychosom Obstet Gynaecol, 32*(1), 35–41. doi:10.3109/0167482x.2010.545457

Stalhandske, M. L., Makenzius, M., Tyden, T., & Larsson, M. (2012). Existential experiences and needs related to induced abortion in a group of Swedish women: A quantitative investigation. *J Psychosom Obstet Gynaecol, 33*(2), 53–61. doi:10.3109/0167482x.2012.677877

Stanford, J. B. & Mikolajczyk, R. T (2002). Mechanisms of action of intrauterine devices: update and estimation of postfertilization effects. *Am J Obstet Gynecol, 187*(6):1699-708.

Sulmasy, D. P. (2008). What is conscience and why is respect for it so important? *Theor Med Bioeth, 29*(3), 135–149.

Tanfer, K., & Horn, M. C. (1985). Contraceptive use, pregnancy and fertility patterns among single American women in their 20s. *Fam Plann Perspect, 17*(1), 10–19.

Tarzian, A. J., & ASBH Core Competencies Update Task Force. (2013). Health care ethics consultation: An update on core competencies and emerging standards from the American Society for Bioethics and Humanities' Core Competencies Update Task Force. *Am J Bioeth, 13*(2), 3–13.

Tomkins, A., Duff, J., Fitzgibbon, A., Karam, A., Mills, E. J., Munnings, K., . . . Yugi, P. (2015). Controversies in faith and health care. *Lancet, 386*(10005), 1776–1785.

United States Conference of Catholic Bishops. (2009). *Ethical and religious directives for Catholic health care services. Fifth Edition.* Washington, D.C.: USCCB.

Upchurch, D. M., & Chyu, L. (2005). Use of complementary and alternative medicine among American women. *Women's Health Issues, 15*(1), 5–13. doi:10.1016/j.whi.2004.08.010

Van Berckelaer, A., DiRocco, D., Ferguson, M., Gray, P., Marcus, N., & Day, S. (2012). Building a patient-centered medical home: Obtaining the patient's voice. *J Am Board Fam Med, 25*(2), 192–198. doi:10.3122/jabfm.2012.02.100235

Vaughan, B., Trussell, J., Kost, K., Singh, S., & Jones, R. (2008). Discontinuation and resumption of contraceptive use: Results from the 2002 National Survey of Family Growth. *Contraception, 78*(4), 271–283. doi:10.1016/j.contraception.2008.05.007

Vu, H. H. (1996). Cultural barriers between obstetrician-gynecologists and Vietnamese/Chinese immigrant women. *Tex Med, 92*(10), 47–52.

Yoon, J. D., Rasinski, K. A., & Curlin, F. A. (2010). Moral controversy, directive counsel, and the doctor's role: Findings from a national survey of obstetrician-gynecologists. *Acad Med, 85*(9), 1475–1481. doi:10.1097/ACM.0b013e3181eabacc

Zaleski, E. H., & Schiaffino, K. M. (2000). Religiosity and sexual risk-taking behavior during the transition to college. *J Adolesc, 23*(2), 223–227. doi:10.1006/jado.2000.0309

CHAPTER 3

RELIGION AND SPIRITUALITY IN PEDIATRICS

Sarah Jean Barton, Lucy Selman, Gary Maslow, and Raymond Barfield

Among adult populations, ample evidence demonstrates that spirituality is associated with improved quality of life, hope, and patient satisfaction (McNeil, 2015; Balboni et al., 2013; Reynolds, 2008; Richardson, 2012; Surbone & Baider, 2010). However, there is a dearth of similar evidence within pediatric populations. Existing pediatric studies focus on the provision of spiritual care by chaplains and nurses, with little investigation of the role of physicians and other medical professionals in addressing the spiritual needs of pediatric clients. In addition, there is sparse evidence on the impacts of spirituality and religious practice in pediatrics, especially how these relate to children and families coping with chronic illness (Drutchas & Anandarajah, 2014).

Despite the scant evidence in pediatrics, especially in comparison to adult populations, the existing evidence affirms spirituality and religious beliefs as "key organizing principles" for children and families within medical contexts (Barnes et al., 2000). Pediatric-specific definitions of spirituality include "the ability to derive personal value and transcend beyond the self through relationships with others," a "passion or wonder for living" (Barros Meireles et al., 2015), and a "capacity for encountering mystery" (Burkhardt, 1991). Belonging and membership emerge as key factors that characterize spirituality among children (Pfund, 2000). Elkins & Cavendish (2004) carefully underscore that issues of spirituality do not only arise among ill or dying children, but also that nearly all children consistently engage in spiritually fueled processes of meaning-making. Mercer (2006) describes "children's spirituality" as "the aspect of children's lives connecting them to a wider sense of meaning-making, to relationships with others and to relationships with the sacred/transcendent." For Mercer, pediatric spirituality is both narrative and symbolic in nature. The central influence of parental spirituality, religious practices, and beliefs in pediatric care makes it a particularly unique clinical setting. In pediatrics, "family-based spiritual care" (Knapp et al., 2011; Rolim Lima et al., 2013), which emphasizes the provision of collaborative parental spiritual care (Smith & McSherry, 2004), is central to addressing the spiritual and religious needs of sick children (Elkins & Cavendish, 2004). For example, medical professionals might address family spiritual and religious needs by connecting both children and their caregivers with non-medical and community-based sources of spiritual and religious support (Barnes et al., 2000).

In this chapter, we first review a range of pediatric populations in which spiritual concerns frequently surface. We then address the "state of the science" regarding spirituality and religion among pediatric populations in medical contexts. We next explore "best practices" among medical professionals to address spirituality in pediatric populations, from theoretical approaches to embodied practices. We conclude the chapter with reflection on salient areas for future research.

COMMON CASES OF SPIRITUAL NEED IN PEDIATRICS

The search for spiritual support often springs from the experience of *isolation* among families and children in medical settings. This isolation arises from a child's removal from his or her typical contexts of play, school, and community activities and is often most strongly apparent among adolescents (Purow et al., 2011). Even more powerfully, isolation from one's religious community, especially when hospitalization prevents physical participation and presence in a community of faith, can lead to pediatric spiritual needs associated with belonging and cultivating a feeling of belovedness by a Higher Power (Elkins & Cavendish, 2004). Consider, for example, the case of a young adolescent boy preparing for his Bar Mitzvah while receiving a bone marrow transplant. The patient and his family face isolation as they realize that the celebration will have to be relocated to his hospital room where large numbers of visitors are prohibited. Similarly, consider the isolation of a pediatric patient whose family's participation in *Salat* (daily prayers) is disrupted as the patient's mother and father are ushered out of her hospital room to make space for a code team rushing in to attend to the other patient sharing the room.

In addition to the spiritual needs related to experiences of isolation, *fearfulness* and *anxiety* associated with experiences of disability and pain, end-of-life decisions and parental distress often indicate a need for spiritual and religious attention (Yates, 2011). Pediatric patients and families report a desire to respond to psychosocial needs related to fear and anxiety with practices such as prayer, thus highlighting the need for health care providers to consider how they might engage patients and families in this area of common religious and spiritual need (Yates, 2011). For example, families navigating difficult medical decisions benefit from medical professionals assisting the family to identify sources of spiritual and religious meaning. In our pediatric clinical settings, this has manifested in everything from familiar gospel music to traditional Jewish prayers of blessing. These familiar sources of religious practice serve as antidotes to fear and anxiety in the medical setting. Physicians and other medical professionals can play a key role in encouraging families to identify and use these kinds of religious practices as a means of addressing spiritual needs.

Profound spiritual needs often arise after children and families receive a significant diagnosis, especially if it is chronic, devastating, or progressive in nature (Cadge et al., 2009; Pehler & Craft-Rosenberg, 2009). The context of a significant change in a child's medical status or a notable loss of function are also times of significant spiritual need (Elkins & Cavendish, 2004). In one case example, a toddler who received a successful heart transplantation but suffered a neurologically devastating stroke just one week after transplant left the toddler's family with significant questions about divine control, new depths of spiritual lament, and a deepened need for religious sensitivity from medical providers as the family more fervently desired prayer from medical practitioners before all interventions.

Research on spiritual and religious needs in pediatric oncology settings highlights the frequency of spiritual distress in this population (Hart & Schneider, 1997; Rolim Lima et al., 2013). Specific spiritual challenges in pediatric oncology may include the fear of body disfigurement (e.g. weight loss, alopecia, loss of limb) and unpredictable prognosis (Hart & Schneider, 1997; Baldacchino et al., 2012). Within the pediatric oncology setting, there is evidence that spirituality acts as a source of hope and comfort—a "protective factor for enhancing resilience and quality of life" (Barros Meireles et al., 2015). For example, we have found that engagement of physicians in spiritually focused discussions with young women facing the loss of their fertility secondary to chemotherapy helps meet the spiritual needs associated with the deep loss experienced by these patients.

The pediatric intensive care unit (PICU) represents another context of common spiritual distress (Longden, 2012; Meert et al., 2005; Robinson et al., 2006). Robinson et al. (2006) found that for many parents, the PICU is viewed as a context for their child's "spiritual journey." A central aspect of this journey is considering the location of a child's death, either in the PICU, or with assistance to transition to home or hospice care during the dying process (Longden, 2012). Robinson et al. (2006) found that the parents of children who died in the PICU commonly understood faith as synonymous with seeking wisdom and discernment from Scripture in order to engage in medical decision making on behalf of their child. This same study identified that for parents whose children died in the PICU, the most important spiritual supports from medical professionals included prayer, facilitation of access to clergy, and help to cultivate a "belief in the transcendent quality of the parent-child relationship that endures beyond death." In addition to these kinds of spiritual support, we have witnessed the positive implications of physicians acting to coordinate spiritually and culturally appropriate space and time for a child's family after a child's death to participate in religious practices of lament as well as ritual religious practices associated with the child's body.

PROVIDER AND PARENTAL PERSPECTIVES ON SPIRITUALITY IN PEDIATRICS

Historically, the primary context for engagement with spirituality and religion between pediatric clinicians and parents has been parental religious objections to their child's medical care (Armbruster et al., 2003). The American Academy of Pediatrics (2013) identifies the following as potentially harmful invocations of parental spirituality into pediatric medical care: parental refusal to medically treat their child, the presence of "religious exemptions to child abuse and neglect laws, and the availability of public funding for the use of 'alternative unproven religious or spiritual healing practices.' "

This historical reality leads many current pediatric clinicians to perceive religion and spiritual convictions as problematic factors in parental medical decision-making. Providers must navigate these situations with wisdom and patience, particularly in the face of power dynamics that strongly favor physicians (Barnes et al., 2000). It is important for providers to remain aware of the heightened vulnerability felt by families as they discuss the spiritual contours of their medical decision making, especially in relationship to "giving bad news in a life-threatening illness and dealing with death and dying" (Siegel et al., 2002). Parents often hesitate to share spiritually influenced beliefs with providers (especially physicians) due to their wishes to maintain their sources of spiritual comfort without physician disruption. Parents also fear rejection and negativity from medical teams if they share their spiritual beliefs (Kemper & Barnes, 2003). This understandable parental hesitancy complicates the provision of spiritual care and can lead to negative outcomes due to a lack of shared understanding between parents and providers.

In light of the common complaints and frustrations regarding religion in the pediatric setting, Siegel et al. (2002) were surprised to find a majority of overwhelmingly positive feelings among pediatric providers regarding the importance of engaging issues of spirituality and religion in pediatric care. Unfortunately, even in clinical contexts where pediatric spirituality is prioritized, parental spiritual needs are often neglected. In settings where parental spirituality is engaged, it is often only at the time of diagnosis and not after a child's death (Meert et al., 2005; Davies et al., 2002).

Parents and caregivers provide critical insights on spiritual and religious needs in pediatric clinical settings. In order to provide best practices, medical professionals must more attentively listen to the spiritual and religious needs of the parents of ill children. Meert et al. (2005) found that in contrast to others involved in a child's medical care, parents identified their primary spiritual concern as maintaining connection with their child, especially during the process of dying, at the time of death, and after their child dies. Medical providers can facilitate this kind of spiritual connection by explicitly facilitating parental participation in the care of their child. For example, physical and occupational therapists might provide parents with recommendations on how to comfortably hold their child who is supported by mechanical ventilation, in order to provide both a child and parent with physical touch during religious practices such as prayer or singing. This kind of facilitation by medical professionals can also continue after a child's death, as when clinicians present parents with spiritually meaningful objects such as a lock of hair, their child's hospital gown, or hand prints (Meert et al., 2005).

Meert et al. (2005) also identified the positive and meaningful impact on parents of receiving truthful and easily understood information from physicians regarding their child's condition. This kind of communication decreased parental spiritual distress. At the same time, Meert et. al (2005) stressed that parents also need providers to offer true compassion, especially when communicating particularly difficult medical updates, or at the time of a child's death.

THE STATE OF SCIENCE IN PEDIATRICS

THE NEGLECT OF SPIRITUAL CARE
AND NEED FOR TRAINING

Though recognized as an important domain in clinical settings, spiritual and religious interventions are often neglected in pediatric practice. In a survey of 90 pediatricians, Armbruster et al. (2003) found that most believed "spirituality and religious issues have health implications, strengthen the therapeutic relationship, warrant appropriate referral, and are a source of support for patients and their families." Over three-quarters of participants believed that pediatricians should "facilitate contact between patients and religious support services." Despite this belief, most study participants did not routinely inquire about spiritual and religious needs with new patients; fewer than one third took a spiritual history at the time of a health crisis.

Similarly, in a questionnaire completed by 737 pediatricians, Grossoehme et al. (2007) found a discrepancy between provider beliefs regarding the relevance of spirituality to clinical practice and the lived reality of only a minority of pediatricians dedicating attention to the spiritual practices and religious needs of their patients. This study identified the following characteristics as significantly associated with practitioners who engaged families and children about spiritual concerns: increased age, Christian religious heritage, self-description as religious and/or spiritual, formal instruction regarding role of spirituality in medical settings, and relative comfort asking about a family's spiritual beliefs and practices.

Medical schools, alongside residency and fellowship programs, offer little to no formal training on issues of spirituality and religion in the pediatric context (Cadge et al., 2009; Davies et al., 2002). Though pediatricians report inadequate training and discomfort in addressing spiritual needs, Child Life professionals represent a part of the medical team specifically trained to care for pediatric spiritual and religious needs in the hospital context. Child Life professionals view spirituality as a source of solace for children and families facing "surgery, chronic illness, disability, trauma, and hospitalization" (Sira & McConnell, 2008). Child Life professionals can also play key roles in addressing sibling spirituality, especially in times of bereavement (Sira & McConnell, 2008). Similarly, community clergy members possess significant training regarding spirituality and religion in the medical context and can serve as helpful allies in making medical communication spiritually accessible to children and parents (Hexem et al., 2011).

ASSESSMENTS

Most pediatric spiritual assessments have been developed from measures originally used in adult populations (Barnes et al., 2000). Unfortunately, there is currently no standard tool for evaluating spirituality among adolescents in medical contexts (McNeil, 2015). The sparse research on spiritual assessment with adolescents heavily overlaps with developmental research (Pehler & Craft-Rosenberg, 2009). However, Pendleton's Classification of Pediatric Spiritual/Religious Coping Strategies provides one useful approach to assessment of spiritual and religious needs in pre-adolescent pediatric populations (see Table 2 in Drutchas & Anandarajah, 2014).

McEvoy (2003) highlights the importance of evaluating, assessing, and understanding a child's and family's "daily practices," including prayer, meditation, and diet, as central to their spiritual and cultural expression. Pfund (2000) echoes the importance of integrating cultural understanding into pediatric spiritual and religious assessment. Purow et al. (2011) highlight the great care that must be taken to not conflate a parent's or family's spiritual beliefs and coping practices with those of the child. They suggest enlisting "the expertise of a spiritual counselor" to both assess and respond to the beliefs and spiritual needs of children.

Walco (2007) argues that future development of "a standardized methodology" may not serve to assess pediatric spirituality justly. Walco makes this claim based on the amount of speculation required in developing a religious and spiritual assessment tool for pediatric populations. Since a strictly psychometric approach may not be appropriate for evaluating religious and spiritual needs in pediatric populations, rigorous work on narrative assessment proves promising. Barnes et al. (2000) present a series of seven questions to assess the impact of language use in pediatric spiritual assessment, including how the child's illness/sickness/disease is understood and explained, who is seen as qualified to address healing, and what the child and family mean by healing. Davies et al. (2002) also offer a series of evaluation questions for exploring spirituality among children and their family members in the medical context. Their study emphasizes the importance of differentiating questions of psychosocial assessment and spiritual assessment. The study does not promote avoidance of integrative care, but rather serves as an important warning to resist conflation of psychosocial and spiritual issues, especially in the assessment of pediatric spiritual and religious needs.

Completion of a spiritual assessment by pediatric medical professionals is vital. Take, for instance, the case of a medical crisis arising without the presence of a hospital chaplain or a clergy member trusted by the child and their family. In this common scenario, the onus is upon the medical team to appropriately address the spiritual and religious needs of the child and their loved ones.

DEVELOPMENTAL FRAMEWORKS

Understanding spiritual and religious needs in the context of pediatrics is often helpfully considered in light of pediatric developmental frameworks, such as those of Piaget, Erikson, Fowler, and Kohlberg (Burkhardt, 1991; Moore et al., 2015; Mueller, 2010; Pehler & Craft-Rosenberg, 2009; Pfund, 2000; Smith & McSherry, 2004). However, Barnes et al. (2000) note that the distinction between spirituality and religious practices among children—especially when understood within a developmental framework— is often blurred. This blurring is particularly noticeable among pediatric populations receiving medical treatment in the religiously plural context of the United States. Contributing to this blurring is the paucity of research on children's spirituality and religious practices, including little research on how to distinguish children's spiritual development from their processes of socialization (Smith & McSherry, 2004). These blurred boundaries challenge physicians and other health care professionals to make ad hoc decisions regarding whether and how to introduce spirituality into evaluative and intervention processes, including whether or not their "jurisdiction" ought to include addressing spiritual and religious concerns (Cadge et al., 2009). In addition, secondary to their developmental and cognitive development, children and adolescents themselves may have difficulties differentiating between religious expression and their own spiritual identity (Pehler & Craft-Rosenberg, 2009). Despite these difficulties arising from blurred boundaries, Drutchas & Anandarajah (2014) argue that spirituality and religion still serve as a significant means of coping for children facing disease, disability, and death.

BEST PRACTICE IN SPIRITUAL CARE IN PEDIATRICS

Current literature suggests a number of "best practices" for clinicians to alleviate spiritual and religious distress in the pediatric context. Purow et al. (2011) suggest the benefit of professional training in both childhood development and spiritual care skills for clinicians working with pediatric populations. McEvoy (2003) stresses the interrelatedness of culture and spirituality, arguing that best practices in addressing spirituality include training clinicians to resist making ill-founded assumptions regarding their patient's spiritual beliefs and practices. Meneses et al. (2011) also describe the interconnections between culture and spirituality, underscoring the importance of making inquiry into a patient's or family's understanding of a disease's "spiritual aspects." These best practices are most naturally embraced by clinicians who have thoroughly explored their own cultural, spiritual, and religious backgrounds (Elkins & Cavendish, 2004) toward ends that "enrich, clarify, deepen, and improve effectiveness" of clinical practice (Kemper & Barnes, 2003).

Part of creating an environment of pediatric care where spiritual needs can be acknowledged and supported involves the practice of explicitly addressing not only a child's spiritual needs, but also those of their parent and/or caregiver (Gillespie et al., 2012). The Association of Pediatric Hematology Oncology Nurses proposes a best practice of evaluating and responding to the spirituality and spiritual traditions of a family, alongside their child, throughout the duration of the child's intervention (Nelson & Guelcher, 2014).

PHYSICAL PRESENCE

One of the simplest yet most profound practices that clinicians can cultivate relies upon the kinds of knowledge found within a patient's physical room, whether in the clinic, hospital, or home (Barfield & Selman, 2014). For example, we have found that shifting medical team rounding from outside a child's room to inside the room, with clinicians seated at the child's eye level, allows for greater communication and comfort with the child and their family. This kind of shift can allow families and children to more fully participate in daily conversations about medical care and decision making. This kind of shift in the physical location and availability of pediatricians also often grants clinicians a new perspective on the child's spiritual and religious experience. For example, while kneeling beside a child's bed, a pediatrician might notice an object or toy of particular spiritual importance to the child or their family. In addition, a clinician's postural change, increasing their physical proximity to a child, allows opportunities to more carefully listen and attend to the child. Davies et al. (2002) nuance the important nature of this physical presence with a child, calling for special attention to a child's "way of being in the world" as a central avenue to build trust with a child. As clinicians seek to become more attuned to a child's experience of illness or disability, interventions such as pain control and relief often increase, providing the child with not only spiritual support but additional positive outcomes in their care.

LISTENING

A closely related best practice is active engagement in listening (Pfund, 2000). Intentionally engaging in listening allows providers to avoid the common pitfall of ignoring children and speaking only with parents or other caregivers (Moore et al., 2015). As clinicians intentionally choose to listen and be present to the suffering of a child, they not only participate in work to prevent death and eliminate suffering, they also work to engage a child's meaning-making of their illness or disability (Barfield & Selman, 2014).

The practice of listening, argue Hart & Schneider (1997), serves as an essential key to identifying spiritual distress among pediatric patients, offering a practice that expands opportunities to improve medical team responsiveness to spiritual and religious needs (Smith & McSherry, 2004). Practices of listening not only help identify distress, but also enable clinicians to identify sources of hope for pediatric patients and their families. Moore et al. (2015) stress that a clinician's act of listening to a child telling his or her own story, without interjection or interruption, helps facilitate a child's honest and full expression of his or her spirituality.

Careful listening also enables clinicians to become more aware of when pediatric patients, particularly adolescents, may be providing cues regarding a desire to spiritually reflect and to form further spiritual connections with their families, providers, and/or the divine (Pehler & Craft-Rosenberg, 2009). Clinicians seeking to engage in active listening with their patients embody this practice best by creating a safe environment, as well as by establishing a collaborative relationship with a child or adolescent in which mutual authenticity and respect are emphasized (Spurr et al., 2013). As clinicians seek to provide caring and appropriate responses to their patients, Stuber & Houskamp (2004) stress the centrality of providing a compassionate presence that eschews "false reassurance of platitudes," especially to children and adolescents who are dying. The goal of listening is a de-centering of the clinician with a simultaneous centering of the spiritual experiences and needs of a child and their family (Stuber & Houskamp, 2004).

SPIRITUAL AND RELIGIOUS ROUTINES

Another best practice for clinicians concerned with incorporating a child's spiritual needs into ongoing intervention includes clinician support of spiritual and religious routines for a child (Elkins & Cavendish, 2004). These kinds of routines often include prayer and other religious or spiritual practices such as meditation or singing. Hart & Schneider (1997) found that the maintenance of these kinds of spiritual routines by children and their families, with support from clinicians, is especially important for infants who are ill, in order to prevent unnecessary challenges and rapid changes in state regulation that may occur when spiritual routines are (often inadvertently) disrupted by clinicians. Pediatricians might support these kinds of routines by collaborating with other members of the medical team, particularly case managers, Child Life specialists, and occupational therapists, to prioritize space and time for a child's participation in daily religious and spiritual practices. Pediatricians can also support these kinds of spiritual routines by consistently checking in with children and their families during rounds about the status of the routine. We have found it helpful to use visual cues outlining a child's religious and spiritual practices, in order to provide the child with a greater sense of control and participation in processes of spiritual meaning-making, as well as to alert all persons involved in the child's care about the importance of the child's spiritual routine. This best practice is supported by Hart & Schneider who emphasize the centrality of maintaining spiritual routines for preschoolers, citing the importance of spiritual practices and ritual in allowing a child to experience a "predictable environment" in the face of illness and/or disability.

PLAY

Play is unarguably one of the most important experiences of childhood. Integrating formal and informal applications of play therapy as a means of probing a child's spiritual needs and responding to these needs stands out as a central embodied practice for clinicians striving to address issues of spirituality with children (Hart & Schneider, 1997; Elkins & Cavendish, 2004; Davies et al., 2002). Play often opens a context in which children's spirituality can be explored in a more natural and candid manner. Play therapy, especially when it includes robust parental or caregiver participation, offers another embodied practice through which to support and meet the spiritual needs and expression of children in the midst of illness, disability, or dying (Hart & Schneider, 1997). In this area of best practice, pediatricians might help foster collaboration between clinicians (such as physical, occupational, and speech therapists) who regularly integrate play into their medical interventions with other pediatric providers such as chaplains and physicians to more fully support a holistic understanding of the child's spiritual needs through the perspective of the child's engagement in play.

TOUCH

Another best practice widely used in addressing pediatric spirituality and religious participation is physical touch (Hart & Schneider, 1997; Elkins & Cavendish, 2004). Examples include clinicians holding the hands of children (Gillespie et al., 2012) during rounds or at other times when care and/or updates are provided to a child and family. A clinician's modeling of therapeutic touch to facilitate discussions of embodied spirituality and religious practices creates an invitation for caregivers as well as interdisciplinary medical professionals, such as chaplains, to practice these kinds of embodied ways of caring. Engaging in therapeutic touch in the context of spiritual and religious practices, such as prayer, work not only to meet a child's potential spiritual need, but also provide non-medicalized opportunities for touching a child's body. Milstein & Little (2000) especially encourage clinicians to model touch among critically ill populations, particularly newborns in the intensive care unit, who must navigate the challenges of a sensitive nervous system and poor overall regulation. Pediatricians who engage in the practice of therapeutic touch often allay parental fears of touching their critically ill child and open spiritually beneficial interactions and connections between children and parents that can be severed by critical illness and/or lines and tubes.

ARTISTIC ENGAGEMENT

Children's emotions associated with spiritual longing and desire often find embodied expression through the arts, including means such as dance, singing, and movement. Mueller (2010) argues that these embodied practices allow children to express complex emotions such as despair, joy, and wonder, as well as question and explore the spiritual meanings surrounding their experience of illness. Yates (2011) suggests integrating material objects into embodied practices of spirituality, such as by allowing a child ready access to religious relics or sacramental objects from their hospital bed.

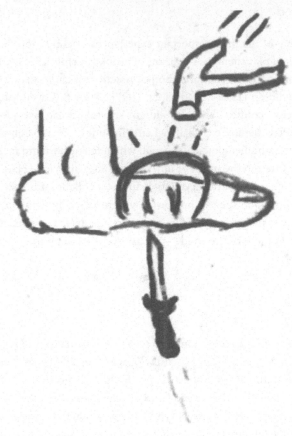

FIGURE 3.1: Drawing of a foot tumor by a teenage boy who had his foot amputated.

Art, and drawing in particular, provide means by which clinicians can help children to access spiritual and emotional concerns. Drawings can provide an opportunity for discussions of illness and meaning. In our own work we will often ask children to "draw your illness." These drawings provide an opportunity to discuss meaning and help children and clinicians to have open discussions regarding the physical and spiritual challenges of illness. As an example, the image in Figure 3.1 was drawn by a teenage boy who had had a foot tumor and was treated by having his foot amputated. In his drawing he illustrates the pain that the tumor had caused him. The drawing provided an opportunity to discuss the loss of his foot, the relief of the pain that he had been experiencing, and also to discuss the meaning of his illness in his broader life. In relationship to spirituality, the drawing facilitated conversations about both opportunity and loss in relationship to the teenager's sense of his life's meaning and arc.

STORYTELLING

Storytelling is a critical best practice at the center of providing spiritual care to children and their families (Elkins & Cavendish, 2004). Pediatric clinicians can work toward integrating story telling by mirroring a child's use of language to process and reflect on pain, illness, disability, and dying

(Purow et al., 2011). Elkins & Cavendish (2004) encourage pediatric clinicians to use pictures to accompany storytelling practices alongside children. For adolescents, Purow et al. (2011), as well as McNeil (2015) and Suzuki & Beale (2006), highlight the role of social media, blogs, and/ or personal websites for adolescents to process spiritual and religious experiences associated with their illness. These contexts also provide opportunities for adolescents to forge deeper spiritual connections with their families and friends, as well as with peers facing similar illness experiences and/or spiritual challenges.

A particularly powerful use of storytelling in connection to pediatric spirituality is its invitation to both children and parents to offer a more holistic perspective on the spiritual components of a pediatric illness experience (Kemper & Barnes, 2003). Rolim Lima et al. (2013) suggest that storytelling is especially important among patients with cancer diagnoses, as realities of suffering become more integrated into the personal narratives of children and families. Moore et al. (2015) encourage the use of "definitional ceremonies" or storytelling performances by children that help them express their identity, culture, and spirituality to both insiders (family, peers, and community members) and outsiders (medical professionals). Following this kind of practice, both "outsiders" and "insiders" are invited to share the portions of the child's story that struck them most deeply and why. Moore et al. (2015) view this kind of practice as key to better understanding children's spiritual perspective on their illness. Mueller (2010) argues that practices of storytelling can also be a means of intervention to alleviate spiritual distress among children.

PRAYER

Engaging prayer as a best practice often occurs in the context of intervention for spiritual distress when explicitly requested by a family or child (Armbruster et al., 2003; Mueller, 2010). Grossoehme et al. (2010) identify prayer as the primary practice for coping with the stresses of pediatric illness and hospitalization. This same study highlights the power of pediatric patients writing prayers to God, focused not only on requests for healing, but also on giving thanks. Similarly to practices of storytelling and narrative sharing, prayer is a best practice that assists pediatric patients in forming a "coherent narrative of experience" (Grossoehme et al., 2010). Hexem et al. (2011) stress the particular salience of prayer in response to acutely stressful medical events, such as a code. Prayer offers a way forward during times of crisis when medicine alone fails to alleviate suffering or fails to provide the spiritual meaning that children and their families seek in times of deep distress (Robinson et al., 2006). In addition, Hexem and colleagues argue for the combination of prayer practices with reading Scripture or other sacred texts.

Practices of prayer can facilitate a renewed sense of connection with the divine for children and adolescents. In the 2010 study by Kamper et al., nearly 80% of children with cancer reported that engaging in prayer made them "feel closer to God." McNeil (2015) found that practices of prayer and meditation were central expressions of spirituality and coping among adolescents with cancer diagnoses. Pehler & Craft-Rosenberg (2009) noted a similar centering of these spiritual practices among adolescents with Duchene Muscular Dystrophy. Though many clinicians anecdotally report discomfort or a lack of experience with identifying the appropriateness of prayer, Siegel et al. (2002) found that 90% of surveyed pediatricians considered it appropriate to pray with patients and families upon their request. In 2011, Yates reported that prayer at the bedside is a common spiritual and religious practice among clinicians serving pediatric populations.

FUTURE RESEARCH

Robustly incorporating best practices and theoretical frameworks regarding spirituality and religion in pediatric care depends on future research trajectories. The widespread belief that spirituality and religion act as barriers in pediatric care, despite strong evidence to the contrary, makes further investigation in this area an urgent endeavor (Cadge et al., 2009). Longitudinal studies are needed to understand the role of spirituality in illness and how spiritual well-being changes throughout the illness trajectory in pediatrics. Studies of religious needs outside the Judeo-Christian traditions are also needed (Pehler & Craft-Rosenberg, 2009). Further work is also needed to interrogate the accuracy and effectiveness of spiritual evaluations and interventions currently used in adult populations when applied to adolescents and children (Drutchas & Anandarajah, 2014).

In addition to these general needs for future research, we have identified four specific areas for future investigation. The first area includes studies that investigate the effects of physician power in relationship to pediatric spirituality (Milstein & Little, 2000). Physician approval, or dismissal, of a child's or family's expressed spirituality often exercises tremendous power over families in medical settings. A second area for future research is the development of interprofessional training opportunities for the development of competencies and practices related to the evaluation of spiritual and religious needs, as well as the provision of spiritual care in pediatric medical contexts. This kind of formational program, inclusive of both physician and non-physician providers, promises to also expand interdisciplinary collaborative efforts across the spectrum of pediatric care (Barnes et al., 2000; Cadge et al., 2009). How to best integrate spiritual care training into pediatric residency programs is another avenue for future research. King et al. (2013) argue that a multi-hour workshop program focused on issues of religion and spirituality may be more effective in training clinicians with already established pediatric practices.

A third priority area for future research includes attention to the cultivation of spiritual practices for children (Mercer, 2006). This kind of research will be best embedded in embodied, collaborative practices shared between pediatric patients, their loved ones, and pediatric clinicians, in order to suggest practices that arise from the actual contexts of encounter within the pediatric context (Grossoehme et al., 2007). The fourth and final area for future investigation is improved research efforts, both quantitative and qualitative, investigating the spiritual and religious needs of pediatric populations on the margins. These populations include infants and children with profound disabilities. This research will include the investigation of concrete lived examples of how spiritual and religious practices are both supportive and detrimental to children and families facing significant illness, disability, and/or the process of dying. Meert et al. (2005) point to the helpfulness of qualitative research in assisting clinicians to move beyond merely abstract discussions of spirituality that neglect reflection on lived religious practices in pediatrics.

CONCLUSION

Responding to the individual experiences of illness, disability, pain, and dying among pediatric patients requires an enormous imaginative engagement with the experience of a patient's life as it is actually lived, not as a mere abstraction (Barfield & Selman, 2014). Much work has been done to give clinicians the foundational tools to begin to meaningfully evaluate and engage with spiritual needs in pediatrics. However, so much more work needs to be done. No child experiences illness, suffering, or death in purely biological terms. For pediatric patients and their families, these are fundamentally spiritual experiences. While contemporary medicine has been dominated by the language of biology, children who are least acquainted with this kind of language remind us that we are more than our biology. Engaging the spiritual and religious needs in the pediatric population reminds us of the deep necessity of wrestling with lived experiences in deeply spiritual practices and vocabularies. We hope that our explorations in this chapter will spur pediatric clinicians onward toward new and more holistic care for the spiritual and religious needs of children and families in medical contexts.

REFERENCES

American Academy of Pediatrics, Committee on Bioethics. (2013). Conflicts between religious or spiritual beliefs and pediatric care: Informed refusal, exemptions, and public funding. Policy statement. *Pediatrics, 132*(5), 962–965.

Armbruster, C. A., Chibnall, J. T., & Legett, S. (2003). Pediatrician beliefs about spirituality and religion in medicine: Associations with clinical practice. *Pediatrics, 111*(3), 227–235.

Balboni, M. J., Sullivan, A., Amobi, A., Phelps, A. C., Gorman, D. P., Zollfrank, A., . . . Balboni, T. A. (2013). Why is spiritual care infrequent at the end of life? Spiritual care perceptions among patients, nurses, and physicians and the role of training. *Journal of Clinical Oncology, 31*, 461–467.

Baldacchino, D. R., Borg J., Muscat C., & Sturgeon, C. (2012). Psychology and theology meet: Illness appraisal and spiritual coping. *Western Journal of Nursing Research, 34*(6), 818–847.

Barfield, R. C., & Selman, L. (2014). Spirituality and religion. In T. Jones, D. Wear, & L. D. Friedman (Eds.), *Health humanities reader* (pp. 376–386). New Brunswick, NJ: Rutgers University Press.

Barnes, L. L., Plotnikoff, G. A., Fox, K., & Pendleton, S. (2000). Spirituality, religion, and pediatrics: Intersecting worlds of healing. *Pediatrics, 104*(6), 899–908.

Barros Meireles, C., Chaves Maia, L., Linhares Miná, V. A., Cardoso Novais, M. D. S. M., Cartaxo Peixoto, J. A. C., Sampaio Cartaxo, M. A. B., . . . Rolim Neto, M. L. (2015). Influence of spirituality in pediatric cancer management: A systematic review. *International Archives of Medicine, 8*(35), 1–13.

Burkhardt, M. A. (1991) Spirituality and children: Nursing considerations. *Journal of Holistic Nursing, 9*(2), 31–40.

Cadge, W., Ecklund, E. H., & Short, N. (2009). Religion and spirituality: A barriers and a bridge in the everyday professional work of pediatric physicians. *Social Problems, 56*(4), 702–721.

Davies, B., Brenner, P., Orloff, S., Sumner, L., & Worden, W. (2002). Addressing spirituality in pediatric hospice and palliative care. *Journal of Palliative Care, 18*, 59–67.

Drutchas, A., & Anandarajah, G. (2014). Spirituality and coping with chronic disease in pediatrics. *Rhode Island Medical Journal*, 26–30.

Elkins, M., & Cavendish, R. (2004). Developing a plan for pediatric spiritual care. *Holistic Nursing Practice*, 179–184.

Fowler, J. W., Nipkow, K. E., & Schweitzer, F. (1991). *Stages of faith and religious development: Implications for church, education, and society.* New York: Crossroad.

Gillespie, G. L., Hounchell, M., Pettinichi, J., Mattei, J., & Rose, L. (2012). Caring in pediatric emergency nursing. *Research and Theory for Nursing Practice: An International Journal, 26*(3), 216–232.

Grossoehme, D. H., Ragsdale, J. R., McHenry, C. L., Thurston, C., DeWitt, T., & VandeCreek, L. (2007). Pediatrician characteristics associated with attention to spirituality and religion in clinical practice. *Pediatrics, 119*(1), 117–123.

Grossoehme, D. H., VanDyke, R., Jacobsen, C. J., Cotton, S., Ragsdale, J. R., & Seid, M. (2010). Written prayers in a pediatric hospital: Linguistic analysis. *Psychology of Religion and Spirituality, 2*(4), 227–233.

Hart, D. & Schneider, D. (1997). Spiritual care for children with cancer. *Seminars in Oncology Nursing, 13*(4), 263–270.

Hexem, K. R., Mollen, C. J., Carroll, K., Lanctot, D. A., & Feudtner, C. (2011). How parents of children receiving pediatric palliative care use religion, spirituality, or life philosophy in tough times. *Journal of Palliative Medicine, 14*(1), 39–44.

Kamper, R., Van Cleve, L., & Savedra, M. (2010). Children with advanced cancer: Responses to a spiritual quality of life interview. *Journal for Specialists in Pediatric Nursing, 15*, 301–306.

Kemper, K. J., & Barnes, L. (2003). Considering culture, complementary medicine, and spirituality in pediatrics. *Clinical Pediatrics, 42*(3), 205–208.

King, S. D. W., Dimmers, M. A., Langer, S., & Murphy, P. E. (2013). Doctors' attentiveness to the spirituality/religion of their patients in pediatric and oncology settings in the Northwest USA. *Journal of Health Care Chaplaincy, 19*, 140–164.

Knapp, C., Madden, V., Wang, H., Curtis, C., Sloyer, P., & Shenkman, E. (2011). Spirituality of parents of children in palliative care. *Journal of Palliative Medicine, 14*(4), 437–443.

Longden, J. (2012). Paediatric palliative care and paediatric intensive care. *Nursing in Critical Care, 17*(4), 167–168.

McEvoy, M. (2003). Culture and spirituality as an integrated concept in pediatric care. *The American Journal of Maternal/Child Nursing, 28*(1), 39–43.

McNeil, S. B. (2016). Spirituality in adolescents and young adults with cancer: A review of the literature. *Journal of Pediatric Oncology Nursing, 33*(1):55–63.

Meert, K. L., Thurston, C. S., & Briller, S. H. (2005). The spiritual needs of parents at the time of their child's death in the pediatric intensive care unit and during bereavement: A qualitative study. *Pediatric Critical Care Medicine, 6*(4), 420–427.

Meneses, V., Vanderbilt, D., Barnes, L., & Augustyn, M. (2011). "Footprints in the bathroom": The role of spirituality in patient diagnosis. *Journal of Developmental & Behavioral Pediatrics, 32*(2), 169–171.

Mercer, J. A. (2006). Capitalizing on children's spirituality: Parental anxiety, children as consumers, and the marketing of spirituality. *International Journal of Children's Spirituality, 11*(1), 23–33.

Milstein, J. M., & Little, T. H. (2000). Invoking spirituality in medical care. *Alternative Therapies in Health and Medicine, 6*(6), 118–120.

Moore, K., Talwar, V., & Moxley-Haegert, L. (2015). Definitional ceremonies: Narrative practices for psychologists to inform interdisciplinary teams' understanding of children's spirituality in pediatric settings. *Journal of Health Psychology, 20*(3), 259–272.

Mueller, C. R. (2010). Spirituality in children: Understanding and developing interventions. *Pediatric Nursing, 36*(4), 197–208.

Nelson, M. B., & Guelcher, C. (Eds.). (2014). *Scope and standards of pediatric hematology oncology nursing practice.* Chicago, IL: Association of Pediatric Hematology/Oncology Nurses.

Pehler, S., & Craft-Rosenberg, M. (2009). Longing: The lived experience of spirituality in adolescents with Duchenne Muscular Dystrophy. *Journal of Pediatric Nursing, 24*(6), 481–494.

Pfund, R. (2000). Nurturing a child's spirituality. *Journal of Child Health Care, 4*(4), 143–148.

Purow, B., Alisanski, S., Putnam, G., & Ruderman, M. (2011). Spirituality and pediatric cancer. *Southern Medical Journal, 104*(4), 299–302.

Reynolds, M. A. (2008). Hope in adults, ages 20-59, with advanced cancer. *Palliative & Supportive Care, 6,* 259–264.

Richardson, P. (2012). Assessment and implementation of spirituality and religiosity in cancer care: Effects on patient outcomes. *Clinical Journal of Oncology Nursing, 16,* E150–E155.

Robinson, M. R., Thiel, M. M., Backus, M. M., & Meyer, E. C. (2006). Matters of spirituality at the end of life in the pediatric intensive care unit. *Pediatrics, 118*(3), 719–729.

Rolim Lima, N. N., Nascimento, V. B. D., Carvalho, S. M. F. D., Rolim Neto, M. L. R., Moreno Moreira, M. M., Quental Brasil, A., . . . Advíncula Reis, A. O. (2013). Spirituality in childhood cancer care. *Neuropsychiatric Disease and Treatment, 9,* 1539–1544.

Siegel, B., Tenenbaum, A. J., Jamanka, A., Barnes, L., Hubbard, C., & Zuckerman, B. (2002). Faculty and resident attitudes about spirituality and religion in the provision of pediatric health care. *Ambulatory Pediatrics, 2*(1), 5–10.

Sira, N., & McConnell, M. (2008). Attitudes toward spirituality and child life services. *The Journal of Pastoral Counseling, 43,* 32–49.

Smith, J. & McSherry, W. (2004). Spirituality and child development: A concept analysis. *Journal of Advanced Nursing, 45*(3), 307–315.

Spurr, S., Berry, L., & Walker, K. (2013). The meanings older adolescents attach to spirituality. *Journal for Specialists in Pediatric Nursing, 18,* 221–232.

Stuber, M. L., & Houskamp, B. M. (2004). Spirituality in children confronting death. *Child & Adolescent Psychiatric Clinics of North America, 13,* 127–136.

Surbone, A., & Baider, L. (2010). The spiritual dimension of cancer care. *Critical Review in Oncology/Hematology, 73,* 228–235.

Suzuki, L. K., & Beale, I. L. (2006). Personal web home pages of adolescents with cancer: Self-presentation, information dissemination, and interpersonal connection. *Journal of Pediatric Oncology Nursing, 23,* 152–161.

Walco, G. A. (2007). Religion, spirituality, and the practice of pediatric oncology. *Journal of Pediatric Hematology and Oncology, 29*(11), 733–735.

Yates, F. D. (2011). Religion and spirituality in pediatrics. *Pediatrics in Review, 32*(9), 91–94.

CHAPTER 4

RELIGION AND SPIRITUALITY IN FAMILY MEDICINE

Timothy P. Daaleman

"Not a week passes in the practice of the ordinary physician but he is consulted about one or more of the deepest problems in metaphysics and religion—not as a speculative enigma, but as part of human agony."

Richard C. Cabot, 1918 (Cabot, 1918)

There is greater awareness among contemporary family physicians and other health care providers of the intersection of religion and spirituality with health care (Cadge, 2012). Multiple factors have contributed to this recognition and it validates a forecast, made many years ago, which projected the adoption of a global understanding of health that placed spiritual factors alongside physical, psychological, and social determinants (Institute for the Future, 2000). Two trends illustrate this notion of spiritually inclusive health. The first is interest in exploring the process and efficacy of religious and spiritual interventions, such as intercessory prayer and meditation, through biomedical models, and is represented in cognitive neuroscience and psychoneuroimmunology (Bottaccioli et al., 2014; Kiecolt-Glaser et al., 2010; Synder, 2008). Researchers at the University of Pennsylvania, for example, have used single photon emission computed tomography (SPECT) to image the brains of meditating Buddhists and Franciscan nuns and have observed localized neural activity during this practice (Newberg, D'Aquili, & Rause, 2001).

A second trend is a push to reclaim and frame the illness experience in less reductionist and more patient-centered ways (Fan et al., 2015). Traditionally, many physicians have considered physical, psychological, social, and spiritual elements as separate components constituting the human condition. However family physicians have an intellectual tradition that is oriented to treating the whole person, by viewing health and disease through the integration of mind, body, and spirit, largely within the context of family and community (Martin et al., 2004). Anthropologists often refer to explanatory models (EMs) as ways in which patients collectively appraise all of these factors to interpret and understand their health and illness

(Kleinman, 1988). Although there is a rich literary tradition of incorporating religious and spiritual perspectives into patient EMs, particularly when suffering is involved (Tolstoy, Pevear, & Volokhonsky, 2012), physician narratives have become more comfortable with and inclusive of language that touches upon the religious and spiritual. For example, a prominent AIDS and cancer researcher authored a collection of stories with the subtitle of "a spiritual exploration of illness"(Groopman, 1997).

At a time of remarkable change in health care, these larger movements suggest a new way of practicing medicine that not only considers, but is actively responsive to, the needs of body, mind, and spirit (Daaleman, 2004). There are, however, considerable practical and ethical challenges for physicians who are attentive to the spiritual and religious concerns of their patients. For the ordinary family physician, a primary challenge lies in not only comprehending the evidence base in this area, but also being responsive to the movements of this unique human dimension across health and illness in their patients, and in themselves (Daaleman, 2004). In consequence, this chapter will frame the intersection of religion and spirituality within the culture of medicine in a way that is relevant and actionable to family physicians, and it will offer evidence-based recommendations that can assist clinicians in their patient care.

EVIDENCE BASE OF RELIGION/ SPIRITUALITY AND HEALTH

Many patients and physicians continue to be drawn to research that looks at the effects of religious/spiritual practices on health outcomes. This attraction is best represented in intercessory prayer studies. A 2009 *Cochrane Review* examined the effects of intercessory prayer as an additional intervention for patients who had identified health problems, such as heart disease, and were already receiving standard medical care (Roberts & Davison, 2009). A systematic search identified 10 studies with over 7,500 patients and found that was no clear effect of intercessory prayer on mortality, when comparing intercessory prayer plus standard care to standard care alone (Roberts & Davidson, 2009). There was also no significant difference between the intervention (i.e., prayer) and standard care group in overall health/clinical status. Four studies in the review found no effect on the outcome of hospital admission and two other studies reported that intercessory prayer had no effect on re-hospitalization (Roberts & Davidson, 2009). The review concluded that the evidence did not support a recommendation either for or against the use of intercessory prayer but that further studies and resources should be used to investigate other areas of health care (Roberts & Davidson, 2009).

One highly relevant area of investigation, and growing evidence base in religion/spirituality, may be found in the clinical settings at the end of life. The Institute of Medicine (IOM), the National Hospice and Palliative Care Organization, and the Joint Commission have all consistently advocated for addressing and meeting the spiritual care needs of seriously ill and dying patients, and their caregivers, as a standard of high-quality, patient-centered care (Field & Cassel, 1997; Institute of Medicine, 2014; National Hospice and Palliative Care Organization, 2009; The Joint Commission, 2008a, 2014). An IOM report on dying in America reaffirmed that the journey toward death awakens and encourages a uniquely spiritual dimension in the final phase of life, although the processes by which religion and spirituality impact the quality of life and quality of care at this critical time are poorly understood (Institute of Medicine, 2014).

Prior to the IOM report, another Cochrane Review assessed spiritual and religious interventions for adults at the end of life (EOL), and evaluated the effectiveness of these interventions on the outcome of well-being (Candy et al., 2012). The search criteria in this review included randomized controlled trials that involved adults at the EOL, and if the trial examined outcomes for interventions that had a religious or spiritual component. The primary outcomes were overall well-being, coping, and quality of life (Candy et al., 2012). Five trials with over 1,100 participants were included; two studies evaluated meditation and the others looked at multi-disciplinary palliative care interventions that involved a chaplain or spiritual counselor as part of the intervention team. The studies that evaluated meditation found no overall difference in effect between patients receiving meditation or usual care on quality of life or well-being (Candy et al., 2012). In addition, the palliative care intervention studies found no significant difference in quality of life outcomes between the trial and control groups. Although the review found inconclusive evidence that interventions with spiritual or religious components impacted well-being for terminally ill adults, it did acknowledge the lack of quality research and the need for more rigorous studies (Candy et al., 2012).

The most rigorous review of empirical evidence at the population level, one that was not focused on end-of-life care, evaluated several hypotheses that ground most of the research assumptions about plausible linkages between religion/spirituality and health outcomes (Powell, Shahabi, & Thoresen, 2003). A standardized approach was used to identify, select, and exclude studies that were considered for review, and an evaluation process determined the strength of each hypothesis (Powell et al., 2003). Using this approach, the review concluded that religion/spirituality: (1) does not protect against cancer mortality; (2) does not protect against disability; (3) does not slow the progression of cancer; and (4) does not improve recovery from acute illness. However, the review reported a strong, consistent, prospective, and often graded risk reduction in mortality of approximately 25% among church/religious service attenders, even after adjustment for demographic, socioeconomic, and health-associated confounders. (Powell et al., 2003) The authors proposed several inferences for the protective impact that church/religious service attendance may have on mortality in this population: (1) healthy lifestyle behaviors; (2) religious social support; (3) positive emotional experience; (4) modeling of positive and caring behaviors, attitudes, and beliefs; and (5) access to material, emotional, and social resources (Powell et al., 2003).

This body of research points to the mediating effect of behavioral and social factors on health outcomes and the utilization of health services (Koenig, King, & Carson, 2012; Marmot & Wilkinson, 2000). Religious and/or spiritually related factors may be considered as some of these larger contextual factors, which are features of the social world and account for many differences in health outcomes at the population level (Berkman & Kawachi, 2000; Dartmouth Medical School Center for the Evaluative Clinical Sciences, 1999). For example, community-dwelling older adults who report greater spirituality also appraise their overall health as good (Daaleman, Perera, & Studenski, 2004). In addition, critically ill patients who have high levels of religious coping are likely to choose more intensive, life-prolonging care near the end of life (Phelps et al., 2009).

IMPORTANT AREAS FOR FUTURE RESEARCH

Exploring the interface of religion/spirituality and health outcomes continues to be hampered by methodological challenges, such as the use of small, non-generalizable samples and, more importantly, the lack of plausible conceptual models (Sloan, Bagiella, & Powell, 1999). These conceptual shortcomings significantly limit empiric research and subsequent evidence-based approaches that support the incorporation of religion/spirituality into practice. A systematic review, for example, concluded that the concept of spirituality was still under development, and that until a common understanding of this concept is brought forth, clinical applications will be difficult to implement (Pike, 2011). The absence of such common understanding contributes to the paucity of plausible models that depict mechanism and causality, which in turn, inform research and practice. In addition, prior approaches to the examination of spirituality and health-related outcomes have been largely confined to the individual level of hypothesis, research design, and implementation and evaluation (Koenig et al., 2012).

Health services research offers a more applied orientation to understanding religion/spirituality within clinical practice. This multidisciplinary field takes a multi-level view—individuals, families, organizations, institutions, communities, and populations—to examine how social factors, financing systems, organizational structures and processes, health technologies, and personal behaviors impact outcomes such as access to health care, the quality and cost of health care, and ultimately health and well-being (Lohr & Steinwachs, 2002). Quality is a key concern within health services research, and a widely recognized framework classifies quality under 3 categories: structure, process, and outcome (Donabedian, 1988). Structure examines the characteristics of the care setting, such as capital resources (e.g., facility, equipment), human resources (e.g., personnel), and the organizational structure (e.g., staffing). Process describes what actually transpires during the delivery and receipt of care, incorporating both patient and provider activities and perspectives (Donabedian, 1988). Finally, outcome examines the effects of care on patient-centered outcomes including satisfaction with care and quality of life.

Our research group at the University of North Carolina at Chapel Hill has used a health services framework in a series of studies to understand how spiritual care at the end of life is delivered and experienced by dying patients and family caregivers (Daaleman, Usher, Williams, Rawlings, & Hanson, 2008; Daaleman, Williams, Hamilton, & Zimmerman, 2008; Hanson et al., 2008). We began our work by conducting interviews with seriously ill patients and family caregivers in order to describe their experience of spiritual care. This approach provided primary data on who provides spiritual care, what is provided, and how well spiritual care satisfied the needs of seriously ill patients and family caregivers. Of the spiritual care providers identified by recipients, 41% were family or friends, 17% were clergy, and 29% were health care providers. Between 66-78% of participants reported various types of spiritual care that helped their relationships with loved ones or God (Hanson et al., 2008). Somewhat smaller percentages of participants (45–73%) reported types of spiritual care that helped with understanding an individuals' sense of self and the illness experience. In response to open-ended questions about spiritual care activities, participants reported activities related to help with insight into dying and comfort. Most notably, the most frequently reported type of spiritual care was help in coping with illness (87%) and the least common was intercessory prayer (4%; Hanson et al., 2008).

Just over half (55%) of spiritual care recipients were very satisfied or somewhat satisfied with the care that they received. Most recipients (72%) felt that the spiritual care they had experienced was very valuable in helping them to meet their spiritual care needs, but smaller percentages felt that it was very valuable as a resource to find inner peace (54%), or to help them make meaning (52%). Most provider characteristics showed no correlation with the recipient's report of satisfaction and their perceived value of spiritual care. To be more specific, the perceived value and satisfaction with spiritual care did not differ according to the spiritual care provider's age, race, gender or frequency of visits, and did not differ if the provider was family or friend, clergy, or health care provider. An interesting finding was that satisfaction tended to be lower if the spiritual care provider shared the recipient's faith tradition. However, the perceived value of care was higher if spiritual care included help with understanding, spiritual care practices, relationships, or with coping with illness (Hanson et al., 2008).

To gain further insight into the health care provider perspective, we conducted a qualitative study to explore the experience of spiritual caregiving (Daaleman et al., 2008). There were several themes identified by providers who were nominated as spiritual care providers by dying patients and their family members. Presence was a predominant theme, marked by physical proximity and intentionality, or the deliberate ideation and purposeful action of providing care that went beyond medical treatment. A second theme was "opening eyes," the process by which providers became aware of their patient's storied humanity and the individualized experience of their current illness. Participants also described another course of action, one that we termed co-creating, which was a mutual, iterative activity between patients, family members, and care providers that began with an affirmation of the patient's life experience, and led to the generation of a holistic care plan that focused on maintaining the patient's humanity and dignity (Daaleman et al., 2008).

We also conducted after-death interviews with family members of residents who died in long-term care facilities across 4 states, to understand organizational-level factors contributing to spiritual care. The focus here was to determine how structural and process elements of spiritual care impacted the quality-of-care at the end-of-life (Daaleman, Williams et al., 2008). A large majority of decedents (87%) received support with their spiritual needs from multiple sources including clergy (85%), family and friends (62%), facility staff (37%), and others (17%). Clergy were more likely to be identified as a source of spiritual care among female decedents (88% vs. 75% for male decedents) and in facilities with a religious affiliation (96% vs. 82%). Long-term care staff (e.g., nurses) were reported as a source of spiritual support more often among non-white decedents (43% vs. 36%), for those in religiously affiliated facilities (63% vs. 30%), and in nursing homes when compared to new-model assisted living facilities (42% vs. 21%; Daaleman, Williams, et al., 2008).

Most noteworthy was the finding that family members of decedents who received spiritual care rated the quality of overall care in the last month of life more highly, when compared with those decedents who did not receive spiritual care (Daaleman, Williams, et al., 2008). In addition, among those receiving support for their spiritual needs, care was rated more highly among those who received support from facility staff, such as nurses, than those who did not. There were no differences observed based on the presence of other sources of support (i.e., clergy). These findings have been corroborated in a later multi-site study of patients with advanced cancer, which reported that support of patients' spiritual needs was associated with enhanced quality of life (Balboni et al., 2010).

Our body of work points to a health services framework as a way to understand religion/spirituality in a rapidly changing health care environment. The most immediate and direct application of this framework may be found in hospice and palliative care programs in the United States, which include religious/spiritual components, and are focused on quality improvement strategies and measures (Durham, Rokoske, Hanson, Cagle, & Schenck, 2011). The Centers for Medicare and Medicaid Services (CMS) issued the Hospice Conditions of Participation Final Report in 2008, requiring all Medicare-certified hospices to implement Quality Assessment and Performance Improvement (QAPI) processes to monitor and ensure quality care (Centers for Medicare and Medicaid Services, 2008). These regulations require hospice providers to use a systematic, data-driven approach to measure the quality of care that they deliver, identify areas of improvement, and develop strategies to enhance care (Durham et al., 2011; Schenck, Rokoske, Durham, Cagle, & Hanson, 2010).

The ongoing shift to value-based health care is promoting a systematic approach to document, measure, and analyze quality indicators (Institute for Healthcare Improvement, 2003). Unfortunately, current approaches to health care quality do not include structured ways to gauge spiritual care (Durham et al., 2011), as evidenced by a technical expert panel that concluded that the spiritual care domain was among the least developed quality measure at the end of life (Schenck et al., 2010; Schenck et al., 2014).

RELIGION/SPIRITUALITY AND PATIENT-PHYSICIAN INTERACTIONS

Most Americans hold positive attitudes and beliefs about the efficacy of spiritually-related interventions, such as prayer for healing, although many remain skeptical about the place of spirituality in clinical encounters (Daaleman, 2004). A *USA Weekend* poll reported that 79% of respondents believe that spiritual faith can help recovery from disease, but only 56% said that their faith had actually helped in their recovery (McNichol, 1996). Another multi-center survey found that only a small proportion of primary care outpatients preferred that physicians address spiritually related matters during routine office visits (MacLean et al., 2003). The study also reported that the context of the visit was important, since patients desired greater physician involvement with their spiritual and religious concerns when the severity of their illness was more life-threatening (i.e., when hospitalized or near death; MacLean et al., 2003).

Exploratory studies at the patient level illuminate some of the nuances in these survey findings. When asked to describe spirituality in the context of well-being, patients in focus-group interviews depicted positive thinking and self-efficacy beliefs, and agency beliefs or their capacity for self-efficacy (Daaleman, Kuckelman Cobb, & Frey, 2001). Agency beliefs are empowering beliefs, viewing individuals as active participants constructing their own life course through the actions that they take (Daaleman et al., 2001). Patients also outlined an ongoing process of finding meaning in the face of illness and of placing their illness experience within a larger life context. These qualitative data point to a patient understanding of spirituality as the capacity to construct an empowering interpretative framework, an explanatory model so to speak, through which health, illness, and life events are viewed, a lattice of meaning and self-identity eloquently captured by one patient as "that kind of harmonious blending of the entire" (Daaleman et al., 2001).

Despite acceptance of a more spiritually inclusive view of health, family physicians and other primary care physicians still grapple with understanding the interplay of religion and spirituality within the context of providing care and, more importantly, ways of negotiating their interactions with patients when they surface (Daaleman, 2004). A recent systematic literature review found that these types of interactions occur predominantly in end-of-life settings, that there are mismatched perceptions between patients and physicians around what constitutes religion and spirituality. In addition, a lack of time, knowledge, and training, were identified as barriers to engaging patients in this area (Best, Butow, & Olver, 2015). Mismatched perceptions also arose in a survey that described the viewpoints of primary care physicians around medically unexplained symptoms—those viewed to be either spiritual in nature or resulting from biomedical conditions— which found wide variation as to how physicians attributed these symptoms (Shin et al., 2013). Physicians who reported greater religiosity/ spirituality were more likely to believe that a medically unexplained symptom reflected a spiritual problem, and that patients with these problems would benefit by attending to their spiritual life (Shin et al., 2013).

A prior national survey reported that most physicians found it appropriate to discuss religious/ spiritual issues if the patient raises them, and that a majority of respondents noted that they affirm their patients' own beliefs and practices during a clinical encounter (Curlin, Chin, Sellergren, Roach, & Lantos, 2006). Physicians who self-identify as being more religious/spiritual are more likely to endorse greater engaged behaviors with patients, such as praying with patients and sharing their own beliefs and experiences, when compared with physicians who have less self-reported religious/spirituality (Curlin et al., 2006). Physician beliefs and attitudes around religion/spirituality go beyond patient communication and interactions since such attitudes have been found to influence physician decision-making around patient care. For example, a national survey of physicians found that more religious physicians were less likely to report that they needed to disclose information about, or refer patients for, morally charged medical treatments, such as terminal sedation and abortion (Curlin, Lawrence, Chin, & Lantos, 2007).

The body of this research points to the practical and ethical issues that family physicians need to consider in their care of patients. To begin, physicians may conceptually consider spirituality as the way in which patients are empowered to find meaning and maintain their self-identity, a process which involves selecting and editing their own narrative amid a diversity of options and possibilities (Giddens, 1991). A patient's self-identity provides a sense of control or mastery, but when there are threats to self-identity and personal meaning, patients may engage in reconstructing and rewriting their life story (Giddens, 1984). Here the primary practical work for family physicians involves engaging their patients in the ongoing process of maintaining self-identity in the face of illness.

From an ethical perspective, theological and normative issues may not be far off from the beliefs and values that guide human action and behavior. There is a moral fabric that ties together patient care encounters, specifying what ought to be done to maintain health, avoid illness, and promote healing (Veatch, 2001). Approaching spirituality from an ethical perspective would consider how the intersecting spiritualities of patient and physician are negotiated, and any approach must be concordant with existing principles in medicine (Beauchamp & Childress, 1994). The concept of power is useful for family physicians who are ethically considering religion/spirituality in patient care encounters and there are several guidelines for power's use (Brody, 1992). First, the physician and patient should utilize all of their power to effect a good patient outcome, which is determined by the patient's definition of the presenting problem, and by the physician's contextual understanding of the patient's life course (Brody, 1992; Weiner, Barnet, Cheng, & Daaleman, 2005). Physicians should also be supportive of the patient's own sense of power, as long as it is consistent with a good outcome and the patient's goals and interests (Brody, 1992). As noted earlier, a patient's sense of power can be manifested in their agency beliefs, and may directly reflect the tenets of their faith, or practices from their religious traditions, such as belief in faith healing or prayer. Physicians should be supportive of these sources of patient empowerment, as long as they are consistent with a good outcome and are concordant with the patient's goals and interests (Brody, 1992).

When a conflict arises between the patient's use of power and those ends, it should be handled with negotiation and persuasion, and with attention to the patient's vulnerability (APA Committee on Religion and Psychiatry, 1990). Physicians should share their power with patients by informing them about the nature and treatment of the disease, or the presenting problem if it is undifferentiated (Brody, 1992). Power is also made manifest in the contextual interpretations that are generated, such as cultural scripts that are conveyed to patients through clinical impressions and in the recommendations of selected therapeutic interventions (Daaleman, 2004). Implicitly or explicitly, physicians wield power through their respective frameworks and in the selection of cultural scripts and illness trajectories that are presented to patients (Daaleman, 2004). For example, in a young adult with recurrent non-cardiogenic chest pain that is triggered by existential concerns and school-related stressors, an assessment of a mood disorder and consultation with a psychiatrist frames the diagnosis in a traditional medical model. However other interpretations may take into account the larger social and cultural issues which may be at play, such as gender identity and social networks. The power wielded here can be mitigated by having physicians offer more than one template to patients, who may in turn choose to incorporate or discard proffered scripts as they construct or reconstruct their self-identity.

Patient care not only engages family physicians as subject matter experts, but also presents the concurrent challenge of maintaining their own personally meaningful world. The day-to-day work of patient care can confront and sometimes threaten a physician's sense of self through the disability, serious illness, or death of those that they care for. Yet the spiritualities offered through patient narratives can contribute to a physician's sense of self—who they are, the integration of their outward practice with their inner lives—by presenting and affirming the human condition in its entirety (Daaleman, 2004). For some physicians, spiritualities may be inclusive of practices that are common to patients, such as prayer, reflection, and self-awareness (Epstein, 1999). For others, spiritualities may arise as philosophical or religious belief systems; beliefs that may be held or shared with their patients and that provide a foundation of purpose (Saba, 1999). However, for all physicians, spiritualities that are brought forth by patient encounters are responsive to a basic human desire to find meaning in an integrated way (Daaleman, 2004).

SUGGESTED BEST PRACTICES
FOR FAMILY PHYSICIANS

Recommendations from a family medicine consensus panel on patient-centered spiritual care can help further guide physicians in their care encounters (Anandarajah et al., 2010). The panel identified a series of assessment and therapeutic skills for physicians who may choose to engage in spiritual care. Assessment skills included: (1) identifying spiritually relevant elements in history-taking and carrying out a spiritual assessment in a culturally sensitive, patient-centered way; (2) using patient narratives to gather information about spiritual beliefs, values, and concerns; and (3) summarizing and communicating relevant information, including patients' identified spiritual needs and concerns and potential resources (Anandarajah et al., 2010). The panel also recommended the following therapeutic skills for physicians: (1) demonstrating empathy and attentiveness; (2) formulating a whole person care plan that is inclusive of spiritual factors; (3) including pastoral and other spiritual care specialists in the care plan; and (4) identifying and addressing concordant and discordant beliefs and values when they arise (Anandarajah et al., 2010).

The Joint Commission has recommended spiritual assessments—a process of discerning an individual's spiritual needs and determining what resources are available to meet those needs—for all hospitalized patients (Joint Commission, 2008b). However, providers should be cautious about using structured spiritual assessment tools, since a recent randomized trial found no effect of spiritual history taking with the *ars moriendi* model (i.e., an approach to dying) on quality of life, patient-provider trust, or pain in palliative home care patients (Vermandere et al., 2015). As noted, well-developed clinical skills are the foundation for more broad-based assessments: empathic and active listening; open-ended questioning; validating, restating, or clarifying information that the patient provides; and determining whether a directed physical or mental status examination is necessary (Daaleman, 2005).

The 7 X 7 Model is one tool that incorporates such a multidimensional, contextual approach to a spiritual assessment, since it includes medical, psychological, and spiritual domains (Fitchett, 1999; Fitchett & Handzo, 1998). The model encourages family physicians to consider seven areas: belief and meaning, vocation and obligations, experience and emotions, courage and growth, ritual and practice, community, authority and guidance (Fitchett, 1999; Fitchett & Handzo, 1998). Equally important, it provides a way for physicians to effectively communicate with other spiritual caregivers and experts, such as community clergy, hospital chaplains, family members, or other sources of spiritual support.

A case study of 69-year-old patient named Mary, who had been newly diagnosed with metastatic colon cancer and reported feeling hopeless during a follow-up visit with her family physician, illustrates how some of these best practices may be employed. For the physician, is Mary's disclosure simply a symptom of depression or is it a concomitant part of her illness trajectory (Breitbart et al., 2000)? Is hopelessness representative of a larger, as yet undisclosed, religious or spiritual problem and, if so, should this be probed for further information? From a treatment standpoint, should pharmacotherapy be initiated or, if Mary reveals a religious or spiritual issue, should an intervention that has been clinically proven to be effective be recommended? As part of his/her data gathering, the physician selectively uses the 7 X 7 Model (Fitchett, 1999; Fitchett &

Handzo, 1998) and learns that Mary is not clinically depressed, that her work and her family are the primary sources of meaning in her life, and that she has a nominal belief in God and no ties to a specific faith tradition or community. As part of this assessment, Mary's physician starts to gain further insight to a lifetime of accumulated beliefs, stories, and practices (i.e., her *background spiritualities*; Shea, 2000).

For Mary, the diagnosis and treatment of cancer have already confronted her with the specter of death, a functional limitation, or a compromised quality-of-life, which are all threats to her self-identity. Her hopelessness is due to the threat of not being able to continue working and being seen as vulnerable and frail by her family. During her history, Mary emphasizes a narrative that she has always been the "strong one" in the family on whom everybody has relied over the years; she even cared for her mother for several years before her death. Mary's functional status is still very good and her physician reviews treatment options that have already been outlined by her cancer team, but with a focus on how each will impact the trajectory of her functioning and her overall goals of care. In addition, he follows up on Mary's story of caring for her mother and explores some of her memories and feelings around that event in her life, which were positive and meaningful. The physician asks Mary to reflect on this experience and how it may relate to her current relationships with her family members, who she has not allowed to be involved in her care. In addition, he suggests consultation with a member of the pastoral care staff, since Mary's disclosure of hopelessness may be tied to a larger existential concern. At the end of the encounter, Mary chooses a specific course of treatment for her cancer that has clear endpoints, and she agrees to meet with the chaplain at the hospital.

Mary is accompanied by her daughter at her follow up visit, one month later, and is receiving treatment for her cancer that still allows her to work. Although she gets fatigued by the end of the day, her daughter and granddaughter have started to help out at home. Mary also reports that she has been meeting weekly with the chaplain, and they have been discussing her image of God—which has been one of a taskmaster—and how her self-identity and work-driven focus are tied to this image. The physician asks about her hopelessness. Although Mary notes that it is still present, it is much less intense and overwhelming since she is starting to have new ways of thinking about her life in the face of her current illness (i.e., her *foreground spiritualities*; Shea, 2000).

FINAL COMMENTS: A SPIRITUALITY OF PRACTICE WITHIN THE PLACE OF HEALTH CARE

Robert Wuthnow has proposed that spirituality in the United States over the last 50 years can be understood as moving from a spirituality of dwelling to a spirituality of seeking, and he introduces the notion of a practice-oriented spirituality (Wuthnow, 1998). This orientation has promise for not only for family physicians, but for all health care providers. A spirituality of practice would build upon the current ways in which physicians develop the knowledge base, attitudes, and skills that are required for patient care. Such a practice would maintain a focus on formation by developing the personal habits and dispositions—the virtues (MacIntyre, 1984)— by which physicians can recognize, traverse, and reflect upon the spiritualities (i.e., the stories, beliefs, and practices) that reside just outside of their care encounters, but are central to the lived experience that they share with patients (Shea, 2000). These virtues would resonate with the clinical dictum that physicians should regard the patient-physician relationship as a primary therapeutic tool (Brody, 1992). It is still during the clinical moments, however—when patients seek help from physicians—that the moral work of medicine is laid bare, work which has historically provided the foundation for sustained therapeutic activity between patients and physicians (Green, Graham, Frey, & Stephens, 2001).

A spirituality of practice within health care has the potential to enlarge and sustain the inner life of not only patients, but physicians as well. Such a vision would enrich the capacity of hospitals, medical homes, and other health care settings as places of healing, each filled with a creative, transformative tension that is generated by lives linked to a present clinical moment, but with uncertainty as to how the story will continue to unfold. In this way of thinking, believing, and relating, a spirituality of practice is powerfully embodied as caring within a much larger enterprise; authentic human interactions in which ongoing meaningful lives—moments of incandescence, both human and divine—are co-created, nurtured, and shared (Daaleman, 2004).

REFERENCES

Anandarajah, G., Craigie, F., Jr., Hatch, R., Kliewer, S., Marchand, L., King, D., . . . Daaleman, T. P. (2010). Toward competency-based curricula in patient-centered spiritual care: Recommended competencies for family medicine resident education. *Academic Medicine*, 85(12), 1897–1904. doi: 10.1097/ACM.0b013e3181fa2dd1

American Psychiatric Association. (2006). Resource Document on Religious/Spiritual Commitments and Psychiatric Practice. https://www.psychiatry.org/File%20Library/Psychiatrists/Directories/Library-and-Archive/resource_documents/rd2006_Religion.pdf; accessed August 13, 2016.

Balboni, T. A., Paulk, M. E., Balboni, M. J., et al. (2010). Provision of spiritual care to patients with advanced cancer: Associations with medical care and quality of life near death. *Journal of Clinical Oncology*, 28(3), 445–452.

Beauchamp, T. L., & Childress, J. F. (1994). *Principles of biomedical ethics* (4th ed.). New York: Oxford University Press.

Berkman, L. F., & Kawachi, I. (2000). *Social epidemiology*. New York: Oxford University Press.

Best, M., Butow, P., & Olver, I. (2015). Doctors discussing religion and spirituality: A systematic literature review. *Palliative Medicine*, 30(4), 327–337.

Bottaccioli, F., Carosella, A., Cardone, R., Mambelli, M., Cemin, M., D'Errico, M. M., . . . Minelli, A. (2014). Brief training of psychoneuroendocrinoimmunology-based meditation (PNEIMED) reduces stress symptom ratings and improves control on salivary cortisol secretion under basal and stimulated conditions. *Explore (NY)*, 10(3), 170–179. doi: 10.1016/j.explore.2014.02.002S1550-8307(14)00030-5 [pii]

Breitbart, W., Rosenfeld, B., Pessin, H., et al. (2000). Depression, hopelessness, and desire for hastened death in terminally ill patients with cancer. *Journal of the American Medical Association*, 284, 2907–2911.

Brody, H. (1992). *The healer's power*. New Haven, CT: Yale University Press.

Cabot, R. C. (1918). *Training and rewards of the physician*. Philadelphia, PA: JB Lippincott.

Cadge, W. (2012). *Paging God, religion in the halls of medicine*. Chicago: University of Chicago Press.

Candy, B., Jones, L., Varagunam, M., et al. (2012). Spiritual and religious interventions for well-being of adults in the terminal phases of disease. In The Chochrane Collaboration (Eds.), *Cochrane database of systematic reviews*, Vol. 5. Hoboken, NJ: John Wiley & Sons.

Centers for Medicare and Medicaid Services. (2008). Medicare and Medicaid programs: hospice conditions of participation: final rule. Retrieved March 10, 2012, from http://edocket.access.gpo.gov/2008/pdf/08-1305.pdf.

Curlin, F. A., Chin, M. H., Sellergren, S. A., Roach, C. J., & Lantos, J. D. (2006). The association of physicians' religious characteristics with their attitudes and self-reported behaviors regarding religion and spirituality in the clinical encounter. *Medical Care*, 44(5), 446–453. doi: 10.1097/01.mlr.0000207434.12450. ef00005650-200605000-00009 [pii]

Curlin, F. A., Lawrence, R. E., Chin, M. H., & Lantos, J. D. (2007). Religion, conscience, and controversial clinical practices. *New England Journal of Medicine*, 356(6), 593–600. doi: 356/6/593 [pii]10.1056/ NEJMsa065316

Daaleman, T. P. (2004). Religion, spirituality, and the practice of medicine. *Journal of the American Board of Family Practice*, 17, 370–376.

Daaleman, T. P. (2005). *Spirituality assessment.* AAFP Home Study and Self-Assessment Program (Audiotape 316). Kansas City, MO: American Academy of Family Physicians.

Daaleman, T. P., Kuckelman Cobb, A., & Frey, B. B. (2001). Spirituality and well-being: An exploratory study of the patient perspective. *Social Science & Medicine*, 53(11), 1503–1511.

Daaleman, T. P., Perera, S., & Studenski, S. A. (2004). Religion, spirituality, and health status in geriatric outpatients. *Annals of Family Medicine*, 2, 49–53.

Daaleman, T. P., Usher, B. M., Williams, S. W., Rawlings, J., & Hanson, L. C. (2008). An exploratory study of spiritual care at the end of life. *Annals of Family Medicine*, 6, 406–411.

Daaleman, T. P., Williams, C. S., Hamilton, V. L., & Zimmerman, S. (2008). Spiritual care at the end of life in long-term care. *Medical Care*, 46, 85–91.

Dartmouth Medical School Center for the Evaluative Clinical Sciences. (1999). *Quality of medical care in the United States: A report on the medicare program: Dartmouth atlas of healthcare.* Chicago, IL: American Hospital Association.

Donabedian, A. (1988). The quality of care. How can it be assessed? *Journal of the American Medical Association*, 260, 1743–1748.

Durham, D. D., Rokoske, F. S., Hanson, L. C., Cagle, J. G., & Schenck, A. P. (2011). Quality improvement in hospice: Adding a big job to an already big job? *American Journal of Medical Quality*, 26, 103–109.

Epstein, R. M. (1999). Mindful practice. *Journal of the American Medical Association*, 282, 833–839.

Fan, J., McCoy, R. G., Ziegenfuss, J. Y., Smith, S. A., Borah, B. J., Deming, J. R., . . . Shah, N. D. (2015). Evaluating the structure of the Patient Assessment of Chronic Illness Care (PACIC) survey from the patient's perspective. *Annals of Behavioral Medicine*, 49(1), 104–111. doi: 10.1007/s12160-014-9638-3

Field, M. J., & Cassel, C. K. (1997). *Approaching death.* Washington, DC: National Academy Press.

Fitchett, G. (1999). Screening for spiritual risk. *Chaplaincy Today*, 15, 1–12.

Fitchett, G., & Handzo, G. (1998). Spiritual assessment, screening, and intervention. In J. K. Holland (Ed.), *Psycho-oncology* (pp. 790–808). New York: Oxford University Press.

Giddens, A. (1984). *The constitution of society.* Berkeley, CA: University of California Press.

Giddens, A. (1991). *Modernity and self-identity.* Stanford, CA: Stanford University Press.

Green, L. A., Graham, R., Frey, J. J., & Stephens, G. G. (2001). *Keystone III. The role of family practice in a changing health care environment: A dialogue.* Washington, DC: The Robert Graham Center and the American Academy of Family Physicians.

Groopman, J. (1997). *The measure of my days, a spiritual exploration of illness.* New York: Penguin.

Hanson, L. C., Dobbs, D., Usher, B., Williams, S. W., Rawlings, J., & Daaleman, T. P. (2008). Providers and types of spiritual care during serious illness. *Journal of Palliative Medicine*, 11, 907–914.

Institute for Healthcare Improvement. (2003). The breakthrough series: IHI's collaborative model for achieving breakthrough improvement. *Innovation series white paper.* Boston, MA: Institute for Healthcare Improvement.

Institute for the Future. (2000). *Health and health care 2010, the forecast, the challenge.* San Francisco, CA: Jossey-Bass.

Institute of Medicine. (2014). *Dying in America: Improving quality and honoring individual preferences near the end of life.* Washington, DC: National Academies Press.

Joint Commission. (2008a). Spiritual assessment. Retrieved August 22, 2014, from http://www.jointcommission.org/standards_information/jcfaqdetails.aspx?StandardsFaqId=290&ProgramId=47

Joint Commission. (2008b). Spiritual assessment. Retrieved July 2, 2015, from http://www.jointcommission.org/standards_information/jcfaqdetails.aspx?StandardsFaqId=290&ProgramId=47

Joint Commission. (2014). Facts about the advanced certification program for palliative care. Retrieved August 22, 2014, from http://www.jointcommission.org/certification/palliative_care.aspx

Kiecolt-Glaser, J. K., Christian, L., Preston, H., Houts, C. R., Malarkey, W. B., Emery, C. F., & Glaser, R. (2010). Stress, inflammation, and yoga practice. *Psychosomic Medicine, 72*(2), 113–121. doi: 10.1097/PSY.0b013e3181cb9377PSY.0b013e3181cb9377 [pii]

Kleinman, A. (1988). *The illness narratives: suffering, healing, and the human condition.* New York: Basic Books.

Koenig, H. G., King, D. E., & Carson, V. B. (2012). *Handbook of religion and health* (2nd ed.). Oxford, England; New York: Oxford University Press.

Lohr, K. N., & Steinwachs, D. M. (2002). Health services research: An evolving definition of the field. *Health Services Research, 37,* 15–17.

MacIntyre, A. (1984). *After virtue: A study in moral theory.* Notre Dame, IN: University of Notre Dame Press.

MacLean, C. D., Susi, B., Phifer, N., Schultz, L., Bynum, D., Franco, M., et al. (2003). Patient preference for physician discussion and practice of spirituality. *Journal of General Internal Medicine, 18,* 38–43.

Marmot, M., & Wilkinson, R. G. (2000). *Social determinants of health.* Oxford, England: Oxford University Press.

Martin, J. C., Avant, R. F., Bowman, M. A., Bucholtz, J. R., Dickinson, J. R., Evans, K. L., . . . Weber, C. W. (2004). The future of family medicine: A collaborative project of the family medicine community. *Annals of Family Medicine, 2 Suppl 1,* S3–32.

McNichol, T. (1996, April 5-7, 1996). The new faith in medicine. *USA Weekend,* pp. 4–5.

National Hospice and Palliative Care Organization. (2009). *Guidelines for spiritual care in hospice* (2nd ed.). Alexandria, VA: NHPCO.

Newberg, A., D'Aquili, E. G., & Rause, V. (2001). *Why God won't go away: Brain science and the biology of belief.* New York: Ballentine.

Phelps, A. C., Maciejewski, P. K., Nilsson, M., Balboni, T. A., Wright, A. A., Paulk, M. E., . . . Prigerson, H. G. (2009). Religious coping and use of intensive life-prolonging care near death in patients with advanced cancer. *Journal of the American Medical Association, 301*(11), 1140–1147. doi: 10.1001/jama.2009.341301/11/1140 [pii]

Pike, J. (2011). Spirituality in nursing: A systematic review of the literature from 2006-10. *British Journal of Nursing, 20,* 743–749.

Powell, L. H., Shahabi, L., & Thoresen, C. E. (2003). Religion and spirituality. Linkages to physical health. *American Psychology, 58*(1), 36–52.

Roberts, L. I. A., & Davison, A. (2009). Intercessory prayer for the alleviation of ill health. In The Chochrane Collaboration (Eds.), *Cochrane database of systematic reviews.* Hoboken, NJ: John Wiley & Sons.

Saba, G. W. (1999). What do family physicians believe and value in their work? *Journal of the American Board of Family Practice, 12,* 206–213.

Schenck, A. P., Rokoske, F. S., Durham, D. D., Cagle, J. G., & Hanson, L. C. (2010). The PEACE Project: Identification of quality measures for hospice and palliative care. *Journal of Palliative Medicine, 13,* 1451–1459.

Schenck, A. P., Rokoske, F. S., Durham, D. D., et al.. (2014). Quality measures for hospice and palliative care: Piloting the PEACE measures. *Journal of Palliative Medicine, 17*(7), 769–775.

Shea, J. (2000). *Spirituality and health care, reaching toward a holistic future.* Chicago, IL: The Park Ridge Center.

Shin, J. H., Yoon, J. D., Rasinski, K. A., Koenig, H. G., Meador, K. G., & Curlin, F. A. (2013). A spiritual problem? Primary care physicians' and psychiatrists' interpretations of medically unexplained symptoms. *Journal of General Internal Medicine, 28*(3), 392–398. doi: 10.1007/s11606-012-2224-0

Sloan, R. P., Bagiella, E., & Powell, T. (1999). Religion, spirituality, and medicine. *The Lancet, 353*, 664–667.

Synder, S. H. (2008). Seeking God in the brain: Efforts to localize higher brain function. *New England Journal of Medicine, 358*, 6–7.

Tolstoy, L., Pevear, R., & Volokhonsky, L. (2012). *The death of Ivan Ilyich* (1st Vintage classics ed.). New York: Vintage Books.

Veatch, R. M. (2001). The impossibility of a morality internal to medicine. *Journal of Medicine and Philosophy, 26*, 621–642.

Vermandere, M., Warmenhoven, F., Van Severen, E., et al. (2015). Spiritual history taking in palliative home care: A cluster randomized controlled trial. *Palliative Medicine*, 1–13. doi: 10.1177/0269216315601953

Weiner, S. J., Barnet, B., Cheng, T. L., & Daaleman, T. P. (2005). Processes for effective communication in primary care. *Annals of Internal Medicine, 142*, 709–714.

Wuthnow, R. (1998). *After heaven: Spirituality in America since 1950*. Berkeley, CA: University of California Press.

CHAPTER 5

RELIGION AND SPIRITUALITY IN PSYCHIATRY

Dan G. Blazer

Empirical study of the association between measures of religion/spirituality (R/S) and mental health outcomes begs a more general and emotionally charged question, "Can the benefits of religious beliefs and practices for health (if there be benefits) be studied, much less proven, via empirical research?" (Blazer, 2007). The question has clear clinical implications in that the answer provides evidence (or a lack thereof) that can be used to guide our clinical practice. However, the question is polarizing, with the extremes of the two poles exemplified by Larry Dossey (1997) and Richard Sloan (2006). Dossey asserts that the question has been clearly answered in the positive and that, for example, prayer is as effective as medication or surgery. Sloan, in contrast, challenges the entire enterprise of research on religion and health. He asserts that contaminating evidence-based clinical practices with unproven "spiritual" approaches cannot be substantiated by any clinical or epidemiological studies.

Today we increasingly conform our practices to what is considered "evidence-based." Therefore our understanding of the evidence for the benefits of our inquiries about our patients' R/S beliefs and practices, for the role of R/S as protective against emotional suffering, and for the efficacy of religiously-oriented interventions is ever more important for clinicians. How is a clinician to negotiate the wide-ranging and conflicting views expressed by Drs. Dossey and Sloan? One important (but certainly not the only) approach is to consider what evidence has accrued over the past few years that can inform us regarding the association between R/S, emotional suffering, and disordered behavior.

This question, however, has a much longer history that precedes what we may consider as empirical. For example, Freud in his famous paper "The Future of an Illusion" (1927/1990)] stated that religion represents a "defense against helplessness" and concluded that "surely [such] infantilism is destined to be surmounted." Freud was intrigued by religion (Kung, 1990), and one of his most amicable relationships was with a Swiss Presbyterian minister, Oscar Pfister (Meng and Freud, 1963). Nevertheless, Freud never ceded his position that religion was detrimental to the emotional well-being of his patients and society at large. That firm stance set up a longstanding antagonism (which does not necessarily persist to this day) between psychiatry and religion. For the purposes of this review it is useful to recognize that Freud based his stance on what he viewed at the time as empirical research, namely the observations of his patients and society at large. Few today would accept such a broad generalization from a small collection of case studies.

In his book *Psychoanalysis and Religion*, Gregory Zilboorg (1962) softened the tension: "Aggression; ambivalence; the constant clash between love and hate;. . .A number of devout [religious] scholars are busy restudying these problems with the upmost care. . .and profound faith. The aid and insight which psychoanalysis provides them proves invaluable... to the...development of religious scholarship and the deeper understanding of the faith."

Yet the tension continued in the literature well into the 1960s. Sanua, in an article published in the *American Journal of Psychiatry* in 1969, wrote, "The contention that religion as an institution has been instrumental in fostering general well-being, creativity, honesty, liberalism, and other qualities is not supported by empirical data. . .there are no scientific studies which show that religion is capable of serving mental health" (Sanua, 1969). Paradoxically, about this same time the number of empirical studies exploring the relationship between R/S and health was expanding at a rapid pace. Already in the five-year period between 1965 and 1969, the topic had received much attention with over 1,000 articles published during this time (though most were not empirical studies). By the five-year interval between 2005 and 2009, that number had increased to over 8,000. The proportion of empirical studies had increased dramatically as well (Koenig et al., 2012). Most of these studies confirm a positive relationship between R/S and both physical and mental health.

Recent studies have provided conflicted results, though methodological problems have lessened the potential for generalization from any particular study. For example, Koenig and colleagues found a clear association between measures of religiosity and remission from depression in the medically ill (Koenig et al., 1998). In contrast, Vaillant and colleagues did not find that the mental health of Harvard University graduates over 65 years was associated with religious involvement (except for a small group of men with major depression or multiple life events) (Vaillant et al., 2008). The Koenig study was performed in the Bible Belt and among a population in the midst of a serious illness. The Vaillant study concentrated on highly educated, politically liberal men centered in the northeastern Unites States. This contrast illustrates the need for a careful reading of empirical studies before jumping to generalizations.

Although the value of R/S for physical and psychological well-being will be debated for years to come, I will discuss epidemiological and clinical studies as well as one imaging study, that explore the association between R/S and psychiatric disorders. This is an important discussion. There has been an explosion over the past 25 years of such studies, which have been commented upon widely in the lay press. I will not discuss the association between neurophysiological function (except tangentially in the imaging study) and self-reports of spirituality (such as those reviewed in Andrew Newberg's *Why God Won't Go Away*) or near-death experiences as associated with brain function (such as popularized recently by Eben Alexander's *Proof of Heaven*) (Newberg et al., 2002; Alexander, 2012). Empirical study will not answer many hotly contested questions, such as "Does God exist?" or "Is religious belief a delusion?" (Blazer, 2007).

To appropriately begin this discussion we need to establish some definitions. Empirical for the purposes of this chapter simply means capable of being proved or disproved by observation or experimentation. R/S is a complex topic. Some demarcate religion from spirituality, suggesting that religion implies a particular faith tradition which includes acceptance of a metaphysical or supernatural reality, whereas spirituality does not and is not bound to any particular religious tradition. The boundaries are blurred and depend on definitions from specific studies. For the studies I review, operational definitions are used as probes for R/S. In other words, R/S means no more and no less than the specific probe used to assess this construct.

When we discuss the mind/brain (or even the soul/mind/brain) relationship, especially within the context of R/S, we traverse a wide range of disciplines—philosophy, theology, perspectives from many faith traditions, neuroscience, alternative approaches to traditional medicine, and individual case studies/reports as well as empirical studies. Each of these disciplines and methodological approaches contribute to the conversation. For the clinician, they provide a context for the clinical encounter. And given the importance and breadth of R/S within societies across the globe, some guidelines have emerged.

Perhaps the most significant and widespread is the recommendation from many sources that a spiritual history be taken during the initial psychiatric evaluation (Moreira-Almeida, 2014). Taking a spiritual history is a commonsense approach by the mental health provider, and empirical studies will not inform clinicians about its value—the value should be self-evident. However, empirical evidence has emerged suggesting the value of the spiritual history. For example, in one study, cancer patients who received a spiritual history inquiry in contrast to usual care after three weeks exhibited less depression, a better quality of life, and had a greater sense of interpersonal caring from their physicians (Kristeller et al., 2005).

Empirical studies are valuable because they are based on observations that can be replicated (from brain scans to epidemiologic studies). Yet they represent only one approach to understanding a complex yet deeply felt aspect of personhood. Even so, these studies are an important base for our clinical practice, and any good clinician must have the knowledge and skill to evaluate the implications of research for her/his practice.

Our movement toward building an "evidence base" for the study and practice of psychiatry/psychology, etc. is reflected in the move from the narrative format of DSM-II to the operational format of DSM-III (APA 1968, 1980). So questions such as "Is regular attendance at religious gatherings associated with better health and longer life?" or "Is a spiritually enhanced psychotherapy as efficacious or more so than a non-enhanced therapy?" can be potentially answered *if* we accept the assessments as adequate probes. For example, questions about self-rated health have been strong predictors of mortality even in studies controlling for a variety of other health indicator (Schoenfeld et al., 1994). In other words, these questions are operational, and we accept the answers to these probes as responses to operational definitions (in the format of probes).

Should persons with strong religious convictions be afraid of empirical study? No. In fact, the Hebrew Scriptures insist that, "The heavens are telling the glory of God and the firmament proclaims his handiwork" (Psalms 19:1, RSV). It is not a stretch to suggest that the behaviors of individuals and society, as well as the behavior of the cosmos and the geophysical characteristics of earth, are not available to our senses only to be admired but to be explored as well. By their very nature, the behaviors of individuals remain impossible to predict exactly, nor can we easily impute the motives of these behaviors. Nevertheless, this should not discourage empirical scientists who wish to explore psychological and social behaviors, nor should it discourage those who wish to test interventions that may have spiritual components. Yet when empirical studies are undertaken by persons of faith, the rules and methods of empirical science must not be violated. And persons of faith must not overgeneralize or exaggerate the benefit of such studies if they are positive nor dismiss them out of hand if negative. The converse is true for persons who do not believe R/S is of value to physical and mental health.

Clinicians must likewise be wise and prudent when reading this literature as a way to inform their clinical practice. In the future, perhaps the near future, studies may emerge that will challenge and/or support our traditional views of how clinical practice by mental health workers should proceed. The evidence base will expand and perhaps change directions. New paradigms will emerge. Clinicians from various faith traditions must be flexible in their thinking yet cautious in their application of these new paradigms.

In this chapter I review and critique studies from four approaches to establish the association between R/S and psychiatric disorders. This critique is not in the service specifically of pointing out methodological flaws, yet persons using such studies to challenge or defend the value of R/S for its positive mental health benefits must be aware of the strengths and weaknesses of the specific design and statistical analyses employed in these studies. Rather, I focus on interpreting the findings given the design and probes used. These four approaches are as follows:

- **Participation**
  Attendance at services, participation in activities such as prayer groups or service projects (Hayward et al., 2012)
- **Salience**
  How important is R/S to you? (Miller et al., 2012; Miller et al., 2014)
- **Intervention**
  Comparative efficacy of religious and non-religious cognitive behavioral therapy for depression (Probst et al., 1992)
- **Affiliation**
  Mainline, conservative, and Pentecostal Protestant (Meador et al., 1992)
  Protestants, Catholics, and Jews (Durkheim, 1951)

PARTICIPATION

The first study to be critiqued is a cross-sectional analysis of a clinical sample intended to determine the association between religious participation and unipolar depression (Hayward et al., 2012). 476 psychiatric patients with a current episode of unipolar major depression, and 167 non-depressed comparison subjects, ages 58 years or older, were assessed from a clinical sample participating in a longitudinal study in North Carolina (mean = 70 years, SD = 7). The presence of depression was related to less frequent worship attendance, more frequent private religious practice, and moderate subjective religiosity. These results were only partially explained by effects of social support and stress buffering in a controlled analysis.

This study is typical and straightforward in terms of a probe (How often do you attend religious services?). As noted, simple probes are the usual means by which R/S is assessed in both community and clinical samples. Perhaps one of the more objective measures is the simple assessment of the self-reported frequency of church attendance. The assumption is that respondents report accurately how often they attend, though this has been disputed (Hadaway et. al., 1993).

However, many external factors must be taken into account when evaluating the results of this study. First, the subjects were older adults. Older adults are more likely to attend religious services if health and functional status permit.

Second, the setting was the southeastern United States (the section of the country which has been labeled the "Bible belt"), where persons are more likely to attend religious services. A significant proportion of persons in this section of the country are evangelical Protestants; attendance at religious services is generally expected of these individuals within the culture of the faith tradition, and therefore they may experience more social pressure to attend services. In addition, attendance at religious services may reflect a lifelong habit rather than a true measure of R/S.

Third, the study is cross-sectional. Therefore we do not know the direction of the effect. For example, does attending religious services prevent depression or does the absence of depression lead to a greater likelihood of attending religious services? A longitudinal design would assist in sorting out this question. Finally, the authors controlled for health but not for functional status. An older adult may rate her health as good, but chronic non-fatal disabilities may prevent that individual from easily attending services.

The primary challenge for clinicians in determining the application of such studies to their practices is interpreting the value of attendance and participation in faith communities. Is the faith community the primary source of social support for the individual? Does the individual gain a sense of communal identity from participation in the faith community? How do expectations of attendance and participation vary across faith communities? Would participation in a secular activity, such as a weekly sporting event (bowling, basketball) provide the same value as participation in activities provided by the faith community? Does geographic location, especially urban versus rural residence, contribute to the perceived value of attendance and participation in the faith community? Does attendance easily translate into active participation? Most studies to date do not answer these questions but simply report an association or lack thereof. This is typical of early epidemiological studies in a particular focus of inquiry.

Despite these challenges to interpretation, studies of participation are the easiest to evaluate. The findings are usually quite clear. In other words, we know what we see in these studies. We have a clear idea of the methods and control variables (especially potential confounders such as health and functional status). And of course, we can then interpret the findings accordingly. For example, some may view this association as a clear endorsement of the value of participation in religious services. Others may see so many flaws in the methodology that they discount the findings. Still others may accept the findings but suggest that attendance at religious services tells us very little in and of itself about the association of R/S and depression. Whatever interpretation one suggests, the basis of this interpretation should be clear to any reader of the study.

SALIENCE

The second study I explore is more complex in terms of methodology (Miller et al., 2012). In this study, 114 adult offspring (mean age 29) of depressed and non-depressed parents drawn from the Greater New Haven, Connecticut area were followed over a twenty-year period. At the ten year follow-up, R/S was measured using three probes: personal importance of religion or spirituality, frequency of attendance, and religious affiliation. The probes read as follows: "How important to you is religion or spirituality?" "How often, if at all, do you attend church, synagogue, or other religious or spiritual services (from never to once a week or more)?" "How would you describe your current religious belief? Is there a particular denomination or religious organization that you are a part of?" Sex, age, and history of depression were controlled. 85% were Catholic and 15% Protestant (other religious groups were excluded).

Given the predominance of the Christian faith in the United States, samples that are exclusively or predominantly Christian tend to populate these studies, although in some areas other faith traditions are more frequent (such as Jewish neighborhoods in New York City). In evaluating such studies, the location of the sample is critical. National samples tend to wash out the unique characteristics of some faith traditions that are underrepresented.

The historical subdivisions of the Christian faith—Catholic, mainline, and evangelical—are still used in most studies, although these boundaries are increasingly blurred. Affiliation may be less important today than in times past. In studies of older adults, religious attendance is more important than salience. Therefore if the clinician asks this question, she/he may wish to probe further to better determine the essence of the actual faith community to which the patient adheres.

The probe "How important is R/S?" is a valuable one despite its apparent simplicity and subjectivity. Consider the powerful predictive value of someone's subjective rating of their health as a predictor of mortality even in highly controlled studies. "How important is R/S to you?" is the same probe as used by the Gallup Poll to determine the pulse of the nation (56% of respondents nationwide felt religion to be very important in the Gallup poll, whereas in the New York City sample 25% reported religion to be of high importance, again emphasizing the importance of the geographic location of the sample) (Miller et al., 2012). Clinicians in busy practices can easily ask this question.

Younger generations are characterized as less active in structured religious activities but nevertheless continuing to view their spirituality as important. The spirituality they describe, however, is quite different from that of their parents (Gallup, 2013). Smith and Snell (2009) describe the current expression of R/S in younger generations as moral therapeutic deism, quite a distance from traditional Protestant and Catholic views. "Moral" suggests an orientation toward being good and nice, "therapeutic" suggests being primarily concerned with one's own happiness, and "deism" suggests a view of God as present though not normally involved. For this reason, the importance of R/S depends not only upon intensity of feelings but also how R/S is conceived, and these conceptions can vary significantly across generations. Therefore the distinction between Catholics and Protestants is probably much less today than in the past (Durkheim, 1951), as I will discuss.

The measured outcome was major depression at twenty-year follow-up. Offspring who reported at year 10 that R/S was highly important had about one quarter of the risk of experiencing depression between years 10 and 20. Religious attendance and denomination did not predict outcome.

Miller et al. used the same sample and design in a second study (2014), yet in this study they explored imaging data as a predictor of protection from depression. As noted, religious or spiritual importance and church attendance were assessed. In this study, cortical thickness was measured on anatomical images of the brain acquired with magnetic resonance imaging (MRI). Salience but not frequency of attendance was associated with thicker cortices in the left and right parietal and occipital regions, the mesial frontal lobe of the right hemisphere, and the cuneus and precuneus in the left hemisphere independent of familial risk. The effects of importance on cortical thickness were stronger in the high-risk compared to the low-risk group, particularly along the mesial wall of the left hemisphere. A thinner cortex at mesial wall of the left hemisphere was associated with a familial risk of developing depressive illness. In other words, salience was associated with thicker cortices in the left hemisphere, and a thinner cortex of the left hemisphere was associated with a familial risk of developing depression.

We might consider this study "state of the art." Yet the state of the science at present is very preliminary. We should not be surprised to find R/S associated in some form with neuroanatomical and functional imaging of the brain. Yet such studies are cross-sectional (in terms of the brain imaging). To my knowledge we do not have any longitudinal studies of import that trace changes in the brain with changes in R/S, and this would be a very difficult study to design and implement. In addition, we must remember that R/S may supervene upon brain function in ways that we cannot directly connect in a 1:1 relationship between R/S and brain structure and function. This in no way undermines the concept of an "embodied" R/S. It does challenge a strictly deterministic or materialistic explanation of R/S. Time will tell how these studies proceed, and we should see many other increasingly refined studies emerge in future years. For the present, imaging studies probing R/S and mental health outcomes do not have clinical relevance, yet in the future they well might.

INTERVENTION

I next consider a randomized control trial of the efficacy of cognitive behavioral therapy (CBT). The goal of therapy was to evaluate the efficacy of religiously-enhanced CBT to reduce the symptoms of depression compared to traditional CBT and pastoral counseling (Probst et al., 1993). The Christian version gave Christian rationales for the procedures, gave religious arguments to counter irrational thoughts, and used religious imagery in the service of cognitive restructuring. Religious and non-religious therapists were involved in each CBT arm of the study. Two additional arms were included, a waitlist arm and an arm using pastoral care (which was also structured via a manual and which focused upon non-directive listing [75%] and Bible verses [25%]). Subjects were recruited from the community via advertising that the study was a program for teaching Christians between the ages of 18 and 65 how to cope with depression. All subjects labeled themselves as Christian. Fifty-nine total subjects completed the study with approximately equal distribution across the treatment groups. Standard measures of depression were used at baseline and in follow-up.

The two arms of CBT both used religious and non-religious therapists whereas the pastoral care arm used only religious therapists. The religious therapists were graduate students in a religiously-oriented clinical psychology program, and the nonreligious therapists were graduate students from a more traditional counseling psychology training program, yet all therapists had similar clinical and academic backgrounds. The investigators further subdivided the two CBT groups by whether there was a match between the religious orientation of the therapist and the type of therapy (religious CBT paired with religious therapist, religious CBT paired with a non-religious therapist, usual CBT with a religious therapist, and usual CBT with a non-religious therapist).

The investigators found that all three treatment arms improved compared to the waitlist controls. Yet at three-month and two-year follow-up there was no difference across the three treatment groups. Surprisingly, in an analysis of covariance, the investigators found that the pairing of religious CBT with non-religious therapists was the most effective mode of treatment (though the numbers were small).

This study was well-designed though it suffered in part from too many comparisons given the number of subjects, yet I will put that methodological critique aside. Using manualized therapies has become increasingly standard and to develop such therapies using religious orientation is an appropriate step to test empirically as these types of psychotherapy are most adaptable to randomized trials. Clinicians can therefore adapt a religiously-oriented manualized form of therapy if acceptable to both clinicians and patients, and see whether such a therapy proves efficacious. A strength of the study is that it can be controlled; mixing the orientations of therapists with the different types of therapies further maximizes the ability to control for bias. Some studies of R/S and mental health outcomes may attempt controlled trials on interventions that simply cannot be controlled, such as intercessory prayer (we cannot control who is praying for whom). Therefore, researchers should assess how well any R/S intervention under study can be controlled in the intervention trial.

Yet there are some hazards that should be considered. First, therapists are not value-free. The counterintuitive finding that non-religious therapists were somewhat superior using religious CBT is interesting yet probably cannot be generalized to the therapeutic community as a whole. Therapists are not usually going to adopt an approach to therapy that conflicts with their value systems. In this study, the willingness of non-religious therapists to participate might indicate a more accepting view of religiously-oriented therapy among these therapists even if they don't personally subscribe to the religious background per se. Another concern is that the entire study may have been impacted by a halo effect given the context and setting in which the study was conducted and the nature of the recruitment of participants (both concerns acknowledged by the authors). A third question is whether religiously-oriented therapies might be developed for other religious affiliations. A study is under way evaluating just this question in which CBT is modified for a variety of religious belief systems (Koenig, 2014). No results are available from this trial at present, however.

AFFILIATION

Studies of affiliation as related to mental health date back over a century. In this section I will consider a more recent study as well as the classic study of Emile Durkheim on religious affiliation and suicide.

In the first study, the authors examined the relationship between religious affiliation and psychiatric disorder among Protestant members of the baby-boomer generation (those born between 1945 and 1966) who resided in the Piedmont area of North Carolina (Meador et al., 1992). Data were obtained on six-month and lifetime rates of major psychiatric disorders among 853 Protestant baby boomers. Participants were grouped into three categories based on religious affiliation: mainline Protestants, conservative Protestants, and Pentecostals. Rates of disorder were compared across denominational groups, controlling for sex, race, physical health status, socioeconomic status, and frequency of church attendance.

Among the baby boomers, Pentecostals had significantly higher six-month and lifetime rates of depressive disorder, anxiety disorder, and any DSM-III disorder. Mainline Protestants had the lowest six-month and lifetime rates of anxiety disorder and the lowest six-month rates of any DSM-III disorder, whereas conservative Protestants fell between the first two groups. The authors concluded that young adult Pentecostals in the Piedmont area experienced high rates of psychiatric disorder, which was not generally true for Pentecostals who were middle-aged or older. Infrequent churchgoers appeared to be at greatest risk, although they seldom sought professional help for their problems.

The study is cross-sectional and therefore we cannot attribute causality; herein lies the major difficulty in interpreting the study. Most such studies show very little relationship between identification with a faith tradition and mental health (e.g., Blazer, 2012). As noted, affiliation may be of less importance today than in the past. Many persons do not adhere to an "organized" or "institutional" religious group. In addition, using affiliation, especially with large categories that aggregate a range of faith traditions, loses much power.

Pentecostal affiliation in the South may be associated with a unique type of support group to which individuals with mental illness gravitate and in which environments they are able to function better on average. In other words, the nature of the Pentecostal worship and social network ties may be more welcoming to individuals who feel somewhat different from the populace as a whole. Free expression of feelings may also play a role. This interpretation is, of course, speculation, yet one must never assume a unidirectional view of causality from a cross-sectional study.

By far the most famous study of the association between religious group affiliation and mental illness was the study of suicide over a century ago by Emile Durkheim (1951). This study has been used by teachers of epidemiology for decades as an example of the potential for what is labeled the "ecological fallacy." The ecological fallacy is the bias that may occur because an association observed between variables on an aggregate level does not necessarily represent the association that exists on an individual level. For example, a study during a hot summer day of the sale of cold drinks and increased watching of television could conclude that the consumption of cold drinks, perhaps because of caffeine, may increase the desire to watch television. In fact, the hot weather probably contributes to both increased consumption of cold drinks and the choice to remain indoors and watch television.

The study by Meador and colleagues described would not by strict definition suffer from the ecologic fallacy, yet asking individuals to group themselves into large categories loses much information in terms of religious affiliation. But Durkheim's study definitely does qualify. Durkheim, in 1897, studied the association of religious affiliation in German states in Europe (by provinces or cantons) with overall national suicide rates. He used population data collected by others. For example, in Austria, he found suicide rates per one million to be 79.5 for Protestants, 51.3 for Catholics, and 20.7 for Jews. He then made many pronouncements about the reason for this discrepancy (e.g., Protestants were more likely to suffer from anomie [moral confusion and lack of social direction] than Catholics and Jews).

This study has therefore been a prime target of criticism for drawing individual conclusions from aggregate data. Historical factors (this was pre-World War I and the milieu of affiliation has changed dramatically in Europe, as well as in the United States) rather than religious affiliation may have shaped Durkheim's results. Remember the findings of Smith and colleagues about younger generations in the United States today (2009).

What renders this study methodologically suspect? First, there are assignment factors (e.g., the asumption that all persons in a Catholic-majority province were necessarily Catholic);the assignment of affiliation was by province, not by individual acknowledgment of religious affiliation. Second, there are case finding factors. The study assumes that suicide assessment was equally valid across all cantons. However, suicide at the time was considered a mortal sin by Catholics. Therefore, assignments of death by suicide may have been underreported or intentionally misreported in these cantons. And finally, the conclusion that anomie is a major contributor to increased frequency of suicide is a conjecture by Durkheim, not an actual finding of the study.

Studies of affiliation are frequently found in the literature; however, the probes in these studies are usually multiple, as affiliation is usually not considered of value independently in our current smorgasbord of religious groups, which cannot be easily categorized by types used in the past. Clinicians would be much better advised to explore the particular milieu and practices within a congregational setting to gain greater insight about affiliation rather than simply asking persons if they identify with, for example, a Protestant, Catholic, Jewish, or Muslim faith tradition.

CONCLUSIONS

The empirical study of R/S has become mainstream within the medical literature, and our understanding of the association between R/S and mental health has been greatly enhanced by these studies. Unfortunately, the topic often devolves into a heated debate between proponents and opponents of religion, those who are most fervent about their views and most unwilling to look at the data objectively. I have attempted in this chapter to provide some guidelines for evaluating these studies—guidelines far from comprehensive but hopefully useful. All empirical studies deserve a thorough critique, and none should be overgeneralized in terms of findings. Therefore what conclusions can we draw from this review?

Measures of religion spirituality fall along a spectrum. Virtually all depend upon self-report. Nevertheless, at one end of the spectrum are the measures that are more quantifiable (religious service attendance) and at the other end are subjective inquires such as, "How important is R/S to you?" All of these measures may have value. Yet they must be taken at *face value* and we cannot read more into the responses than what we observe

When performing such studies, age is critical as a control variable. Many studies have been performed among the elderly. Yet patterns of religious practice and basic belief structures have changed significantly over the past 50 years. Older adults are more likely to equate R/S with active participation, either private or public (service attendance, scripture reading, regular prayer) than younger adults. Younger adults are more likely to equate R/S with an individualistic and subjective perspective, which may not be easily synchronized with observable behaviors.

Studies of spiritual intervention must be thought through in terms of generalizability, and they range dramatically in the information that can be generalized to the population at large. For example, studies of the effectiveness of prayer would be almost impossible to perform for the reasons I have suggested here. In the future we will have available more intervention studies of "spiritually enhanced" types of therapy. If controlled well, they could be generalized to larger populations. Yet these studies must be carefully designed. The fitting of psychotherapies to specific faith traditions within the framework of CBT is in its infancy.

Finally, we must recognize that in some, perhaps most, faith traditions, there is no promise that faithfulness to that tradition improves health and relieves suffering. We must consider factors such as the martyrs of many faith traditions: for example, the apostle Paul's thorn in the flesh and the tortured life of Job. Adherence to some faith traditions may make the promise of health, wealth, and happiness, yet this has not historically been the message from sacred scriptures and the lives of the models of faith from the past. Therefore, empirical studies cannot be interpreted outside the historical context of that tradition. This in no way should discourage the undertaking of such studies, but should add a level of caution and reality. Of course, studies of R/S and health are far from unique. All empirical studies must proceed with caution. The process is iterative and always will be.

APPLICATIONS TO CLINICAL PRACTICE

The first application to clinical practice is a clear one, namely that any good mental health professional must critically read the literature about the association of R/S and mental health as well as the literature about specific faith communities to determine what findings might be of value to her or his practice. From the extant research, it appears to me that enough evidence has emerged such that any clinician who does not inquire about patient R/S is losing essential contextual data upon which to make informed clinical decisions with some assurance that those decisions will be implemented by the patient. For example, a clinician who does not inquire about the beliefs in a faith community regarding the use of psychotropic medications may prescribe such medications in peril of noncompliance in use because other factors beyond the advice of the clinician could be informing the decision of the patient. In addition, mental health professionals may be called upon by faith communities to instruct them in the latest thinking about psychiatric disorders. When asked, these professionals should make every effort to comply, for this audience may be essential for helping the members of the patient's social network to better understand these apparently mysterious, disordered beliefs and behaviors.

Moreira-Almeida and colleagues (2014) have suggested some general principles to guide clinicians as they explore the interface between R/S and psychiatric disorders. These include maintaining appropriate ethical boundaries; taking a person-centered approach; recognition of the potential for countertransference given that all clinicians bring spiritual or anti-spiritual values into the clinical encounter; remaining open minded; and taking a careful approach as a clinician regarding one's personal faith tradition (though when faith traditions are concordant, self-disclosure may enhance the clinical encounter). These guidelines begin with taking a spiritual history, as discussed previously.

Yet the implications for a good clinician go beyond simply reviewing the empirical literature and obtaining a spiritual history from patients. Clinical practice, of course, is driven by many factors beyond empirical research. Faith communities can teach the clinician about various aspects of a disorder and its care which fall outside the standard investigative articles and standard textbooks.

Consider what faith communities can teach mental health professionals about depression. To begin, faith communities have been caring for the depressed far longer than current mental health disciplines. What have they learned? When a faith community is functioning as a support for its members, how does that support translate into care for the depressed? I suggest the following as lessons the mental health professional can learn from faith communities:

- Depression is at once biological and spiritual. Humans are embodied souls from the perspective of almost all religious traditions and there is no room for either Cartesian dualism or a total materialistic approach to the patient. If the clinician does not accept this, she/he should recognize that this is the perspective of most of our patients.

- Patients tell stories. Mental health professionals may go through a checklist to determine whether a patient suffers from a disorder or not according to DSM-5 (APA, 2013). There is nothing wrong with diagnosis, yet there is a story behind the symptoms, and patients want their doctors (and their pastors, rabbis, and priests) to hear the story. Faith communities are repositories of stories.

- Faith communities help the depressed search for meaning in their depression. Depression is an emotion in search of a meaning. Yet that meaning may never be found in the midst of severe depression. At times the meaning is more or less apparent, at other times not apparent at all. It is the search that counts and an environment that encourages searching. A faith community that is non-judgmental and patient with the congregant, a community that can tolerate uncertainty and futility in search of meaning yet adapting nevertheless, can be of great value to the depressed.

- Faith communities help us name our depression. We all search for a name for our infirmities, in what has been called the Rumpelstiltskin phenomena (Torrey, 1972). (The maiden in this fairy tale is captured by a terrible little creature who promised freedom if she could name him.) When we seek help from doctors we want a diagnosis. Yet for emotional suffering a diagnosis often falls far short of giving us control over our pain (in contrast to a pain in the abdomen, which can be better tolerated once we identify it as a gallbladder attack that can be cured by removal of the gallbladder). How can faith communities help? They can provide different names and descriptions for what might seem a sterile term such as depression: "The Dark Night of the Soul" (though not actually the depression that psychiatrists see, was described by St. John of the Cross as a deep despair as part of the spiritual journey), a pilgrims' progress, fellow strugglers (such as Job), growth through pain toward something better (though care must be taken not to suggest that all suffering has an apparent reason), etc. These names evoke a sense of community in that all within the community are walking the same path, slogging through the same tough times (1959).

- Faith communities teach that hope and purpose are critical to healing depression. Depression seals off the sense of hope for many people. They see no future and they lose hope. Our society does not always provide messages of hope. Faith communities almost invariably look to a future that is better than the present and find hope in that future. Faith communities also provide, if they are true to human flourishing, a purpose. Not a purpose from someone else but rather a finding of purpose individually. To put this another way, one finds one's unique mission within the overall mission of the faith community.

REFERENCES

Alexander E: Proof of Heaven. New York, Simon & Schuster, 2012

APA: Diagnostic and Statistical Manual of Mental Disorders (DSM-5), Fifth Edition. Washington, DC, American Psychiatric Publishing, 2013

APA: Diagnostic and Statistical Manual of Mental Disorders, 2nd Edition. Washington, DC, American Psychiatric Association, 1968

APA: DSM-III: Diagnostic and Statistical Manual of Mental Disorders, III. Washington, DC, American Psychiatric Association, 1980

Blazer D: Religious beliefs, practices and mental health outcomes: what is the research question? American Journal of Geriatric Psychiatry 2007; 15:269–272

Blazer D: Religion/spirituality and depression: what can we learn from empirical studies? American Journal of Psychiatry 2012; 169:10–12

Dossey L: Healing Words: the Power of Prayer and the Practice of Medicine, New York, HarperCollins, 1997

Durkheim E: Suicide: a Study in Sociology. New York, The Free Press, 1951

Freud, Sigmund: The Future of an Illusion, 500 Fifth Avenue. New York, NY: W.W. Norton and Company, 1990 (original in German in 1927)

Gallup: Religion, http://www.gallup.com/poll/1690/religion.aspx#1, 2013

Hadaway C, Marler P, Chaves M: What the polls don't show: a closer look at church attendance. American Sociological Review 1993; 58:741–752

Hayward RD, Owen AD, Koenig HG, et al: Religion and the presence and severity of depression in older adults. American Journal of Geriatric Psychiatry 2012; 20:188–192

Koenig H, George L, Peterson B: Religiosity and remission from depression in medically ill older patients. American Journal of Psychiatry 1998; 155:536–542

Koenig H, King D, Carson V: Handbook of Religion and Health. New York, Oxford University Press, 2012

Koenig HG: Depression in chronic illness: does religion help? Journal of Christian Nursing: A Quarterly Publication of Nurses Christian Fellowship 2014; 31:40–46

Kristeller J, Rhodes M, Cripe L, et al: Oncologist assisted spiritual intervention study (OASIS): patient acceptability and initial evidence of effects. International Journal of Psychiatry in Medicine 2005; 35:329–347

Kung H: Freud and the Problem of God. New Haven, Yale University Press, 1990

Meador KG, Koenig HG, Hughes DC, et al: Religious affiliation and major depression. Hosp Community Psychiatry 1992; 43:1204–1208

Meng H, Freud E (eds.): Psychoanalysis and Faith: The Letters of Sigmund Freud and Oskar Pfister. New York, Basic Books, 1963

Miller L, Wickramaratne P, Gameroff MJ, et al: Religiosity and major depression in adults at high risk: a ten-year prospective study. Am J Psychiatry 2012; 169:89–94

Miller L, Bansal R, Wickramaratne P, et al: Neuroanatomical correlates of religiosity and spirituality: a study in adults at high and low familial risk for depression. JAMA Psychiatry 2014; 71:128–135

Moreira-Almeida A, Koenig HG, Lucchetti G: Clinical implications of spirituality to mental health: review of evidence and practical guidelines. Revista Brasileira di Psiquiatria 2014; 36:176–182

Newberg A, D'Aquili E, Rause V: Why God Won't Go Away: Brain Science and the Biology of Belief, New York, Random House, 2002

Propst LR, Ostrom R, Watkins P, Dean T, Mashburn D: Comparative efficacy of religious and nonreligious cognitive-behavioral therapy for the treatment of clinical depression in religious individuals. Journal of Consulting and Clinical Psychology 1992; 60(1):94–103

St. John of the Cross: Dark Night of the Soul. New York, Image Books, 1959

Sanua V: Religion, mental health, and personality: a review of empirical studies. American Journal of Psychiatry 1969; 125:1203–1213

Schoenfeld D, Malmrose L, Blazer D, et al: Self-rated health and mortality in the high-functioning elderly—a closer look at healthy individuals: MacArthur Field study of successful aging. Journal of Gerontology: Medical Sciences 1994; 49:M109–M115

Sloan R: Blind Faith: The Unholy Alliance of Religion and Medicine. New York, St. Martin's Press, 2006

Smith C, Snell P: Souls in Transition: The Religious Lives of Young Adults in America. New York, Oxford University Press, 2009

Torrey E: The Mind Game: Witchdoctors and Psychiatrists. New York, Emerson Hall, 1972

Vaillant G, Templeton J, Ardelt M, et al: The natural history of male mental health: health and religious involvement. Soc Sci Med 2008; 66:221–231

Zilboorg G: Psychoanalysis and Religion, New York, Farrar, Straus & Cudahy, 1962.

CHAPTER 6

RELIGION AND SPIRITUALITY IN INTERNAL MEDICINE

Lydia S. Dugdale and Daniel P. Sulmasy

The task of general internal medicine is to provide primary medical care to adult patients, both in and out of the hospital. The internal medicine doctor in the United States sometimes is also called a "general internist" or an "internist." In the United Kingdom, such physicians are called "general practitioners" or "GPs" in the outpatient setting, with the term "internist" reserved for inpatient adult medical doctors. A new internal medicine subspecialty of "hospitalists" has now emerged in the US, however, that more closely emulates the British system. Internists are distinguished from family medicine doctors, who receive additional training to care for obstetric, gynecologic, and pediatric patients. As primary providers of general medical care to adult patients, internists are uniquely positioned to know their patients and their patients' communities thoroughly, including faith communities.

The integration of religion and spirituality into practices of internal medicine, then, might be said to arise naturally from the cultivation of patient-physician relationship over time and circumstance. As with any relationship, the commitment of two people (that is, doctor and patient) to a common purpose (the health of the patient) lends itself to the building of trust and to increasing knowledge of one another, especially as various pitfalls challenge and shape both parties over a lifetime. Many patients bring a religious or spiritual framework into the clinic, and many doctors approach patient care with the same degree of formation by a spiritual community.

COMMON SCENARIOS

Numerous scenarios can help to illustrate how patients might carry religion and spirituality into the clinical encounter. Sometimes religious sentiments are expressed in passing. Patients might say, "God will help me through it" or, "The Lord is looking after me." Some patients offer a "God bless you" to their doctor on the way out the door. Other patients will correlate the onset of symptoms with a particular religious or spiritual experience. For example, a patient might report, "The dizziness started during a church service." Still others point to religion or spirituality as a method of coping with illness. Meditation and mindfulness reduce stress; prayer and reading the Bible increase faith and hope. For some, religion explicitly affects medical choices, such as when the bleeding Jehovah's Witness patient refuses a blood transfusion, or a Muslim patient refuses a vaccination derived from a porcine cell line. Some patients become more spiritual or religious in the face of a life-threatening diagnosis or as they are actively dying. They might call for a chaplain, or ask their physician to pray, or ask existential questions that they had not previously considered.

Like their patients, doctors also take their own religious and spiritual lives into the clinical environment. In some schools, medical students are taught to ask a patient about his or her spiritual background as part of taking a "social history." This means that in addition to asking a patient about substance use, sexual practices, and employment, the medical professional invites a patient to talk about religious or spiritual commitments and the role that a faith community plays in the patient's life. Sometimes a physician's religious views can affect treatment recommendations. For instance, doctors opposed to physician-assisted suicide on religious grounds might refuse to provide the intervention if requested by a terminally-ill patient. Furthermore, internists who know that they share a faith tradition with a patient might draw on the resources of the tradition to help a patient make sense of illness or grief.

Such examples highlight a few of the many ways that religion and spirituality enter into the space where internist and patient meet. These briefly described clinical scenarios suggest that discussions of religion or spirituality often occur naturally and effortlessly as an expression of the authenticity of two individual persons, unfolding in the clinical and interpersonal history of a particular patient-physician relationship.

EMPIRICAL EVIDENCE

While a number of empirical studies have addressed the intersection of medicine and religion, we present data only from those studies most relevant to general internal or primary care medicine. This empirical evidence might be usefully divided into studies representing the views of patients and the views of physicians, including physicians in training. We will consider these in turn.

THE PATIENT PERSPECTIVE

Many of the studies performed with adult medicine patients found that spirituality and/or religion help patients to cope with illness or to achieve better health. Treloar, for example, explored how spirituality helps people affected by disabilities to find meaning for what she calls their "lived experiences" with disability (Treloar, 2002). She interviewed 30 adults who either live with disability or are the primary caretakers of a child with disability. Interviewees were ages 22 and above, would be classified as a population that seeks medical care from an internist, and all self-identified as evangelical Christian. While the sample size was too small to make the findings generalizable to a larger population, Treloar found that disability creates difficulties that challenged the spirituality of participants, and that increased their reliance upon and strengthened their faith in God. Spiritual beliefs helped to stabilize the lives of those affected by disability and provided a framework for meaning despite adverse circumstances. Christian faith enabled study participants to choose to live with thankfulness and joy. Despite the benefits conferred by faith, study participants expressed a need for the church to promote a theological understanding of disability and to provide increased assistance, including emotional, spiritual, social, and practical support.

A number of studies have shown that patient spiritual or religious variables are associated with improved health care outcomes. Multiple well-designed studies (that control for confounding factors such as the fact that religions often proscribe unhealthy behaviors) have demonstrated that patients who attend religious services, independent of denomination, have better long-term somatic health care outcomes and even live longer (Hummer et al, 1999; Koenig et al, 1999; McBride et al, 1998; Oman & Reed, 1998; Strawbridge et al, 1997; Gillum et al, 2008). Religiosity and spiritual experiences are especially associated with better mental health outcomes (McCauley et al, 2008; Koenig, 2007).

Paranjape and Kaslow (2010) assessed the role of spirituality (but not religion) as a "culturally relevant determinant" of health status for African American women. The researchers preferred the term "spirituality" because of the way it assists "individuals through times of adversity by helping them develop a sense of meaning and purpose" (1900). Study participants were ages 50 and over in two urban primary care practices. The researchers found that higher levels of spirituality were associated with better mental and physical health status as assessed by a validated scoring system that rates a variety of dimensions of health which they transformed into two summary scores of physical and mental health.

McFadden and colleagues (2011) assessed the relationship between spiritual beliefs and tobacco use among adult medicine patients. They used the five-item Duke Religion Index (DUREL) to assess spirituality. They found that nonsmokers were more likely to engage in religious activities such as prayer, Bible study, and regular church attendance. After adjusting for demographic factors, however, they found no significant difference in intrinsic spirituality between smokers and nonsmokers.

Other studies attempt to assess what sort of religious or spiritual service patients would like in the clinical environment. MacLean and colleagues (2003) conducted a survey of adult patients' preferences for physician discussion and practices of spirituality. Seventy percent of survey respondents were Protestant or Catholic Christian. One-third of patients wanted their doctors to ask about their religious beliefs during routine office visits, and two-thirds thought that their physicians should be aware of their spiritual or religious beliefs. Respondents' interest in religious or spiritual interaction with their doctors was inversely proportional to the intensity of the activity: one-third welcomed a simple discussion of religion or spirituality, 28% agreed to physician silent prayer, but only 19% agreed to physician prayer with a patient. Patients were more likely to agree to their doctors' prayers if they were hospitalized or close to death. Despite such interest, only 10% of patients were willing to trade time spent on medical issues for a religious or spiritual discussion with their physicians. After controlling for other variables, African American respondents were more likely to make this trade-off.

Other studies, such as one by Ellison and colleagues (2012), have explored whether religious or spiritual individuals were more likely to use complementary and alternative medicine. After controlling for demographic, mental, and physical health factors, religious and spiritual identities were independent predictors of the use of certain types of alternative medicine. Respondents who self-identified as spiritual and religious were more likely to pray, meditate, participate in spiritual healing, and take biologically-based therapies such as vitamins. Those who described themselves as only spiritual were more likely to use other sorts of body-mind therapies and energy therapies like Reiki, and acupuncture. Those who self-identify as only religious are less likely to use complementary and alternative medicines.

Taken together, these studies suggest that religion and spirituality do play a role in how patients cope with illness and think about health. On the whole they suggest that religion or spirituality or a combination of the two have a positive impact on the health of patients. The study by MacLean and colleagues, however, suggests that while patients have an interest in their doctors' engagement of religious or spiritual questions, they typically do not value a doctor's counsel on these matters above medical advice. With this in mind, it is worth next considering the views of physicians on matters of religion and spirituality.

THE PHYSICIAN PERSPECTIVE

Studies of physicians' perspectives on religion and spirituality might be further divided between studies of physicians in training (or "residents") and physicians in practice.

TRAINEES

Luckhaupt and colleagues (2005) conducted a survey of primary care (including, but not limited to internal medicine) residents' beliefs about the role of religion and spirituality in medical contexts. Nearly half of residents felt that physicians should play a role in the spiritual or religious lives of their patients. Residents who reported greater frequency of participation in organized religious activity, a higher personal level of spirituality, and an older age were more likely to favor incorporating spiritual and religious activity into the clinical environment. Overall, as patients became sicker, residents were more likely to agree with incorporating religion and spirituality into the care of those patients. When compared with family practice residents, however, internal medicine residents were less likely to agree that the physician should play a role in patients' spiritual and religious lives (33% versus 46–74% of other primary care residents), less likely to agree that a physician should be aware of patients' spiritual and religious beliefs (79% versus 88–96% of others), and less likely to favor silent prayer in an office visit (20% versus 27–41% of others).

Yi and colleagues (2006) performed a different analysis of the same survey data of primary care residents to assess for depression and spiritual coping. Their 2006 paper reports that the prevalence of significant depressive symptoms was more than 25%, highest among residents in the combined internal medicine and pediatrics residency program and lowest among family medicine residents. They also found that religion and spirituality greatly enhanced residents' abilities to discriminate between the presence and absence of significant depressive symptoms. Those who adopted negative religious coping (through spiritual discontent or spiritual abandonment), who sought greater spiritual support, or who reported poorer spiritual well-being were more likely to have significant depressive symptoms. The authors posit that the relationship between spiritual support seeking and depression might reflect residents at higher risk for mood disorders or those who are seeking spiritual support as a way of coping with their problems. Overall, the authors suggest that despite a growing emphasis on teaching medical trainees to incorporate religion and spirituality into the patient-doctor relationship, deliberate attention to physicians' own spiritual needs has not been well emphasized.

In a subsequent analysis of the same data, Yi and colleagues (2007) report that resident physicians rate their health lower than might be expected for a young presumably healthy population. Internal medicine residents rated their health lower than other primary care residents. Higher self-rated levels of depressive symptoms and lower levels of spiritual well-being also correlated with lower self-rated health.

Spirituality has also been shown to be associated with less burnout among physicians, especially those in high stress settings in which patients frequently die, such as oncology and palliative care, whether as trainees or as physicians in practice (Kash et al, 2000; Holland & Neimeyer, 2005; Clark et al, 2007; Krasner et al, 2009).

Physicians in training, in sum, have much the same views on religion and spirituality as do patients. Religion and spirituality help residents to cope well with the difficulties of training, and higher individual religiosity tends to be associated with greater overall levels of health. Many residents would agree with patients that religion and spirituality have a role, if minimal, in the clinical encounter. We next turn to physicians in practice.

PRACTICING PHYSICIANS

Some of the earliest studies of physicians' attitudes and preferences regarding religion and spirituality in the clinical environments come from the family practice literature. Monroe and colleagues (2003) performed one of the first survey studies that sought specifically to include general internists together with family practice doctors. They included residents together with practicing physicians. They found that even though most physicians believed that they should be aware of the spirituality of their patients, internists—when compared with family practitioners—were consistently less likely to agree with asking about patients' spiritual beliefs in all clinical settings and less likely to agree to silent prayer for hospitalized and dying patients.

Curlin and colleagues (2005) performed the largest study of religious characteristics of US physicians. One-third of respondents identified as internal medicine doctors or as a subspecialist in internal medicine. In their seminal paper, they report that 55% of physicians say that their religious beliefs influence their practice of medicine. They also describe how the religiosity of US physicians differs from the general population. Physicians, when compared with the population at large, are equally likely to report religious affiliation but more likely to identify with underrepresented religious traditions in the US. They are more likely to attend regular religious services but less likely to carry their religious beliefs over into all other aspects of life. Physicians are twice as likely to consider themselves spiritual but not religious, and twice as likely to cope with major life difficulties without relying on God. This study confirms earlier findings that family physicians and pediatricians are generally more religious and psychiatrists are generally less religious than other medical specialties, but the researchers acknowledge that such relationships between religiosity and clinical specialty require further exploration.

In a subsequent analysis of the same data, Curlin and colleagues (2006) report that almost all physicians agree that it is appropriate to discuss religion and spirituality when a patient brings it up, and about three-quarters encourage patients' own religious or spiritual beliefs and practices when issues of religion or spirituality surface during the clinical encounter. Fewer physicians actually initiate discussions of such themes with patients, talk about their own religious or spiritual ideas and experiences, or pray with patients. Physicians who identify as being more religious and more spiritual (particularly those who are Protestant) are more likely to incorporate spiritual activities into the patient visit. This study did not analyze responses by medical specialty, thus, we cannot know whether internal medicine doctors were more or less likely than their colleagues to participate in conversations about religion and spirituality or to pray with patients.

Subsequent works by Curlin and colleagues also do not differentiate based on medical specialty, but they do add further insight to the empirical research on the role of religion and spirituality in the medical environment. A 2007 paper (Curlin et al.) looked at physicians' views of the influence of religion and spirituality on health. In accordance with other studies, most physicians believed that religion and spirituality help patients to cope, and provide patients with a positive state of mind and emotional support. The higher the physician's degree of religiosity, the more likely he or she was to report that patients often mention issues of religion and spirituality, believe that they strongly influence health, and interpret their influence in positive ways.

Another study by Curlin and colleagues (2007) considered whether religious physicians were more likely to report practice among the poor. Although about one-quarter of US physicians responded that their patient populations are considered underserved, physicians who were generally more religious—as measured by intrinsic religiosity scales or frequency of religious service attendance—were not more likely to report practice among the underserved. They were, however, more likely to view the career of medicine as a calling. Those who were more likely to report practice among the underserved included those who described themselves as highly spiritual, those who strongly agreed that their religious beliefs influenced their practice of medicine, and those who strongly agreed that the family in which they were raised prioritized service to the poor. Again, these researchers did not discriminate based on medical specialty.

A final study by Curlin and colleagues (2009) sought to compare religious characteristics of general internists, rheumatologists, naturopaths, and acupuncturists, as well as to examine associations between physicians' religious characteristics and their openness to integrating complementary and alternative medicine. They found that naturopaths and acupuncturists were three times as likely as internists and rheumatologists to report no religious affiliation, but they were more likely to describe themselves as very spiritual and to report that they try to carry their religious beliefs into other areas of life. Among physicians, increased spirituality and religiosity coincided with more personal use and a greater willingness to integrate complementary and alternative medicine into a treatment program.

Thus, broad themes that emerge from the empirical literature point to the notion that both resident physicians and doctors in practice feel that religion and spirituality can help patients as well as themselves to cope with stress or illness. Although the largest studies do not differentiate by medical specialty in detail, internal medicine physicians on the whole tend to report lower levels of spirituality or religiosity than family medicine physicians but not levels as low as psychiatrists report.

The empirical research only ever tells part of the story. Issues of religion and spirituality within the clinical space are often much more complicated. Empirical research might suggest that doctors and patients are more comfortable engaging religious questions the closer a patient approximates death, but the content of an existential conversation does not lend itself to analysis with a survey tool. It would thus be helpful to consider how conceptual scholarship on the subject might contribute.

CONCEPTUAL ARGUMENTS

Religion is the oldest form of medical practice (Sulmasy, 2009). Whether appealing to a shaman or to God, most of the world's religions, East and West, have intricately linked religion with healing. Although Americans increasingly define themselves as "spiritual but not religious," sickness and death raise questions for patients that are at once spiritual and religious. Thus, we argue that physicians have a moral obligation to attend to their patients' spiritual needs. This is true for several reasons. First, the care of and respect for the whole patient demands consideration of their religious or spiritual views. Second, clinicians are uniquely positioned in their relationships to patients to elicit concerns that are spiritual. Third, religious or spiritual factors may be directly relevant to patient care—for instance, by interfering with a proposed therapy--a conflict that might be avoided or mitigated by seeking to understand a patient's religious or spiritual beliefs.

Curlin and Moschovis (2004) further the case for the relevance of religious conversations to the doctor-patient relationship. They argue that the secularist critique—which asserts that physicians who make space for religion or spirituality in a clinical encounter lack qualification to do so and might abuse their position of authority—is artificially neutral. Instead, they propose an enriched dialectic between doctor and patient in which faith has relevance. Recognition of faith should enhance, rather than diminish, care of patients. "Physicians who are devoutly religious should recognize the particularities of their perspective, and begin to empathically engage their patients' spiritual concerns," they write. "Even in the case where physician and patient speak from religiously discordant perspectives, the physician can compassionately and sensitively engage the patient on the patient's terms, rather than forcing the patient to address difficult questions within a foreign moral framework." In contrast to the secularist critique, this approach strengthens rather than threatens the clinician's relationship with the patient.

Curlin and Hall (2005) take this idea of an enriched dialogue between doctor and patient one step further. They argue that there are two techniques by which clinician and patient might interact. What they have dubbed the "stranger-technique" framework focuses on questions of the doctor's competence and the patient's autonomy. Under such a rubric, religion is neutral, which potentially hampers doctor-patient dialogue. They argue instead for "an ethic of moral friendship that seeks the patient's good through wisdom, candor, and respect." This framework promotes a robust moral discourse between doctor and patient, which does not disregard religious commitments but takes them into consideration when deliberating with patients over moral choices in health care. Curlin and Hall do not propose a particular tool, as some have, for approaching these conversations.

Writing for family physicians, Anandarajah and Hight (2001) suggest that physicians might employ the HOPE spiritual assessment tool in order to discern patients' spiritual and religious views. They note that the strength of this tool is that "it allows for an open-ended exploration of an individual's general spiritual resources and concerns and serves as a natural followup to discussion of other support systems." Each letter of the HOPE tool represents a particular domain for questioning. The H of HOPE refers to a patient's basic spiritual resources, including sources of hope, meaning, comfort, and connection; it does not focus immediately on religion or spirituality. The O and P pertain to areas of inquiry regarding the importance of organized religion for patients and to the specific aspects of their personal spirituality and practices that they find to be most helpful. E represents the effects of a patient's spirituality and beliefs on medical care and end-of-life issues. The information gleaned from use of the HOPE tool might in some cases direct physicians toward further incorporation of spirituality or religion into preventative care, adjuvant therapy, or treatment plans.

D'Souza (2007) proposes an alternative tool for investigating patients' spirituality, "what they hold to be the purpose of their lives." He holds with others that physicians should not exercise their position of authority to impose or prescribe their own religious or spiritual beliefs to patients. Rather, he commends for the purposes of taking a spiritual history the four basic questions that were formulated by a consensus panel of the American College of Physicians:

1. Is faith (religion, spirituality) important to you?
2. Has faith been important to you at other times in your life?
3. Do you have someone to talk to about religious matters?
4. Would you like to explore religious, spiritual matters with someone?

D'Souza's conclusions echo those of Curlin, Moschovis, and Hall: such questions convey that the clinician cares about the whole person, thereby strengthening the doctor-patient relationship.

Rather than an assessment tool, Winslow and Wehtje-Winslow (2007) adopt a principled approach to spiritual care of patients. They put forth a set of five normative principles, which center on respect for the patient and professional integrity. The first holds that clinicians who aim to provide "respectful care" should attempt to achieve a basic understanding of their patients' spirituality. They propose approaching this through four questions developed by Puchalski and colleagues (2010). Using this "FICA" tool, a clinician asks a patient whether she considers herself to be spiritual or religious; how important such beliefs are and whether they influence how she cares for herself; whether she belongs to a spiritual community; and how health care professionals might address such needs. The second normative principle is that clinicians must respect and follow their patients' wishes with regards to spiritual care. Third, clinicians should not prescribe specific spiritual practices nor discourage patients from exercising their own religious or spiritual beliefs. Fourth, clinicians who provide spiritual care for patients should likewise seek to understand their own spiritual beliefs. Fifth, participation in spiritual care should be commensurate with professional integrity. The authors argue that physicians who are uncomfortable with spiritual care should not do it; "feigning spirituality would be a regrettable failure of integrity and a breach of patients' trust." For those clinicians who strive to provide comprehensive care for patients, these normative principles might help to frame an ethic of spiritual care.

Rumbold (2007) is somewhat wary of the aforementioned techniques, assessments, and approaches; he is concerned that health care will subsume spirituality in order to resolve the dissonance between them. Furthermore, he maintains that health frameworks misrepresent and misinterpret the way spirituality is understood by society more broadly, and this may even do harm: "Clinical spiritual care, based on expert assessments, may be experienced as invasive and presumptuous or—worse—may immobilize patients by depriving them of a resource they need to cope or survive." He maintains that spiritual assessment tools inevitably omit much of what brings coherence to a patient's life. Such tools should not impose their own definitions but should be designed such that they elicit and clarify the patient's beliefs. Rumbold then provides guidelines for how he thinks spiritual assessments could be relocated within a patient's spiritual framework:

1. Respect patients' perspectives and do not infringe on privacy
2. Involve all members of the interdisciplinary team to the extent that they are able and willing to contribute
3. Permit clear documentation of needs, strategic responses to these needs, resources required, and outcomes
4. Integrate strategies into an overall care plan in ways that are readily understood by all members of the interdisciplinary team
5. Provide a shared framework for continuity of care between community agencies and inpatient services
6. Provide a place for religious care but do not conflate spiritual issues with religious practice. While spiritual care in general may be provided by a team, specific religious care is best provided by a person from the same faith community, preferably one willing to participate in the team.

Once situated within the patient's framework, spiritual assessments then should be understood not as events but processes—processes which lead to the development of a spiritual care plan for a patient. Ultimately, Rumbold seems to return to making a place for spiritual assessments within the clinical encounter or, at least, to making space for ongoing conversations regarding the implications of patients' spiritual and religious beliefs on health.

All of these tools are merely aids that are often most useful to novice learners. More experienced clinicians will learn to ask open-ended questions, listen carefully, and follow the patient's lead. For example, in the inpatient setting, sitting down next to the patient and asking, "How are you doing?" can be the most important aspect of spiritual assessment (Sulmasy, 2006). In the outpatient setting, one question such as, "What role does spirituality or religion play in your life?" both normalizes inquiry about religious and spiritual needs and can open a discussion that leads to the disclosure of all the information that these tools are designed to elicit (Sulmasy, 2006).

Whether describing a formal "spiritual assessment tool" or a rich dialogue between doctor and patient, these scholars underscore the findings elucidated by the empirical research: it is a disservice to patients to prohibit discussions of religion and spirituality within the context of the clinician-patient relationship.

BEST PRACTICES FOR INTERNAL MEDICINE

Having reviewed the empirical and conceptual literature relevant to medicine and religion within the context of internal medicine practice, we will now attempt to distill out what might be considered the best practices for attending to questions of religion and spirituality within the context of the practice of internal medicine. We will take as a foundational assumption that medicine must include such conversations.

Before proceeding, however, we must note a word of caution. Just because the evidence points to an association between religion/spirituality and health does not mean that the former causes the latter. For example, no one is certain whether religious practice makes people healthy or whether healthy people are more inclined to be religious. And one need look no further than Jesus or Gandhi to see that religion can actually be bad for one's health. Moreover, physicians should refrain from exploiting the power differential in the doctor-patient relationship through proselytizing, just as they should refrain from instrumentalizing religion by advertising its health benefits. Finally, some sensitive and personal choices ought to be outside of the domain of health—even for physicians. Just because married people live longer doesn't mean doctors should tell all single people to get married for the health benefits! With these ethical principles in mind, we turn now to the best practices for addressing religion and spirituality within the medical environment.

First, as with any aspect of patient care, physicians have a professional obligation to familiarize themselves with the medical literature pertinent to medicine and religion/spirituality. This includes physicians who for themselves reject religion and spirituality. Such literature is central to care of patients and thus should be integrated into the ongoing training of clinicians.

Second, recognizing that most patients and most physicians report some degree of intrinsic religiosity and that religion and spirituality have an impact on health, the spiritual history should be incorporated into the taking of a patient's complete social history. This should be done in both the inpatient medical ward and the outpatient clinic as part of a comprehensive review of the patient's health.

Third, physicians should make time to address spiritual concerns. Just as patients might be asked to return in two weeks for a blood pressure check after the introduction of a new medication for poorly-controlled blood pressure, so too a patient might be brought back to clinic to discuss further spiritual or religious concerns brought up in an earlier visit. On a practical note, doctors might be relieved to find that they can sometimes bill for such services: ICD-9 and ICD-10 codes exist for diagnoses such as "religious or spiritual problem" (V62.89 and Z65.8, respectively) and "spiritual or religious counseling" (V65.49 and Z71.81, respectively).

Fourth, physicians should see themselves as part of a broader team that exists to address patients' needs. Internists are not experts in everything and rely on many specialists for assistance. Just because some doctors might feel ill-equipped to provide solutions to specific religious or spiritual problems does not mean that they should avoid such conversations. Taking a careful history is part of working toward any diagnosis and solution. If a patient's discontent is found to be due to a religious problem beyond the expertise of the health care professional, the patient's own clergy or chaplain services may be summoned.

Fifth, for non-clinicians who might read this volume, it is worth emphasizing that laypeople, perhaps, have as much responsibility to voice concerns to their physicians as physicians have to ask. Jehovah's Witnesses, for example, are typically quite clear when they do not want blood transfusions. Why should Roman Catholics, for example, be any less clear about wanting to receive Viaticum?

Sixth, patients and doctors alike need to think broadly about what the spiritual and religious content of the doctor-patient encounter might look like. In survey tools, questions often refer to prayer or taking a spiritual inventory, but there is no reason that the conversation can't push toward deeper questions. An older patient with acute worsening of a chronic illness might develop anxiety at the thought of death's approach. Would the internist appropriately care for such a patient by prescribing an anxiolytic? Or might the doctor ask about the source of the anxiety, whether the patient has made his peace in this life, and whether the patient has thought about an afterlife? If the patient then acknowledges his anxiety as being related to death and its aftermath, shouldn't the physician then ask whether the patient has a religious or spiritual framework to help him make sense of this, or whether there are other resources on which he might draw? Good care requires that we push toward deeper conversations with patients and not hastily plaster over existential concerns.

Finally, clinicians need to become more conscious of their own spiritual and/or religious values, needs, and resources. Better spiritual care is likely to be delivered by clinicians who have cultivated their own spiritual lives (Sulmasy, 1999). Moreover, it is helpful for clinicians to be conscious of the ways in which their spiritual and religious commitments affect their recommendations to patients and clinical practice styles.

FUTURE RESEARCH

Having attempted to review the literature germane to the practice of internal medicine, it has become evident that very little of this research to date has distinguished approaches to religion and spirituality by medical specialty. The relationships between religiosity and clinical specialty will therefore require further exploration. Additionally, the time has come in this field to push the research questions deeper than asking whether clinicians talk about religion or pray with patients. If this first set of research questions has strengthened the patient-physician relationship then we can expect that a deeper and richer discourse will further the same.

CONCLUSION

Internal medicine physicians have a unique place in patients' lives, caring for them from early adulthood through to death. Such relationships not only can endure a lifetime, but they can develop a depth that might otherwise be impossible for other medical specialists. It is not surprising that many internists come to know of their patients' religious or spiritual beliefs.

The majority of doctors and patients endorse some sort of spiritual or religious belief. Internal medicine doctors tend to be less religious or spiritual than family medicine doctors but more so than psychiatrists. Although many internists feel religious and spiritual beliefs have a place in health care settings, and most studies show a positive correlation between religion and health, only the minority of patients express interest in specific practices, such as prayer, with their doctors.

As the oldest form of medical practice, religion is central to the belief systems of many patients. Physicians therefore have a moral obligation to address their patients' spiritual and religious concerns. While various tools might be employed to further this aim, they might ultimately fall short of the rich dialogue that can substantively deepen and meaningfully enhance the doctor-patient relationship. We suggest that physicians should respectfully inquire about their patients' spiritual and religious beliefs, make time to address spiritual concerns as they would physical concerns, and make use of the team approach to medical care, drawing on the assistance of chaplains and lay clergy as needed. Patients might be encouraged to articulate for themselves how they would like to bring their religious or spiritual practices into the clinical environment, and physicians must be encouraged to cultivate their own spirituality. Together, doctor and patient alike might further and deepen conversations and relationships, thereby strengthening the therapeutic alliance.

REFERENCES

Treloar LL. Disability, spiritual beliefs and the church: the experiences of adults with disabilities and family members. *J Adv Nursing.* 2002; 40: 594–603.

Hummer RA, Rogers RG, Nam CB, Ellison CG. Religious involvement and U.S. adult mortality. *Demography* 1999; 36: 273–285.

Koenig HG, Hays JC, Larson DB, George LK, Cohen HJ, McCullough ME, Meador KG, Blazer DG. Does religious attendance prolong survival? a six-year follow-up study of 3,968 older adults. *Journal of Gerontology, Series A,* 1999; 54(7): M370–376.

McBride JL, Arthur G, Brooks R, Pilkington L. The relationship between a patient's spirituality and health experiences. *Family Medicine* 1998; 30: 122–126.

Oman D, Reed D. Religion and mortality among the community-dwelling elderly. *American Journal of Public Health* 1998; 88: 1469–1475.

Strawbridge WJ, Cohen RD, Shema SJ, Kaplan GA. Frequent attendance at religious services and mortality over 28 years. *American Journal of Public Health* 1997; 87: 957–961.

Gillum RF, King DE, Obisesan TO, Koenig HG. Frequency of attendance at religious services and mortality in a U.S. national cohort. *Ann Epidemiol* 2008; 18:124–129.

McCauley J, Tarpley MJ, Haaz S, Bartlett SJ. Daily spiritual experiences of older adults with and without arthritis and the relationship to health outcomes. *Arthritis Rheum* 2008; 59:122–128.

Koenig HG. Religion and remission of depression in medical inpatients with heart failure/pulmonary disease. *J Nerv Ment Dis* 2007; 195:389–395.

Paranjape A, Kaslow N. Family violence exposure and health outcomes among older African American women: do spirituality and social support play protective roles? *J Womens Health (Larchmt)* 2010; 19: 1899–1904.

McFadden D, Croghan IT, Piderman KM, Lundstrom C, Schroeder DR, Taylor Hays J. Spirituality in tobacco dependence: A Mayo clinic survey. *Explore* 2011; 7:162–167.

MacLean CD, Susi B, Phifer N, et al. Patient preference for physician discussion and practice of spirituality. *J Gen Intern Med* 2003; 18: 38–43.

Ellison CG, Bradshaw M, Roberts CA. Spiritual and religious identities predict the use of complementary and alternative medicine among US adults. *Prev Med.* 2012 January; 54(1): 9–12.

Luckhaupt SE, Yi MS, Mueller CV, et al. Beliefs of primary care residents regarding spirituality and religion in clinical encounters with patients: a study at a midwestern U.S. teaching institution. *Acad Med.* 2005; 80: 560–570.

Yi MS, Luckhaupt SE, Mrus JM. Religion, Spirituality, and Depressive Symptoms in Primary Care House Officers. *Ambulatory Pediatrics.* 2006; 6: 84–90.

Yi MS, Mrus JM, Mueller CV, et al. Self-rated health of primary care house officers and its relationship to psychological and spiritual well-being. *BMC Medical Education.* 2007; 7:9

Kash C, Holland JC, Breitbart W, Berenson S, Dougherty J, Ouellette-Kobasa S, Lesko L. Stress and burnout in oncology. *Oncology* 2000; 14:1621–1633.

Holland J, Neimeyer R. Reducing the risk of burnout in end-of-life care settings: The role of daily spiritual experiences and training. *Palliat Support Care* 2005; 3: 173–181.

Clark L, Leedy S, McDonald L, Muller B, Lamb C, Mendez T, Kim S, Schonwetter R. Spirituality and job satisfaction among hospice interdisciplinary team members. *J Palliat Med* 2007; 10:1321–1328.

Krasner MS, Epstein RM, Beckman H, Suchman AL, Chapman B, Mooney CJ, Quill TE. Association of an educational program in mindful communication with burnout, empathy, and attitudes among primary care physicians. *JAMA* 2009; 302:1284–1293.

Monroe MH, Bynum D, Susi B, et al. Primary care physician preferences regarding spiritual behavior in medical practice. *Arch Intern Med* 2003 Dec 8–22; 163(22): 2751–2756.

Curlin FA, Lantos JD, Roach CJ, Sellergren SA, Chin MH. Religious characteristics of U.S. physicians: a national survey. *J Gen Intern Med* 2005; 20:629–634.

Curlin FA, Chin MH, Sellergren SA, Roach CJ, Lantos JD. The association of physicians' religious characteristics with their attitudes and self-reported behaviors regarding religion and spirituality in the clinical encounter. *Med Care* 2006; 44: 446–453.

Curlin FA, Sellergren SA, Lantos JD, Chin MH. Physicians' observations and interpretations of the influence of religion and spirituality on health. *Arch Intern Med.* 2007 April 9; 167(7): 649–654.

Curlin FA, Dugdale LS, Lantos JD, Chin MH. Do religious physicians disproportionately care for the underserved? *Ann Fam Med* 2007; 5: 353–360.

Curlin FA, Rasinski KA, Kaptchuk TJ, Emanuel EJ, Miller FG, Tilburt JC. Religion, clinicians, and the integration of complementary and alternative medicines, *J Alt and Compl Med* 2009; 15: 987–994.

Sulmasy DP. Spirituality, religion, and clinical care. *Chest* 2009; 135:1634–1642.

Curlin FA, Moschovis PP. Is religious devotion relevant to the doctor-patient relationship? *J Fam Pract* 2004; 53: 632–636.

Curlin FA, Hall DE. Strangers or Friends? A proposal for a new spirituality-in-medicine ethic, *J Gen Intern Med* 2005; 20: 370–374.

Anandarajah G, Hight E. Spirituality and medical practice: using the HOPE questions as a practical tool for spiritual assessment. *Am Fam Physician* 2001; 63: 81–89.

D'Souza R. The importance of spirituality in medicine and its application to clinical practice. *Med J Australia* 2007; 186: S57–S59.

Winslow GR, Wehtje-Winslow BJ. Ethical boundaries of spiritual care. *Med J Australia* 2007; 186: S63–S66.

Borneman T, Ferrell B, Puchalski CM. Evaluation of the FICA Tool for spiritual assessment, *J Pain Symptom Manage* 2010;40:163–173.

Rumbold BD. A review of spiritual assessment in health care practice. *Med J Australia.* 2007; 186: S60–S62.

Sulmasy DP. Spiritual issues in the care of dying patients: ". . . it's okay between me and god." *JAMA* 2006;296:1385–1392.

Sulmasy DP. *The rebirth of the clinic: an introduction to spirituality in health care.* Washington, DC: Georgetown University Press, 2006: 138.

Sulmasy DP. Is medicine a spiritual practice? *Acad Med* 1999;74:1002–1005.

CHAPTER 7

RELIGION AND SPIRITUALITY IN SURGERY

John Tarpley and Margaret Tarpley

RESEARCH

WHAT IS THE STATE OF THE SCIENCE OF R/S IN SURGERY?

The influence of religion and spirituality (R/S) on surgeons dates back to the early history of modern surgery and continues into the 21st century. Ambroise Paré, a father of modern surgical practice in the 16th century, brought to surgery a view of practice involving gentle treatment of tissue and compassion for the injured. Paré declared: "I dressed him and God healed him" (Paré, 1921). Alexis Carrel, arguably one of the most influential and innovative surgeons of the 20th century, investigated miraculous healings attributed to the spring waters of Lourdes, France, and publically supported validity for some of the claims. This exercise derailed his academic career in France when he was accused of being either fooled or a promoter of the Roman Catholic Church. He relocated to the U.S. where he won the Nobel Prize in Physiology or Medicine in 1912 but did not pursue further public research in religion. His two small books, one on prayer (Carrel, 1948) and the other about Lourdes (Carrel, 1950), were published posthumously in 1948 and 1950.

In any discussion of R/S and surgery, wide variability of beliefs and practices, even within a particular world religion, denomination, ethnic group, or cultural community, must be acknowledged. Excellent resources such as Setta and Shemie's "An Explanation and Analysis of How World Religions Formulate Their Ethical Decisions on Withdrawing Treatment and Determining Death" (Setta and Shemie, 2015) and Healthcare Chaplaincy Network's *Handbook (of) Patients' Spiritual and Cultural Values for Health Care Professionals* (Wintz and Handzo, 2015) offer starting points rather than universally applicable answers. This chapter presents numerous reports on R/S and surgical practice with each study offering a glimpse into a particular group or institution at a particular time. Two consistent themes emerge: (1) the vital significance of R/S to patients, families, and many surgeons; and (2) the paucity of medical education and training concerning R/S.

Prayer plays a central role in most world religions. In 1988, the Byrd study of intercessory prayer (IP) effects on post-cardiac surgery patients in the coronary care unit (CCU) helped ignite discussion as well as research on the role of prayer and religious practices for surgical patients (Byrd, 1988). Over 70% of PubMed articles on prayer in surgery have been published since 1988. R/S research takes place in academic teaching institutions across North America and in international settings as well. Because of the numerous aspects of R/S open to study, the peer-reviewed literature offers reports relating to effects on health and healing of spiritual practices including IP, social cohesion, coping, study of holy texts, communal worship, singing, meditating, the role of chaplains, clergy or faith leaders as well as behavioral practices involving dietary restrictions, intervention prohibitions, and tobacco and alcohol abstention.

The 2009 Cochrane Review concerning efficacy of intercessory prayer concluded (1) the results were equivocal; (2) evidence was not convincing that further trials of this intervention should be undertaken; and (3) any resources available for such a trial should be used to investigate other health care questions. A widely quoted Cha paper from 2001 on efficacy of prayer for successful in vitro fertilization was subsequently withdrawn as controversial from the *Journal of Reproductive Health* website with Cochrane excluding it from the review while stating it had no proof the study was bogus (Roberts, Ahmed, and Davison, 2009; Cha and Wirth, 2001). These Cochrane conclusions provoked mixed responses and did not curtail research. A 2012 Australian randomized, blinded study on efficacy of IP for spiritual well-being in patients with cancer reported a small but significant positive impact (Olver and Dutney, 2012).

Religiosity and spiritual practices appear to assist persons in coping with recuperation from surgical procedures (Ai et al., 2013), as well as chronic medical issues in Western (McCauley et al., 2005) and non-Western settings (Steglitz et al., 2012); these are all relevant for members of the surgical community who frequently deal with co-morbidities, the elderly, and long recuperations. Addressing and promoting aspects of spiritual well-being are recommended because separating the power of social support from R/S practices is almost impossible due to the communal nature of much R/S practice.

Matthew Walker, chairman of surgery from 1944 to 1973 at Meharry Medical College in Nashville, insisted that medical students and physicians needed to be in touch with their own mortality if they were to assist patients and their families in dealing with end-of-life (EOL) (Organ and Kosiba, 1987). Surgical training currently encourages self-reflection that could involve consideration of how one's personal beliefs that may affect surgical decisions (Stern, Rasinski, and Curlin, 2011; Curlin et al., 2005) as well as technical practice and treatment options.

EXAMPLES OF THE STATE OF SCIENCE IN R/S RESEARCH

TRAUMA

Influenced by research demonstrating that religious affiliation is associated with reduced mortality (Strawbridge et al., 1997), a Howard University group studied 2303 patients admitted to their Level I trauma center in 2009 but did not note a statistically significant association between religious affiliation and mortality or length of stay. (Khoury et al., 2012) In burn patients, utilization of pastoral care appears to be linked to size of burn, financial charges, and length of stay, with religious affiliation serving as a possible marker for improved survival, suggesting that plastic surgeons and burn teams should consider addressing the spiritual needs of burn patients as a component of recovery (Hultman et al., 2014).

CANCER SURGERY

Many aspects of beliefs and background relating to cancer treatment have been considered. Several studies focused on the role of R/S for coping with colorectal cancer including a Kaiser Permanente study recommending that quality of life (QOL) interventions for colorectal cancer survivors with ostomies should involve elements that promote spiritual well-being including inner peace, interconnectedness and belonging. (Bulkley et al., 2013) Attempting to discern the role of R/S in psychological distress before urologic surgery, Biegler et al. found that R/S was associated with engagement coping but not with any of the measures of distress, thus requiring further study (Biegler et al., 2012). The coping-mechanism benefits of religion in patients undergoing craniotomies for tumors were validated in a Toronto qualitative case study of 36 randomly selected adults (Ravishankar and Bernstein, 2014). In Iran, narrative interviews were conducted with 8 post-mastectomy women who reported religion related to both acceptance and hope (Sadati et al., 2015). All aspects of the surgeon's background—experience, regional culture, and training—impacted treatment and palliation of pancreatic head adenocarcinoma (Hurdle et al., 2014).

END-OF-LIFE DECISIONS

The major world religions house myriad beliefs and teachings concerning death and how death is determined. Decisions relating to the extent to which treatment is continued when death seems imminent or if brain death is declared can be strongly influenced by the religious sensibilities of the family or surrogate. Knowing the patient's religious or spiritual background is often vital for navigating EOL decision making that includes determining an appropriate level of care, consulting palliative medicine, transitioning to comfort care, determining death, and donating organs (Setta and Shemie, 2015). A 2014 study revealed that religiously-affiliated intensive care unit (ICU) patients receive more aggressive EOL care, in part because they or their families requested it. Although survival rates were the same, Shinall et al. at Vanderbilt found that religiously affiliated patients in the EOL group incurred 23% ($P = 0.030$) more hospital charges, 25% ($P = 0.035$) more ventilator days, 23% ($P = 0.045$) more hospital days, and 30% ($P = 0.036$) longer time until death than their non-religiously affiliated counterparts (Shinall, Ehrenfeld, and Guillamondegui, 2014). The studies of Balboni et al. and of Epstein-Peterson and colleagues showed that nurses and physicians sometimes desire to provide spiritual care (SC) within the setting of terminal illness in an advanced cancer environment. They surveyed 75 patients (Response Rate [RR], 73%) and 339 nurses and physicians (RR 63%) and found SC was infrequently provided: 20% encouraged or affirmed beliefs; 16% made chaplain referrals; and 10% took a spiritual history. Forty percent of nurses/physicians offered SC less often than they would have liked. Most nurses and physicians had no SC training and training was the strongest predictor of SC provision (Epstein-Peterson et al., 2014; Balboni et al., 2013).

EOL care involves a team of professionals; the surgeon may consult internal medicine, palliative care, and others. The physician's religiosity as well as that of the patient may affect treatment recommendations (Curlin et al., 2005). A survey of 443 Jewish physicians at four Israeli hospitals reported that religiosity was not related to withholding most life-sustaining treatments; however very religious physicians, compared to moderately religious and secular physicians, were much less likely to believe that life-sustaining treatment should be withdrawn (11% vs. 36% v. 51%, $p < 0.001$) or to approve of prescribing needed pain medication if it could hasten death (69% vs. 80% vs. 85%, $p < 0.01$) (Wenger and Carmel, 2004).

USE OF BLOOD AND BLOOD PRODUCTS

Driven primarily by adapting to the Jehovah's Witnesses' (JW) refusal of blood products, bloodless surgery has made extraordinary strides with a number of surgeons who specialize in JW care. A 2014 study from Johns Hopkins with a control group to compare to the blood-free procedural group revealed that appropriate blood conservation measures for patients who do not accept allogeneic blood transfusion (ABT) result in similar or better outcomes and are associated with equivalent or lower costs (Frank et al., 2014). A retrospective study of pancreas and liver resections performed at Memorial Sloan-Kettering Cancer Center found the procedures could be performed safely in JWs. (Konstantinidis et al., 2013)

BODY INTEGRITY INCLUDING ORGAN DONATION AND AMPUTATION

A number of cultural and religious communities believe the body must remain intact as the person passes from life to death; this belief will influence whether a patient will accept an amputation or stoma or the family allow organ donations (Wintz and Handzo, 2014). Although a marked diversity between different countries and even within individual countries exists, in Asia the overall low rate of deceased donation is due largely to social, cultural, religious, and economic factors (Lo, 2012). One example of attitudes is from Islam. Muslims are allowed to donate their organs for transplant providing that they are not compromising their own lives. They are also allowed to receive organs. However, opinions differ, so tact is necessary; some Muslims believe that the physical body should not be "mutilated," but should remain "intact" in order to pass easily into the next life. Muslims have no objections to blood transfusions (Nursing with Dignity. Part 8: Islam, 2002). A small South Dakota report and a survey of medical, law, divinity, nursing, and communication students in Turkey suggest that education might improve organ donation in the Muslim community (Hafzalah et al., 2014; Kocaay et al., 2015).

COSMETIC SURGERY

A British study to discern factors, including religious beliefs and attitudes, that motivate persons to seek cosmetic surgery concluded that religious persons consider body alteration for cosmetic purposes to be counter to teachings of Christian religious scriptural authority but advocated for further research into the attitudes of all religions concerning cosmetic surgery (Furnham and James Levitas, 2012).

PROCEDURES SOMETIMES INVOLVING SURGEONS

Male circumcision, rooted in cultural practice and religious ceremonies rather than medical necessity, is likely the most commonly practiced elective surgical procedure in the United States and perhaps in the world, with a third of men worldwide being circumcised (Savulescu, 2013), although a variety of non-surgeons perform most of the procedures. Historical evidence for circumcision predates the Abrahamic biblical record and has been documented in numerous communities around the globe but is not a universal practice. Concluding that current evidence indicates that the health benefits of newborn male circumcision outweigh the risks, the American Academy of Pediatrics (AAP) validated this procedure in its 2012 Technical Report and Policy Statement on male circumcision. However, physicians in other countries, including Europe, Canada, and Australia, do not agree that the evidence is convincing for the prophylactic benefits cited by the AAP involving reductions in urinary tract infections, penile cancer, some traditional sexually transmitted diseases, and HIV/AIDS (Frisch et al., 2013). An American critic of the AAP report cited insufficient data concerning surgical complications as well as lack of attention paid to the possible benefits of a foreskin to an individual and the ethics involved in removing that foreskin from a non-consenting child (Darby, 2015).

Female circumcision is referred to as female genital mutilation/cutting (FGM/C) by those who view it as an unwarranted and violent practice against women. A Norwegian systematic review of 21 studies revealed that complex cultural and religious beliefs and practices contributed to the practice but concluded on a positive note stating: "The results showed that within this intricate web of cultural, social, religious, and medical pretexts for FGM/C, conditions hindering its continuance existed, such as a legal framework and national discourse against FGM/C" (Berg and Denison, 2013).

Regarding *gender, transgender,* and *sex change,* R/S teachings are often cited as the basis for negative and even hostile attitudes toward the lesbian, gay, bisexual, and transgendered (LGBT) population. Surgery is frequently required for gender reassignment, and in one study over 41% of female to male (FTM) participants reported verbal harassment, physical assault, or denial of equal treatment in a doctor's office or hospital (Shires and Jaffee, 2015). LGBT medicine has not been a strong part of the medical curriculum, but guidelines are being established (Wilczynski and Emanuele, 2014). A sequela of deficiencies in clinical education, in addition to negative biases, is failure to perform adequate histories and physicals on LGBT patients, with the transgendered not receiving procedures such as breast cancer or prostate screening or PAP smears when birth-assigned gender is not immediately recognizable, that may lead to late presentation of disease.

WHAT ARE IMPORTANT AREAS
FOR FUTURE RESEARCH?

Ethics, economics of care, education, EOL issues, international collaboration, and patient autonomy provide fertile fields of R/S research in surgical practice.

Surgical morbidity, mortality, and improvement (M&M) conferences provide frequent examples of adverse events and unfortunate outcomes related to operations on patients with poor prognoses, thus offering research opportunities for the intersection of R/S and ethics. Historically, a procedure-driven medical specialty such as surgery faces a conflict-of-interest with every patient because—unless the surgeon is salaried with no bonus incentives—performing an operation offers higher remuneration than offering an opinion or providing medical advice. Reimbursement models based on flat fees for bundles of care may alleviate but not solve the dilemma. Decisions become even more complex when the patients are elderly, have multiple comorbidities, or are quite frail regardless of age. The ethical issues of justice and equity surface when making EOL choices for fragile, elderly, or near-death persons projecting long stays in ICUs incurring huge daily bed charges with consumption of blood and expensive (even scarce) drugs coupled with palliative procedures of questionable efficacy. A 2015 Harvard study revealed surgeons were less likely to refer patients with poor-prognosis cancers for hospice than other physicians such as medical oncologists (Obermeyer et al., 2015).

Strategies for increasing surgeon-chaplain cooperation whenever patients and families may be experiencing spiritual stress deserve attention. Several studies reported that chaplains are often consulted late, shortly before death rather than when patients are admitted to ICUs. The 2015 Duke University Hospital study reported chaplain visits in the ICU were uncommon and most frequently documented right before death rather than soon after admission (Choi et al., 2015).

With evidence demonstrating high religiosity associated with family/surrogate insistence on continued intervention for patients extremely unlikely to return to quality living (Shinall et al., 2014), research involving the impact of an education program for clergy on EOL decision making regarding the social, psychological, and economic impact of prolonged dying is worth pursuing because these religious leaders are in positions to influence their faith communities.

Cultural practices cannot be divorced from the R/S conversation because many persons base their medical decision making on their own cultural norms combined with tenets of their faith. Research is warranted concerning the ethical aspects of insisting on patient autonomy as persons from non-Western cultures bring to the surgical encounter a sense of family/community decision making wherein the patient may have little or no say in the discussion (Morita et al., 2015).

As more US surgeons participate in international surgical humanitarian missions, opportunities exist to examine the impact of R/S on surgical outcomes globally in cooperation with medical professionals in host countries. Lucchese and Koenig looked at published quantitative research on the relationship between R/S and cardiovascular disease (CV) and found that, although R/S is vital to many Brazilians, as of 2013, no published research from Brazil on R/S and CV was located (Lucchese and Koenig, 2013).

PRACTICE

HOW DOES RELIGION/SPIRITUALITY COMMONLY ARISE IN THE PATIENT ENCOUNTER WITHIN SURGERY?

Worldwide, about 80% of people claim some sort of religious faith and the US percentage is similar (Pew Research Center, 2012). Although surgeons made up less than 10% of the responders to the Curlin survey on physician characteristics, they offered responses similar to other physicians and were not outliers as stereotype sometimes suggests. Curlin's data show that 62% of surgeons express intrinsic religiosity (meaning R/S has some degree of importance for them). About 25% of surgeons sometimes pray with patients, about 40% sometimes discuss religious experiences, and virtually all thought that R/S contributed to a hopeful attitude. Over half thought their beliefs affected their medical practice and about a third believed that beliefs caused patients to refuse or even stop treatment. Only 20% thought the physician should never pray with patients (Curlin et al., 2005; Curlin et al., 2006; Curlin et al., 2007; Stern, Rasinski, and Curlin, 2011). In a number of studies physicians reported that lack of training in medical school or residency provokes feelings of inadequacy to address the issues of religion/spirituality when they arise in patient/surgeon encounters.

SCENARIOS

Asking the surgeon to pray

As the surgeon and the rounding team enter the patient's room, the surgeon sits down by the bed and inquires about how the patient is feeling and if there are any questions concerning the procedure scheduled for later that morning. The patient expresses confidence in the hospital and the surgeon and then says, "Dr. Doe, do you mind if we pray right now for you and the team and for my successful outcome?" In some regions of the United States, particularly in the South, religious practices occupy public as well as private space in the culture. In a secular Western context wherein a sneeze invokes a blessing, should surgeons express surprise if a patient or a family member asks the physician to join them in prayer or even pray for a successful operation and healing? Being mentally prepared to offer a respectful response to a request involving prayer would likely come from personal experience if the surgeon is religious/spiritual, having had prior experience working with persons who express faith or spirituality, or having formal R/S instruction during training. No one, including the surgeon, is required to participate in a religious practice that is uncomfortable or perhaps offensive, but a refusal should be worded in such a manner as to honor the request without accepting the offer, just as one might refuse a drink or food or gift. Conversely, if the surgeon is willing to pray with or for the patient, there appear to be no boundaries violated as long as both parties participate without coercion.

Decision making at end of life

The family is gathered around the unconscious patient in the surgical ICU cubicle. After reviewing the medical records that reveal a very poor prognosis, the surgeon involved in the patient's care requests a family conference to discuss medical decision making as well as the recommendations from the palliative care team's consultation. In the conference room, the surgeon explains the patient's condition and the very low likelihood of any return to normal function or QOL, a significant chance for a prolonged stay in the ICU, and possible nursing home care needed if the patient survives. Because no advance directives were found in the records, the surgeon gently suggests implementing the palliative care team's recommendations for a transition to comfort care and possible hospice. With the patient unable to participate in the conversation, the family and surgeon discuss the proposed options. A member of the health care team may offer to contact the chaplaincy service or inquire if the family wants to involve someone from their faith community such as a rabbi or priest or imam in this conversation. Studies show that often persons with strong religious beliefs such as evangelical Christians and Orthodox Jews push for every procedure that might extend life, even life with a projected poor outcome. A corollary scenario occurs when the surgical or ICU team declares the unconscious patient brain dead but breathing and circulation continue. The family or responsible adult is queried about withdrawal of life support and someone says that their religious beliefs do not permit "euthanasia." Keeping in mind that each patient and family is unique and may not fit neatly into the category ascribed to a particular faith system, Setta and Shemie (Setta and Shemie, 2015) offer a valuable guide concerning how the major world religions decide about withdrawing treatment and determining death. If organ donation is a consideration, involving a religious professional from the faith community of the patient and family might be advisable because lay persons may not be aware of official religious faith policy concerning these issues.

Looking for a miracle

The couple in their mid-sixties sit down in the surgeon's office to discuss a treatment plan for the man's newly-diagnosed esophageal cancer. Workup revealed adenocarcinoma with transmural extension. Given the patient's performance status and scant co-morbidities, the surgeon recommends neo-adjuvant therapy followed by an esophagectomy if no progression is seen. The wife confidently states that she has been praying and has a vision that operation is not warranted and that her husband will receive a "miraculous healing" if they seek care involving herbs and rituals in Mexico that she has learned of via the internet. The surgeon shares that she has not heard of this particular place or treatment and offers articles that show the lack of effectiveness for complementary and alternative medicine (CAM) for this particular cancer. The wife states, "We are people of faith and our church is praying for complete healing." After discussing various options for therapy, allopathic vs. CAM, the surgeon comments: "We provide information, answer questions, and make recommendations. The patient makes decisions." The surgeon then respectfully replies that she hopes he will continue to come to her for follow-up even as he pursues other avenues for healing. Comment: The hope for a miracle is pervasive among many people of strong R/S faith; faith may include belief in allopathic medicine, alternative therapies, and prayer simultaneously. One study of cardiac surgery patients shows correlation between high religiosity and use of CAM (Nicdao and Ai, 2014).

WHAT ARE THE BEST PRACTICES FOR SURGERY AS THEY PERTAIN TO R/S?

One of the best surgical R/S practices involves inclusion of chaplains on rounds, in the ICU, and in the trauma bay. Unfortunately, some hospitals have actually retreated from this practice, possibly for financial reasons. Spiritual care providers may even be considered integral parts of interdisciplinary teams such as in the ICU/critical care (Adhikari et al., 2010; Ott, 2010) and on the trauma service (Perechocky et al., 2014; Oklahoma University Medical Center. Pastoral Care Service, 2015). A Des Moines, Iowa team including trauma surgeons as well as nurses and allied health staff decided to allow parents to be present during pediatric trauma resuscitations; they approached chaplains who agreed to be trained to serve as family support persons during the resuscitations (Meeks, 2009).

Taking a spiritual history and having it as part of the medical record would add significantly to the surgeon's understanding of the patient and decision making. Embedding R/S in the hospital culture requires a team approach. The Joint Commission (formerly known as Joint Commission on Accreditation of Healthcare Organizations) requires that spiritual issues be addressed (not resolved) (The Joint Commission, 2010) and hospital intake/history forms frequently contain questions relating to religious affiliation or request for a chaplain/clergy visit; but those items may not always be filled in, likely due to time constraints or lack of appreciation for importance. On the nursing assessment intake form for the VA health care system is the question: "Are there religious practices or spiritual concerns you want the chaplain, your physician or other health care team members to know about?" If they answer "Yes," a referral form for a chaplain visit appears.

Taylor and colleagues at University of South Alabama "argue that religiosity and spirituality are inherent perspectives of patient-surgeon relationships." Their survey found that 83% of the 361 (RR, 97%) general and orthopedic surgical outpatient respondents agreed that surgeons should be aware of their patients' beliefs; 63% thought surgeons should take a spiritual history; and 64% said it would increase their trust in the surgeon (Taylor, 2011). Several spiritual history templates are available such as FICA (Puchalski, 2014) and the chaplain-developed FACT (Larocca-Pitts, 2008).

Advocates for taking a spiritual history have been around for years, but the practice has not been universally adopted by any medical specialty. While the most recent Cochrane review suggests researching the role of prayer in surgical practice may not be warranted, patients may not agree as demonstrated in the University of Oklahoma ophthalmology survey where over 90% of patients (overwhelmingly Christian) were positive about prayer before an elective procedure (Siatkowski et al., 2008).

The religiosity of cardiac surgery candidates correlated positively with their use of CAM (Nicdao and Ai, 2014); therefore, surgeons are advised to be aware that patients may not think of health supplements or alternative therapies as warranting report.

Interpersonal communication skills are critical. Surgeons should know how to talk to patients and families about treatment plans, should be skilled in delivering bad news such as adverse outcomes or poor prognoses in an honest, yet sensitive manner, and assist with EOL decision making. The 2014 Institute of Medicine (IOM) report on EOL experiences, *Dying in America*, reported that apparently many health care professionals do not know how to have EOL conversations and recommended that one strategy to insure that physicians are trained in discussing EOL issues would be to tie it in with their requirements for relicensure and certification (Institute of Medicine, 2014).

WHAT IS THE ROLE OF CLERGY, FAITH COMMUNITIES, AND CHAPLAINS IN SURGERY?

Events such as heart attacks, road traffic crashes, falls with head injuries, or other disastrous events create emotional, psychological, and even spiritual crises that may require training beyond that of medical school and residency. Routine operations occasionally incur adverse outcomes. Hospital chaplains play a vital role of support in stressful situations wherein patients and families are faced with challenges ranging from temporary inconvenience and limited activities to permanent disabilities or even impending death. The rise of outpatient surgery could affect the spiritual well-being of patients who have less hospital time for care and counseling (Griffin, 2013).

Communicating bad news is an art and is often a unit of medical student and resident education curriculum. US medical centers serve patients from around the world. A number of cultures do not share the Western tradition of forthright explanations to the patient about a poor prognosis or when EOL decisions need to be made. An example is Nigeria, where surgeons may choose to disclose worsening conditions to clergy or the patient's children or family members rather than the patient (Ogundiran and Adebamowo, 2012). Clergy hospital visitation is a time-honored practice. Even in the United States, the patient's own clergy may become an unofficial go-between for the surgeon and the patient when health literacy or even language comprehension deficiencies occur due to emotional and spiritual distress.

Care for the care giver is a critical component of the health care system. In some institutions chaplains and clergy may also be involved in providing support for surgeons and other medical professionals who frequently find themselves overwhelmed by the severity of a disease process or emotional exhaustion of dealing with difficult patients and families or the sheer work load.

R/S communities often provide physical as well as spiritual support of patients and their families through visitation, transportation, food, worship opportunities, and volunteer service in the hospital.

SPECIFICALLY, HOW SHOULD PHYSICIANS FACILITATE CONNECTIONS WITH THESE RESOURCES TO PROVIDE SPIRITUAL CARE OR WORK TO OVERCOME MEDICAL-SPIRITUAL CONFLICTS?

Surgeons have an opportunity to address R/S issues and call for consults when appropriate but need training in order to recognize situations wherein spiritual support is required whether in a trauma situation, diagnosis of disease, or EOL. The Joint Commission states, "Cultural, religious, or spiritual beliefs can affect a patient's or family's perception of illness and how they approach treatment. In addition, patients may have unique needs associated with their cultural, religious, or spiritual beliefs that staff should acknowledge and address." (The Joint Commission, 2010)

A common theme recurs in the literature past and present: lack of training remains a significant barrier to involvement with R/S in care. Instruction concerning the role of R/S in health and healing in medical school, residency, and continuing education should (1) raise awareness of how frequently these issues influence patients and families in decision making, compliance, acceptance, and coping; (2) increase the comfort level for discussing these issues with patients and families or even colleagues; (3) assist physicians in recognizing the influence of their own R/S (or lack thereof) in treatment plans; and (4) provide information about the roles played by chaplains or clergy in order for them to consider involving these persons when appropriate (McCauley et al., 2005; Perechocky et al., 2014; Balboni et al., 2014; Rodin et al., 2015; Balboni et al., 2013; Mason, 2015).

Patient-centered medical school curricula should address how disease, trauma, and mortality raise religious and spiritual issues and should include instruction concerning the role played by chaplains. The hospital chaplains provide a first line of response; however, including chaplains on surgical services for provision of support and spiritual care usually requires that a physician or nurse request a chaplaincy consult unless the intake history requests a visit. The surgeon who is sensitive to R/S issues may ask the patient/family if they wish to have their own clergy involved.

HOW SHOULD CLINICIANS PROVIDE SPIRITUAL CARE WHEN THERE ARE NO CLERGY OR CHAPLAINS AVAILABLE?

Having surgeons recognize the need to address spiritual concerns of patients and families requires education as described. Training in R/S is associated with having R/S discussions with patients (Rasinski et al., 2011). Sulmasy provides educational advice for taking a spiritual history, observing ethical boundaries, deciding whether to pray with patients, and discerning when to refer patients to chaplains or to their own personal clergy (Sulmasy, 2009). Many hospitals, even secular or government institutions, have chapels or prayer rooms that offer quiet spaces for reflection or prayer as well as occasional services. Surgeons should be aware of the chapel or prayer room location and inform the patient/family about the spaces. All surgeons—regardless of their beliefs or lack thereof—can provide a "ministry of presence" by being there bodily and mentally with a patient or family who are suffering physically or spiritually and by offering concern without invoking religious language.

Acknowledgments: Farr Curlin for provision of the raw data from the physician characteristics survey.

REFERENCES

Ambroise Paré, *Life and Times of Ambroise Paré, 1510-1590,* trans. Francis R. Packard (New York: P.B. Hoeber, 1921) 160.

Alexis Carrel, *Prayer.* (New York: Morehouse-Gorham, 1948).

Alexis Carrel, *The Voyage to Lourdes.* (New York: Harper, 1950).

Susan Setta and Sam Shemie, "An Explanation and Analysis of How World Religions Formulate Their Ethical Decisions on Withdrawing Treatment and Determining Death," *Philosophy, Ethics, and Humanities in Medicine* 10, no. 6 (2015), accessed 9 June 2015, http://www.peh-med.com/content/pdf/s13010-015-0025-x.pdf.

Susan Wintz and George Handzo, *Handbook Patients' Spiritual And Cultural Values For Health Care Professionals,* Healthcare Chaplaincy Network, 2014, accessed June 8, 2015, http://www. healthcarechaplaincy.org/docs/publications/landing_page/cultural_sensitivity_handbook_from_healthCare_chaplaincy_network_8_15_2014.pdf..

Randolph C. Byrd, "Positive Therapeutic Effects of Intercessory Prayer in a Coronary Care Unit," *Southern Medical Journal* 81, no. 7 (July 1988):826–829.

Leanne Roberts, Irshad Ahmed, and Andrew Davison, "Intercessory Prayer for the Alleviation of Ill Health (Review)." *Cochrane Database Systematic Reviews* 15, no. 2 (April 2009):CD000368, accessed 23 June 2015, http://onlinelibrary.wiley.com/doi/10.1002/ 14651858.CD000368.pub3/pdf.

K. Y. Cha and Daniel P. Wirth, "Does Prayer Influence the Success of In Vitro Fertilization-Embryo Transfer? Report of a Masked, Randomized Trial," *Journal of Reproductive Medicine* 46, no. 9 (September 2001): 781–787. Erratum in: *Journal of Reproductive Medicine* 49, no. 10 (October 2004): 100A, Rogario Lobo [removed as author from 2001 paper].

Ian N. Olver and Andrew Dutney, "A Randomized, Blinded Study of the Impact of Intercessory Prayer on Spiritual Well-Being in Patients with Cancer," *Alternative Therapies in Health and Medicine* 18, no. 5 (September-October 2012): 18–27.

Amy L. Ai et al., "Posttraumatic Growth in Patients Who Survived Cardiac Surgery: The Predictive and Mediating Roles of Faith-Based Factors," *Journal of Behavioral Medicine* 36, no. 2 (Apr 2013): 186–198.

Jeanne McCauley et al., "Spiritual Beliefs and Barriers Among Managed Care Practitioners," *Journal of Religion and Health* 44, no. 2 (Summer 2005): 137–146.

Jeremy Steglitz et al., "Divinity and Distress: The Impact of Religion and Spirituality on the Mental Health of HIV-Positive Adults In Tanzania," *AIDS and Behavior.* 16, no. 8 (November 2012): 2392–2398.

Claude C. Organ C Jr. and Margaret M. Kosiba, *A Century of Black Surgeons: The USA Experience,* vol. 1. (Norman, OK: Transcript; 1987):109–133.

Robert M. Stern, Kenneth A. Rasinski, and Farr A. Curlin, "Jewish Physicians' Beliefs and Practices Regarding Religion/Spirituality in the Clinical Encounter, "*Journal of Religious Health* 50, no. 4 (December 2011): 806–817.

Farr Curlin et al., "Religious Characteristics of U.S. Physicians: A National Survey," *Journal of General Internal Medicine* 20, no. 7 (July 2005): 629–634.

William J. Strawbridge et al., "Frequent Attendance at Religious Services and Mortality Over 28 Years," *American Journal of Public Health* 87, no. 6 (June 1997): 957–961.

Amal Khoury et al., "Living on a Prayer: Religious Affiliation and Trauma Outcomes," *American Surgeon* 78, no. 1 (January 2012): 66–68.

Charles S. Hultman et al., "To Heal and Restore Broken Bodies: A Retrospective, Descriptive Study of the Role and Impact of Pastoral Care in the Treatment of Patients with Burn Injury," *Annals of Plastic Surgery* 72, no. 3 (March 2014): 289–294.

Joanna Bulkley et al., "Spiritual Well-Being in Long-Term Colorectal Cancer Survivors with Ostomies," *Psychooncology.* 22, no. 11 (November 2013): 2513–2521.

Kelly Biegler et al., "The Role of Religion and Spirituality in Psychological Distress Prior to Surgery for Urologic Cancer," *Integrative Cancer Therapies* 11, no. 3 (September 2012): 212–220.

Nidhi Ravishankar and Mark Bernstein, "Religion Benefiting Brain Tumour Patients: A Qualitative Study," *Journal of Religion and Health* 53, no. 6 (December 2014): 1898–1906.

Ahmad K. Sadati et al., "Religion as an Empowerment Context in the Narrative of Women with Breast Cancer," *Journal of Religion and Health* 54, no. 3 (June 2015): 1068–1079.

Valerie Hurdle et al., "Does Regional Variation Impact Decision-Making in the Management and Palliation of Pancreatic Head Adenocarcinoma? Results from an International Survey," *Canadian Journal of Surgery* 57, no. 3 (June 2014): E69–74.

Myrick C. Shinall, Jr., Jesse M. Ehrenfeld, and Oscar D. Guillamondegui, "Religiously Affiliated Intensive Care Unit Patients Receive More Aggressive End-Of-Life Care," *Journal of Surgical Research* 190, no. 2 (August 2014): 623–627.

Zachary D. Epstein-Peterson et al., "Examining Forms of Spiritual Care Provided in the Advanced Cancer Setting," *American Journal of Hospice & Palliative Care* http://www.ncbi.nlm.nih.gov/pubmed/25005589 32 (July 8, 2014): p. ii: 1049909114540318.

Michael J. Balboni et al., "Why Is Spiritual Care Infrequent at the End of Life? Spiritual Care Perceptions among Patients, Nurses, and Physicians and the Role of Training," *Journal of Clinical Oncology* 31, no. 4 (February 2013): 461–467.

Neil Wenger and Sara Carmel, "Physicians' Religiosity and End-Of-Life Care Attitudes and Behaviors," *Mt Sinai Journal of Medicine* 71, no. 5 (October 2004): 335–343.

Steven N. Frank et al., "Risk-Adjusted Clinical Outcomes in Patients Enrolled in a Bloodless Program," *Transfusion* 54, no. 10, pt. 2 (October 2014): 2668–2677.

Ioannis T. Konstantinidis et al., "Pancreas and Liver Resection in Jehovah's Witness Patients: Feasible and Safe," *Journal of the American College of Surgeons* 217, no. 6 (December 2013): 1101–1107.

Chung-Mau Lo, "Deceased Donation in Asia: Challenges and Opportunities," *Liver Transplantation* 18, Suppl 2:S5–7 (November 2012): doi: 10.1002/lt.23545.

Nursing with Dignity. Part 8: Islam. *Nursing Times* (16 April 2002), accessed 25 June 2015, http://www.nursingtimes.net/nursing-with-dignity-part-8-islam/206284.article..

Mina Hafzalah et al., "Improving the Potential for Organ Donation in an Inner City Muslim American Community: The Impact of a Religious Educational Intervention," *Clinical Transplantation* 28, no. 2 (February 2014): 192–197.

A.F. Kocaay et al., "Brain Death and Organ Donation: Knowledge, Awareness, and Attitudes of Medical, Law, Divinity, Nursing, and Communication Students," *Transplantation Proceeding* 47, no. 5 (June 2015): 1244–1248.

Adrian Furnham and James Levitas, "Factors That Motivate People to Undergo Cosmetic Surgery," *Canadian Journal of Plastic Surgery* 20, no. 4 (Winter 2012): e47–e50.

Julian Savulescu. "Male Circumcision and the Enhancement Debate: Harm Reduction, Not Prohibition," *Journal of Medical Ethics* 39, no. 7 (July 2013): 416–417.

Morten Frisch et al., "Cultural Bias in the AAP's 2012 Technical Report and Policy Statement on Male Circumcision," *Pediatrics* 131, no. 4 (April 2013): 796–800.

Robert Darby, "Risks, Benefits, Complications and Harms: Neglected Factors in the Current Debate on Non-Therapeutic Circumcision," *Kennedy Institute Ethics Journal* 25, no. 1 (March 2015): 1–34.

Rigmor C. Berg and Eva Denison, "A Tradition in Transition: Factors Perpetuating and Hindering the Continuance of Female Genital Mutilation/Cutting (FGM/C) Summarized in a Systematic Review," *Health Care for Women International* 34, no. 10 (October 2013):837–859.

Deirdre Shires and Katy F. Jaffee, "Factors Associated with Health Care Discrimination Experiences among a National Sample of Female-to-Male Transgender Individuals," *Health & Social Work* 40, no. 2 (May 2015): 134–141.

Cory Wilczynski and Mary Ann Emanuele, "Treating a Transgender Patient: Overview of the Guidelines," *Postgraduate Medicine* 126, no. 7 (November 2014): 121–128.

Ziad Obermeyer et al., "Physician Characteristics Strongly Predict Patient Enrollment in Hospice," *Health Affairs* 34, no. 6 (June 2015): 993–1000.

Philip J. Choi, Farr A. Curlin, and Christopher E. Cox, "The Patient Is Dying, Please Call the Chaplain: The Activities of Chaplains in One Medical Center's Intensive Care Units," *Journal of Pain and Symptom Management* 49 (May 26, 2015): S0885-3924 (15)00245-6.

Tatsuya Morita et al., "Palliative Care Physicians' Attitudes Toward Patient Autonomy and a Good Death in East Asian Countries," *Journal of Pain and Symptom Management* 49 (March 28, 2015): S0885-3924(15)00157-8.

Fernando A. Lucchese and Harold G. Koenig, "Religion, Spirituality and Cardiovascular Disease: Research, Clinical Implications, and Opportunities in Brazil," *Revista Brasileira de Cirurgia Cardiovascular* 28, no. 1 (March 2013): 103–128..

Pew Research Center. "Table: Religious Composition by Country, in Numbers. 18 Dec 2012," accessed 19 June 2015, http://www.pewforum.org/2012/12/18/table-religious-composition-by-country-in-numbers/.

Farr A. Curlin et al., "The Association of Physicians' Religious Characteristics with Their Attitudes and Self-Reported Behaviors Regarding Religion and Spirituality in the Clinical Encounter," *Medical Care* 44, no. 5 (May 2006): 446–453.

Farr A. Curlin et al., "Physicians' Observations and Interpretations of the Influence of Religion and Spirituality on Health." *Archives of Internal Medicine* 167, no. 7 (April 2007): 649–654.

Robert M. Stern, Kenneth A. Rasinski, and Farr A. Curlin, "Jewish Physicians' Beliefs And Practices Regarding Religion/Spirituality in the Clinical Encounter," *Journal of Religion and Health* 50, no. 4 (December 2011): 806–817.

Ethel G. Nicdao and Amy L. Ai, "Religion and the Use of Complementary and Alternative Medicine (CAM) among Cardiac Patients," *Journal of Religion and Health* 53, no. 3 (June 2014): 864–877.

Neill Adhikari et al., "Critical Care and the Global Burden of Critical Illness in Adults," *Lancet* 376, no. 9749 (October 16, 2010): 1339–1346.

Barbara B. Ott, "Progress in Ethical Decision Making in the Care of the Dying," *Dimensions of Critical Care Nursing* 29, no. 2 (March-April 2010): 73–80.

Andrew Perechocky et al., "Piloting a Medical Student Observational Experience With Hospital-Based Trauma Chaplains," *Journal of Surgical Education* 71, no. 1 (January-February 2014): 91–95.

Oklahoma University Medical Center. Pastoral Care Services. University of Oklahoma, accessed 9 June 2015, https://www.oumedicine.com/oumedicalcenter/medical-services-and-departments/pastoral-care/pastoral-care-services.

Reylon A. Meeks, "Parental Presence in Pediatric Trauma Resuscitation: One Hospital's Experience," *Journal of Pediatric Nursing* 35, no. 6 (November-December 2009): 376–380.

The Joint Commission: *Advancing Effective Communication, Cultural Competence, and Patient- and Family-Centered Care: A Roadmap for Hospitals*. Oakbrook Terrace, IL: The Joint Commission, 2010, accessed 25 June 2015. http://www.jointcommission.org/assets/1/6/ARoadmapforHospitalsfinalversion727.pdf.

Dan Taylor, "Spirituality within the Patient-Surgeon Relationship," *Journal of Surgical Education* 68, no. 1 January-February 2011): 36–43.

Christina M. Puchalski, "The FICA Spiritual History Tool #274," *Journal of Palliative Medicine* 17, no. 1 (January 2014): 105–106.

Mark A. Larocca-Pitts, "FACT: Taking a Spiritual History in a Clinical Setting," *Journal of Health Care Chaplaincy* 15, no. 1 (2008): 1–12.

R. Michael Siatkowski, Sterling L. Cannon, and Bradley K. Farris, "Patients' Perception of Physician-Initiated Prayer Prior to Elective Ophthalmologic Surgery," *Southern Medical Journal* 101, no. 2 (February 2008): 138–141.

Institute of Medicine. *Dying in America: Improving Quality and Honoring Individual Preferences Near the End of Life* (Washington, DC: The National Academies Press, 2014), 228, accessed 25 June 2015, http://www.nap.edu/catalog.php?record_id=18748.

Andrew Griffin, "The Lived Spiritual Experiences of Patients Transitioning Through Major Outpatient Surgery," *AORN Journal* 97, no. 2 (February 2013): 243–252.

T. O. Ogundiran and C. A. Adebamowo, "Surgeon-Patient Information Disclosure Practices in Southwestern Nigeria," *Medical Principles and Practice* 21, no. 3 (April 2012): 238–243.

Michael J. Balboni et al., "Nurse and Physician Barriers to Spiritual Care Provision at the End of Life," *Journal of Pain and Symptom Management* 48, no. 3 (September 2014): 400–410.

Danielle Rodin et al., "Whose Role? Oncology Practitioners' Perceptions of Their Role in Providing Spiritual Care to Advanced Cancer Patients," *Supportive Care in Cancer* 23 (Jan 28, 2015).

Michael J. Balboni et al., "Why Is Spiritual Care Infrequent at the End of Life? Spiritual Care Perceptions Among Patients, Nurses, and Physicians and the Role of Training," *Journal of Clinical Oncology* 31, no. 4 (February 2013): 461–467.

Diane J. Mason, "Conversations About How We Die," *Journal of the American Medical Association* 313, no. 19 (May 19, 2015): 1895–1896.

Kenneth A. Rasinski et al., "An Assessment of US Physicians' Training in Religion, Spirituality, and Medicine," *Medical Teacher* 33, no. 11 (November 2011):944–945.

Daniel P. Sulmasy, "Spirituality, Religion, and Clinical Care," *Chest* 135, no. 6 (June 2009):1634–1642.

CHAPTER 8

RELIGION AND SPIRITUALITY IN GERONTOLOGY

Harold G. Koenig

T he field of gerontology has become center stage with reports that those over age 65 are the fastest growing age group in the world, and that by 2030, 13% of the 8.3 billion people on the planet will be in this demographic (Sepulveda & Murray, 2014). As people advance in age, losses of friends and family and changes in health, independence, and mobility begin to mount, often occurring one after the other or simultaneously. This is where religion really begins to take life and often separates those who are able to cope from those who end up despairing (or settling for a life that is less than it could be). Much of this chapter, then, has to do with the role that religion/spirituality (R/S) plays in adapting to the aging process. The ability to cope in older age has consequences for all aspects of health—mental, social, behavioral, and physical.

This chapter describes the state of the science regarding the relationship between R/S and health in older adults as it applies to coping with illness, mental health, and physical health. It then describes important avenues for future research, examines how R/S commonly arises during the patient encounter (with a case example), and finally discusses "best practices" on how to assess and address the spiritual needs of older adults.

STATE OF THE SCIENCE

While the focus here is on quantitative research, the reader should be aware of the vast research base involving qualitative studies that illustrates case by case the role that R/S plays in the lives of older adults—especially those with chronic, disabling, or terminal medical illnesses. As an example, I collected a number of qualitative reports of patients using religion to cope during my geriatric medicine fellowship at the Durham VA Hospital in North Carolina between 1986 and 1989. I systematically collected 68 stories from male veterans age 65 or older who were admitted to the medical and neurological inpatient services of the hospital (Koenig, 1994). To these men, religious coping meant prayer, reading the Bible, and personal belief in and surrender to the Divine as understood by them, and all of these seemed to help. These findings are consistent with hundreds of other qualitative studies reporting how people cope with disabling or life-threatening health problems, deal with loss of loved ones, or have survived through natural disasters (see elsewhere for literature reviews) (Pargament, 1997; Koenig, 2012).

I turn now, however, to the quantitative research—peer-reviewed studies conducted between 1940 and 2010 in older adults, which can be found in the appendices of two editions of the *Handbook of Religion and Health* (Koenig et al., 2001; 2012) This systematic review covers an estimated 75% of all the peer-reviewed research published in the English language during that period. Studies were identified from online databases (Medline, PsychInfo, Soclit, HealthStar, Cancerlit, CINAHL, etc.) and the reference lists contained in these reports. Because of the massive number of studies (over 3,000), I limit the present review to a few important areas of mental health (well-being, depression) and physical health (coronary heart disease and hypertension, dementia, all-cause mortality). Following this summary, I briefly discuss selected studies published since 2010 that illustrate the types of findings reported in recent years.

MENTAL HEALTH

WELL-BEING

Our 2010 systematic review identified 69 studies conducted in older adults that examined relationships between R/S and well-being. Of those, 60 studies (56 statistically significant at $p < 0.05$ and four at a statistical trend level, i.e., $0.05 < p < 0.10$) reported positive relationships between R/S and greater well-being, life satisfaction, or happiness (87%); seven studies found no association, and two reported mixed results (positive and negative findings). No studies reported a significant relationship between R/S and lower well-being or even a trend in that direction.

DEPRESSION

At least 96 studies examined R/S and depression in older adults (generally over age 55) from 1940 through 2010. Of those, 61 (63%) found a significant inverse relationship between R/S and depression (one at a trend level), seven (7%) reported positive relationships with greater depression, 12 (13%) indicated mixed results, and 16 (17%) reported no association. These studies were primarily observational in design (cross-sectional or prospective). To our knowledge, there were no randomized clinical trials examining R/S interventions for treating depression in older adults.

PHYSICAL HEALTH

CORONARY HEART DISEASE

Most studies examining R/S and coronary heart disease (CHD) were conducted in middle-aged or older adults, so I summarize the findings here for all ages. We identified 19 studies that examined relationships between R/S and CHD up through 2010. Of those, 12 (63%) reported inverse relationships and one reported a positive relationship. In addition, if one includes the 16 studies examining R/S and biological risk factors for CHD (i.e., cardiovascular reactivity, inflammatory markers such as C-reactive protein and fibrinogen, heart-rate variability, and outcomes following cardiac surgery), then this increases the number of studies to 35. Of those, 23 (66%) reported significant relationships between R/S and less CHD or lower levels of physiological risk factor for CHD. Many other studies have examined relationships between R/S and health behaviors that influence CHD risk, such as exercise/physical activity and cigarette smoking; 68% of 37 studies for physical activity, and 90% of 137 studies for smoking indicate reported a positive CHD profile in the more religious.

HYPERTENSION

As with CHD, the vast majority of studies examining R/S and blood pressure or hypertension have been conducted in middle-aged or older adults, so I also summarize results here for all age groups. Our systematic review identified 63 studies that examined relationships with R/S, of which 36 (57%) reported lower blood pressure or less hypertension in the more religious.

DEMENTIA/COGNITION

Not surprising, all studies we identified in our review of R/S and memory, cognition, or dementia were conducted in older adults. At least 21 studies had examined this relationship up through 2010. Of those, 11 (52%) reported slower cognitive decline with aging or better cognitive function in those with dementia among those who were more R/S, whereas three (14%) reported a significant positive relationship, two reported mixed findings, and five (24%) indicated no association. Of the seven prospective cohort studies, five (71%) reported that religious involvement at baseline predicted less cognitive decline over time, a finding especially strong in those with high depression scores at baseline.

Psychosocial and physiological reasons exist to explain why memory may decline more slowly among those who are more R/S. First, R/S activities (listening to sermons, reading religious scriptures) may actually "exercise" frontal cortical functions involved in dealing with religious concepts, areas of the brain that may be adversely affected by aging. Second, the social interaction that goes with participation in a faith community may have a positive influence on the retention of cognitive functions, given the etiological role that social disengagement may play in cognitive decline among older adults (Bassuk et al., 1999; Barnes et al., 2004). Third, if coping with life stress is improved, well-being is greater, and depression is less, then stress hormones (cortisol, epinephrine, and norepinephrine) will be lower. High levels of these stress hormones have been shown to adversely affect memory areas of the brain in both animal and humans (Sapolsky, 2001; Yaffe et al., 2010). Finally, individuals who have greater purpose in life (associated with greater R/S in 93% of 45 studies) and those who are more conscientious (associated with R/S in 63% of 30 studies) may be at lower risk for both cognitive decline and dementia (Wilson et al., 2007; Boyl et al., 2010).

MORTALITY

As with CHD and hypertension, studies of R/S and mortality are almost all relevant to older adults since they have usually been conducted across the lifespan or in older adults specifically. Mortality is one of the best indicators of the cumulative effect that a psychosocial-behavioral construct such as religiosity has on physical health. We identified 121 studies (almost all prospective) that examined effects of baseline R/S on later mortality. Of those, 82 (68%) reported that R/S (three at a trend level) predicted greater longevity net of confounders, seven (6%) reported shorter longevity, 13 (11%) reported mixed or complex findings, and 19 (17%) found no association. Of the 17 best designed studies (largest sample sizes, longest follow-up, multiple controls), 13 (76%) reported greater longevity among the more religious; in fact, of the 12 studies that examined frequency of religious attendance, 11 (92%) indicated this finding, with several studies reporting a dose-effect response.

Based on this review of studies through 2010, then, older adults who are more engaged in religious activity are more likely (in general) to have higher well-being, less depression, less coronary heart disease, lower blood pressure, a slower decline in cognition with age, and live significantly longer than persons who are less R/S.

LATEST RESEARCH

Within the last five years, many studies have been published examining the relationship between religion, spirituality, and health in older adults. This section presents a selection of recent studies that were published within the past two years that illustrate the kinds of findings now being reported.

QUALITY OF LIFE

To examine the relationship between religious involvement and quality of life (QOL) in stressed caregivers, Koenig and colleagues (2016) surveyed 251 female family caregivers ages 40 to 75 of those with severe disability (often dementia or a debilitating neurological illness). Participants were recruited in Durham County, North Carolina ($n = 151$), and Los Angeles County, California ($n = 100$). QOL was conceptualized as adaptation to the caregiver role, and was assessed by low levels of depressive symptoms (measured by the 20-item CES-D), perceived stress (Cohen's 10-item Perceived Stress Scale), and caregiver burden (Zaret's 22-item Burden Interview). Religious involvement was measured by a 41-item scale that combined organizational and non-organizational religiosity items from the Duke Religion Index, the 10-item Hoge Intrinsic Religiosity Scale, the 10-item Belief into Action Scale, the 12-item Krause Religious Support Scale, and the 7-item Negative RCOPE (overall alpha = 0.93). Results indicated a significant inverse association between religious involvement and poor caregiver adaptation (B =−0.09, SE = 0.04, t = −2.08, $p = 0.038$), independent of age, race, education, caregiver health, cared-for person's health, social support, and health behaviors. Effects were strongest in older caregivers (ages 58–75) and in spouse caregivers.

Investigators in the department of sociology at the University of Stockholm, Sweden, surveyed a random sample of 214 persons age 55 or over in Addis Ababa, Ethiopia, examining relationships between religion, spirituality, social support, and QOL (Hamren et al., 2014). The religious composition of participants was Orthodox Christian (86%), Protestant (13%), and Catholic (1%). R/S was measured using the Brief Multidimensional Measure of Religiousness/Spirituality; social support by the 12-item Multidimensional Scale of Perceived Social Support; and quality of life by the 12-item CASP-12, which assesses control, autonomy, pleasure, and self-realization. Results indicated that Protestants scored highest on QOL, followed by Catholics and then Orthodox Christians. QOL scores were significantly and positively correlated with R/S ($r = 0.42$) and with social support ($r = 0.44$). After controlling for age, gender, marital status, religious denomination, education, financial status, pension income, number of children, need for financial aid, and social support, R/S remained significantly and positively correlated with QOL. The effect size was similar to the association between social support and QOL (after controlling for social support). Researchers concluded that "Both religiousness/spirituality and social support are positively associated with quality of life and might be important buffers against deprivation." To my knowledge, this is one of the few studies (perhaps the only study) of R/S, social support, and QOL in a random sample of older adults from Ethiopia. The findings are similar to those reported in the West, as might be expected since Ethiopia is largely a Christian nation (76% vs. 79% in the United States).

DEPRESSION

Researchers examined the onset and recovery from depression in a sample of 7,732 older adults (mean age 68) participating in the US Health and Retirement Study, a nationally representative sample of adults over age 50 (Ronneberg et al., 2014). The aim of this report was to examine the effect of religiosity on the development of depression and recovery from depression between 2006 and 2008. Depression was assessed using the 8-item CES-D, where a cutoff of 3 or higher indicates an increased likelihood of clinical depression. Religious characteristics assessed at baseline included frequency of religious attendance, number of friends and relatives in one's congregation, importance of religiosity, a four-item index of intrinsic religiosity, and frequency of private prayer. Covariates included age, gender, ethnicity, chronic health problems, social support, somatic events in past two years, self-reported health, and physical functioning (instrumental and physical ADLs), as well as alcohol abuse, history of psychiatric illness, stressful life events, and current residence in the community vs. nursing home. Controlling for covariates, researchers found that among 5,740 participants not depressed at baseline, those who attended religious services frequently were 35% less likely to develop depression over the 2-year follow-up period ($OR = 0.65$, $p = 0.001$). Among the 1,992 persons depressed at baseline, those who engaged frequently in private prayer were significantly less likely to remain depressed when followed up two years later ($OR = 0.93$, $p = 0.015$). Investigators concluded that "both organizational and non-organizational forms of religiosity affect depression outcomes in different circumstances (i.e., onset and recovery, respectively)."

In another recent study (with different results), Dutch researchers analyzed data from the Longitudinal Aging Study of Amsterdam to examine associations between depression, feelings about God, and religious coping during a 12-year follow-up (Braam et al., 2013). In this population-based sample of 3,107 community-dwelling individuals ages 55–85, participants were interviewed at baseline in 1992/1993, and then again at three, six, and nine years later. In 2005, twelve years from baseline, 206 participants who scored high on depressive symptoms at any of the four time-points plus 137 never depressed respondents were interviewed a final time ($n = 343$, ages 67–97). Depression at each time point was assessed using the 20-item CES-D, with scores 16 or higher indicating significant depression. Participants were also categorized as (1) never depressed, (2) depressed in past, but remitted before 2001, (3) depressed in past, but recently remitted (2001–2005), (4) depressed in past and currently (depressed at all time-points), and (5) depressed only recently (2001–2005).

In 2005 (last follow-up), feelings about God were assessed using a 34-item Questionnaire on God Image that measured (1) positive feelings (thankfulness, proximity, trust, security, love), (2) fear of God (fear of being not being good enough, fear of punishment, uncertainty, guilt, shame), and (3) feeling wronged by God (disappointment, anger, oppression, loneliness, need of more freedom, dissatisfaction, desolation). A 9-item brief RCOPE was also used to measure religious coping (RC), with 5 items assessing positive RC and 4 items assessing negative RC. The religious characteristics of participants were 35% no religious affiliation, 32% Catholic, and 33% Protestant; frequency of religious attendance was 30% attended weekly or more and frequency of prayer was 49% daily or more.

After controlling for age, gender, marital status, and education, depression was associated with lower scores on positive feelings about God, higher scores on fear of God, higher scores on feeling wronged by God, and higher scores on negative religious coping. No association was found with positive religious coping. Depression was especially associated with feelings of uncertainty about God, feelings of desolation, and feelings of being abandoned by God. Researchers concluded that "Religious feelings may parallel the symptoms of anhedonia or a dysphoric mood and could represent the experience of an existential void." The study provides further evidence of an association between negative religious coping (feelings of punishment, abandonment, desolation by God) and depression. Since religious measures were obtained only in 2005, however, this study does not address the question of whether depression leads to such feelings about God, whether such feelings about God lead to depression, or both.

A third study explored the relationship between general religiousness, positive and negative religious coping, and depressive symptoms in 34 older inpatients with major depression or bipolar disorder admitted to Harvard's McLean psychiatric hospital (Rosmarin et al., 2014). Participants were ages 55 to 89 years (mean age 71), 53% were female, and 85% had education beyond high school; 47% had bipolar disorder and 53% major depression. Religious affiliation was reported as Catholic (38%), other (29%), and none (33%). Less than half (47%) reported certain belief in God (vs. 60% in surrounding community); 21% attended religious services weekly (vs. 30% in community); and 18% indicated they prayed at least once a day (vs. 41% in community). The Brief RCOPE was used to measure negative religious coping (NRC) and positive religious coping (PRC). Depressive symptoms were assessed using the clinician-rated Montgomery-Asberg Depression Rating Scale (MADRS) and the self-rated Geriatric Depression Scale (GDS); mania symptoms were rated using the Young Mania Rating Scale (YMRS). Results indicated that NRC (feeling punished or abandoned by God) was strongly correlated with all measures of depression ($r = 0.37$ with MADRS, $r = 0.41$ with GDS) and mania ($r = 0.35$ with YMRS). NRC, however, was not related to having a religious affiliation, belief in God, frequency of religious attendance, or frequency of prayer or scripture study. Controlling for other factors, NRC explained a significant proportion of the variance in observer-rated depression severity (19.4%), self-rated depression severity (17.7%), and observer-rated mania severity (12.5%). Private religious activity (prayer and scripture reading), in contrast, was inversely related to both observer-rated and self-rated depressive symptoms ($r = -0.34$ with MADRS, $r = -0.42$ with GDS). As in the study described earlier, researchers concluded that NRC in older adults is an important risk factor for depression.

Despite the small sample and relatively low statistical power to detect relationships, this study found strong connections between feeling abandoned or punished by God and symptoms of depression or mania. Private religious activity (one of the best indicators of being religiously devout), in contrast, was significantly and inversely related to depressive symptoms. Finally, religious belief and practices reported by mood-disordered older adults in this study were less frequent compared to those of healthy elders living in the community.

HEALTH BEHAVIORS

Volunteering is a health behavior that is known to be connected with better mental and physical health in later life (Lum & Lightfoot, 2005). Data were analyzed from 8,148 persons ages 64 to 67 participating in the 2004 wave of the Wisconsin Longitudinal Study to examine relationships between religiosity, spirituality, the value given to voluntarily assisting others, and rates of actual volunteering (Okun et al., 2014). Religiosity was measured using a three-item index that assessed frequency of religious attendance, level of involvement in church groups other than church itself, and level of involvement in church/temple/other places of worship. Spirituality was assessed by two questions: "How spiritual are you?" and "How important is spirituality in your life?" Results indicated that both religiosity and spirituality were positively correlated with value-expressed volunteer motivation (the value placed on voluntarily assisting others) ($r = 0.28$ for both). These correlations were the strongest correlates in a field of 23 other predictors. With regard to actual volunteering, religiosity was again the strongest predictor of all variables included in a logistic regression model, with an odds ratio of 2.61 ($p < 0.001$). Interestingly, when religiosity and value-expressed volunteer motivation were both included in the model, spirituality was significantly and *inversely* related to actual volunteering ($OR = 0.85$, $p < 0.001$). Authors explained that "spirituality [apart from religion] is associated with a preference for solitary and self-focused pursuits. . ."

DIABETIC CONTROL

Analyzing data from the US Health and Retirement Study, researchers examined cross-sectional and longitudinal relationships between religious involvement, depression, and diabetic control in 2,539 diabetics (Dzlvakwe & Guarnaccia, 2014). Data collected during Wave 8 (2008) and Wave 10 (2010) were examined. Cross-sectional analyses revealed that religiosity in 2010 was related to fewer depressive symptoms ($r = -0.04$, $p < 0.05$), fewer number of weeks depressed ($r = -0.05$, $p < 0.05$), and was positively associated with perceptions of diabetic control ($r = 0.04$, $p < 0.05$). In longitudinal analysis, religiosity in 2008 predicted fewer depressive symptoms in 2010 ($r = -0.04$, $p < 0.05$). Religiosity was also found to moderate the relationship between perceived diabetic control and number of weeks depressed. Among those with high religiosity, perceptions of diabetic control were not as strongly related to number of weeks depressed as in those with lower religiosity. Authors concluded that, "Understanding how these constructs [religiosity and depressive symptoms] jointly influence diabetes management and psychological functioning is critical in that medical professionals may utilize such knowledge to enhance treatment outcomes." Although the correlations reported here are pretty weak, this is an important study because of the high quality of the data (Health Retirement Study), large sample size, and because both cross-sectional and longitudinal analyses were reported.

ALLOSTATIC LOAD

Researchers analyzed data from a US national random sample of 1,450–2,934 adults ages 57 to 85 (National Social Life, Health, and Aging Project) to examine relationships between religious attendance and a wide range of physiological functions (Hill et al., 2014). Religious attendance was measured on a scale from 0 (never attend) to 3 (attend every week or several times a week). Physiological functions included body-mass index (BMI), diastolic blood pressure (DBP), systolic blood pressure (SBP), pulse rate, C-reactive protein (CRP), hemoglobin A1c (HbA1c), Epstein Barr Virus titers (EBV), dehydroepiandrosterone (DHEA), and overall allostatic load (created by summing all the variables together). After controlling for age, gender, race, education, and income in regression analyses, frequency of religious attendance was associated with lower overall allostatic load ($B = -.19$, $p < 0.05$), lower diastolic blood pressure ($B = -0.03$, $p < 0.05$), lower pulse rate ($B = -0.01$, $p < 0.001$), lower BMI ($B = -0.001$, $p < 0.05$), and lower CRP ($B = -0.09$, $p < 0.01$). No relationships were found with DHEA, SBP, HbA1c, or EBV. Researchers concluded that "religious attendance is associated with healthier biological functioning in later life." This study adds to the growing evidence of a link between religious involvement and physiological factors known to influence disease risk in later life. Because of this study's cross-sectional nature, future longitudinal studies are needed to help identify direction of causation (i.e., does religious attendance have a positive influence on biological risk factors, or do these biological markers influence the capacity to attend religious services).

AVENUES FOR FUTURE RESEARCH

These studies support a connection between R/S involvement and health in older adults. Much more research, however, is needed to better understand how religious involvement affects health and whether this relationship is causal. Qualitative studies in older adults experiencing a wide range of stressful situations consistently report that R/S helps to cope with stress and loss. There are also many cross-sectional studies demonstrating positive associations between religious involvement and health, along with a number of well-designed prospective studies as well. Randomized clinical trials (RCTs) involving R/S interventions, however, are almost non-existent in older adults. There are a few clinical trials involving meditation, but these have been typically small and not rigorously controlled. There is a dire need, then, for clinical trials that test R/S interventions adapted to the religious or spiritual beliefs of older adults to determine impact on mental, social, behavioral, and physical health outcomes. The challenge is that clinical trials are difficult to do and are very expensive to do well. They are not impossible, however.

When conducting a R/S intervention in older adults with depression, anxiety, or physical conditions such as chronic pain, potential participants are first screened to determine whether they are at least somewhat religious, informing them that there is a 50% chance that they will receive a religious intervention (and describing what that intervention will consist of). For those who indicate that they are religious and are willing to receive a R/S intervention like the one described (and after signing informed consent), they are randomized to receive either the R/S intervention or a standard/control treatment after a baseline evaluation is completed. Effects over time on the outcome are then compared in those receiving the R/S intervention with those in the control group, wehre assessments are conducted in a "blinded" fashion. R/S interventions are always patient-centered, based on the R/S tradition of the participant. For example, consider the RCT conducted by Koenig and colleagues that utilized a religious intervention in the treatment of major depressive disorders in the setting of chronic medical illness (Koenig et al., 2015). Many of the 132 participants in this study from central North Carolina and Southern California were older (since having a chronic illness was among the inclusion criteria, as was being at least somewhat spiritual or religious). All participants were to receive ten 50-minute sessions of cognitive-behavioral therapy (CBT) remotely by telephone. Participants were randomized to receive either conventional secular (CCBT) or religiously integrated CBT (RCBT). Christian, Jewish, Muslim, Hindu, and Buddhist therapy manuals were developed so that those randomized to RCBT would receive it based in their own religious tradition (for manuals that describe the content of RCBT interventions, see website http://www.spirituality-andhealth.duke.edu/index.php/religious-cbt-study/therapy-manuals).

Results indicated that both treatments were equally effective in reducing depressive symptoms on the Beck Depression Inventory, with the overall effect slightly favoring the RCBT group (group by time interaction $B = 0.50$, $SE = 0.55$, $t = 0.91$, $p = 0.36$, Cohen's $d = 0.10$) although this study was not powered as a non-inferiority trial. There was also an interaction between baseline religiosity and treatment group, such that RCBT was particularly effective (vs. CCBT) in those who were more religious. Furthermore, religious participants tended to be more likely to comply with treatment if they were assigned to the RCBT arm. Thus, RCTs with religious interventions can be done.

Critics of such RCTs say that religion is being used in a utilitarian manner to achieve outcomes it was not intended to. Really? Every major world religion has developed out of the people's needs to make sense of the social, emotional, physical, and existential suffering that they confront as part of the human condition. Members of every world religion seek to have compassion with those who experience pain and misfortune. How are recognition of R/S as a positive resource and efforts made to utilize it to relieve human distress contrary to such goals? Are not many sermons preached from pulpits around the world focused on utilizing listeners' faith to affect the quality of their lives and relationships with others? Indeed, they are. Is this utilitarian? How is this different from a treatment for depression that strengthens a person's faith and religious practice, over one that involves taking a medication and ignoring religion?

I will now describe a number of other high priority studies that could be done in older adults.

Given the associations reported thus far between R/S and mental health, more research is needed to substantiate these connections and establish the time order of effects through prospective cohort studies. Studies in common disorders with high public health impact are a priority.

EMOTIONAL DISORDERS

In 1990, depression was the leading cause of disability in the world and in 2020 is expected to be the world's second leading cause, second only to cardiovascular disease (Murray & Lopez, 1996; Lopez & Murray, 1998). Depression and anxiety are common in later life, especially in those with medical illness and functional disability that interfere with independence and self-care. With improvements in sanitation, health care, and social changes, people are living longer, but often with chronic illness. Rates of emotional disorder related to chronic illness, then, will be likely increase over time. This is likely to be especially true in aging baby boomers, a population group where rates of depression and anxiety are quite high (Maples et al., 2006). What will happen as 76 million baby boomers move into later life and develop chronic illness that affects the independent lifestyles this generation has so cherished? Thus, a high priority for future research is identifying R/S characteristics that improve coping with chronic illness, and then developing R/S interventions for clinicians to use in religious patients. Studies are also needed on the development and course of emotional disorders in those with dementia, given projections of a dramatic increase in dementia rates worldwide during the next 25 years—estimated to exceed 80 million by 2040 (Ferri et al., 2005).

CAREGIVER COPING

As older adults living with chronic illness and disability increase in number, the burden on family caregivers will also increase. Simply placing older adults in nursing homes will be more and more difficult in the future, and caring for elders at home will become a necessity in most cases (Schneider, 1999). Information, then, is needed on the role that R/S plays in helping family members care for loved ones. Research so far suggests that many family caregivers depend on religious beliefs to cope (70%), and that greater religiosity predicts caregiver adaptation over time (Haley et al., 2004). Research is needed to better understand this phenomenon and to develop R/S interventions that may help family members shoulder the caregiving burden. This issue has huge public health importance, since the costs of caring for chronically ill elders is projected to overwhelm the capacity of the government to provide health care and other social programs as well (Editorial, 2005).

CHRONIC MENTAL DISORDERS

There is almost no information about the relationship between R/S and chronic mental disorders in older adults. Because of the schism between religion and psychiatry (beginning with Freud), few researchers in psychiatry have invested time, talents, and resources on this topic. By chronic mental disorders, I mean mental disorders such as schizophrenia, schizoaffective disorder, bipolar disorder, delusional disorder, and severe personality disorders (antisocial, borderline, etc.). Does R/S protect against such disorders, or does it cause or exacerbate them? Can R/S moderate the course of these disorders? Might R/S treatments, either individual or group therapies, be developed to improve prognosis or reduce need for mental health services? What is the role of religious organizations in supporting older adults with chronic mental disorder? Research like this is needed in persons from different ethnic, cultural, and religious backgrounds.

INTERACTIONS WITH TREATMENT

How might R/S moderate the response to conventional treatments in older adults with acute or chronic mental disorders such as depression, anxiety, psychotic disorder, or substance abuse? In other words, does religious involvement improve or worsen response to psychotherapy, antidepressants, benzodiazepines, anti-psychotics, naltrexone or acamprosate (for alcohol abuse), methadone (for drug maintenance), or other psychotropic medication? How does R/S influence the response to electro-convulsive therapy or transcranial magnetic stimulation? There are many ongoing and planned studies to test the efficacy of these treatments in older adults. Why not simply add a short measure of R/S to the baseline evaluation and then see how R/S interacts with treatment response? Such studies would require very little funding since these clinical trials are already funded; only time, access to the data, and ability to analyze the results and write the paper would be needed. There is already some evidence that those who are more R/S respond more quickly to conventional psychological therapy, although that research does not focus on older adults (Bowen et al., 2006).

NEGATIVE EFFECTS

Although I focus in this chapter on the positive effects of R/S on health, it is also important to realize that R/S can also have (or at least appear to have) negative effects as well. At a minimum, persons with mental disorder (or those with anti-social tendencies) can distort R/S in such a way that it appears associated with mental illness. Examples are persons with religious delusions (present in about 20–25% of those with schizophrenia or in the manic phase of bipolar disorder); emotionally sensitive individuals who are disabled by guilt due to failure to live up to religious teachings; those whose religious pride alienates them from friends and family; and persons with a distorted view of devout religious beliefs as exemplified by suicide bombers who kill themselves and others for purportedly religious reasons. There has been almost no systematic research on how R/S may harm, especially among older adults, and this side of the story also needs to be told—if there is one.

PHYSICAL HEALTH

There is great need for research on R/S and physical illness (besides mortality) in older adults. Most (80%) of the research has focused thus far on mental health, leaving much to be done on studying relationships with physical disorders that are influenced by psychological, social, or behavioral factors (the mechanism by which R/S affects health).

STRESS-RELATED DISEASES

Many of the diseases in later life are stress-related, in that stress either contributes to the etiology of the illness or affects its course. Stress-related diseases include coronary artery disease, cardiac arrhythmias, hypertension, renal disease, stroke, vascular dementia, certain types of cancer, chronic fatigue syndrome, fibromyalgia, asthma, and a wide range of gastrointestinal disorders including irritable bowel syndrome, peptic ulcer disease, Crohn's disease, and inflammatory bowel disease. Better understanding of relationships between these diseases and R/S beliefs and activities may lead to the development of R/S interventions to prevent or treat these diseases.

COGNITIVE DISORDERS

Given the research reviewed here that suggests R/S can slow age-related memory decline, delay the onset of dementia, or slow the progression of dementia, studies are needed to better understand the physiological basis for these relationships. If studies continue to show a buffering effect of R/S on cognitive decline, as a number of studies have already documented (Kaufman et al., 2007; Zhang et al., 2010; Coin et al, 2010; Inzelberg et al., 2013) then R/S interventions tailored to a person's religious background could be developed and tested in clinical trials. Religious beliefs and practices are widespread and easily accessed by most of the population. If utilizing this resource could even slightly reduce the increase in Alzheimer's disease or related dementia, the impact on public health and on the cost of caring for those with dementia would be huge.

DISABILITY AND CHRONIC PAIN

As physical disability and chronic pain become more prevalent as the population ages and must live with chronic illness, there will be an increasing need for strategies to deal with these problems. To what extent might R/S help to delay the onset of physical disability with age or reduce chronic pain? There is some research that suggests an effect for R/S in terms of delaying the onset of disability (Idler & Kasl, 1997; Hybels et al., 2012) and buffering pain (Wachholtz & Pearce, 2009) in older adults, although well-designed prospective studies are needed to replicate these findings and improve our understanding of the mechanisms involved.

CHANGES WITH AGING

R/S may alter the speed at which physiological functions decline with increasing age, as suggested by studies examining cardiovascular reactivity (Masters et al., 2004) and inflammatory markers (cytokine levels, C-reactive protein, etc.) (Koenig et al., 1997; For et al., 2006). Given the research reviewed that indicates religious involvement is associated with greater longevity in the vast majority of studies (particularly the higher quality studies), research is needed to better understand how R/S affects physiological changes associated with aging. Might R/S involvement actually slow the aging process? There is basis for this possibility given the relationship between psychosocial stress and cellular aging (Epel et al., 2004). Again, if religious beliefs help older adults to cope and increase social support, then lower stress levels may affect biological processes within the cell. Although research is now being done to examine such possibilities (Koenig et al., 2016), more studies of this type are needed, especially longitudinal studies.

FAITH-BASED PROGRAMS

Many older adults today, and in the future, will be members of faith communities. Faith communities with a high proportion of older congregants are beginning to develop health ministries that focus on disease detection and prevention through health education, on increasing compliance through individual counseling, and on preventing hospitalization through mobilization of community support, activities often coordinated by a parish or congregational nurse (Cantanzaro et al., 2007). These programs are especially prevalent now in minority communities where health disparities abound, although they seldom focus on older adults (Wingood et al., 2013; Bopp et al., 2013). With an increasing number of older adults with chronic illness falling through cracks in the government-funded health system, religious organizations are left to pick up the pieces (as they have done throughout human history and are currently doing in many developing countries). Almost no studies have systematically examined the effectiveness or cost of faith-based health programs over time, despite the fact that such research will be crucial in guiding the development of future programs of this type (Dehaven et al., 2004).

INTERACTIONS WITH TREATMENT

As I suggested for studies in mental health, research is needed to understand how religious involvement moderates the effects of medication, surgery, radiation therapy, and other biological treatments for physical diseases. Does higher R/S activity improve response rate (or reduce side-effects) to cardiac medications, anti-hypertensive drugs, antibiotics, or chemotherapy? Given associations between R/S, immune, endocrine, and cardiovascular functions, might greater R/S act synergistically with these natural healing systems and antibiotic drugs to slow the spread of infection or eliminate it? The same kind of research is needed for cancer drugs, where there is at least preliminary evidence that R/S affects both response and side-effects to chemotherapy (Lissoni et al., 2008a; Lissoni et al., 2008b). Also needed are studies that examine the moderating effects of R/S on surgical interventions in terms of wound healing and recovery time. If R/S helps older adults to cope better with the stress of surgical procedures, and psychological stress slows wound healing and increases infection rates in older populations, (Kiecolt-Glaser et al., 1996) then R/S may be associated with better surgical outcomes. This has already been demonstrated in at least two studies of older adults (Oxman et al., 1995; Contrada et al., 2004), although needs replication in prospective studies in different populations.

For a more comprehensive and detailed discussion of future research, with studies prioritized by need and by funding requirements, the reader is referred elsewhere (Koenig, 2011).

RELIGION IN THE PATIENT ENCOUNTER

How does R/S manifest itself during interactions with older patients? Spiritual needs related to medical illness are widespread among older adults (Hodge et al., 2011; Pearce et al., 2012). However, older patients often do not bring up the subject themselves because of concern that this is not something appropriate to bring up with their physician. Prompting by the clinician, then, is often necessary.

CLINICAL CASE

Mrs. Smith is an 84-year-old widowed female with multiple medical problems impairing her mobility and forcing her to move about using a walker. Of particular concern has been a problem with her larynx that both interfered with her breathing and left a constant sensation of fullness in her throat. Unfortunately, multiple medical and surgical consultations have not revealed a problem that can be corrected. She has struggled with this problem day-in and day-out, with no relief except when she falls asleep at night. After several months without improvement, she became very depressed, prompting her primary care physician to prescribe antidepressant and anti-anxiety medication. After several months of treatment without response, she was finally referred to me. She was clearly depressed and the medication was not working. During my initial evaluation I learned that she lived alone in her own home, and in order to stay there, she had to hire in-home help for 6 hours per day five days per week. The cost of such care, however, was rapidly using up savings that she had hoped to leave to her three children. She was feeling very guilty about this, despite the fact that none of her children offered to help care for her.

Toward the end of the evaluation, she indicated to me that she was just tired of living and wished that "God would just take me." This prompted me to perform a brief "spiritual history" from which I learned that while she was a deeply religious person and had always been so, lately she had begun struggling with her faith. Over and over again she had prayed that God would heal her, but to no avail. She wondered whether God still cared about her, or maybe was punishing her for past sins she had committed. I listened to her talk about her religious struggles, and after adjusting her psychotropic medications, tried to encourage and support her. After several months, her physical health had not improved and she continued to suffer with breathing and swallowing problems. The medications I had prescribed had little effect on her depression, and I was at a loss on how to help her. During one clinic visit when she was particularly distraught, I told her that I would pray for her each day on my own. I asked her what she would like me to pray for. She said, "Doctor, please pray for contentment and peace concerning my problems breathing and swallowing, even if it doesn't improve, and pray that I wouldn't feel guilty about spending my children's inheritance." I said I would do that.

BEST PRACTICES

No "best practices" have been widely recognized in dealing with R/S issues that come up during clinical encounters with older adults. However, there are some commonsense guidelines that I would suggest. First and foremost, is to take a brief spiritual history. This can be done as part of the social history during an initial new patient evaluation, during a well-patient exam (when more time is available), and/or at the time of hospital admission.

The spiritual history serves several purposes. First, it provides information about the patient's religious background and whether he or she has religious or spiritual support; second, it helps identify R/S beliefs that might influence medical decisions and compliance with treatment; third, it may uncover unmet spiritual needs related to medical illness; and fourth, it will create an atmosphere where the patient feels comfortable talking with their physician about spiritual needs affecting medical care. If spiritual needs are identified, then the patient is referred to a chaplain or pastoral counselor to address those needs.

Although many different formats for the spiritual history have been proposed, I now recommend three questions (shortened from the five originally reported in my article published in JAMA) (Koenig, 2002). After identifying the patient's religious affiliation (if any), the physician asks (1) "Do you have a religious or spiritual support system to help you in times of need?" (2) "Do you have any religious beliefs that might influence your medical decisions?" (3) "Do you have any other spiritual concerns that you would like someone to address?" Based on pilot studies, this spiritual history (including responses) takes an average of 1–2 minutes.

Taking the spiritual history, supporting the religious or spiritual beliefs of the patient (as part of the patient-centered spiritual history), and referring to chaplains to address spiritual needs comprise the primary responsibility of the physician. If this is done routinely with older adults, particularly those with life-threatening diseases, disabling chronic illnesses, chronic pain, depression, or other conditions that challenge coping, then the "best practices" goal will have been met. Besides this minimum, what else might physicians do if they have the time or the desire? Here are a few:

1. *Listen.* Listen to and try to understand the patient's spiritual concerns. This involves taking the time to sit with the patient and just let them talk—not providing advice or trying to find solutions.
2. *Support.* Support the patient's religious or spiritual beliefs, even if beliefs appear to conflict with the medical care plan; the payoff is a better doctor-patient relationship and better compliance with whatever treatment plan is agreed on.
3. *Pray.* Pray for or with the patient. Praying privately for the patient during the physician's own time requires no consent; however, praying aloud "with" the patient does require consent and should not be done unless the patient initiates the request for prayer or provides uncoerced permission to receive prayer (Balboni et al., 2011).
4. *Accommodate.* In acute hospital or other inpatient settings, accommodate the environment to meet the patient's spiritual needs, such as ensuring that someone provides a prayer rug to a Muslim patient or delivers Holy Communion to a Catholic patient.

There are also boundaries that physicians and other health professionals should seldom cross: don't prescribe religion to non-religious patients; don't force a spiritual history if the patient is not religious; don't pray with a patient before taking a spiritual history and unless the patient asks; don't spiritually counsel patients (always refer to trained chaplains or pastoral counselors); and don't do any activity that is not patient-centered and patient-directed. For a more detailed description of best practices with regard to integrating spirituality into the care of older patients, the reader is referred elsewhere (Koenig, 2013; Koenig 2014).

CONCLUSIONS

Much research has now been published on relationships between religion, spirituality, and health in older adults. The vast majority of that research suggests that religious or spiritual involvement is associated with better mental, social, behavioral, and physical health. New research is appearing regularly that supports these earlier findings and expands on them. While much research has been done, these studies barely scratch the surface of what needs to be known. This chapter identifies a few of the many studies needed to determine if R/S actually affects health in later life and how it does so. Based on what is already known however, a number of sensible clinical applications exist that will allow clinicians to better care for the holistic needs of older adults, especially those struggling with complex medical and psychiatric issues.

REFERENCES

Balboni MJ, Babar A, Dillinger J, Phelps AC, George E, Block SD, Kachnic L, . . . Balboni TA (2011). "It depends": Viewpoints of patients, physicians, and nurses on patient-practitioner prayer in the setting of advanced cancer. *J Pain Symptom Manage* 41(5):836–847.

Barnes LL, Mendes de Leon CF, Wilson RS, Bienias JL, Evans DA (2004). Social resources and cognitive decline in a population of older African Americans and whites. *Neurology* 63: 2322–2326.

Bassuk, SS, Glass, TA, Berkman, LF (1999). Social disengagement and incident cognitive decline in community-dwelling elderly persons. *Ann Intern Med.* 131:165–173.

Bopp M, Baruth M, Peterson JA, Webb BL (2013). Leading their flocks to health? Clergy health and the role of clergy in faith-based health promotion interventions. *Family & Community Health* 36 (3): 182–192.

Bowen R, Baetz M, D'Arcy C (2006). Self-rated importance of religion predicts one-year outcome of patients with panic disorder. *Depress & Anxiety* 23(5):266–273.

Boyle PA, Buchman AS, Barnes LL, Bennett DA (2010). Effect of purpose in life on risk of incident Alzheimer disease and mild cognitive impairment in community-dwelling older persons. *Arch Gen Psychiatry* 67:304–310.

Braam AW, Schaap-Jonker H, van der Horst MH, Steunenberg G, Beekman AT, van Tilburg W, Deeg DJ (2013). Twelve-year history of late-life depression and subsequent feelings to God. *Am J Geriatr Psychiatry* 22(11):1272–1281.

Catanzaro AM, Meador KG, Koenig HG, Kuchibhatla M, Clipp EC (2007). Congregational health ministries: A national study of pastors' views. *Pub Health Nurs* 24(1):6–17.

Coin A, Perissinotto M, Najjar A, Giaradi EM, Inelmen G, Enzi EM, Sergi G (2010). Does religiosity protect against cognitive and behavioral decline in Alzheimer's dementia? *Curr Alzheimer Res* 7 (5):445–452.

Contrada RJ, Goyal TM, Cather C, Rafalson L, Idler EL, Krause TJ (2004). Psychosocial factors in outcomes of heart surgery: the impact of religious involvement and depressive symptoms. *Health Psychol* 23(3): 227–238.

DeHaven MJ, Hunter IB, Wilder L, Walton JW, Berry J (2004). Health programs in faith-based organizations: are they effective? *Am J Pub Health* 94(6): 1030–1036.

Dzivakwe VG, Guarnaccia C (2014). Religiosity as a coping resource for depression and disease management among older diabetic patients. *Ann Behav Med* 47 (1 Supplement, A-055): s17.

Editorial (2005). Report on Health Care Congress (sponsored by the Wall Street Journal and CNBC, Washington, DC). *Clin Psychiatry News* 33 (4):86.

Epel ES, Blackburn EH, Lin J, Dhabhar FS, Adler NE, Morrow JD, Cawtrhorn RM (2004). Accelerated telomere shortening in respoinse to life stress. *Proc Nat Acad Sci*

Ferri CP, Prince M, Brayne C, Brodaty H, Fratiglioni L, Ganguli M, Hall K, Hasegawa K, . . . Scazufca M; Alzheimer's Disease International (2005). Global prevalence of dementia: A Delphi consensus study. *Lancet* 366(9503):2112–2117.

Ford ES, Loucks EB, Berkman LF (2006). Social integration and concentrations of C-reactive protein among US adults. *Ann Epidemiol* 16(2):78–84.

Haley WE, Gitlin LN, Wisniewski SR, Mahoney DF, Coon DW, Winter L, Corcoran M, Schinfeld S, Ory M (2004). Well-being, appraisal, and coping in African-American and Caucasian dementia caregivers: findings from the REACH study. *Aging & Mental Health* 8(4):316–329.

Hamren K, Chungkham HS, Hyde M (2015). Religion, spirituality, social support and quality of life: Measurement and predictors CASP-12 (v2) amongst older Ethiopians living in Addis Ababa. *Aging & Mental Health.* 19(7):610-21.

Hebert RS, Dang Q, Schulz R (2007). Religious beliefs and practices are associated with better mental health in family caregivers of patients with dementia: Findings from the REACH study. *Am J Geriatr Psychiatry* 15: 292–300.

Hill TD, Rote SM, Ellison CG, Burdette AM (2014). Religious attendance and biological functioning: A multiple specification approach. *J Aging and Health* 26 (5): 766–785.

Hodge DR, Horvath VE (2011). Spiritual needs in health care settings: a qualitative meta-synthesis of clients' perspectives. *Social Work* 56(4):306–316.

Hybels CF, Blazer DG, George LK, Koenig HG (2012). The complex association between religious activities and functional limitations in older adults. *Gerontologist* 52(5):676–685.

Idler EL, Kasl SV (1997). Religion among disabled and nondisabled persons II: Attendance at religious services as a predictor of the course of disability. *J Gerontology* 52B (6):S306–316.

Inzelberg R, Afgin A, Massarwa M, Schechtman E, Israeli-Korn S, Strugastsky R, . . . Friedland R (2013). Prayer at midlife is associated with reduced risk of cognitive decline in Arabic women. *Curr Alzheimer Res* 10(3):340–346.

Kaufman Y, Anaki D, Binns M, Freedman M (2007). Cognitive decline in Alzheimer disease: Impact of spirituality, religiosity, and QOL. *Neurology* 68(18):1509–1514.

Kiecolt-Glaser JK, Marucha PT, Malarkey WB, Mercado AM, Glaser R (1996). Slowing of wound healing by psychological stress. *Lancet* 346(8984):1194–1196.

Koenig HG (1994). *Aging and God: Spiritual Pathways to Mental Health in Midlife and Later Years.* Binghamton, NY: Haworth Press, pp 189–217.

Koenig HG (2002). An 83-year-old woman with chronic illness and strong religious beliefs. *J Am Med Assoc* 288(4): 487–493.

Koenig HG (2011). *Spirituality and Health Research: Methods, Measurement, Statistics, and Resources.* Philadelphia, PA: Templeton Foundation Press, pp 47–71

Koenig HG (2012). Religion, spirituality and health: the research and clinical implications. *ISRN Psychiatry.* Article ID 278730 (doi:10.5402/2012/278730)

Koenig HG (2013). *Spirituality in Patient Care*, 3rd ed. Philadelphia, PA: Templeton Foundation Press.

Koenig HG (2014). The spiritual care team: Enabling the practice of whole person medicine. *Religions* 5(4): 1161–1174.

Koenig HG, Cohen HJ, George LK, Hays JC, Larson DB, Blazer DG (1997). Attendance at religious services, interleukin-6, and other biological indicators of immune function in older adults. *Int J Psychiatry in Med* 27:233–250.

Koenig HG, Cohen HJ, Nelson B, Shaw SF, Saxena S (2016). Religious involvement and telomere length in women family caregivers. *J Nerv Ment Dis* 204(1):36-42.

Koenig HG, King DA, Carson VB (2012). *Handbook of Religion and Health*, 2nd ed. New York, NY: Oxford University Press.

Koenig HG, McCullough ME, Larson DB (2001). *Handbook of Religion and Health*, 1st ed. NY, NY: Oxford University Press.

Koenig HG, Nelson B, Shaw SF, Saxena S, Cohen HJ (2016). Religious involvement and adaptation in female family caregivers. *J Am Geriatr Soc* 64(3):578-83

Koenig HG, Pearce MJ, Nelson B, Shaw SF, Robins CJ, Daher N, Cohen HJ, . . . King MB (2015). Religious vs. conventional cognitive-behavioral therapy for major depression in persons with chronic medical illness. *J Nerv & Mental Dis* 203(4):243–251.

Lissoni P, Messina G, Balestra A, Colciago M, Brivio F, Fumagalli L, Fumagalli G, Parolini D (2008a). Efficacy of cancer chemotherapy in relation to synchronization of cortisol rhythm, immune status and psychospiritual profile in metastatic non-small cell lung cancer. *In Vivo: Int Inst Anticancer Res* 22(2): 257–262.

Lissoni P, Messina G, Parolini D, Balestra A, Brivio F, Fumagalli L (2008b). A spiritual approach in the treatment of cancer: Relation between faith score and response to chemotherapy in advanced non-small cell lung cancer patients. *In Vivo: Int Inst Anticancer Res* 22(5):577–582.

Lopez AD, Murray CC (1998). The global burden of disease, 1990–2020. *Nature Med* 4: 1241–1243.

Lum TY, Lightfoot E (2005). The effects of volunteering on the physical and mental health of older people. *Research on Aging* 27:31–55.

Maples MF, Abney PC (2006). Baby boomers mature and gerontological counseling comes of age. *J Counsel & Develop* 84(1):3–9.

Masters KS, Hill RD, Kircher JC, Lensegrav Benson TL, Fallon JA (2004). Religious orientation, aging, and blood pressure reactivity to interpersonal and cognitive stressors. *Ann Behav Med* 28(3):171–178.

Murray C, Lopez A (1996). *The Global Burden of Disease*. Cambridge, MA: Harvard University Press.

Okun MA, O'Rourke HP, Keller B, Johnson KA, Enders C (2015). Value-expressive volunteer motivation and volunteering by older adults: relationships with religiosity and spirituality. *J Gerontology* (Psychological and Social Sciences). 70(6):860-70.

Oxman TE, Freeman DH, Manheimer ED (1995). Lack of social participation or religious strength and comfort as risk factors for death after cardiac surgery in the elderly. *Psychosom Med* 57: 5–15.

Pargament K (1997). *The Psychology of Religion and Coping*. New York, NY: Guilford Press.

Pearce MJ, Coan AD, Herndon JE 2nd, Koenig HG, Abernethy AP (2012). Unmet spiritual care needs impact emotional and spiritual well-being in advanced cancer patients. *Supp Care Cancer* 20(10):2269–2276.

Ronneberg CR, Miller EA, Dugan E, Porell F (2016). The protective effects of religiosity on depression: A 2-year prospective study. *Gerontologist* 56(3):421-31

Rosmarin DH, Malloy MC, Forester BP (2014). Spiritual struggle and affective symptoms among geriatric mood disordered patients. *Int'l J Geriatr Psychiatry*. 29(6):653–660.

Sapolsky RM (2001). Depression, antidepressants, and the shrinking hippocampus. *Proc Nat Acad Sci.* 98:12320–12322.

Schneider EL (1999). Aging in the third millennium. *Science* 283(5403):796–797.

Sepulveda J, Murray C (2014). The state of global health in 2014. *Science.* 345 (6202):1275–1278.

Wachholtz AB, Pearce MJ (2009). Does spirituality as a coping mechanism help or hinder coping with chronic pain? *Curr Pain & Headache Rep* 13:127–132.

Wilson RS, Schneider JA, Arnold SE, Bienias JL, Bennett DA (2007). Conscientiousness and the incidence of Alzheimer Disease and mild cognitive impairment. *Arch Gen Psychiatry* 65:1204–1212.

Wingood GM, Robinson LR, Braxton ND, Er DL, Conner AC, Renfro TL, Rubtsova AA, Hardin JW, DiClemente RJ (2013). Comparative effectiveness of a faith-based HIV intervention for African American women: Importance of enhancing religious social capital. *Am J Pub Health* 103 (12): 2226–2233.

Yaffe K, Vittinghoff E, Lindquist K, Barnes D, Covinsky KE, Neylan T, Kluse M, Marmar C (2010). Posttraumatic stress disorder and risk of dementia among US veterans. *Arch Gen Psychiatry* 67(6):608–613.

Zhang A (2010). Religious participation, gender differences, and cognitive impairment among the oldest-old in China. *J Aging Research* Article ID 160294, doi:10.4061/2010/160294

CHAPTER 9

RELIGION AND SPIRITUALITY IN ONCOLOGY

Alan B. Astrow

Patients with cancer may confront the possibility of their own mortality for the first time. This experience may evoke a variety of concerns related to life's meaning and purpose that go beyond the physical or psychological and that have been termed "spiritual." Some patients will address these concerns through some form of organized religion; others will access the spiritual dimension through a purely secular, existential path. Whatever route patients choose to take, oncologists ought to be aware that spiritual matters may affect their patients' experience of illness and quality of life and the decisions that patients make about their medical treatment. Oncologists are often face to face with patients as they grapple with spiritual questions. Many patients wish to be able to discuss their hopes and fears with their oncologist and to relate to their oncologist in a more human way and may be more satisfied with the care that they receive when oncologists are able to do so.

In their efforts to address the spiritual dimension to the struggle with illness, oncologists face three tasks: to acknowledge that some patients have spiritual questions, to recognize when spiritual concerns are contributing to feelings of distress, and to develop an approach that helps them engage with their patients about spiritual issues without feeling pressured to answer the unanswerable or solve the unsolvable. These tasks require specific skills: to listen to and talk with patients in an atmosphere of equality, to respect differing approaches to life's fundamental questions, and to be aware and be present for their patients when they are in deepest need. Oncologists need to conduct themselves in this sensitive arena without a hint of proselytizing, any suggestion of a hidden agenda or attempt to impose their own views, other than to counsel patients to act in the best interests of their own health and well-being. These are challenging professional obligations and require reflection and training, inner personal discipline, and external support.

THE STATE OF SCIENTIFIC UNDERSTANDING

The diagnosis of cancer may initiate an existential crisis for patients, even those with early stage disease (Burt, 2003; Astrow, 2008) which may lead to a variety of psychiatric disturbances such as anxiety and depression that require the oncologist's attention (Derogatis, 1983). But clinical terminology often does not do justice to the profound human distress that a cancer diagnosis may evoke. Existential dread and a sense of impending doom, alienation, shame, despair, rage, a sense of loss, resentment, hopelessness—these kinds of concerns can lead patients to questions about the purpose of life and whether or not one has lived a worthy life, what one ought to do with the time that one has, whether one needs to reconcile with family and friends, what happens after we die, and whether or not there is a God that gives our lives meaning (Groopman, 1997).

Many Americans had traditionally turned to organized religion seeking answers to questions of that sort. With the increasing cultural diversity of the United States population, however, along with growth in the number of Americans unaffiliated with any specific religion but still seeking some overarching purpose to their lives beyond the strictly material, attention has focused on "spirituality" as a broader heading under which to consider existential themes. This section reviews empirical studies that address spiritual issues in oncologic medical and nursing care. While at the current stage of research into religion and spirituality in oncology, there are more questions than answers, some tentative recommendations to guide clinical practice will follow.

Some have noted the evolving definition of the term "spiritual," moving over time from overtly religious connotations and connection with notions of transcendence and Divinity (Sulmasy, 1997) to one that sees the spiritual wherever people locate ultimate meaning, "having to do with "a person's sense of peace, purpose, connection to others, and beliefs about the meaning of life" (National Cancer Institute, 2015). Critics have wondered whether the terminology itself in its effort to be inclusive has drained the term spiritual of specific value, while at the same time surreptitiously casting existential questions about life's significance in Western and specifically Christian terms (Salander, 2005).

Other critics have questioned the validity of measures of "spirituality" or "spiritual well-being" outside the specific context in which these have been developed and expressed. In the view of these critics, the attempt to quantify qualitative dimensions of life such as spirituality or its ecclesiastical counterpart "religiousness" or "religiosity" for research purposes distorts the subjects of interest by reducing complex systems of human experience to check-lists of measurable behaviors or alternatively to subjective and unverifiable reports of inner states. Instruments that distinguish numerically between the "religious" and the "non-religious" overly simplify both categories, and gloss over profound differences within each group, or even the extent to which some of these measures may be fluid within an individual. More fundamentally, efforts to document the health benefits of religious practices and spiritual beliefs threaten to focus attention on an intermediate endpoint, health, and to treat spirituality as a form of therapy in service of health as the ultimate end. The true purpose of most spiritual traditions is to equate the good with some form of right living in relationship with a source of ultimate meaning and to pursue this good for its own sake (Hall et al., 2008).

The counter-argument sees spirituality as a reproducibly measurable dimension to quality of life. While health in most spiritual traditions may not rank as the ultimate good, it is seen as a substantial good that facilitates the pursuit of higher goods and so healthy living practices and pursuit of high quality medical care are endorsed by most spiritual traditions. People across a range of cultures are able to identify concerns that through consensus comprise what is meant by the term spiritual. These address issues of ultimate meaning, purpose, and faith, and one's relationship to God or to values above and beyond oneself and are distinct from the psychological or philosophical (Moadel, 1999; Gijsberts, 2011). Instruments have been validated that measure "spiritual well-being" and "spiritual needs" in the context of illness. The Functional Assessment of Chronic Illness Therapy Spiritual Well-being subscale (FACIT-Sp) consists of eight items that measure existential well-being and the Faith subscale that consists of four items that measure religious well-being (Brady et al, 1999; Munoz et al, 2015). While the FACIT-Sp has been faulted for confusing emotional states with the spiritual, its defenders respond that its measures capture a distinctive human need, separate from the emotional, to find meaning and purpose by living in accord with our highest values.

An alternative approach is to focus less on how spirituality feels ("well-being") than on how it functions. The RCOPE (Pargament et al, 2000) and the brief RCOPE (Pargament et al, 2011) examine how patients use religion to cope with the stress of illness, and have identified a range of spiritually grounded coping styles, from "self-directing" to "deferring." The SNAP (Spiritual Needs Assessment for Patients) measures a group of 13 needs which patients have agreed comports with their understanding of the term "spiritual" including "finding meaning in the experience of illness," "finding hope," "relationship to God or something beyond oneself," "coping with suffering" "finding peace of mind" and "finding forgiveness" (Sharma et al, 2011). The SNAP has been translated into and validated in Chinese, Russian, and Spanish. While there are cultural differences in terminology, the need to place one's life experience in some larger overall context appears to be universal (Astrow et al, 2012).

Better health may not be the ultimate purpose of religion, it is a core goal of medicine. Physicians, working in cooperation with their patients, need to use all the tools at their disposal in the interest of restoring patients to health, or if that is not possible, alleviating symptoms. The unsettled state of research measures of spirituality notwithstanding, from the standpoint of oncology practice, it is often crucial to come to know something about a patient's underlying spiritual belief system in order to work with that patient. In a study of 100 South Carolina patients with newly diagnosed lung cancer, patients ranked faith in God just below their oncologist's recommendations as the most important factor in their decisions about treatment (Silvestri, 2003). Americans hold differing views of who or what God is and how God relates to human life: authoritative, benevolent, critical, or distant according to one recently constructed typology (Froese & Bader, 2010). These sorts of views may influence a patient's approach to medical care and relationship with the medical team. Some patients will see God as an active partner who supports those with illness through loving concern. They may seek to access God's healing power through prayer and other ritual practices.

Others who relate to the Divine primarily as awesome and overwhelming power may be less hopeful about their ability to change the course of their illness. For instance, a recent study from the Netherlands of cultural and religious differences among 61 women during breast cancer treatment found that non-native Dutch women, predominantly Muslim, were less active during their treatment and more likely to gain weight due "to doubts about their own influence on their disease" (Kruif et al, 2015). The physician might utilize knowledge and respect for the patient's spiritual outlook, gained through attentive listening, as a means toward forming a healing alliance (Schenck, 2012) A patient might see her own efforts as insignificant and beside the point and yet by the mere fact of presenting to a physician might indicate a degree of openness toward a more active approach to her illness. The point would not be to challenge the patient's belief system but instead to be aware of it, and then work within that system of belief, enlisting the help of others in the medical team, including clergy if the patient so wished, in the interest of more productive attitudes toward human efforts to treat illness.

Several studies have shown that quantitative measures of spiritual well-being correlate with overall quality of life in patients with advanced cancer. Although subject to concerns about the validity of generic measures of spiritual well-being, these studies support the common sense suspicion that the ability to find meaning and purpose in life despite serious illness provides a degree of comfort and reassurance, along with the strength to carry on, to many with incurable illness. One cross-sectional study of 163 Indiana outpatients with advanced cancer showed that spiritual well-being correlated with quality of life measures (Fisch, 2003). Among 883 outpatients at the University of California San Francisco Comprehensive Cancer Center, spiritual well-being (measured using the single item Steinhauser screening scale, "I feel at peace") was associated with greater quality of life, greater general well-being, less anxiety, less fatigue, and less pain (Rabow & Knish, 2015). 200 of 3212 potentially eligible patients in a New York City palliative care hospital were more likely to report end-of-life despair if they also reported low spiritual well-being (McClain, 2003).

Spiritual needs and concerns appear to be common in patients receiving treatment for cancer. In a study of 69 patients receiving palliative radiation therapy, 86% reported one or more spiritual concerns, including 57% "seeking a closer connection to God or your faith" and 51% "finding meaning in the experience of your cancer" (Winkelman et al., 2011). Unmet spiritual needs are associated with lower quality of life and psychological adjustment. In one study of 313 patients in a Manhattan out-patient cancer center, 18% of patients reported that their spiritual needs were not being met (Astrow at al., 2007). In another study of 230 patients with advanced cancer treated at a cooperating group of academic cancer centers, where the question regarding spiritual needs was framed differently from the Manhattan study, 47% reported that their spiritual needs were minimally or not being met by their religious community and 72% not being met by the medical system (T. Balboni et al., 2007).

Specific approaches to spiritual concerns may ameliorate or conversely exacerbate patient distress. Religious coping may provide support and comfort but has also been associated with painful feelings of guilt and shame. Constellations of religious and spiritual attitudes may predict for increased distress or alternatively may support patients when faced with a spiritual crisis. Negative religious copers" (identified through high negative scores on the RCOPE survey instrument) in one exploratory study of 114 patients with cancer drawn from the waiting room of a mid-Western oncology practice were at increased risk for depression while patients whose coping style used a high degree of religion and spirituality (based upon high scores on the faith and the meaning/peace subscales of the FACIT-Sp) were at low risk (Kristeller et al., 2011). Provision of spiritual care, "care that supports a patient's spiritual health," has been associated with increase in hospice use and decrease in aggressive medical interventions at the end of life (T Balboni et al.,

2010), while in contrast patients who report a higher degree of "religious coping" have a greater likelihood of receiving aggressive care at the end of life (Phelps et al., 2009). These seemingly contradictory findings highlight the degree to which spiritual matters influence crucial quality of care measures in cancer treatment and deserve more attention in cancer research and efforts to improve cancer care.

Many seriously ill cancer patients would welcome physician expression of interest in their core beliefs and values. A majority of patients favor discussion about their spiritual concerns with their physician in the setting of life threatening illness or the threatened loss of loved ones, though not as much when seeing the doctor in less dire circumstances (Ehman et al., 1999; McCord et al., 2004). Patients from the southeast, and from rural areas, are more desirous of frank acknowledgment of their religious and spiritual practices (King & Bushwick, 1994) but even urban secular-minded patients have spiritual needs. In the lower Manhattan cancer center study, 58% of patients believed it appropriate for their physician to inquire about spiritual needs, 52% about their religious beliefs (Astrow et al., 2007). All studies agree that physicians seldom inquire about their patients' spiritual needs, beliefs, or religious affiliation.

While patients want oncologists to focus on practical medical issues, patients also want to be respected as individuals and not seen as numbers or cases (Sered & Tabory, 1999). Knowing patients as individuals in America means knowing that Americans tend to be religious but that in urban areas many people (67% in the lower Manhattan cancer center) now identify themselves as "spiritual but not religious" (Sered & Tabory, 1999). Unaddressed spiritual needs may diminish a patient's satisfaction with medical care and their perception of the quality of their medical care (Astrow et al., 2007). Oncologists as a group are aware that these issues are important to patients. A substantial percentage in one study acknowledged responsibility for addressing spiritual distress with their patients but they also reported that they did not routinely do so because of perceived lack of time or expertise (Kristeller et al., 1999).

National palliative care guidelines define the "domain of care in the setting of advanced illness that recognizes that religious and spiritual concerns of the patient and family and attends to spiritual needs" as "spiritual care" (Vallurupalli et al., 2012; Peteet & Balboni, 2013). In a study conducted in a group of cancer centers in Boston of 75 patients with advanced cancer and 339 cancer physicians and nurses, most patients (77.9%), physicians (71.6%), and nurses (85.1%) believed that routine provision of spiritual care would benefit patients. Participants who viewed spiritual care in a positive light suggested that it might enhance patient well-being and improve the patient-clinical relationship. Among the minority of participants who were critical, concerns expressed included the fear that some patients might take offense and that for physicians, spiritual care was outside the scope of their training or expertise (Phelps et al., 2012). Nurses were more likely than physicians to perceive medical practitioners as having a role in the delivery of spiritual care (Rodin et al., 2015). Provision of spiritual support by the medical team (doctors and nurses) was associated with better patient quality of life near death among 343 patients with advanced cancer in a group of northeastern academic cancer centers (Winkelmann et al., 2011). Lack of adequate training of physicians and nurses appears to be a major barrier to provision of spiritual care services (Rodin et al., 2015).

Several small studies have attempted to improve patient quality of life by specifically addressing the spiritual concerns of cancer patients. A randomized trial conducted at the Mayo Clinic assigned a group of 131 patients with advanced stage cancer receiving radiation therapy to either an intervention arm consisting of six 90 minute in-person sessions based on the physical, emotional, social, or spiritual domains of quality of life or a control arm that received standard medical care. Three sessions in the intervention arm, led by board-certified chaplains, included the spiritual component and covered spiritual themes such as life review, meaning and purpose, and grief and acceptance. The intervention group showed improved spiritual quality of life (or spiritual well-being) as measured by the FACIT-Sp at 4 weeks but not by the Linear Analog Self-Assessment (LASA), a quality of life measurement tool constructed at the Mayo Clinic for use in cancer patients. One item in the LASA instrument addressed spiritual well-being: "How is your spiritual well-being over the past week?" on a 0 to 10 scale. The FACIT-Sp improvement was not maintained at weeks 27 or 52 (Piderman et al., 2014).

A study involving 475 patients with a diagnosis of stage I-IV non-small cell lung cancer and 354 family caregivers was conducted at the City of Hope Cancer Center in Southern California. This was a non-randomized, sequential intervention trial where patients received standard treatment first followed by the intervention. The intervention comprised three components: first, a baseline quality of life assessment including assessment of spiritual well-being using the FACIT-Sp-12 scale. Results of this assessment led to the creation of a personalized palliative care plan, including a spiritual well-being section. Second, patients and their family caregivers were discussed at weekly interdisciplinary case meetings, guided by the personalized palliative care plan. The meetings led to specific referrals for patients and their family caregivers, including chaplaincy referrals when this seemed warranted. Third, four sessions led by two advanced practice nurses were conducted for each patient and family caregiver. For those patients or their family caregivers in which spiritual well-being was a major concern, sessions might focus on such topics as hope, inner strength, uncertainty, purpose and meaning in life, positive changes, redefining self and priorities, and spirituality/religiosity. Main findings from this study were that religiously affiliated patients reported better scores on the Faith subscale of the FACIT-Sp-12 and that patients who received the intervention showed significantly improved scores for the Meaning/Peace subscale. For the family caregivers, however, spiritual well-being was higher in the usual care group than after the intervention. Whether any of these measured differences is clinically meaningful is unknown (Sun et al., 2015).

An alternative approach to provision of spiritual care by the medical team involves various forms of existential psychotherapy. Though not specifically focused on the patient's spirituality, these forms of therapy all seek to improve spiritual well-being as one of several endpoints. Supportive-expressive group therapy focuses on "social and emotional support for discussions of death and dying and reordering of life priorities in the face of death" (Classen et al., 2001; Kissane et al., 2007). "Dignity therapy" is a form of brief psychotherapy that provides patients with the opportunity "to reflect on things that matter most to them or that they would most want remember." Patients are asked to respond to questions such as: "Are there specific things that you would want your family to know about you? What are your most important accomplishments? What are your hopes and dreams for your loved ones? What have you learned about life that you would want to pass along to others?" Answers are audiotaped and transcribed with the final transcription given to the patient to be passed on to a recipient of the patient's choice. A 441 patient three-arm randomized trial of dignity therapy failed to show any advantage to dignity therapy in the primary endpoint of lessening distress levels, though it did show improvement in secondary endpoints such as improving a patient's self-reported spiritual well-being (Chochinov et al., 2011).

Meaning-Centered Group Psychotherapy is an eight-session psychotherapy intervention based upon the work of Holocaust survivor Viktor Frankl, author of *Man's Search for Meaning*, and that focuses on helping patients with advanced cancer develop an increased sense of meaning in their lives. A psychiatrist, clinical psychologist, or social worker with experience treating patients with advanced cancer leads the sessions. 253 patients with advanced cancer enrolled in a randomized controlled trial of Meaning-Centered Group Psychotherapy at Memorial Sloan-Kettering Cancer Center (Breitbart et al, 2015). Participants in the intervention group who attended three or more sessions showed greater improvement in quality of life and in spiritual well-being compared with controls and greater reductions in depression, hopelessness, and desire for hastened death. Intent to treat analysis showed significant benefit for treatment group only in quality of life, depression, and hopelessness but not for other outcome variables.

The strength of the study is its rigorous randomized design. Limitations include a high drop-out rate and lack of threshold level of distress as a requirement for entry with the likelihood that many patients had only modest levels of need at entry. This also made it difficult to ascertain how effective this form of therapy was for those with the highest levels of spiritual distress. Somewhat limited information about patient demographics raises the possibility that these results may not be broadly generalizable.

An underlying question might be whether spiritual need is best addressed through psychotherapy, either individual or group. A cancer diagnosis is often a lonely and frightening experience. To what extent is the communal and ritual dimension that religion provides, and the transcendent system of moral values that religion offers, a crucial element to meeting spiritual need in the broad population of cancer patients? Given the documented decline in allegiance to mainstream religious dominations in contemporary America and the rise of more fundamentalist versions, are religions themselves up to the task (Pew Research Group, 2015)?

When patients indicate in surveys that they wish their medical team to provide spiritual care, perhaps they are hoping that their doctors and nurses will function in part as a quasi-religious community, a community that voluntarily holds itself to high standards of interpersonal behavior, that cares about them and will sacrifice for them. Physicians and nurses, though, may already feel under strain meeting their primary responsibility to provide competent medical and nursing care in the face of increasing productivity expectations and the substantial new documentation requirements placed on them by electronic medical records. What are reasonable professional expectations for physicians and nurses in the presence of spiritual need and where will they find the community that supports their efforts to take on this vital but weighty assignment? These are crucial challenges for the fields of medicine and nursing if they are to live up to the highest aspirations of their professions and care for the sick in their full humanity.

AREAS FOR FUTURE RESEARCH

Studies of religion and spirituality in oncology have been limited by selection bias, small sample sizes, varying definitions of spirituality and spiritual care, lack of validated instruments, and geographic clustering. While this situation has been improved somewhat by the development of survey instruments such as the FACIT-Sp-12, the Fetzer Multidimensional Measure of Religiousness/

Spirituality, the RCOPE and the SNAP, and by the careful studies of spiritual care in the Coping with Cancer Study, the numbers of patients enrolled in these sorts of studies is modest and the field lacks consensus on the very nature of what is being measured.

Even the association between spirituality and well-being has been questioned because of the cross-sectional (in contrast to longitudinal) design of validating studies, the self-referential questions (i.e. many items in the scale refer to well-being) in the commonly used FACIT-Sp, and the fact that many items deemed "spiritual" inevitably overlap with the emotional or existential since the field of action for all three is the human brain (Groopman, 1997; Visser et al., 2009). "Peace of mind" for instance is partly an emotional state, yet in the context of spiritual search might refer beyond the mere feeling to a person's sense of relationship with values outside the self connected to that person's ultimate source of meaning. Ideally, studies of patient spiritual need and spiritual well-being ought to be based upon widely-agreed upon definitions and be large enough and sufficiently demographically inclusive to be able to offer cross-cultural comparisons.

Key questions for research on spirituality and religion in oncology are as follows:

1. What is meant by spirituality in the context of illness and can it be measured outside the context of some specific spiritual tradition, religious or secular? Can we devise survey instruments that reproducibly measure the dimension of experience that we can agree through consensus represents the spiritual and that differs from the psychological or philosophical? How does spiritual well-being, and which specific aspects, influence patient quality of life across the disease spectrum?

2. What is the role for religious faith and for religious communities in supporting the bodily and spiritual needs of cancer patients? How can we incorporate religious perspectives in a way that respects the diversity of viewpoints and practices around spiritual and existential issues in contemporary American life? How might physicians and nurses best respond to forms of spirituality that appear to be counter-productive from the standpoint of patient health? How can we best understand and evaluate the increasing subjectivism and individualism of spirituality in American life?

3. What specific dimensions of spiritual need do cancer patients express most often, from diagnosis and initial treatment, through survivorship, to treatment for recurrent disease, and including end-of-life care? Are there ethnic/cultural differences in spiritual needs?

4. Which spiritual needs can we reasonably expect the medical care system to meet? Who ought to address spiritual concerns with patients? What do we mean by "spiritual care" and who ought to provide it?

5. If patients are able to discuss their spiritual concerns and have their spiritual needs addressed in the context of their medical care, will they report higher perceptions of quality of care and/or greater satisfaction with care?

6. How important is the spirituality of physicians and nurses in the care of the seriously ill? Are some forms of spirituality in health care professionals more effective than others in warding off burnout and demoralization? Are there specific changes in the work environment for physicians and nurses that might be conducive to the development of a more caring atmosphere for patients?

7. How can we best educate physicians, nurses, and social workers to address patients' spiritual concerns?

8. What is the role of non-denominational chaplains in our system of cancer treatment and care, and what source of funding is there to support chaplaincy services?

9. What role can community clergy play? If we are going to involve community clergy to a greater extent, what sort of training would they need? Where will they receive the needed training?

The growing importance of palliative care provides a potential locus for studies of patient spirituality and spiritual needs and for potential therapeutic interventions (Kelley & Morrison, 2015). The risk to this approach is that attention to patient spirituality will be seen as largely connected with end-of-life care needs and relegated to the palliative care consultant. Spiritual concerns appear to affect patient decision-making throughout the course of cancer treatment, not only at the end of life. Oncologists risk losing an opportunity to deepen their relationship with their patients if patient spirituality is seen as primarily a concern of palliative care specialists.

COMMON CLINICAL SCENARIOS

When spiritual issues arise in the course of oncology care, there is no announcement that this is a spiritual moment. Instead, it is up to the physicians and nurses caring for the patient to recognize when the patient may have spiritual concerns or be experiencing spiritual distress. The following are a few representative scenarios and the questions that these patient scenarios raise. The responses are the author's own based upon his reflections on over 30 years clinical practice of hematology and medical oncology and his familiarity with the relevant literature and are meant to stimulate discussion. Certainly other physicians and nurses will hold different views.

CASE 1

A 79-year-old man has metastatic prostate cancer to bone. He has disease progression through maximal hormonal treatment. He has developed increasing weakness and pain to the point where it is difficult for him to walk.

At a recent visit he was informed that his blood tests had worsened and that the cancer had progressed.

When he was informed he became visibly fearful and overwhelmed. He looked as if he were so frightened that he couldn't absorb any information.

After the patient's physician left the exam room, the patient's nurse practitioner said to the patient, "You look scared."

The patient replied, "Of course I'm scared, look at the PSA." He refused to say anything more.

The patient is a widower. He is Catholic. He has no children. He has two living brothers. He lives alone. He has a close friend male friend who often accompanies him to doctor visits.

CASE 2

A 62-year-old woman has advanced ovarian cancer, which has progressed through all available chemotherapeutic treatments. She is now hospitalized and is to be transferred to an in-patient hospice for terminal care.

On the morning of the planned discharge, her physician noticed that she was upset and asked her what she was feeling.

"Fear," she replied. "Fear of the unknown."

The patient was Catholic and had taught in Catholic elementary school. She was very involved with her local church.

QUESTIONS

1. From a religious or a secular standpoint, how does one address existential dread in the setting of illness? What can one say? What can one do?

In both cases, the role of the clinician is to recognize and acknowledge the patient's fears, listen, and then express support. "I can understand how frightening this must be for you. Please tell me what you are thinking right now." Simply sitting and listening can express empathy and help relieve the patient's distress.

2. Whose role is it to address the patient's fearfulness? How important is it for a physician to be aware of a patient's fears? If a physician becomes aware that a patient is deeply fearful about the prospect of impending death, what should the physician do? If the physician or nurse has a different spiritual outlook, what is the proper stance to take?

It is the clinician's role to address the patient's fearfulness. Fear of death is a concern shared by all people, though most of us prefer not to think about it. Many patients draw strength from their relationships with their physicians and nurses, and at these moments of deepest dread for a patient, it may be crucial for physicians and nurses to express a sense of human solidarity. If the clinician is unaware of the patient's fear, the patient may feel isolated and unsupported and may fall into a state of hopelessness Once aware, the physician may conclude that referral to a clinical psychologist or chaplain is appropriate. The physician's spiritual beliefs should not be the issue here aside from the extent to which these beliefs remind the physician to focus on the patient's needs. The required task is to elicit and support the patient's feelings and spiritual resources in the interest of the patient's well-being.

3. What does the physician or nurse do about his/her own fears or doubts in this realm?

The physician or nurse needs to recognize his or his own fears and doubts. A degree of self-awareness is needed so that physicians and nurses can overcome their own fears and be present for patients when they are in profound need. This may require that physicians and nurses draw upon their own spirituality, though they do not need to let their patients know that they are doing so.

For physicians and nurses who are finding that they lack the inner resources to support their frightened patients, additional study, reflection, or counseling may be helpful.

4. Is it important for a physician or nurse to be aware of the patient's religious beliefs concerning the possibility of an afterlife? If the physician or nurse believes in an afterlife, would it be appropriate to use this belief in order to reassure the patient?

Patients appreciate it when their physicians and nurses take an interest in who they are as persons, including their work, family, outlook on life, and personal philosophy. It may be helpful for a physician or nurse to know something of a patient's beliefs about eternal life but only if the patient initiates the discussion. While some patients may wish to engage physicians in conversation about existential matters and physicians may choose to respond depending upon their level of comfort, it would be disrespectful of a physician or nurse to press on a patient his or her views in this realm, or about religious, political or philosophical doctrines in general.

Patients may not often ask their physicians about the afterlife, understanding that this is more the realm of clergy. They do often express to their physicians a sense of bewilderment or disbelief at what has befallen them, and anger at the unfairness of it all. If they are from a religious background, they may relate in anger or in sorrow a sense that God has abandoned them.

One possible response is simply to acknowledge the unfairness, reassure the patient that he or she has not done anything wrong to deserve the illness, sit quietly with the patient, and demonstrate through presence and concern that you will not abandon the patient. A caring human environment may give the patient hope and even help restore a religious patient's relationship with God, without directly attempting to do so.

CASE 3

A 50-year-old man has lung cancer metastatic to liver. He is six foot four inches tall and has a physically large frame. He is a professional writer, has been married for 25 years, and lives in Greenwich Village. He has no children.

The patient prides himself on having been independent throughout his life and having control over his surroundings and self. He sees himself as an intellectual and greatly values his ability to project an appearance of confidence and command. The staff knows much of this from talking with him and reading parts of his will. For example, he wrote, "Death is as much a reality as birth, growth, maturity, and old age—it is the only certainty of life."

He was born Presbyterian but currently practices no religion and describes himself as an Atheist. He does not believe in any life beyond this one. For that reason, the quality of his life carries ultimate significance and his continued physical decline has been not only physically but also spiritually deeply troubling to him. His sense of self-worth has been challenged by a disease process that is making him increasingly dependent on others.

On several trips to the cancer center, he appeared extremely weak and in need of assistance. However, he refused to request or accept any kind of assistance. This at times placed him in unsafe situations. At home, he was having difficulty accepting help with his activities of daily living from even his wife or family. The medical team has faced a quandary in wanting to assure his safety but also wants to respect the patient's own deeply felt need to remain independent and in control.

CASE 4

A 60-year-old woman has metastatic cervical cancer. The cancer has invaded her bladder and rectum and as a result, she has persistent severe pain in her pelvis, constantly leaks urine and has a foul smelling vaginal discharge.

She has worked most of her life as a cleaning woman for local theaters, though most recently she has been employed as a switchboard operator. She has continued to work throughout her illness, though co-workers have complained about her absence from her job because of illness.

She is divorced with two children, whom she has raised largely on her own. Her daughter accompanies her on most of her visits to the cancer center. She is fiercely independent, does not want to see herself as "a burden," and has refused all forms of assistance offered by the Cancer Center social worker, including home care and hospice referral. "I don't want someone in here doing what I can do for myself," she has explained. She sees herself as a very proud person. It appears that the patient is refusing to accept help because to do so would be to admit that she is becoming progressively ill. This has been difficult for her daughter who loves her mother and wants to care for her but is also engaged to be married and is ready to move on with her own life.

The patient is a devout Catholic who has asked to receive communion in the Cancer Center and is involved with her local parish.

QUESTIONS:

5. For many patients, maintaining their sense of dignity requires that they remain independent. Serious illness, though, often frustrates this wish, making us dependent on the assistance of others. When patients face loss of those aspects of themselves that help define their own sense of uniqueness how might professional staff best respect patients' wishes but also need to address the reality of their need for care?

The key in both cases is to acknowledge the patient's system of values and show respect for who the patients are and for the choices they have made in their lives. There is no simple solution to the problem of assuring the safety of patients as their physical capacities decline when they express an understandable wish to maintain their independence. We can certainly show support and admiration for their efforts and try to work with them as much as is humanly possible, tipping the balance toward independent functioning, going the extra mile to find solutions for them within the context of resources that are available. It is fair, though, to remind patients who take pride in their independence that the need to accept help does not lessen one's value as a person and suggest that it is likely that they have helped others before and now might be a time when they may need to accept some assistance.

Even when patients are in decline, physicians need to respect their dignity by consulting with them and deferring to them regarding decisions about their care, rather than turning to family members to decide for them, unless patients have explicitly stated that they prefer to leave decision-making to others.

6. Placing the issue in a larger context, individual autonomy is a highly prized value in our democratic society. Religious traditions are often associated with an emphasis on

dependence and paternalistic deference to authority but may also offer structures of communal support to needy patients and families What sources of wisdom can we draw upon that speak to the balance between autonomy and dependence in the maintenance of individual human dignity?

Religious wisdom may provide an excellent source for reflection on how to balance dependence and independence over the course of our lives. While most religious traditions have structures of communal support for the sick, they may also sustain belief in the intrinsic dignity of each individual human being, and encourage believers to treat one another with respect, no matter what the circumstances.

BEST PRACTICES

1. TALKING WITH PATIENTS

Oncologists are present with people as they struggle with life's fundamental mysteries in a way that few other professionals are. They have no particular expertise about these matters and have more than enough to do dealing with the day-to-day issues of keeping up with the literature and taking care of their patients. Still, an emerging literature suggests that patients look to their oncologists not necessarily for answers, but for a level of emotional engagement about the core issues of living and dying that they do not usually expect from other physicians. As a result, their ability to acknowledge patients' spiritual concerns affects patients' satisfaction with care, and physicians without some sort of spiritual grounding may be at higher risk for burnout.

Several groups have proposed algorithms that might help physicians subtly inquire about whether a patient is experiencing spiritual distress. The Oasis algorithm proposes open-ended questions about a person's spirituality: "Religious or spiritual beliefs sometimes influence how people deal with illness. I would be interested to learn your views about this" (Kristeller et al., 2005). FICA, another system, stands for Faith, Importance, Community, Address/Action in care (Puchalski & Romer, 2003). However one chooses to go about it, the physician needs to develop a relationship with his or her patients that encourages open conversation about the patient's underlying beliefs and values. As part of an initial interview, some oncologists will ask patients if they have any specific spiritual beliefs or practices that they would like known and some will generally ask if their patients practice any religion.

The key is to get to know a patient over time, to create an atmosphere in which the patient feels comfortable speaking about these matters, and then to pay attention to any signs that a patient may be in distress. One might, for instance, take note of what a patient is reading. A patient waiting in the exam room might have open the book of Job or the book of Psalms. An observant physician ought readily to surmise what might be on the patient's mind and might deepen the physician-patient relationship by asking the patient about the reading matter. The point is not to lecture or debate, or to pry when a patient does not want to talk, but simply to express interest in who the other is, what that person is about, to listen, and to be able to express human concern. A patient's symptoms out of proportion to the nature of the actual medical problem may represent anxiety but may also be a clue to underlying spiritual distress. A patient with early stage breast cancer and a good prognosis presenting for an urgent visit about a brief minor nosebleed might have concerns beyond the nosebleed. Gentle exploration might lead to the admission that the patient's father had died soon after a major nosebleed, and that yes, she had been concerned that she might be dying.

Failure to acknowledge that a patient is in an existential crisis can lead to a breakdown in communication between doctor and patient. Journalist David Rieff recounted the harrowing experience of his mother, Susan Sontag, as she sought medical care for her fatal leukemia. After she had left the hematologist's office, she couldn't recall what the hematologist had said (Rieff, 2008). As reviewers Diane Johnson and John Murray comment: "Almost anyone who has dealt with some grave medical situation will feel that doctors are either too frank or not forthcoming enough; and sometimes we feel both things at once. . ." (Johnson & Murray, 2008). Sometimes, all that is called for is a kind and understanding word, expressed simply and without condescension that acknowledges what it is that the patient is going through. "Yes, this is a terribly difficult position to be in. And yes, it is totally unfair that you have to face this now after all that you've been through."

Requests from patients that the doctor participate in any specific religious practices, handled sensitively, can strengthen the relationship between doctor and patient. Oncologist-author Jerome Groopman several years ago wrote about an elderly Catholic woman with metastatic breast cancer who asked him to pray with her. Rather than simply reject the request, he took note that the patient was clearly frightened by the course of her illness, drew upon his own Jewish tradition, and found a creative way to meet her need by eliciting her wish that he pray "for God to give my doctors wisdom" (Groopman, 2004). On the other hand, proselytizing by patients or by staff is clearly disrespectful to others and unprofessional. Cancer Center staff may have to remind patients and families not to hand out religious literature to other patients who do not share their faith. Lois Ramondetta and Deborah Rose Sills, in *The Light Within*, describe a California nurse's clumsy efforts to offer spiritual support to Sills, who was dying from ovarian cancer. "It breaks my heart to imagine people dying and not having met love and power of Jesus Christ," the nurse tells the Jewish Sills. As Ramondetta observes, this was monologue, when the goal, for patients who want to talk about these matters, ought to be dialogue and the listening that entails (Ramondetta, 2008).

2. HOW TO BE PRESENT

The professional requirement for the physician is to be fully present to suffering humanity in all its variety. Fortunately, that level of engagement is not needed for the average visit but oncologists may unexpectedly find themselves called upon to provide added support to a patient at times when they themselves may feel fatigued, stressed, rushed, generally depleted, or lacking in some capacity that the patient needs. Reaching out to the other often involves a degree of self-awareness and sometimes self-overcoming. How to develop those capacities, how to become a complete person, is a lifelong project that physicians and nurses need to pursue each in his or her own way.

For some the path may be found in secular philosophy and psychology, in humanism, or professionalism (Cassell, 1994; Schapira, 2007; Cohen, 2007). Others may draw strength from a sense of religious calling or the fellowship of a religious community (Sulmasy, 2006; Hauerwas, 1986). Critics who view religions from the outside may presume that their focus is primarily on theological beliefs and ritual observance. Those on the inside respond that the underlying spirit of most religions is about how to be in the world, particularly about how to respond to those in need (Putnam, 2008).

Is it helpful to bring the language of "God" into the care of cancer patients in spiritual distress, when what we want and intend in practical terms is a caring human presence (Buckman, 2002)? Medicine's hard won independence from religion has led to spectacular advances in medical science and far-reaching improvements in public health, though an explanatory framework that can help us accept limits to what medical science can accomplish may be lacking (Astrow et al., 2001). "God" may work in the spirituality of cancer treatment as a path of access to wisdom traditions that balance limits with hope and that serve as unspoken prods to conscience. The spirituality of cancer treatment and care may require that physicians and nurses locate sources of language and community that provide context to our obligations to others, add depth to powerful human experiences, and remind us of the shared personhood of patients from all backgrounds and our neediness and frailty in the face of the vast unknown (Heschel, 1966).

REFERENCES

Burt BA. *Death Is That Man Taking Names: Intersections of American Medicine, Law, and Culture.* Berkeley, CA: University of California Press, 2003.

Astrow AB. Isn't There Someone to Blame? J Clin Oncol. 2008; 26:1560–1561.

Derogatis LR, Morrow GR, Fetting J. The Prevalence of Psychiatric Disorders among Cancer Patients. JAMA. 1983; 249:751–757.

Groopman J. *The Measure of Our Days: New Beginnings at Life's End.* New York: Viking Penguin, 1997.

Sulmasy DP. *The Healer's Calling: A Spirituality for Physicians and Other Health Care Professionals.* Mahway, NJ: The Paulist Press, 1997.

National Cancer Institute (Accessed December 1, 2015). Spirituality in Cancer Care. 2015. http://www.cancer.gov/about-cancer/coping/day-to-day/faith-and-spirituality/spirituality-pdq#link/stoc_h2_0

Salander P. Who Needs the Concept of Spirituality? Psycho-Oncology. 2005; 647–649.

Hall DE, Meador KG, Koenig HG. Measuring Religiousness in Health Research: Review and Critique. J Relig Health. 2008; 47: 134–163.

Moadel A, Morgan C, Fatone A, et al. Seeking Meaning and Hope: Self-Reported Spiritual and Existential Needs among an Ethnically Diverse Cancer Patient Population. Psychooncology. 1999; 8:378–385.

Gijsberts MJ, Echteld MA, van der Steen JT, et al. Spirituality at the End of Life: Conceptualization of Measurable Aspects—A Systematic Review. J Pall Med. 2011; 14: 852–863.

Brady MJ, Peterman AH, Fitchett G, et al. A Case for Including Spirituality in Quality of Life Measurement in Oncology. Psycho-Oncology. 1999; 8:417–428.

Munoz AR, Salsman JM, Stein KD, et al. Reference Values of the Functional Assessment of Chronic Illness Therapy-Spiritual Well-Being: A Report From the American Cancer Society's Studies of Cancer Survivors. Cancer. 2015; 121: 1838–1844.

Pargament KI, Koenig HG, Perez LM. The Many Methods of Religious Coping: Development and Initial Validation of the RCOPE. J Clin Psych. 2000; 56: 519–543.

Pargament K, Feuille M, Burdzy D. The Brief RCOPE: Current Psychometric Status of a Short Measure of Religious Copings. Religions. 2011; 2(1): 51–76.

Sharma RS, Astrow AB, Texeira K, et al. The Spiritual Needs Assessment for Patients (SNAP): Development and Validation of a Comprehensive Instrument to Assess Unmet Spiritual Needs Journal of Pain and Symptom Management. J. Pain Symptom Management, 2012 Jul; 44(1): 44–51.

Astrow AB, Sharma RK, Huang Y, et al. A Chinese Version of the Spiritual Needs Assessment for Patients (SNAP) Survey Instrument. J Palliat Med. 2012; 15(12):1297–1315.

Silvestri GA, Knittig S, Zoller JS, Nietert PJ. Importance of Faith on Medical Decisions Regarding Cancer Care. J Clin Oncol. 2003; 21:1379–1382.

Froese P, Bader C. *America's Four Gods: What We Say About God and What that Says About Us*. New York: Oxford University Press, 2010.

Kruif de A, Derks M, Winkels R, et al. Cultural and Religious Differences During Breast Cancer Treatment Between Dutch and non-Western Immigrant Women. 2015; San Antonio Breast Cancer Symposium, Abstract P1-10-28.

Schenck D, Churchill L. *Healers: Extraordinary Clinicians at Work*. New York: Oxford University Press, 2012.

Fisch MJ, Titzer ML, Kristeller JL, et al. Assessment of Quality of Life in Outpatients with Advanced Cancer: The Accuracy of Clinician Estimations and the Relevance of Spiritual Well-Being—A Hoosier Oncology Group Study. J Clin Oncol. 2003; 21:2754–2759.

Rabow MW, Knish SJ. Spiritual Well-Being among Outpatients with Cancer Receiving Concurrent Oncologic and Palliative Care. Support Care Cancer.; 2015; 23:919–923.

McClain CS, Rosenfeld B, Breitbart W. Effect of Spiritual Well-Being on End-of-Life Despair in Terminally Ill Cancer Patients. Lancet. 2003; 361: 1603–1607.

Winkelman WD, Lauderdale K, Balboni MJ, et al. The Relationship of Spiritual Concerns to the Quality of Life of Advanced Cancer Patients: Preliminary Findings. J Pall Med. 2011; 14: 1022–1028.

Astrow AB, Wexler A, Texeira K, He MK, Sulmasy DP. Is Failure to Meet Spiritual Needs Associated with Cancer Patients' Perceptions of Quality of Care and Their Satisfaction with Care? J Clin Oncol. 2007; 25(36):5753–5757.

Balboni TA, Vanderwerker LC, Block SD, et al. Religiousness and Spiritual Support among Advanced Cancer Patients and Associations with End-of-Life Treatment Preferences and Quality of Life. J Clin Oncol. 2007; 25:555–560.

Kristeller JL, Sheets V, Johnson T, et al. Understanding religious and spiritual influences on adjustment of cancer: individual patterns and differences. J Behav Med. 2011; 32:550–561.

Balboni TA, Paulk ME, Balboni MJ, et al. Provision of spiritual care to patients with advanced cancer: Associations with medical care and quality of life near death. J Clin Oncol. 2010; 28: 445–452.

Phelps AC, Maciejewski PK, Nilsson M, et al. Religious Coping and Use of Intensive Life-Prolonging Care Near Death in Patients with Advanced Cancer. JAMA. 2009; 301:1140–1147.

Ehman JW, Ott BB, Short TH et al. Do Patients Want Physicians to Inquire About Their Spiritual or Religious Beliefs If They Become Gravely Ill? Arch Intern Med. 1999; 159:1803–1806.

McCord G, Gilchrist VJ, Grossman SD, et al. Discussing Spirituality with Patients: A Rational and Ethical Approach. Ann Fam Med. 2004; 2:356–361.

King DE, Bushwick B: Beliefs and Attitudes of Hospital Inpatients about Faith Healing, and Prayer. J Fam Pract 1994; 39:349–352.

Sered S, Tabory E. You Are a Number, Not a Human Being: Israeli Breast Cancer Patients' Experiences with the Medical Establishment. Med Anthropol Q. 1999; 13:223–252.

Gallup G. *Religion in America*. Princeton, NJ: Princeton Religious Research Center, 1990.

Kristeller JL, Zumbrun CS, Schilling RF. "I Would If I Could": How Oncologists and Oncology Nurses Address Spiritual Distress in Cancer Patients. Psycho-oncology. 1999; 8:451–458.

Vallurupalli M, Lauderdale K, Balboni M. et al. The Role of Spirituality and Religious Coping in the Quality of Life of Patients with Advanced Cancer. J Support Oncol. 2012; 10:81–87.

Peteet JR, Balboni MJ. Spirituality and Religion in Oncology. CA Cancer J Clin. 2013; 63:280–289.

Phelps CA, Lauderdale KI, Alcorn S, et al. Addressing Spirituality within the Care of Patients at the End of Life: Perspectives of Patients with Advanced Cancer, Oncologists, and Oncology Nurses. J Clin Oncol. 2012; 30:2538–2544.

Rodin D, Balboni M, Mitchell C, et al. Whose Role? Oncology Practitioners' Perceptions of Their Role in Providing Spiritual Care to Advanced Cancer Patients. Supp Care Cancer. 2015; 23:2543–2550.

Balboni MJ, Sullivan A, Amobi A, et al. Why Is Spiritual Care Infrequent at the End of Life? Spiritual Care Perceptions Among Patients, Nurses, and Physicians and the Role of Training. J Clin Oncol. 2013; 31:461–467.

Piderman KM, Johnson ME, Frost MH, et al. Spiritual quality of Life in Advanced Cancer Patients Receiving Radiation Therapy. Psychooncology. 2014; 23: 216–221.

Sun, V, Kim JY, Irish TL, et al. Palliative Care and Spiritual Well-Being in Lung Cancer Patients and Family Caregivers. Psycho-Oncology. 2015; Published on-line prior to print. 2015.

Classen C, Butler LD, Koopman C, et al. Supportive-Expressive Group Therapy Reduces Distress in Metastatic Breast Cancer Patients: A Randomized Clinical Intervention Trial. Arch Gen Psychiatry. 2001; 58: 494–501.

Kissane DW, Grabsch B, Clarke DM, et al. Supportive-Expressive Group Therapy for Women with Metastatic Breast Cancer: Survival and Psychosocial Outcome from Randomized Controlled Trial. Psychooncology. 2007; 16:277–286.

Chochinov HM, Kristjanson L, Breitbart et al. Effect of Dignity Therapy on Distress and End-of-Life Experience in Terminally Ill Patients: A Randomized Controlled Trial. www.thelancet.com/oncology. 2011; 12:753–762.

Breitbart W, Rosenfeld B, Pessin H, et al. Meaning-Centered Group Psychotherapy: An Effective Intervention for Improving Psychological Well-Being in Patients with Advanced Cancer. J Clin Oncol. 2015; 33: 749–754.

Pew Research Group. America's Changing Religious Landscape. http://www.pewforum.org/2015/05/12/americas-changing-religious-landscape/ Accessed December 7, 2015.

Visser A, Garssen B, Vingerhoets A. Spirituality and Well-Being in Cancer Patients: A Review. Psycho-Oncology. 2009; published on-line in Wiley InterScience.

Kelley AS, Morrison RS. Palliative Care for the Seriously Ill. N Engl J Med 2015; 373:747–755.

Kristeller JL, Rhodes M, Cripe LD, et al. Oncologist Assisted Spiritual Intervention Study (OASIS): Patient Acceptability and Initial Evidence of Effects. Int J Psychiatry Med. 2005; 35:329–347.

Puchalski CM, Romer AL. Taking a Spiritual History Allows Clinicians to Understand Patients More Fully. J Palliat Med. 2003; 3:129–137.

Rieff D. *Swimming in a Sea of Death: A Son's Memoir.* New York: Simon and Schuster, 2008.

Johnson D, Murray JF. Will to Live; Review of *Swimming in a Sea of Death.* New York Review of Books. 2008; 55(2).

Groopman J. God at the Bedside. N Engl J Med. 2004; 350: 176–1178.

Ramondetta LM, Sills DR. *The Light Within: The Extraordinary Friendship of a Doctor and Patient Brought Together by Cancer.* New York. William Morrow. 2008

Cassell EJ. *The Nature of Suffering and the Goals of Medicine.* New York. Oxford University Press. 1994

Schapira L. An Existential Oncologist. J Clin Oncol. 2002; 20:2407–2408.

Cohen JJ. Viewpoint: linking professionalism to humanism: what it means, why it matters. Acad Med. 2007; 82: 1029–1032.

Sulmasy DP. *The Rebirth of the Clinic: An Introduction to Spirituality in Health Care.* Washington, D.C. Georgetown University Press. 2006

Hauerwas S. *Suffering Presence: Theological Reflections on Medicine, the Mentally Handicapped, and the Church.* Notre Dame, Indiana. University of Notre Dame Press. 1986.

Putnam H. *Jewish Philosophy as a Guide to Life: Rosenzweig, Buber, Levinas, Wittgenstein. Bloomington and Indianapolis*. Indiana University Press 2008.

Buckman R. *Can We Be Good Without God? Biology, Behavior, and the Need to Believe*. Amherst, NY. Prometheus Books. 2002

Astrow AB, Puchalski C, Sulmasy DP: "Religion, Spirituality and Health Care: Social, Ethical, and Practical Considerations," Am J Med. 2001; 110: 283–287, 2001.

Heschel AJ. The patient as a person. In: *The Insecurity of Freedom*. New York: Noonday Press/Farrar, Strauss, and Giroux; 24–38, 1966.

CHAPTER 10

RELIGION AND SPIRITUALITY IN PALLIATIVE MEDICINE

Tracy A. Balboni and Michael J. Balboni

Spirituality and medicine frequently intersect within the field of palliative care since patients at the end of life often have multifaceted needs including the psychological (Block, 2006), social (Prigerson, 1992), and spiritual (Alcorn et al., 2010; Steinhauser et al., 2000). Providers in this field thus have an important role in providing for the holistic needs of their patients. Cicely Saunders, an English physician credited for beginning the hospice movement in the mid-1900s (Clemens & Klaschik, 2009) wrote, "Expertise in symptom control is required. . . together with an ability to make sense of the inner concerns and values of the person. Above all, there is a need to engage with "the whole area of thought concerning moral values throughout life"—"the spiritual" (Saunders, 2006). Though patients' religion and spirituality has historically been an integral component of palliative care from its inception and the creation of US palliative care guidelines, the incorporation of palliative care into the larger biomedical community has led to spiritual care becoming controversial. Research remains an important way to engage questions related to how patient care at the end of life intersects with patients' religion/spirituality (R/S). This chapter will review key literature within the field of spiritual care in the palliative setting, provide case examples of common ways that R/S arises within palliative care, and suggest ways that physicians providing palliative treatment can engage their patients.

STATE OF THE SCIENCE

Research in religion/spirituality and palliative care aims to understand its role in the care of patients with advanced illness through observation and measurement of their spiritual experiences. Patients' spirituality, beliefs, and practices often serve as an important mediating factor in the patient's ability to cope with advanced illness, impacting both treatment and decision-making near the end of life. Research conducted in the last few decades has been critical in identifying ways of re-integrating spirituality into advanced illness. Key research findings with regard to R/S and palliative care include data regarding the importance of R/S, its impact on quality of life, the prevalence of spiritual needs, patient opinions on spiritual care from medical professionals, the impact of R/S on medical outcomes, and spiritual care training for medical professionals.

PATIENT-RATED IMPORTANCE OF RELIGION/ SPIRITUALITY IN LIFE-THREATENING DISEASE

Koenig et al., in a 1998 study at Duke University Medical Center involving 542 hospitalized patients, aimed to determine the scope of religious beliefs and practices among patients and how patients' R/S relates to their psychological and social well-being (Koenig, 1998). Results showed that 88% considered their R/S beliefs and faith to be important to them, 59% reported performing daily religious activities (e.g., prayer), and 67% reported that religion was important to coping with illness. While religiosity is clearly dependent on geographic region—such as the variability in R/S characteristics between populations in New York City (Astrow, Wexler, Texeira, He, & Sulmasy, 2007) and Houston (Delgado-Guay et al., 2011)—the United States as a whole, like many other areas in the world, has a highly prevalent R/S population (Pew Research, 2014; "U.S. Religions Landscape Survey," 2008). This is seen in the regionally diverse Coping with Cancer study, where 68% of 343 advanced cancer patients regarded religion to be very important and 88% considered religion to be at least somewhat important (T.A. Balboni et al., 2007). The endorsement of R/S among ethnic minorities within Coping with Cancer was even more notable, with 89% of African Americans and 79% of Hispanics indicating that religion was very important. In a study of 75 advanced cancer patients at four Boston academic centers, 78% reported that R/S was important to them in their cancer experience (Alcorn et al., 2010). In the same patient population, 84% reported that R/S plays a central role in their ability to cope with cancer (Vallurupalli et al., 2012). Furthermore, patients frequently identified R/S beliefs, spiritual practices, and religious communities as having an important role in bringing about transformation through the personal experience of cancer (Alcorn et al., 2010).

Similarly, in a survey-based study of 100 advanced lung cancer patients (Silvestri et al., 2003), patients and family caregivers were asked to rank the importance of seven factors contributing to patients' treatment decision-making. Patients' faith in God was considered by patients and their caregivers to be a key factor in medical decision-making—ranked second behind only the ability of the treatment to cure disease. In a study by Ehman et al. (1999), 45% of patients reported that religious beliefs would influence their medical decisions (Ehman et al., 1999). Likewise, the importance of R/S in medical decision-making is highlighted by a study showing that terminally ill religious patients are more likely to prefer aggressive medical measures to extend life (Phelps et al., 2009). In the Coping with Cancer study, advanced patients who rely on their religious beliefs to cope with illness—high religious coping patients—were found to be nearly three times more likely to receive intensive life-prolonging care near death and less likely to enter hospice during the final week of life (Phelps et al., 2009). Although reasons for this association are not clearly understood, Phelps et al suggested that there are numerous possible explanations: high religious coping patients may be holding out for a miracle (Widera et al., 2011), patients are concerned that they are "giving up on God" (Sulmasy, 2006), and there is an ethical worry that a choice to not pursue medical treatment may somehow be an act of suicide (Phelps et al., 2009).

Together, this evidence indicates that most patients with advanced disease hold R/S to be an important dimension of their experience with life-threatening disease. R/S plays multiple roles in the cancer experience, including as a means for coping and as a catalyst for transformation (Alcorn et al., 2010). Additionally, R/S plays a key role in medical decisions (T. A. Balboni et al., 2007; Silvestri et al., 2003), leading to more aggressive medical interventions at the end of life for some patients (Phelps et al., 2009).

RELIGION/SPIRITUALITY AND QUALITY OF LIFE

In 1999, Brady et al. carried out a multisite, cross-sectional study of 1,610 cancer patients (Brady et al., 1999). After controlling for other predictors of quality of life, higher patient R/S was found to be associated with improved patient quality of life. Furthermore, the patients with higher reported R/S in comparison to less spiritual/religious patients had better quality of life even in the setting of a high burden of physical symptoms (e.g., pain). Likewise, greater patient religious coping and patient spirituality has been reported to be associated with better patient psychological well-being and overall quality of life (Vallurupalli et al., 2012). Similarly, unaddressed spiritual concerns of patients are associated with decreased psychological and overall quality of life within advanced illness (Winkelman et al., 2011). Recently hospitalized patients studied by Steinhauser et al. viewed "being at peace with God" and "freedom from pain" as the two most important elements of quality of life at the end of life (Steinhauser et al., 2000). In contrast, other studies have found associations between spiritual pain and adverse physical and emotional symptoms including increased depression, anxiety, and anorexia (Delgado-Guay et al., 2011). These studies provide initial evidence that R/S plays a key role in the well-being of patients with advanced illness and influences quality of life when facing death. Such evidence has led the National Consensus Project for Quality Palliative Care to include the spiritual, religious, and existential aspects of care among eight domains for quality palliative care ("NCP Clinical Practice Guidelines for Quality Palliative Care. National Consensus Project," 2009). Likewise, the Joint Commission and World Health Organization have called for recognition of patient R/S as part of EOL care ("The Joint Commission," 2011; World Health Organization Palliative Care: Symptom Management and End of Life Care) and require staff training that prepares medical professionals to meet patients' spiritual needs.

PREVALENCE OF PATIENTS' RELIGIOUS/ SPIRITUAL NEEDS AT THE END OF LIFE

Moadel et al. aimed to identify the nature and prevalence of spiritual needs in a convenience sample of 248 ethnically diverse, urban cancer patients (Moadel et al., 1999). The study found that 75% had at least one spiritual need. Among R/S needs surveyed, 51% of patients wanted help to overcome their fears, 42% to find hope, and 40% to find meaning. Hispanics and African American patients more frequently endorsed spiritual needs than Caucasians. In another study of patients at an outpatient cancer clinic in New York City, 73% reported at least one spiritual need (Astrow et al., 2007). In a study by Delgado-Guay et al. among a Houston palliative care population, 44% of advanced patients reported experiencing "spiritual pain" (Delgado-Guay et al., 2011). Patients with spiritual pain had significantly lower self-perceived religiosity and spiritual quality of life. Likewise, in a study by Alcorn et al. of advanced cancer patients receiving palliative radiation therapy in Boston, 85% identified one or more spiritual issues, with a median of 4 issues per patient among 14 spiritual issues assessed (Alcorn et al., 2010). Key spiritual issues among patients included: "seeking a closer connection with God or one's faith," 54%; "seeking forgiveness (of oneself or others)," 47%; and "feeling abandoned by God," 28%. Surprisingly, among the 22% of patients who said that R/S was "not important" to their cancer experience, two-thirds had at least one spiritual issue and 40% reported four or more spiritual issues. The results of these studies suggest that there is a high prevalence of R/S needs among patients facing life-threatening illness, especially ethnic minorities. Further, spiritual needs are frequent even among patients who do not consider themselves particularly religious or spiritual.

PATIENT OPINIONS CONCERNING MEDICAL PROFESSIONAL SPIRITUAL CARE

Multiple studies suggest that patients experiencing life-threatening illness want the medical team to address their R/S as part of medical care. Ehman et al. found that two-thirds of patients desired that their physicians ask about patients' R/S beliefs if they were to become gravely ill (Ehman et al., 1999). In a study of patients seen in a family practice setting by McCord et al, 77% wanted spiritual discussions with their physicians if they were facing life-threatening illness, and majorities of these patients thought that these spiritual discussions would better enable physicians to encourage realistic hope, give better medical advice, and might lead to a change in medical decision-making (McCord et al., 2004). Steinhauser et al., in their study examining factors determining quality of life at the end of life among recently hospitalized patients, reported that 50% found it important to discuss their spiritual beliefs with their physician during the period approaching death (Steinhauser et al., 2000). Similarly, in a multi-regional survey of 456 patients in a primary care setting, MacLean et al. reported that 70% of patients agreed that physicians should ask about R/S when patients were near death, and 50% agreed that physicians should pray with patients if dying (MacLean et al., 2003). In a New York City cancer center where 66% of patients surveyed indicated that they were spiritual but not religious, 58% thought it was appropriate for physicians to inquire about spiritual needs (Astrow et al., 2007). In a report by Winkleman et al. of terminally ill cancer patients, most (87%) agreed it was at least mildly important for physicians and nurses to consider patients' spiritual concerns within the medical setting (Winkelman et al., 2011). Interestingly, this study reported higher rates of patients desiring spiritual care from medical providers in comparison to studies in healthier patients, suggesting that patients with advanced illness are more likely to want their medical caregivers to address R/S concerns in comparison to patients in earlier stages of illness.

In a study comparing terminally ill cancer patients and their oncology nurses and physicians (M. J. Balboni et al., 2013), majorities of patients indicated that spiritual care from nurses and physicians is an important component of cancer care (86% and 87%). Similarly, most nurses and physicians thought that spiritual care should at least occasionally be provided (87% and 80%). Majorities of patients, nurses, and physicians endorsed the appropriateness of eight examples of patient-practitioner spiritual care interactions (averages, 78%, 93%, and 87%, respectively; $P = 0.01$). Among patients reporting spiritual care from either a nurse or physician, most indicated that their spiritual interaction was very positive (M. J. Balboni et al., 2013). The most common form of spiritual care by medical professionals was encouraging or affirming spiritual beliefs (Epstein-Peterson et al., 2015). In addition, physicians hold more negative perceptions of spiritual care than patients ($P < 0.001$) and nurses ($P = 0.008$) (Phelps et al., 2012). The benefits of spiritual care identified by patients and practitioners included supporting patients' emotional well-being and strengthening patient-provider relationships. Objections to spiritual care frequently relate to professional role conflicts. Among those interviewed in the Boston study, most described ideal spiritual care to be individualized, voluntary, inclusive of chaplains/clergy, and based on assessing and supporting patient spirituality (Phelps et al., 2012).

Nonetheless, despite patient preferences and overall positive evaluations, most patients with advanced cancer in the Boston study had never received any form of spiritual care from their oncology nurses or physicians (87% and 94%) (M. J. Balboni et al., 2013). Similarly, other studies report 6–26% of patients report having had their spiritual needs addressed by the medical system (Astrow et al., 2007; T. A. Balboni et al., 2007; Ehman et al., 1999). These studies demonstrate patient preferences concerning medical professionals addressing patients' R/S, and also highlight the importance of sensitivity to the minority of patients who do not want R/S to be addressed in their patient care.

RELIGION/SPIRITUALITY AND MEDICAL OUTCOMES AT THE END OF LIFE

Studies suggest that spiritual care in the medical setting is associated with notable medical outcomes among patients with life-threatening illness. A study of hospitalized patients in Chicago found that patients who reported that their spiritual needs were not being addressed by medical staff were more likely to negatively assess overall quality of care and be less satisfied with their medical care (Williams et al., 2011). Moreover, in a multi-regional study of advanced cancer patients followed through death, patients who reported high support of their spiritual needs by the medical team at baseline had better quality of life near death (T. A. Balboni et al., 2010). Furthermore, patients reporting high support of their spiritual needs by the medical team were three times more likely to enter hospice at the end of life as compared to patients receiving low spiritual support (T. A. Balboni et al., 2010). High religious coping patients whose spiritual needs were well-supported by the medical system were five times more likely to enter hospice and five times less likely to receive aggressive care during the final week of life. Consequently, while high religious copers are more likely to receive aggressive care at the end of life as found in the Phelps et al study (Phelps et al., 2009), subsequent analyses showed that medical system spiritual support reverses this outcome. In a follow-up report, the associations of spiritual care with medical care received at the end of life were found to impact end-of-life medical costs (T. Balboni et al., 2011). The medical care of patients whose spiritual needs were poorly supported cost on average $2,441 more in the final week of life than patients who were spiritually well-supported by the medical team.

By comparison, the Coping with Cancer study also showed that religious/spiritual support from religious communities predicted more aggressive care in the last week of life (T.A. Balboni, 2013), suggesting that collaboration with and education of religious communities may be part of an important strategy to help reduce aggressive care within terminal disease. Certain religious beliefs such as hoping for a miracle (Widera et al., 2011) or the sanctity of life (Sulmasy, 2006) may be correlated with religious patients' medical decisions, and further supported by patients' faith communities (T.A. Balboni, 2013) and ministers (LeBaron et al., 2015). Religious beliefs appear to hold an important role in patient decisions, and on-going studies seek to describe if clergy intend these outcomes and the degree to which they discuss medical issues at the end of life.

These studies demonstrate that spiritual care in the medical setting strongly impacts patient end-of-life outcomes, such as satisfaction with care near or at the end of life, and patient medical decision-making. These outcome studies demonstrate that patients' R/S, patient community supporters, and the medical team's provision of spiritual care are not peripheral to the medical experience, but have a cascading effect measurable within other domains of medicince. Outcome studies highlight the importance of the inclusion of spiritual care as a key component of the palliative care system, particularly among high religious coping patients and ethnic minorities, populations at greater risk of receiving futile, aggressive interventions at the end of life. This evidence points to the need for a comprehensive approach to spiritual care within palliative care of patients.

SPIRITUAL CARE TRAINING OF MEDICAL PROFESSIONALS

The National Consensus Project (NCP) in its Clinical Practice Guidelines for Quality Palliative Care has highlighted spiritual, religious, and existential aspects of care as one of eight key components of quality palliative care ("National Consensus Project, 2009). As a follow-up to the NCP guidelines, leaders within spiritual care convened a consensus conference in 2009 in order to define key questions related to spiritual care, particularly the question of spiritual care roles and organization (Puchalski et al., 2009). Consensus Conference leaders concluded that an "interprofessional spiritual care" model based within a generalist-specialist medical approach was the most appropriate paradigm in engaging patients' R/S within palliative care. This model emphasizes that an initial spiritual screening should be performed by medical professionals such as physicians and nurses. If a spiritual issue or spiritual distress is identified, and is considered to be a complex or unresolved spiritual issue, then health care providers should refer the patient to a board-certified chaplain. As trained R/S specialists, certified chaplains provide a comprehensive spiritual assessment and formulate a spiritual treatment plan, which the healthcare provider can subsequently incorporate within the overall treatment plan.

The Consensus Conference Interprofessional Spiritual Care Model provides an important foundation for providing spiritual care as a component of comprehensive palliative care and aids in clarifying the roles of different medical caregivers in spiritual care provision. However, many practical issues remain regarding spiritual care roles that require further exploration. First, it is not clear how the medical system should interface with patients' spiritual communities and clergy in meeting the spiritual needs of patients (M.J. Balboni & T.A. Balboni, 2010; T.A. Balboni, 2013; LeBaron et al., 2016). In light of the frequent central role of patients' own spiritual communities and clergy in their illness experience, a spiritual care model that includes a central role for spiritual communities—when they are relevant for patients—is required, as reflected by the Joint Commission's spiritual care guidelines (Joint Commission, 2011). Second, data suggests that few medical professionals receive spiritual care training, and that lack of training is the strongest predictor of whether spiritual care is actually provided (M. J. Balboni et al., 2013). Few training programs exist and most are optional, resulting in training of those who are already predisposed to provide spiritual care (M. J. Balboni et al., 2014; Zollfrank et al., 2015). In addition, multiple systemic barriers remain problematic and entrenched in nurse and physician attitudes. Barriers that predict less frequent spiritual care provision include inadequate training, "not my professional role," and "power inequity with patient" (M. J. Balboni et al., 2014). Third, a frequent lack of sufficient funding for hospital chaplaincy (Cadge et al., 2008; Miller-McLemore, 2005) is another clear obstacle, implicating the need for greater chaplaincy funding and greater training of other medical providers (e.g., physicians, nurses, social workers) in generalist spiritual care competencies (M. J. Balboni et al., 2013). Finally, the frequent central role of patient R/S in determining patients' values and medical decisions at the end of life (T.A. Balboni, 2013; Phelps et al., 2009; Steinhauser et al., 2000; Widera et al., 2011) demonstrates the need for greater interaction between spiritual care professionals and medical caregivers in spiritual care provision. This is implied in the 2010 study (T. A. Balboni et al., 2010) which found that spiritual care from the medical system, including physicians and nurses, was associated with higher rates of hospice use and less aggressive care at the EOL, whereas chaplaincy visits alone were not predictive of these outcomes. These issues point to the need for further research to better clarify spiritual care roles and the interaction among medical caregivers, chaplaincy, and spiritual communities in providing palliative care.

SUGGESTIONS FOR FUTURE RESEARCH

Despite current research trends and national guidelines incorporating spiritual care as part of palliative end-of-life care, (Joint Commission, 2011; National Consensus Project, 2009) medical systems often fail to sufficiently address and provide for the spiritual needs of patients facing advanced illness (M. J. Balboni et al., 2013; T. A. Balboni et al., 2007). Given its importance in advanced illness, further research is required in order to more clearly identify the roles of the health care providers and better identify the ways in which spiritual care should be provided. As Steinhauser et al. suggest in a review on the state of the science of palliative care and spirituality, we currently stand at a critical juncture in the research field (Steinhauser, under review). They suggest the need to (1) consistently define the concept of religion/spirituality, (2) advance ways of measurement of religion/spirituality, (3) clarify what the evidence base is for key outcomes in palliative care, (4) standardize procedures to screen and assess spiritual needs, (5) identify interventions that have been successful and those that must be improved, and (6) educate professionals in addressing religion/spirituality among palliative care patients and their families. Conducting research in these areas has the potential to offer further knowledge of the interaction of religion/spirituality within palliative care, and to improve the spiritual, social, psychological, and physical dimensions of patients' experience of advanced illness.

RELIGION AND SPIRITUALITY IN PATIENT ENCOUNTERS

The intimate interplay of spirituality with quality of life (for both patients and family caregivers) and patient medical decision-making and care can be seen in encounters between palliative care physicians and their patients with advanced illness. As noted, religion/spirituality often affects patients' ability to cope with illness and influences their medical decisions. Consider the following four cases illustrating how religion/spirituality can be intertwined within serious illness.

FOUR CASE DESCRIPTIONS

Case #1: Ms. Rodriguez, a 35-year-old Latina with two young children, has been in the ICU for the previous three weeks having suffered traumatic brain injury from an automobile accident. She has shown no signs of improvement and physicians do not believe there is any chance of meaningful recovery. Having been active Pentecostal believers who were also strongly committed to the sanctity of life, the Rodriguez family is surrounded by a caring faith community. Church members are involved by providing child care throughout the ordeal, and many congregational members hold vigils at the hospital praying that God would do a miracle and "wake her from her sleep." The palliative care team attempts to discuss terminal extubation but Mr. Rodriguez refuses, indicating that doctors' knowledge is limited. Both he and his wife firmly believe that once enough people pray, God will certainly do a miracle.

Case #2: Ms. White is a 67-year-old white, retired psychologist, who holds deep convictions about the power of alternative healing for her cancer. She and her partner participate in an all-female healing energy group, and they consider themselves spiritual not religious. Ms. White was discouraged by her group from resorting to Western medicine, but she and her partner ultimately decide to use both methods to address her cancer. Some of the energy healers in her group disagree with her decision and view chemo and radiation therapies as unnatural poisons. Ms. White is referred for a palliative care consult after she indicated to her oncologist that she is "concerned about quality of life and not just being treated with poisons." During her interview with the palliative care doctor, Ms. White mentions that her primary means of coping is through the aura of healing energy. The physician responds with slight discomfort in his expression and posture. "Be careful with some forms of pseudo-science," he warns, "there are a lot of people who will take advantage of you."

Case #3: Mr. R is a 46-year-old white, married man struggling with metastatic throat cancer for the past three years. He is the father of two elementary-school-age daughters, and he is a popular high school science and religion teacher at a conservative Roman Catholic high school. Recently the cancer progressed to the point of causing pain and difficulty with swallowing, prompting a palliative care consult. Mr. R is visited by the palliative care physician, who prescribes long-acting morphine and recommends palliative radiation therapy to improve swallowing. The palliative physician explains to Mr. R that two weeks of "palliative radiation" should give him some relief from his swallowing symptoms. Mr. R then asks, "What does 'palliative' exactly mean?" His physician explains that palliative care and palliative radiation aim to relieve symptoms of his disease and increase his quality of life but not cure the cancer itself. Upon hearing this explanation, Mr. R becomes angry, and states, "I don't like your attitude, doctor. We're going to kick this thing and I expect you to be on my team—or let's find another doctor who will be." After assuring Mr. R. that she will do everything medically possible in fighting the cancer, the palliative care physician asks him what is giving him strength during this difficult time and what is behind his strong will to fight. "I'm not worried about myself. I know where I'll be when I die. It is because of my two daughters." Mr. R replies, "God has given those girls to me as my responsibility and I have to be around at least until they finish high school. If Jesus can heal all kinds of sickness, why not me?" Mr. R. sobs before the physician. The physician, a practicing Roman Catholic herself, holds Mr. R's hand and says. "I am with you." Within moments he regains his composure and she returns to discussing next steps for treating his pain in swallowing.

Case #4: Ms. Watson is a 43-year-old African-American woman living in subsidized housing, diagnosed with Stage III HPV-positive uterine cancer. With aggressive therapy, she has a 32% chance of cure, but requires daily radiation over the course of seven weeks. Unfortunately, Ms. Watson is missing some treatments each week. On two occasions when coming for treatment, she has asked the physician about his faith and told him that she needed prayer. But the physician, who only attends religious services on Jewish holidays, responds that he is not religious himself, that his job is to take care of her illness, and that she should talk to a minister about spiritual topics. Though raised in the church, Ms. Watson got into drugs in her late teens and early twenties, at which time she had her three children from two different fathers, both also drug users. She tried many times to end her drug habit, without success. Then, when she was 29 years old and social services agents were on the verge of taking away her three children, she experienced a profound spiritual conversion. "Jesus saved me from the grip of the devil," she recounts. "When I came to him, I was that sinful woman at his feet, just crying, crying tears on his feet." She then added, "Now, I'm paying for those old sins. Even when the blood first started coming, I knew I was bleeding for my sins."

IMPLICATIONS FOR PALLIATIVE CARE PRACTICE

SPIRITUAL INFLUENCES ON PATIENTS' EXPERIENCE AND TREATMENT

As each case illustrates, the interplay between religion and life-threatening illness is complex. The experience of patients with serious illness is directly shaped by an assortment of particular religious or spiritual beliefs, practices, relationships, and motivations. These issues are multifaceted, which partly explains why a majority of clinicians avoid or sidestep patient spirituality given its challenges. As the cases illustrate, however, neglecting or avoiding religion/spirituality has significant implications for the medical care of patients. In case #1, the patient's proxy believes that his wife will recover from traumatic brain injury through prayer to an all-powerful Healer. In case #2, the physician's negative receptivity to the patient's reliance on alternative spiritual healing therapies undermined the patient's trust in her doctor. The physician's response not only fails to be patient-centered but also could enable future alienation or communication breakdown in the patient-clinician relationship. In case #3, Mr. R's desire to be present for his daughters is supported by his faith-based moral code to take care of one's children as well as a belief that God can heal no matter the odds. The patient is not willing to consider his condition as terminal and is hostile if anyone implies it. In case #4, Ms. Watson has a realistic chance of cure but this partly depends on her not missing seven consecutive weeks of radiation therapy. She misses some treatments for unclear reasons, perhaps connected to her socio-economic status, the practical needs of taking care of her grandchildren, or her interpretation that her cancer is a just discipline or judgment from God for her past life of drugs and illicit sexual activity. In all four cases, particular religious or spiritual beliefs and motivations influence how the patient understands and acts upon illness.

PHYSICIAN RESPONSES TO PATIENT SPIRITUALITY

Each case also illustrates how differing responses from a physician concerning religion/spirituality may impact the course of care. In case #1, the medical team's efforts to discuss continuation of futile treatment are rebuffed by the patient's proxy, who finds support in his beliefs (which he reasonably believes are shared with his wife) and finding additional support from congregants. The palliative care team could respond to the proxy's reliance on a miracle with openness and expressions of support, or alternatively with argumentative and frustrated reactions. In cases #2 and #4 the physician held biases against each patient's spiritual perspective. In case #2 this undermined trust, which created an unhealthy relational environment that could reasonably lead to future miscommunication or dismissal of the physician's medical advice. In case #4, the physician politely declined interaction with his patient who twice initiated a faith discussion. Her initiation suggested that religion was not only important to her, but may also have been part of the reason for her missing treatment. Would her course of treatment have been different if her physician had engaged her faith or knew her story in greater detail? In case #3, by contrast, the physician accidently challenged the patient's assumption that he would be cured. At first the patient became upset with her since "palliative therapy" was a threat to his personal and religious hope. The physician not only successfully reassured Mr. R. that they were on the same team, but she also asked a question about his underlying motives, which uncovered deeper religious motivations driving his care decisions. This not only may inform the physician's future interactions with Mr. R but also creates a closer bond. In time, this bond could enable discussions that assess the unlikeliness of cure or his need to entrust his daughters to God and others.

BEST PRACTICES IN PALLIATIVE CARE

These case scenarios demonstrate ways in which a patient's religion/spirituality can intersect with life-threatening illness, and highlights that deeper discussions about religion/spirituality between palliative care providers and their patients can improve patients' quality of life, care, and medical outcomes. Specifically, the Spiritual Care Consensus Conference in 2009 identified eight key spiritual care competencies that palliative care providers should attain (Table 10.1).

TABLE 10.1. Spiritual Care Competencies in Palliative Care from 2009 Spiritual Care Consensus Conference (Puchalski et al., 2009)

1	Training in spiritual care commensurate with scope of physician's practice
2	Awareness of basic spiritual diagnosis and treatment
3	Awareness of spiritual resources available to patients (e.g., chaplaincy)
4	Training in the tenants of different faiths and cultures to aid in spiritual and cultural competence, enabling better patient care
5	Basic training in the influences that spiritual values and beliefs have on medical decisions, both for patients and their families
6	Awareness of spiritual care roles of various providers, including knowledge of when to refer to each
7	Training in compassionate presence and active listening
8	Training in self-care, spiritual self-reflection, and spiritual self-care

Future research will be critical in validating and further developing each of these competencies. To date, few studies exist that examine the nature of these competencies, how to best develop them, or how to evaluate their impact on patient care. From this vantage point the empirical evidence that would advance best practices in religion/spirituality and palliative care is lacking.

While these key competencies are important to flesh out in research, here we sketch two concepts that are basic to the physician-patient relationship as it pertains to religion/spirituality: (1) Performing a spiritual screening of patients to identify spiritual relevance to illness, and (2) necessary conditions for physician engagement of patient religion/spirituality.

1. SPIRITUAL SCREENING: ASK PATIENT ABOUT R/S IN FIRST MEETING

Spiritual screening is a critical tool for bringing R/S into the context of palliative medicine. Medical care givers should be aware of their patient's faith and how it functions in the experience of illness. This can be achieved through a few, basic questions included as part of a general assessment at the time of initial consultation.

Probably the most cited model for spiritual screening is the FICA model (Puchalski & Romer, 2000), with "FICA" being an acronym for the domains of inquiry, including "F," or faith, asking if patients considers themselves to be spiritual or have a faith that is important to them; "I," or importance, asking about the importance of this faith to a patient's life and/or illness; "C," or community, inquiring about the patient's spiritual community supporters; and "A," or address, asking how a patient would like for their spirituality or spiritual needs to be addressed as part of care, including inquiring about whether they would like a visit from a chaplain. The FICA model has undergone testing in a sample of 76 cancer patients, with findings supporting both its feasibility and concurrent validity using quantitative measures of spirituality (Borneman et al., 2010).

As the case examples suggest, palliative care professionals who have information pertaining to their patients' spiritual understandings will inevitably be better able to understand their patients, communicate with them more clearly, and potentially navigate more skillfully the intersection of faith and palliative care. Asking a few basic spiritual questions of patients lays the foundation within the relationship for future interactions. It allows the physician to have a clearer sense of whether R/S could potentially be a factor in the patient's experience and decision-making. Asking about this subject in the first meeting also allays the patient fear that the question implies that the patient is dying—since it is taking place in the first meeting and part of the larger medical history. Spiritual inquiry also signals to the patient that the physician is open to all aspects of the patient's experience, which patients report to be supportive (M.J Balboni et al., 2013; Phelps et al., 2012). This evidence argues for the need for physicians to incorporate spiritual inquiry within their initial medical history-taking. While few physicians are performing R/S histories in palliative care settings (M. J. Balboni et al., 2013; Epstein-Peterson et al., 2015), case #1 suggests that at times it will be critical to understand and weigh the religious rationales of patients or their proxies, cases #2 and 4 illustrate the problems that arise when these issues are avoided, and case #3 suggests how spiritual inquiry can have a positive impact.

With the understanding gained from an initial assessment, medical professionals create the necessary building blocks to navigate R/S, especially in its clinical relevance to medical decision-making. Discussing R/S in its relationship to palliative medical issues has been classified as an advanced communication skill and physicians should heed warnings to not overstep their expertise (Lo et al., 2002). While complex, our case examples illustrate how avoiding or redirecting away from R/S issues is not always possible (cases #1–3) or best for the patient (case #4). For example, in case #1 the issues of sanctity of life and miracles directly contradict the medical team's prognosis and what they believe to be medically indicated. While there is little data available to guide these circumstances, several commentators have suggested that clinicians in such circumstances should express to the patient/proxy that they will not abandon them, provide them an impartial view of the medical prognosis, inquire about other hopes that the proxy has for the patient (e.g., not to be in pain), and finally, suggest that if a miracle occurs, the palliative care team's actions (e.g. withdrawal of life support) cannot prevent it (Lo et al., 2002; Sulmasy, 2006; Widera et al., 2011). Just as importantly, palliative care professionals should seek a wider collaboration by coordinating support with the patient's clergy and hospital chaplains. This is especially well illustrated in case #4, in which the medical team, being aware of the important role of Ms. Watson's religious community, might consider inviting Ms. Watson to bring spiritual supporters to her appointments to facilitate an integrated discussion and understanding of her illness and the implications of any medical interventions. These supporters might include hospital chaplains, many of whom have considerable training and experience in the context of illness, or might include the patient's pastor, an appropriate congregational member, or another spiritual friend. Integrating religion/spirituality and medical practice by making spiritual inquiries and by referring patients to chaplains requires minimal training and is feasible for any medical care-giver regardless of faith background. We will later suggest that further spiritual training also be given to medical care-givers to facilitate deeper conversations with their patients about the impacts that a patient's spirituality may have on his or her illness, but this model is a good beginning point for palliative care providers to engage their patients' spirituality.

2. CONDITIONS FOR PHYSICIAN-PATIENT ENGAGEMENT

More controversially, there is at least some initial evidence that clinicians may go beyond spiritual inquiry under certain circumstances by engaging their patients in spiritual questions, conversations, or spiritual practices (e.g., prayer). Evidence for or against such engagement is scant. Some initial evidence is from a 2011 multisite, cross-sectional study of advanced, incurable cancer patients, oncology nurses, and oncology physicians (M. J. Balboni et al., 2011). This study found that a majority of palliative care patients, nurses, and physicians view spiritual encounters between the clinician and patient as potentially appropriate, depending on certain conditions. The most frequently noted conditions were that the clinician must have a prior awareness of the patient's spiritual background and a meaningful relationship in place with the patient. Most agree that engaging in spiritual conversations or practices involves relational dynamics that transcend either a utilitarian exchange of goods or a brief meeting of strangers (Curlin & Hall, 2005). The physician-patient relationship that includes a spiritual gesture, conversation, or practice must take place within a growing or established relationship. Additionally, the same study (M. J. Balboni et al., 2011) found that in order for a spiritual encounter to appropriately take place, both patient and clinician needed to feel comfortable and that this was more likely to take place when both sides held some concordant spiritual beliefs. While not always the case, it is more likely that a shared set of beliefs or practices will create positive conditions of spiritual engagement, whereas the greater the difference in spiritual identity or beliefs the more potential for challenges and discomfort. Some have suggested that religion/spirituality functions like a human "language" (Hall et al., 2004). When two people do not share the same language, shared communication is not impossible but more difficult. However, having a shared spiritual "language" allows for a greater set of shared presuppositions, more overlapping of theological beliefs, and potentially, greater familiarity with one another's particular spiritual practices. When clinicians have a relationship with their patients, know something of their spiritual background, and share a level of concordance, then a greater level of engagement beyond spiritual screening may be appropriate, desired, and positively impact outcomes (T.A. Balboni, 2013; Phelps et al., 2012). This principle may also apply to the issue of who may initiate a spiritual encounter. For example, several commentators have suggested that it is ill-advised for a physician to initiate prayer with a patient (Lo et al., 2003). However, a majority of patients, nurses, and physicians in the Boston study indicated that practitioner-initiated prayer was at least occasionally appropriate in the palliative care context (M. J. Balboni et al., 2011), and 80% of patients said that they would find practitioner-initiated prayer personally supportive. This suggests that initiation by palliative care clinicians may at times be warranted, especially if several of the conditions above are met.

In all four cases, the physician-patient relationship is potentially affected by the dynamics of concordance and discordance. In case #1, a physician who believes in a God of miracles or who resonates with the sanctity of life will have a greater ability to directly engage in the language of the patient and proxy, and may have available opportunities to discuss these issues with greater acuity and skill. With discordance there is greater risk of disagreement or alienation. In case #3, Mr. R and his physician share a similar religious tradition. The physician hears about Mr. R's religious motivations, and while she does not reveal her own faith, it likely enables her to more immediately sympathize with Mr. R's motivations and strong hope for a miracle. The situation does not call on her to go further than to regain his trust and express her support of him. There may come a time, however, when it will be especially helpful for him to understand her own faith background, such as when a patient wants futile treatment in the hopes of a miracle. Their shared beliefs may enable her to talk with nuance about his refusal to consider palliative care and hospice, perhaps suggesting a different point of view on how his faith informs the medical decisions he may face.

In cases #2 and 4, there are multiple differences at play including metaphysical beliefs (#2), race, socio-economic background, and religious identity (#4). These factors likely influence each clinician's ability to understand and engage the patient's beliefs and actions. Discordance cannot be changed in most circumstances but certain differences can be mitigated when the physician approaches the patient with intent to understand and empathize (Lo et al., 2002). In addition, navigating differences includes both accommodation whenever possible and a respectful candor in circumstances when an impasse has been reached (Curlin & Hall, 2005). In case #2, the physician clearly is skeptical when it comes to the therapeutic effects of healing energy. It may have been better, however, if he did not express this view immediately to Mrs. White without first understanding the level of importance that spirituality held for her or assessing its potential to undermine clinical treatment. By contrast, in case #4, the physician does not engage, even with multiple invitations, the patient's religious gestures. There is spiritual discordance in two ways. Not only is there denominational discordance with the patient Christian and the physician Jewish, but the level of importance of religion in each of their lives also diverges. A non-religious physician can engage a religious person in at least three ways. First, spiritual inquiry enables the physician to assess how large a role faith holds in the patient's life and its potential to influence treatment. Second, the physician can invite the patient to include her spiritual supporters in her treatment visits and decisions. Third, when available, hospital chaplains should be included as part of care. This is especially important in those cases when the patient is religious and the physician is not.

Upon assessing key conditions for interaction related to religion/spirituality, physicians and nurses will have a clearer understanding of how to handle patients' spiritual issues and be better positioned to sensitively offer interaction regarding patients' religion/spirituality. If nurses and physicians were to more frequently make spiritual inquiries then not only would spiritual issues be frequently identified (Alcorn et al., 2010), but some issues would be seen to directly impinge on palliative decisions as seen in the cases described (Balboni TA, 2013). This recognition has led John Peteet et al. to put forth a "clinical relevance model," which suggests that "the more clearly a religious or spiritual issue is connected to medical treatment, the more clearly a physician is obligated to understand and engage that issue as part of their professional obligation" (Peteet & D'Ambra, 2011, p. 27). For example, Peteet et. al. suggest that if a cancer patient believes that his or her cancer is a result of divine judgment (as illustrated in case #4) a physician should only directly engage this belief when it is interfering with clinical issues. Thus, if the physician came to understand that Ms. Watson believed her cancer to be caused by divine punishment but she continued to adhere to an agreed-upon treatment plan, he should refer her to chaplaincy or encourage her to talk with her pastor. But if the physician suspects that the patient's belief is infringing on willingness to receive treatment, as case #4 implies, then it falls clearly within the orbit of his professional relevance. The manner and depth of engagement will depend on issues of concordance, the physician's relationship with the patient, the physician's comfort level in directly engaging the patient's faith, and the patient's desire to be engaged by the physician. In cases of perceived discordance, the physician should enlist others from the medical team, such as a nurse, social worker, another physician, or hospital chaplain, in order to find ways to navigate and constructively engage the patient's spiritual beliefs and the medical issues being faced. With patient consent, her minister should also be included within the care of the patient. In the case of Ms. Watson, the inclusion of her minister would advance the opportunity for pastoral care to engage her belief of punishment of her sins. If informed about her medical condition and the importance of treatment, the minister would be enabled to discuss with the patient from within their tradition the importance of her not missing future treatment. The minister may also be able to facilitate practical supports from within the community, such as transportation to the clinic or help with childcare for Ms. Watson's grandchildren.

CONCLUSION

Within the field of palliative care, there is a growing body of data demonstrating the importance and impact of religion/spirituality during advanced illness. Clinicians should begin by taking a short spiritual history and by assessing this dimension of illness, especially in its clinical relevance to decision making and quality of life. Training of clinicians remains a critical need within the field. Conditions for engaging in these complex relationships include religious/spiritual concordance and establishing a physician-patient relationship. External supports, including the patient's minister and hospital chaplains, are important.

AUTHORS' NOTE

Portions of this chapter were previously published by the authors:

El Nawawi, N. M., Balboni, M. J., Balboni, T. A. (2012). Palliative care and spiritual care: The crucial role of spiritual care in the care of patients with advanced illness. *Curr Opin Support Palliat Care*, 6(2):269–274.

REFERENCES

Alcorn, S. R., Balboni, M. J., Prigerson, H. G., Reynolds, A., Phelps, A. C., Wright, A. A., . . . Balboni, T. A. (2010). "If God wanted me yesterday, I wouldn't be here today": Religious and spiritual themes in patients' experiences of advanced cancer. *J Palliat Med*, 13(5), 581–588. Retrieved from http://www.ncbi.nlm.nih.gov/entrez/query.fcgi?cmd=Retrieve&db=PubMed&dopt=Citation&list_uids=20408763

Astrow, A. B., Wexler, A., Texeira, K., He, M. K., & Sulmasy, D. P. (2007). Is failure to meet spiritual needs associated with cancer patients' perceptions of quality of care and their satisfaction with care? *J Clin Oncol*, 25(36), 5753–5757. Retrieved from http://www.ncbi.nlm.nih.gov/entrez/query.fcgi?cmd=Retrieve&db=PubMed&dopt=Citation&list_uids=18089871

Balboni, M. J., Babar, A., Dillinger, J., Phelps, A. C., George, E., Block, S. D., . . . Balboni, T. A. (2011). "It depends": viewpoints of patients, physicians, and nurses on patient-practitioner prayer in the setting of advanced cancer. *J Pain Symp Manage*, 41(5), 836–847. doi:10.1016/j.jpainsymman.2010.07.008

Balboni, M. J., & Balboni, T. A. (2010). Reintegrating care for the dying, body and soul. *Harvard Theological Review*, 103(3), 351–364.

Balboni, M. J., Sullivan, A., Amobi, A., Phelps, A. C., Gorman, D. P., Zollfrank, A., . . . Balboni, T. A. (2013). Why is spiritual care infrequent at the end of life? Spiritual care perceptions among patients, nurses, and physicians and the role of training. *J Clin Oncol*, 31(4), 461–467. doi:10.1200/JCO.2012.44.6443

Balboni, M. J., Sullivan, A., Enzinger, A. C., Epstein-Peterson, Z. D., Tseng, Y. D., Mitchell, C., . . . Balboni, T. A. (2014). Nurse and physician barriers to spiritual care provision at the end of life. *J Pain Symptom Manage, 48*(3), 400–410. doi:10.1016/j.jpainsymman.2013.09.020

Balboni, T., Balboni, M., Paulk, M. E., Phelps, A., Wright, A., Peteet, J., . . . Prigerson, H. (2011). Support of cancer patients' spiritual needs and associations with medical care costs at the end of life. *Cancer, 117*(23), 5383–5391. doi:10.1002/cncr.26221

Balboni T. A., Balboni, M., Phelps, A. C., Gallivan, K., Paulk, M. E., Wright, A. A., . . .Prigerson, H. G. (2013). Provision of spiritual support to advanced cancer patients by religious communities and associations with medical care at the end of life. *JAMA Internal Medicine, 173*(12), 1109–1117.

Balboni, T. A., Paulk, M. E., Balboni, M. J., Phelps, A. C., Loggers, E. T., Wright, A. A., . . . Prigerson, H. G. (2010). Provision of spiritual care to patients with advanced cancer: associations with medical care and quality of life near death. *J Clin Oncol, 28*(3), 445–452. Retrieved from http://www.ncbi.nlm.nih.gov/entrez/query.fcgi?cmd=Retrieve&db=PubMed&dopt=Citation&list_uids=20008625

Balboni, T. A., Vanderwerker, L. C., Block, S. D., Paulk, M. E., Lathan, C. S., Peteet, J. R., & Prigerson, H. G. (2007). Religiousness and spiritual support among advanced cancer patients and associations with end-of-life treatment preferences and quality of life. *J Clin Oncol, 25*(5), 555–560. Retrieved from http://www.ncbi.nlm.nih.gov/entrez/query.fcgi?cmd=Retrieve&db=PubMed&dopt=Citation&list_uids=17290065

Block, S. D. (2006). Psychological issues in end-of-life care. *J Palliat Med, 9*(3), 751–772. doi:10.1089/jpm.2006.9.751

Borneman, T., Ferrell, B., & Puchalski, C. M. (2010). Evaluation of the FICA tool for spiritual assessment. *J Pain Symptom Manage, 40*(2), 163–173. Retrieved from http://www.ncbi.nlm.nih.gov/entrez/query.fcgi?cmd=Retrieve&db=PubMed&dopt=Citation&list_uids=20619602

Brady, M. J., Peterman, A. H., Fitchett, G., Mo, M., & Cella, D. (1999). A case for including spirituality in quality of life measurement in oncology. *Psychooncology, 8*(5), 417–428. Retrieved from http://www.ncbi.nlm.nih.gov/entrez/query.fcgi?cmd=Retrieve&db=PubMed&dopt=Citation&list_uids=10559801

Cadge, W., Freese, J., & Christakis, N. A. (2008). The provision of hospital chaplaincy in the United States: a national overview. *South Med J, 101*(6), 626–630. doi:10.1097/SMJ.0b013e3181706856

Clemens, K. E., J. B., Klaschik, E. (2009). The history of hospice. In D. Walsh (Ed.), *Palliative Medicine* (pp. 18–23). Philadelphia, PA: Saunders.

Curlin, F. A., & Hall, D. E. (2005). Strangers or friends? A proposal for a new spirituality-in-medicine ethic. *J Gen Intern Med, 20*(4), 370–374. Retrieved from http://www.ncbi.nlm.nih.gov/entrez/query.fcgi?cmd=Retrieve&db=PubMed&dopt=Citation&list_uids=15857497

Delgado-Guay, M. O., Hui, D., Parsons, H. A., Govan, K., De la Cruz, M., Thorney, S., & Bruera, E. (2011). Spirituality, religiosity, and spiritual pain in advanced cancer patients. *Journal of Pain and Symptom Management, 41*(6), 986–994. doi:10.1016/j.jpainsymman.2010.09.017

Ehman, J. W., Ott, B. B., Short, T. H., Ciampa, R. C., & Hansen-Flaschen, J. (1999). Do patients want physicians to inquire about their spiritual or religious beliefs if they become gravely ill? *Arch Intern Med, 159*(15), 1803–1806. Retrieved from http://www.ncbi.nlm.nih.gov/entrez/query.fcgi?cmd=Retrieve&db=PubMed&dopt=Citation&list_uids=10448785

Epstein-Peterson, Z. D., Sullivan, A. J., Enzinger, A. C., Trevino, K. M., Zollfrank, A. A., Balboni, M. J., . . . Balboni, T. A. (2015). Examining forms of spiritual care provided in the advanced cancer setting. *Am J Hosp Palliat Care, 32*(7), 750–757. doi:10.1177/1049909114540318

Hall, D. E., Koenig, H. G., & Meador, K. G. (2004). Conceptualizing "religion": How language shapes and constrains knowledge in the study of religion and health. *Perspect Biol Med, 47*(3), 386–401. Retrieved from http://www.ncbi.nlm.nih.gov/entrez/query.fcgi?cmd=Retrieve&db=PubMed&dopt=Citation&list_uids=15247504

Joint Commission. (2011). (3.7.0.0 ed., pp. PC.02.02.13): E-dition.

Koenig, H. G. (1998). Religious attitudes and practices of hospitalized medically ill older adults. *Int J Geriatr Psychiatry, 13*(4), 213–224. Retrieved from http://www.ncbi.nlm.nih.gov/entrez/query.fcgi?cmd=Retrieve&db=PubMed&dopt=Citation&list_uids=9646148

LeBaron, V. T., Cooke, A., Resmini, J., Garinther, A., Chow, V., Quinones, R., . . . Balboni, M. J. (2015). Clergy views on a good versus a poor death: Ministry to the terminally ill. *J Palliat Med.* doi:10.1089/jpm.2015.0176

LeBaron, V. T., Smith, P. T., Quinones, R., Nibecker, C., Sanders, J. J., Timms, R., . . . Balboni, M. J. (2016). how community clergy provide spiritual care: Toward a conceptual framework for clergy end-of-life education. *J Pain Symptom Manage, 51*(4), 673–681. doi:10.1016/j.jpainsymman.2015.11.016

Lo, B., Kates, L. W., Ruston, D., Arnold, R. M., Cohen, C. B., Puchalski, C. M., . . . Tulsky, J. A. (2003). Responding to requests regarding prayer and religious ceremonies by patients near the end of life and their families. *J Palliat Med, 6*(3), 409–415. Retrieved from http://www.ncbi.nlm.nih.gov/entrez/query.fcgi?cmd=Retrieve&db=PubMed&dopt=Citation&list_uids=14509486

Lo, B., Ruston, D., Kates, L. W., Arnold, R. M., Cohen, C. B., Faber-Langendoen, K., . . . Tulsky, J. A. (2002). Discussing religious and spiritual issues at the end of life: A practical guide for physicians. *JAMA, 287*(6), 749–754. Retrieved from http://www.ncbi.nlm.nih.gov/entrez/query.fcgi?cmd=Retrieve&db=PubMed&dopt=Citation&list_uids=11851542

MacLean, C. D., Susi, B., Phifer, N., Schultz, L., Bynum, D., Franco, M., . . . Cykert, S. (2003). Patient preference for physician discussion and practice of spirituality. *J Gen Intern Med, 18*(1), 38–43. Retrieved from http://www.ncbi.nlm.nih.gov/entrez/query.fcgi?cmd=Retrieve&db=PubMed&dopt=Citation&list_uids=12534762

McCord, G., Gilchrist, V. J., Grossman, S. D., King, B. D., McCormick, K. E., Oprandi, A. M., . . . Srivastava, M. (2004). Discussing spirituality with patients: a rational and ethical approach. *Ann Fam Med, 2*(4), 356–361. Retrieved from http://www.ncbi.nlm.nih.gov/entrez/query.fcgi?cmd=Retrieve&db=PubMed&dopt=Citation&list_uids=15335136

Miller-McLemore, B. (2005). Pastoral Theology as Public Theology: Revolutions in the "Fourth Area." In R. J. Hunter (Ed.), *Dictionary of Pastoral Care and Counseling* (pp. 1370–1380). Nashville: Abingdon.

Moadel, A., Morgan, C., Fatone, A., Grennan, J., Carter, J., Laruffa, G., . . . Dutcher, J. (1999). Seeking meaning and hope: Self-reported spiritual and existential needs among an ethnically-diverse cancer patient population. *Psychooncology, 8*(5), 378–385. Retrieved from http://www.ncbi.nlm.nih.gov/entrez/query.fcgi?cmd=Retrieve&db=PubMed&dopt=Citation&list_uids=10559797

National Consensus Project. (2009). NCP Clinical Practice Guidelines for Quality Palliative Care. 2nd ed. Retrieved from http://ww.nationalconsensusproject.org/guideline.pdf

Peteet, J. R., & D'Ambra, M. N. (2011). *The soul of medicine: spiritual perspectives and clinical practice.* Baltimore, MD: Johns Hopkins University Press.

Pew Research Center (2014). America's changing religious landscape. http://assets.pewresearch.org/wp-content/uploads/sites/11/2015/05/RLS-08-26-full-report.pdf, Washington, DC: Author.

Phelps, A. C., Lauderdale, K. E., Alcorn, S., Dillinger, J., Balboni, M. T., Van Wert, M., . . . Balboni, T. A. (2012). Addressing spirituality within the care of patients at the end of life: Perspectives of patients with advanced cancer, oncologists, and oncology nurses. *J Clin Oncol, 30*(20), 2538–2544. doi:10.1200/JCO.2011.40.3766

Phelps, A. C., Maciejewski, P. K., Nilsson, M., Balboni, T. A., Wright, A. A., Paulk, M. E., . . . Prigerson, H. G. (2009). Religious coping and use of intensive life-prolonging care near death in patients with advanced cancer. *JAMA, 301*(11), 1140–1147. Retrieved from http://www.ncbi.nlm.nih.gov/entrez/query.fcgi?cmd=Retrieve&db=PubMed&dopt=Citation&list_uids=19293414

Prigerson, H. G. (1992). Socialization to dying: Social determinants of death acknowledgement and treatment among terminally ill geriatric patients. *Journal of health and social behavior, 33*(4), 378–395. Retrieved from http://www.ncbi.nlm.nih.gov/pubmed/1464721

Puchalski, C., Ferrell, B., Virani, R., Otis-Green, S., Baird, P., Bull, J., . . . Sulmasy, D. (2009). Improving the quality of spiritual care as a dimension of palliative care: The report of the Consensus Conference. *J Palliat Med*, 12(10), 885–904. Retrieved from http://www.ncbi.nlm.nih.gov/entrez/query.fcgi?cmd=Retrieve&db=PubMed&dopt=Citation&list_uids=19807235

Puchalski, C., & Romer, A. L. (2000). Taking a spiritual history allows clinicians to understand patients more fully. *J Palliat Med*, 3(1), 129–137. doi:10.1089/jpm.2000.3.129

Saunders, C. (2006). *Cecily Saunders: Selected Writings 1958-2004*. New York, NY: Oxford University Press.

Silvestri, G. A., Knittig, S., Zoller, J. S., & Nietert, P. J. (2003). Importance of faith on medical decisions regarding cancer care. *J Clin Oncol*, 21(7), 1379–1382. Retrieved from http://www.ncbi.nlm.nih.gov/entrez/query.fcgi?cmd=Retrieve&db=PubMed&dopt=Citation&list_uids=12663730

Steinhauser, K. E., Christakis, N. A., Clipp, E. C., McNeilly, M., McIntyre, L., & Tulsky, J. A. (2000). Factors considered important at the end of life by patients, family, physicians, and other care providers. *JAMA*, 284(19), 2476–2482. Retrieved from http://www.ncbi.nlm.nih.gov/entrez/query.fcgi?cmd=Retrieve&db=PubMed&dopt=Citation&list_uids=11074777

Steinhauser, K.E., Fitchett, G., Handzo, G., Johnson, K.S., Koenig, H., Pargament, K., Puchalski, C., Sinclair, S., Taylor, E.J., Balboni, T.A. (under review). State of the Science of Spirituality and Palliative Care Research Part I: Definitions and Taxonomy, Measurement, and Outcomes.

Sulmasy, D. P. (2006). Spiritual issues in the care of dying patients: ". . . it's okay between me and god." *JAMA*, 296(11), 1385–1392. Retrieved from http://www.ncbi.nlm.nih.gov/entrez/query.fcgi?cmd=Retrieve&db=PubMed&dopt=Citation&list_uids=16985231

U.S. Religions Landscape Survey. (2008). Retrieved from http://religions.pewforum.org/maps

Vallurupalli, M., Lauderdale, K., Balboni, M. J., Phelps, A. C., Block, S. D., Ng, A. K., . . . Balboni, T. A. (2012). The role of spirituality and religious coping in the quality of life of patients with advanced cancer receiving palliative radiation therapy. *J Support Oncol*, 10(2), 81–87. doi:10.1016/j.suponc.2011.09.003

Widera, E. W., Rosenfeld, K. E., Fromme, E. K., Sulmasy, D. P., & Arnold, R. M. (2011). Approaching patients and family members who hope for a miracle. *J Pain Symptom Manage*, 42(1), 119–125. doi:10.1016/j.jpainsymman.2011.03.008

Williams, J. A., Meltzer, D., Arora, V., Chung, G., & Curlin, F. A. (2011). Attention to inpatients' religious and spiritual concerns: Predictors and association with patient satisfaction. *J Gen Int Med*. doi:10.1007/s11606-011-1781-y

Winkelman, W. D., Lauderdale, K., Balboni, M. J., Phelps, A. C., Peteet, J. R., Block, S. D., . . . Balboni, T. A. (2011). The relationship of spiritual concerns to the quality of life of advanced cancer patients: preliminary findings. *J Palliative Med*, 14(9), 1022–1028. doi:10.1089/jpm.2010.0536

World Health Organization. (2004). Palliative care: Symptom management and end of life care. (Accessed May 15, 2009, at http://ftp.who.int/htm/IMAI/Modules/IMAI_palliative.pdf).

Zollfrank, A. A., Trevino, K. M., Cadge, W., Balboni, M. J., Thiel, M. M., Fitchett, G., . . . Balboni, T. A. (2015). Teaching health care providers to provide spiritual care: A pilot study. *J Palliat Med*, 18(5), 408–414. doi:10.1089/jpm.2014.0306

CHAPTER 11

RELIGION AND SPIRITUALITY IN THE INTENSIVE CARE UNIT

Alexandra Cist and Philip Choi

Unique aspects of the Intensive Care Unit (ICU)—high mortality, the prominence of prognostic uncertainty, and the high rate of surrogate decision making—create an atmosphere ripe with spiritual and existential angst. The place can be stressful for patients, their families, and the clinical staff (Puchalski, 2001). Professional medical and nursing societies are encouraging increased attention to the religious and spiritual needs of patients and families as part of high quality ICU care, especially around end-of-life decision making and care. The responsibilities of caring for ICU patients and their families can bring emotional and spiritual stresses—as well as rewards—to clinical staff, chaplains, and visiting clergy, who may find the distinctive qualities of the ICU particularly challenging. This chapter will explore the importance of religion and spirituality in ICU medicine, describe unique challenges to providing religious and spiritual support, and offer suggestions for best practices so that ICU clinicians may provide high quality spiritual care for patients and families.

CULTURE OF THE ICU: HIGH MORTALITY

ICU clinicians care for the most critically ill patients. In the United States, about 5 million people are admitted to ICUs each year. Although medical technology has greatly improved over the past several decades and mortality rates have drastically decreased, ICU mortality rates remain relatively high, at 10–29% (www.sccm.org/Communications/Pages/CriticalCareStats.aspx).

Providing high-quality end-of-life care is crucial in the ICU, and an important component of this care is attention to the religious and spiritual needs of patients and families.

CASE 1

A 40 year-old woman with impending respiratory failure secondary to an aspiration event is being admitted to the ICU. She has been battling cancer for 11 years, having undergone multiple surgeries, rounds of chemotherapy, and radiation. The ICU team learns that the patient lives in some sort of "religious community." On the precipice of a decision whether or not to intubate, the attending physician (Protestant) reviews with the patient (Roman Catholic) views on the sanctity of life, God's provision in the face of suffering, and the patient's freedom to forgo interventions whose burdens are disproportionate to their benefits. Following a trans-Atlantic call to her spiritual leader, the patient chooses to forgo intubation. She is transferred to a private room on the Palliative Care service, and dies a few days later, surrounded by members of her community.

Religion and spirituality can help patients prepare for and cope with critical illness. Their beliefs may influence their advance care planning, as well as their acute decisions. In an urban academic medical center, medical inpatients who were highly religious and/or spiritual were more likely than their non-religious/spiritual counterparts to have assigned a surrogate decision maker. The groups had similar rates of preparing an advance directive or having a DNR order (Karches et al., 2012). In one study, a higher degree of religiosity was associated with patients choosing more ICU care (Maciejewski et al., 2012). However, in a separate study by some of the same investigators, they found that, if patients' religious and spiritual needs were addressed, they tended to choose more hospice care and had lower medical costs (T. Balboni et al., 2011; T. A. Balboni et al., 2010). In a study of Jordanian Muslim men in a Cardiac Care Unit, the patients noted that "faith facilitated their acceptance of illness and enhanced their coping strategies, that seeking medical treatment did not conflict with their belief in fate, that spirituality enhanced their inner strength, hope and acceptance of self-responsibility and it helped them to find meaning and purpose in their life" (Nabolsi & Carson, 2011). The importance of religion and spirituality have been recognized to the extent that National Palliative Care guidelines and the Joint Commission have mandated that clinicians address these issues as a part of regular patient care. A Critical Care Medicine task force also stressed the importance of addressing religious and spiritual needs (Davidson et al., 2007). Nevertheless, there remain challenges to making this a reality.

CULTURE OF THE ICU: PROGNOSTIC UNCERTAINTY AND UNALIGNED EXPECTATIONS

The intensive care unit poses particularly unique challenges in medicine. Much of the work on religion and spirituality in medicine has been done in outpatient oncology or palliative care settings. In those clinical situations, clinicians often have the opportunity to develop longitudinal relationships with their patients. Even though those patients may have incurable illnesses, the outpatient environment allows the patient and clinician to build relationships and trust. Conversations regarding end-of-life decisions can develop over the course of time. In contrast, the ICU provides a strikingly different clinical scenario. ICU patients and families are choosing aggressive, invasive, intensive care—or at least, not opting out of it—so there may be inherent bias in terms of how they may approach end of life decision-making. While some patients may have experienced sudden, unforeseen events, many patients who enter the ICU have pre-existing chronic illness. Some may have metastatic cancer, end stage lung disease, or liver disease without a chance for transplant. For these patients, care in the ICU will not necessarily alter the course of their disease. Some may never have had end-of-life conversations with their physicians, or some may simply have been resistant to hearing the truth about their poor prognosis. They enter the ICU with expectations of aggressive care, yet these expectations may not align with what the medical team believes they should reasonably offer. The differing expectations and a short window of time challenge the possibility of developing a therapeutic alliance. ICU clinicians often must work through cultural and religious differences with patients and their families in order to develop and maintain that therapeutic alliance.

CULTURE OF THE ICU: CHALLENGES TO DEVELOPING A THERAPEUTIC ALLIANCE

As an inpatient sub-specialty, ICU medicine is handicapped by existing patient care structures. In large academic centers, physicians quickly rotate on and off service. Medical residents may spend 30 hours on call, then return two days later. While attempts are made to achieve nursing assignment consistency, a given patient may have different nurses day by day. With so many various clinicians caring for a patient throughout an ICU stay, a true therapeutic alliance, one that is able to plumb the depths of a patient's or family's deepest spiritual needs, may be difficult to achieve. While these issues are shared with other inpatient fields of medicine, the acuity and fast-paced nature of the ICU may accentuate problems that challenge clinician-patient relationships.

The pace of ICU care hinders clinicians' ability to address religious and spiritual needs. For critically ill patients, the early stages of care involve piecing together information, often from limited data, in order to understand the etiology of their illness and to develop a plan of care. Initial evaluation may require spending hours performing procedures such as intubation and inserting central and arterial lines simply to stabilize the patients. The ICU context typically necessitates that clinicians focus predominantly on the biomedical issues, since small lapses in care could potentially quickly lead to poor outcomes, including death. *Life and death decisions* in the ICU often need to be made on the order of minutes to hours, creating unique challenges as the clinicians attempt to build trust. Issues regarding religion and spirituality usually receive a lower priority than the medical problems bringing a patient to the ICU.

CULTURE OF THE ICU: FAMILY STRESSES AND SURROGATE DECISION-MAKING

CASE 2

The brother of a critically ill man angrily confronts ICU staff and refuses to engage in discussions about goals of care. Even the brother's wife tearfully leaves a meeting when her husband begins shouting at ICU staff. Following two prolonged meetings between the brother and a chaplain—discussing end-of-life religious beliefs—the brother's tone changes dramatically, and he re-engages in surrogate decision making.

For multiple reasons, many patients who enter the ICU are unable to participate in decisions about their care. They may be intubated for respiratory failure; have brain injury following cardiac arrest, stroke, or trauma; be heavily sedated; or simply be delirious from critical illness. Therefore, the family, through the process of surrogate decision-making, often voices the needs and desires of the patient. Critical illness is an extremely physically, emotionally, and spiritually vulnerable experience for patients and family members; additionally, they generally have no prior relationship with the ICU caregivers. Family members are genuinely afraid they may lose their loved one. When ICU patients are alert, they may fear pain, alienation, and death (Dzul-Church et al., 2010). For surrogates, the responsibility of participating in decision making is extremely stressful—particularly if family members are faced with uncertain prognostic information and don't know what the patient would "want" under the circumstances. Decision-making is even more stressful if family members disagree among themselves. It can be overwhelming if they are asked to consider letting go of their loved one, because it is difficult for surrogates not to feel somehow responsible—or guilty—for the death of their loved one. Family members may be burdened by questions of meaning and unsettled by events that shake their faith, beliefs, or values. ICU family members can be prone to depression, anxiety, PTSD, and financial strain following the patient's ICU admission, which may also lead to spiritual and existential concerns.

MANIFESTATIONS OF RELIGION AND SPIRITUALITY IN THE ICU: VISIBLE AND INVISIBLE

CASE 3

A couple gives birth to their first son: a "blue baby," born with congenital heart disease. Four generations of family gather from across the country into the hospital to celebrate the baptism of the child, fearing his likely early death. His Grandmother has provided him a long white Christening gown.

CASE 4

Life-support is about to be discontinued from a critically ill devout Muslim man who is expected to die. The timing of the withdrawal is delayed so that the man's ihram clothing, which he wore during the Hajj, could be sent from the Middle East. The family emphasized that it would be significant for him to wear this clothing around the time of his death.

Family members also want to, perhaps *need to*, find hope amidst the stress and fear. They may desire opportunities merely to *be with* their loved one; to express love; to reminisce; to be thankful for their loved one's life and influence in their lives. In the setting of strained relationships, family and friends may long for better days or for reconciliation or for absolution (Koenig, 2002).

They may want to say goodbye or come to some sort of closure. They may hope for something transcendent and familiar to find peace and to cope with the stresses of the ICU (Piderman et al., 2010). In a study of parents whose children had died in Pediatric ICUs, nearly half of the parents "identified implicitly spiritual resources that they had found helpful. . . .These included wisdom borne of their experience; guidance according to one's own values; and virtues such as hope, trust, and love"(Robinson et al., 2006). Some seek a specific ritual or practice to address these needs; some may find fulfillment through unscripted interfaith spiritual interventions. Spiritual practices such as prayer, song, meditation, reflection on sacred texts, and various rituals may help patients and families cope with the various stresses of the ICU. Patients and families may make their spiritual needs known and their practices overt. Some bring sacred texts or religious objects to the bedside (crosses, images, holy water, prayer rugs), or drape the patient with items such as rosaries, scapulars, crosses, and prayer shawls. Others may be reluctant to reveal their concerns, beliefs or expressions of faith. Such reluctance may stem from many sources, including: the feeling of burdening medical professionals on topics that may be beyond their expertise; ignorance as to what forms of spiritual support are available within their hospital; difficulty articulating spiritual concerns; uncertainty or shame about their relationship with the divine; or from fear of discrimination based on their beliefs. Even if they don't mention it, patients and families may hope that someone will offer spiritual support. Some experience psychological or existential events that they don't identify as being spiritual or religious, per se (Cadge, 2012; Lo et al., 2002). Additionally, some patients and families may have never considered themselves particularly religious or spiritual, but in the context of life-threatening illness may reach out for deeper meaning and hope.

MANIFESTATIONS OF RELIGION AND SPIRITUALITY IN THE ICU: MIRACLE LANGUAGE

CASE 5

A 78-year-old man suffered a cardiac arrest at home. No CPR was performed until EMS arrived 10 minutes later. After 20 minutes of resuscitative efforts, he had return of spontaneous circulation. He has now been in the ICU for five days. He has persistent myoclonic jerks, no purposeful movements, and remains unresponsive. Despite the ICU team explaining that the prognosis is very poor, with little chance of meaningful recovery, the patient's wife and grown children insist that they believe in God and miracles, that God will provide a miracle, and that Mr. C will walk out of the hospital fully healed.

While religion and spirituality often manifest through rituals and prayers, which may serve to unify family and clinicians, religious expression may also arise through the family's use of miracle language, which may evoke discord between the family and ICU team. Many patients who enter the ICU are incurable. They may have metastatic cancer or multi-organ failure from irreversible processes. Setting realistic expectations by clinicians is a key component of good communication with families. For example, if a patient begins to develop multi-organ failure in the setting of metastatic cancer that has been unresponsive to chemotherapy, life-sustaining measures such as intubation, dialysis, and cardiopulmonary resuscitation would not change the expected poor outcome. However, sometimes in these situations families speak of miracles. "We believe in God, and we believe that God will provide a miracle. He will walk out of this ICU healed." This language often creates communication barriers. Clinicians get caught among conflicting goals: doing what the family wishes, providing realistic beneficial care, and trying to avoid inflicting the harms of non-beneficial invasive interventions. Frequently, communication begins to break down.

A study looking at ICU family meetings at multiple centers found that religious and spiritual topics frequently arose, oftentimes in the form of miracle language. Interestingly, rather than further investigating the miracle language, physicians often change the subject, referring back to objective medical information (Ernecoff et al., 2015). This demonstrates an important challenge for ICU clinicians. Building trust with patients and families is a vital aspect of ICU care. In the study, it was unclear why physicians often brought the topic back to medical language. A large component may be that physicians feel uncomfortable discussing miracles, particularly when the objective data point to a poor prognosis (Cadge, 2012). While physicians are not particularly accurate prognosticators, and patients may occasionally defy odds, truly miraculous recoveries for which families hope are extraordinarily rare. However, in the process of avoiding the subject of "miracles," clinicians lose opportunities to explore further the beliefs and values of the patient and family. Exploring religious or spiritual topics may in fact build trust and allow the patient or family to disclose deeper information that may be influencing their desire for a miracle. The patient may have outlived expectations in the past; there may be underlying conflict within the family; or there may be past emotional trauma from withdrawing treatments from another family member. Disengaging from conversation about spiritually grounded hope for healing, regardless of how unaligned that hope may be with clinical prognostication, may cause clinicians to miss opportunities to help patients and families through emotionally and spiritually distressing times.

When talk of miracles arises—or other language indicating spiritually-grounded hope, meaning, purpose, identity, or value—clinicians should engage directly with the patient or family in these conversations (Delisser, 2009; Sulmasy, 2006). Ideally, the clinicians will have already established a relationship through empathic concern. Building upon that, one can ask open questions such as "What do you mean when you say miracle?" Or: "Is there a religious or spiritual source of your hope?" Or: "Are there religious or spiritual beliefs or practices that help you in times like this?" . . . . "Tell me about that. . . . What other things are you hoping for-for (your loved one) or your family or others? Are you/he/she part of a religious or spiritual community? We can help you/him/her address those spiritual concerns as best as we can here in the ICU. . . . including with the help of our chaplains and your own clergy/spiritual advisor." In addition to asking about their hopes, this might also be an opportunity to ask about their fears: "You have mentioned some things you are hoping for. . .Do you have any fears concerning your loved one?" Such questions are asked to help sort out realistic hopes and fears from unrealistic hopes and fears and set in motion plans for addressing these—usually in the form of ongoing communication and provision of psycho-social-spiritual support. If there are particular ritual or sacred activities which the patient or family desire, or if there are particular questions about theological doctrine, religious practice, or expectations of miraculous intervention, the ICU team should consult with chaplaincy. Although some families and clinicians may interpret various ICU events as miraculous—such as the experiences of peace amidst ICU turmoil, unexpected opportunities to tie up loose ends, long overdue reconciliations within families, and countless acts of compassion—clinicians nevertheless should be cautious about reframing families' hope for miraculous healing into these other forms of "miraculous" events. Endeavoring to do so may come off as disrespectful, disingenuous, or dismissive, especially if families are experiencing a crisis of faith - thinking that their loved one's healing is dependent on their own prayers and expectations for miraculous healing. Hospital chaplains are trained in addressing such matters. Sulmasey and Delisser provide sage practical advice about discussing miracles with patients and their families. While Delisser cautiously advocates for physicians attempting to reframe the meaning or manifestation of miracles, Sulmasey is much more circumspect about this practice by untrained clinicians.

Hospital chaplains are professional spiritual leaders in the inpatient clinical setting, and physicians should regularly include them when advanced spiritual assessment and caregiving are needed. While studies have shown that hospital inpatients would welcome a visit from a chaplain, one study showed that a majority of patients were not seen by one (Piderman et al., 2010). A study at a large academic center looked at how chaplains were incorporated into patient care in the ICU. The study showed that chaplains are primarily called for dying patients, usually in the last 24–48 hours of life (Choi et al., 2015). This way of including chaplains in patient care in the ICU is particularly important, as families generally have higher levels of satisfaction when spiritual care is provided at the end of their loved one's life (Gries et al., 2008). However, it also highlights the fact that medical teams are not only reserving the provision of spiritual support for patients who are dying, but that the care is often being outsourced to the hospital chaplain.

CLINICIANS' APPROACHES TO RELIGION AND SPIRITUALITY IN THE ICU

Regarding religion and spirituality, ICU clinicians have a wide range of interest, desire, understanding, and capability. ICU nurses emphasize the inclusion of spiritual care as integral to whole-person, holistic nursing care (Holt-Ashley, 2000; Kociszewski, 2004; Weiland, 2010). Spiritual care is viewed as instrumental in alleviating existential suffering or "spiritual pain"(Dolan et al., 2011). Spiritual caregiving is noted to be mutually beneficial—to the patient and to the caregiver (Carpenter et al., 2008). In contrast to the nursing literature, there is less written about how physicians specifically approach topics of religion and spirituality (Clark & Heidenreich, 1995; Pettigrew, 1990; Smith, 2006). In Cadge's study, ICU clinicians talked about "objects, rituals, and prayers" when identifying explicit religious and spiritual expression in ICUs; and they viewed religion and spirituality as most relevant "in times of crises, of difficult decisions, and at the end of life"(Cadge, 2012). Cadge also observed that religion and spirituality occasionally influence ICU clinicians in how they cope with and make sense of illness, suffering, and death. Clinicians employ "sense-making practices," such as prayer, exercise, crying, attending patients' funerals, and reflecting with colleagues or family (Cadge, 2012). While the medical literature supports that addressing religion and spiritual needs of patients and families is important, it still appears that ICU physicians have difficulty making this a part of their regular practice.

The barriers preventing ICU clinicians from addressing the spiritual needs of patients remain unclear—and, thus, ripe for investigation. One study of physician trainees showed that discussing religious and spiritual topics was considered a more advanced skill than discussing code status (Ford et al., 2012). Even with changes in medical curricula, which increasingly stress attending to the spiritual aspects of patients, trainees still find that discussing religion and spirituality is more challenging than having a secular end of life discussion. This may help explain why chaplains are brought into care at the end of life, as physicians may not feel sufficiently comfortable to address some of these issues. Interestingly, a study at one academic medical center showed that a majority of ICU physicians and nurses see it as their responsibility to inquire about the religious and spiritual needs of patients; and in fact, they also *report* that they generally feel comfortable asking about these needs. However, most clinicians do not make this a regular part of clinical practice (Choi, P.J. et al., 2015). Why the disconnect between perceived role and actual practice? Could it be that the medical issues are so pressing that emotional or spiritual issues are simply forgotten or forgone until little more is to be done medically? Could it be that clinicians don't truly value the emotional or spiritual needs along with the medical needs?

To be fair to ICU clinicians, it should be noted that the ICU should not be the first place where goals of care, end-of-life, and spiritual discussions occur. Advance care planning and discussing goals of care belong in the ambulatory care setting or in the pre-ICU clinical setting, and can include addressing spiritual concerns. When this is not done, the time-consuming burdens of simultaneously trying to diagnose and treat acute critical illness, establish a trusting relationship, engage in shared decision making, and address life-and-death clinical and spiritual concerns fall on the shoulders of very busy critical care clinicians. Given that point of view, it may not be so surprising that ICU clinicians "outsource" spiritual matters to others. Nevertheless, this is not a justification for overlooking religious and spiritual concerns in the ICU. A collaborative team approach can help diffuse the "burden" of the task of addressing these matters. For spiritually inclined clinicians and for chaplains, doing so is not viewed as burdensome, but, rather, as uplifting.

It remains an interesting problem that in some centers, chaplain visits seem to be reserved for actively dying patients. When surveyed, physicians and nurses in these ICUs were less likely to believe that chaplains would be clinically useful for patients who are recovering from critical illness (Choi, P.J. et al., 2015). ICU clinicians may believe that surviving patients will not require as much spiritual support as those who are dying. In fact, for the actively dying patient, spiritual support becomes focused on grieving family members. Yet patients who survive critical illness are often severely debilitated—sometimes requiring months of rehabilitation. Others may have chronic illnesses that lead to recurrent ICU admissions. ICU survivors may have multiple spiritual or existential concerns, including: their sense of identity and purpose, fluctuating hope and despair, and distress from recurrent episodes of wondering whether they will survive. Opportunities abound for providing spiritual support for survivors in the ICU.

Since ICU clinicians demonstrate varying approaches to incorporating spiritual care into practice, a multidisciplinary method may be the most appropriate means for providing high quality spiritual care. As a parallel example, nursing-driven protocols for recognizing ICU delirium are now standard of care in most ICUs. These nursing assessments are vital to ICU rounds, and are a model of how communication among various members of the ICU team can lead to improved care. While spiritual or existential concerns may be more difficult to quantify, the use of assessment tools may be the start of developing improved communication among nurses, physicians, and chaplains, in order to provide effective multi-disciplinary spiritual care.

BEST PRACTICES: ASSESS AND ADDRESS

Assessing and addressing religious and spiritual needs can be accomplished in a myriad of ways. We describe some "Best Practices" under several domains: asking, listening and discerning, addressing, and training. See Box 11.1.

BOX 11.1 BEST PRACTICES: ASK, LISTEN & DISCERN, ADDRESS, TRAIN

Ask:

About needs and resources
Religious affiliation recorded in patient's demographic profile
Spiritual screen of patient and family at time of admission to ICU
Include assessment in nursing and physician admission notes
Discuss assessment in multidisciplinary rounds
When advanced assessment is required, consider using validated Spiritual
    History or Spiritual Assessment tools
Revisit asking about spiritual needs at important junctures in ICU course
Discuss patient's wishes for end-of-life care

Listen and Discern:

Listen for questions of identity/meaning/purpose, uncertainty, grief, regret, guilt,
    anger, angst, fear, abandonment; and also: expressions of values, virtues,
    legacies, transcendence, meaning, certainty, hope, faith, love, gratitude,
    relationship, reconciliation, resilience, celebration
Don't avoid conversations about religious or spiritual matters
Listen to assess needs and to identify resources/coping strategies/community
Allow chaplaincy documentation in chart
Interdisciplinary verbal communication about significant spiritual matters
Inclusion of chaplaincy or spiritual advisor in ICU Interdisciplinary team
Interdisciplinary reflection rounds to attend to staff needs
Recognize when to consult an advanced spiritual caregiver

Address:

Listen attentively, which itself may be therapeutic
Provide creative opportunities for religious and spiritual expression
Provide access to spiritual advisor/chaplaincy
Facilitate access to spiritual resources: internal or external to hospital
Facilitate religious and cultural practices for patients and families
Provision of quiet and private space
Be proactive: don't reserve only for dying patients and their families
Provide multidimensional end-of-life support and care
Provide bereavement support (even before death, patient and family may grieve)
Use non-judgmental, non-proselytizing approaches

Train:

Screening and assessing skills
Listening and discernment skills
Familiarization of clinicians with needs, resources, and approaches
Facilitation of clinical pastoral training for interested clinicians
Familiarization of clinicians with chaplaincy lingo
Familiarization of chaplains with clinical lingo and ICU culture

ASK

The first intervention is simply to ask ICU patients and their families about their spiritual or religious needs and preferences (Clark & Heidenreich, 1995; Ehman et al., 1999). A non-clergy member of the ICU team, with some brief training, can perform a spiritual screen or history. Two available assessment tools include **FICA** (Borneman et al., 2010; **F**aith/belief/meaning, **I**mportance/**I**nfluence, **C**ommunity, **A**ddress in Care) and **HOPE** (Anandarajah & Hight, 2001; source of **H**ope, involvement in **O**rganized religion, **P**ersonal spirituality and practice, **E**ffects on medical care and end of life issues). Both these assessments provide simple ways to pose three questions: whether religion or spirituality is important to the patient and family, whether personal spirituality or involvement in communities is important, and how spirituality may affect their medical decision-making.

LISTEN AND DISCERN

Listening to the family talk about the patient may be particularly significant—not only for the information gained, but also for the intrinsic value of the relational process. Reminiscing with the family about the patient is important and may lead to improved family satisfaction, particularly at the end of a patient's life (Johnson et al., 2014).

Psychiatrist and priest Edwin Cassem points out that caregivers can feel "impotent" in the face of their dying patient's hopelessness and despair. He emphasizes the importance of the caregiver *listening* to the dying person. Citing Hospice founder Cicely Saunders, Cassem notes, "When no answers exist, one can offer silent attention"(Cassem, 1997). Listening to ICU families is of parallel importance. One can offer ICU families "silent attention," which itself may be comforting. Cassem provides a set of revealing questions one might ask when trying to discern "the uniqueness resume" of a dying patient (Cassem, 2009). Focusing on who this person is and was provides a relational means of dignifying the person's life. Also, by listening, one might discern spiritual or existential needs.

ADDRESS

After assessing patient and family spiritual concerns, the next step is to address those needs. The clinical team, as spiritual "generalists," could address some needs; and other needs might require a spiritual "specialist" such as a chaplain. As mentioned earlier, spiritual care is provided in many ways, tailored to the patient's and family's needs: prayer, song, meditation, silent attention, reflection on sacred texts, various ritual practices, use of religious clothing or objects. An interdisciplinary approach is an effective way to address spiritual needs in the ICU. Nurses, physicians, and chaplains approach religion and spirituality in various ways; and they should communicate with one another about their interventions with particular patients and families. Most medical centers may not have the staff available to provide an ICU chaplain to be part of the interdisciplinary ICU team. In these institutions, all teams should be prepared to address the religious and spiritual concerns of their ICU patients and families. This may involve recognizing patients and families who are at high risk for spiritual distress and developing triggers to provide more robust spiritual care for these patients.

Many patients and families are connected to local pastors and religious communities who may deeply understand their religious, spiritual, and cultural values. ICU teams can access these resources to improve spiritual care, particularly if a patient's religious tradition differs from what is typically provided within the hospital setting.

TRAIN

Providing effective spiritual care must go beyond simply using assessment tools or consulting chaplains. Clinicians can be adequately trained to approach these complex issues. Several authors describe training programs in spirituality for clinicians and clinical students. One academic hospital program had a 2-hour workshop for medical students and residents (Barnett & Fortin, 2006). Another described a program for medical students, shadowing a chaplain in a trauma ICU (Perechocky et al., 2014). Two intensivists describe a 5-month supervised clinical pastoral education program for staff clinicians (Todres et al., 2005). Educational curricula have yet to be standardized, but targeting clinicians-in-training may be the most effective and efficient method of improving the quality of spiritual care provided by clinicians. In addition, training for staff physicians, nurses, and other clinicians could help propagate spiritual care through role modeling.

CONCLUSION

Despite the focus on data, evidence, and technology in the ICU, the critical care setting is nevertheless imbued with a great deal of uncertainty. There are uncertainties about diagnoses, etiologies, prognoses, and choice of therapies. This is unsettling—for patients, their families, and the staff who care for them. Families are threatened by the impending possible loss of a loved one. Families are thrust into surrogate decision making roles, often uncertain about *what their loved one would want*. Clinicians are uncertain about *what is best* for the patient, even as they try to uncover the facts and values that might guide optimal decision making. The unfamiliarity of the ICU can feel alienating and mysterious to families. Families can seem foreign and mysterious to staff. Spirituality and religion tap into a different sort of mystery: a transcendent yet familiar mystery that may bring meaning, purpose, and comfort to those experiencing the stresses of the ICU. Even so, the religious/spiritual beliefs and practices of patients and families may sometimes seem unfamiliar and mystifying to staff—possibly compounding a sense of alienation and discord.

For patients and families, much of their critical care experience can be a stressful time of existential crisis and spiritual turmoil, troubled by grief, guilt, expectant loss, mortality, and questions about meaning. So also, they may have spiritual celebrations of lives saved, relationships restored, and families reconciled. ICU clinicians also experience both stress and celebration. They try to understand patients' and families' needs and resources through a bio-psycho-social-spiritual lens, as part of good patient and family-centered care. Shining a spiritual light through that lens may help ICU teams better "see" spiritual and religious needs and intervene to address them. A spiritual needs assessment may be analogous to a critical needs assessment, in which clinicians simultaneously intervene while searching for causes and reversible problems in order to refine their interventions. ICU clinicians can be trained to assess spiritual and religious needs and to intervene in interdisciplinary and collaborative ways, reaching out to chaplains or other spiritual caregivers when needed. Clinicians and chaplains can tap into resources—earthly and transcendent—to provide spiritual care. The illuminating quality of this approach holds promise for improving patient and family centered care, as well as improving ICU function, utilization, and morale.

REFERENCES

Anandarajah, G., & Hight, E. (2001). Spirituality and medical practice: Using the HOPE questions as a practical tool for spiritual assessment. *American Family Physician, 63*(1), 81–89.

Balboni, T., Balboni, M., Paulk, M. E., Phelps, A., Wright, A., Peteet, J., . . . Prigerson, H. (2011). Support of cancer patients' spiritual needs and associations with medical care costs at the end of life. *Cancer, 117*(23), 5383–5391. doi: 10.1002/cncr.26221

Balboni, T. A., Paulk, M. E., Balboni, M. J., Phelps, A. C., Loggers, E. T., Wright, A. A., . . . Prigerson, H. G. (2010). Provision of spiritual care to patients with advanced cancer: associations with medical care and quality of life near death. *Journal of Clinical Oncology, 28*(3), 445–452. doi: 10.1200/jco.2009.24.8005

Barnett, K. G., & Fortin, A. H. T. (2006). Spirituality and medicine. A workshop for medical students and residents. *Journal of General Internal Medicine, 21*(5), 481–485. doi: 10.1111/j.1525-1497.2006.00431.x

Borneman, T., Ferrell, B., & Puchalski, C. M. (2010). Evaluation of the FICA tool for spiritual assessment. *Journal of Pain and Symptom Management, 40*(2), 163–173. doi: 10.1016/j.jpainsymman.2009.12.019

Cadge, W. (2012). *Paging God: Religion in the halls of medicine*. Chicago: University of Chicago Press.

Carpenter, K., Girvin, L., Kitner, W., & Ruth-Sahd, L. A. (2008). Spirituality: A dimension of holistic critical care nursing. *Dimensions of Critical Care Nursing, 27*(1), 16–20. doi: 10.1097/01.DCC. 0000304668.99121.b2

Cassem, N. (1997). The dying patient. *The Massachusetts General Hospital Handbook of General Hospital Psychiatry*. 4th Edition, pp 623–624.

Cassem, N. (2009). An overview of care and management of the patient at the end of life. In B. W. Chochinov HM (Ed.), *Handbook of Psychiatry in Palliative Medicine*. 2nd Edition, pp 27–31.

Choi, P. J., Curlin, F. A., & Cox, C. E. (2015). "The Patient Is Dying, Please Call the Chaplain": The Activities of Chaplains in One Medical Center's Intensive Care Units. *Journal of Pain and Symptom Management, 50*(4), 501–506. doi:10.1016/j.jpainsymman.2015.05.003

Choi, P.J., Curlin, F.A. & Cox, C.E. (2015). Spiritual Care and Chaplaincy in the Intensive Care Unit: An ICU Clinician Study. *Unpublished Manuscript.*

Clark, C., & Heidenreich, T. (1995). Spiritual care for the critically ill. *American Journal of Critical Care, 4*(1), 77–81.

Davidson, J. E., Powers, K., Hedayat, K. M., Tieszen, M., Kon, A. A., Shepard, E., . . . Armstrong, D. (2007). Clinical practice guidelines for support of the family in the patient-centered intensive care unit: American College of Critical Care Medicine Task Force 2004-2005. *Critical Care Medicine, 35*(2), 605–622. doi: 10.1097/01.ccm.0000254067.14607.eb

Delisser, H. M. (2009). A practical approach to the family that expects a miracle. *Chest, 135*(6), 1643-1647. doi:10.1378/chest.08-2805

Dolan, E. A., Paice, J. A., & Wile, S. (2011). Managing cancer-related pain in critical care settings. *AACN Advanced Critical Care, 22*(4), 365–378. doi: 10.1097/NCI.0b013e318232c6b8

Dzul-Church, V., Cimino, J. W., Adler, S. R., Wong, P., & Anderson, W. G. (2010). "I'm sitting here by myself ...": Experiences of patients with serious illness at an urban public hospital. *Journal of Palliative Medicine, 13*(6), 695–701. doi: 10.1089/jpm.2009.0352

Ehman, J. W., Ott, B. B., Short, T. H., Ciampa, R. C., & Hansen-Flaschen, J. (1999). Do patients want physicians to inquire about their spiritual or religious beliefs if they become gravely ill? *Archives of Internal Medicine, 159*(15), 1803–1806.

Ernecoff, N. C., Curlin, F. A., Buddadhumaruk, P., & White, D. B. (2015). Health care professionals' responses to religious or spiritual statements by surrogate decision makers during goals-of-care discussions. *JAMA Intern Med, 175*(10), 1662–1669. doi: 10.1001/jamainternmed.2015.4124

Ford, D. W., Downey, L., Engelberg, R., Back, A. L., & Curtis, J. R. (2012). Discussing religion and spirituality is an advanced communication skill: An exploratory structural equation model of physician trainee self-ratings. *Journal of Palliative Medicine, 15*(1), 63–70. doi: 10.1089/jpm.2011.0168

Gries, C. J., Curtis, J. R., Wall, R. J., & Engelberg, R. A. (2008). Family member satisfaction with end-of-life decision making in the ICU. *Chest, 133*(3), 704–712. doi: 10.1378/chest.07-1773

Holt-Ashley, M. (2000). Nurses pray: use of prayer and spirituality as a complementary therapy in the intensive care setting. *AACN Clinical Issues, 11*(1), 60-67. http://www.sccm.org/Communications/Pages/CriticalCareStats.aspx Retrieved 12.14.15

Johnson, J. R., Engelberg, R. A., Nielsen, E. L., Kross, E. K., Smith, N. L., Hanada, J. C., . . . Curtis, J. R. (2014). The Association of Spiritual Care Providers' activities with family members' satisfaction with care after a death in the ICU. *Critical Care Medicine, 42*(9), 1991–2000. doi: 10.1097/ccm.0000000000000412

Karches, K. E., Chung, G. S., Arora, V., Meltzer, D. O., & Curlin, F. A. (2012). Religiosity, spirituality, and end-of-life planning: a single-site survey of medical inpatients. *Journal of Pain and Symptom Management, 44*(6), 843–851. doi: 10.1016/j.jpainsymman.2011.12.277

Kociszewski, C. (2004). Spiritual care: a phenomenologic study of critical care nurses. *Heart and Lung, 33*(6), 401–411.

Koenig, H. G. (2002). A commentary: The role of religion and spirituality at the end of life. *Gerontologist, 42* (Spec No. 3), 20–23.

Lo, B., Ruston, D., Kates, L. W., Arnold, R. M., Cohen, C. B., Faber-Langendoen, K., . . . Tulsky, J. A. (2002). Discussing religious and spiritual issues at the end of life: A practical guide for physicians. *JAMA, 287*(6), 749–754.

Maciejewski, P. K., Phelps, A. C., Kacel, E. L., Balboni, T. A., Balboni, M., Wright, A. A., . . . Prigerson, H. G. (2012). Religious coping and behavioral disengagement: Opposing influences on advance care planning and receipt of intensive care near death. *Psycho-Oncology, 21*(7), 714–723. doi: 10.1002/pon.1967

Nabolsi, M. M. & Carson, A. M. (2011). Spirituality, illness and personal responsibility: The experience of Jordanian Muslim men with coronary artery disease. *Scandinavian Journal of Caring Sciences,* 25(4):716–24.

Perechocky, A., DeLisser, H., Ciampa, R., Browning, J., Shea, J. A., & Corcoran, A. M. (2014). Piloting a medical student observational experience with hospital-based trauma chaplains. *Journal of Surgical Education,* 71(1), 91–95. doi: 10.1016/j.jsurg.2013.07.001

Pettigrew, J. (1990). Intensive nursing care. The ministry of presence. *Critical Care Nursing Clinics of North America, 2*(3), 503–508.

Piderman, K. M., Marek, D. V., Jenkins, S. M., Johnson, M. E., Buryska, J. F., Shanafelt, T. D., . . . Mueller, P. S. (2010). Predicting patients' expectations of hospital chaplains: A multisite survey. *Mayo Clinic Proceedings,* 85(11), 1002–1010. doi: 10.4065/mcp.2010.0168

Puchalski, C. M. (2001). The role of spirituality in health care. *Proceedings (Baylor University. Medical Center),* 14(4), 352–357.

Robinson, M. R., Thiel, M. M., Backus, M. M., & Meyer, E. C. (2006). Matters of spirituality at the end of life in the pediatric intensive care unit. *Pediatrics, 118*(3), e719–729. doi: 10.1542/peds.2005-2298

Smith, A. R. (2006). Using the synergy model to provide spiritual nursing care in critical care settings. *Critical Care Nurse, 26*(4), 41–47.

Sulmasy, D. P. (2006). Spiritual issues in the care of dying patients: ". . . it's okay between me and god". *JAMA, 296*(11), 1385-1392. doi:10.1001/jama.296.11.1385

Todres, I. D., Catlin, E. A., & Thiel, M. M. (2005). The intensivist in a spiritual care training program adapted for clinicians. *Critical Care Medicine, 33*(12), 2733–2736.

Weiland, S. A. (2010). Integrating spirituality into critical care: an APN perspective using Roy's adaptation model. *Critical Care Nursing Quarterly, 33*(3), 282-291. doi:10.1097/CNQ.0b013e3181ecd56d

CHAPTER 12

RELIGION AND SPIRITUALITY IN MEDICAL ETHICS

Farr A. Curlin

I suspect that no reader will find it hard to believe that religion matters for medical ethics. Ethics, or *practical* reason, is that domain of reason that has to do with how we ought to act—what we ought to do in any particular case and how we ought to live in the broader sense. Religions obviously make authoritative claims about how we ought to act and how we ought to live. Where we find a medical ethics question, therefore, we will find religious answers, and religious answers will frequently differ from those that emerge from secular frames of reasoning, which, with respect to answering ethical questions, often work analogously to religious traditions. Nor are religious answers all of one piece. There are of course multiple religions, and often there are distinct traditions within a given religion. These will rarely speak with one voice regarding ethical questions. Religious traditions do speak, however, and so religion and medical ethics are caught up and intertwined with one another.

The following analysis starts at the surface—with how religion shows up in everyday clinical ethical disputes. For example, suppose a patient with terminal cancer asks, "Should I seek a physician's assistance in ending my life?" The patient's physician in turn poses the question, "Should I provide such assistance if asked?" In such a case, religion may show up explicitly. The patient may decide that he should seek physician-assisted suicide because there is no God and the remainder of the patient's life will be merely a burden. The patient's physician may decide that she should refuse the patient's request, because there is a God and God has forbidden intentionally cooperating in a person's suicide. Even where not made explicit, however, religion is implicitly entailed. The patient might seek physician-assisted suicide because he wants his pain to end. The physician might refuse because she believes that granting this patient's request would make it harder for other gravely ill patients to trust her with their care. Although neither of these decisions explicitly entails religious concerns, the reasonableness of both depends on questions—Does God exist? Has God made it clear that suicide is wrong even when one is in pain?—to which religions give authoritative answers.

It is not enough to know that religion and medical ethics are inextricably, we might say *intrinsically*, intertwined. The question is what difference does that make for the practice of medicine? To explore that difference, I shall review findings from several studies of US physicians. These studies suggest that religious convictions and practices do more to explain how clinicians reason and act, with respect to ethically disputed clinical practices, than all other social and cultural factors put together. I focus on clinicians because I have spent more than a decade studying religion-associated variations in physicians' clinical practices and clinically-relevant attitudes. I focus on clinicians also because modern medical ethics in its conventional form already acknowledges that *patients'* values and cultural norms should guide clinical decisions. That *clinicians'* practices and clinical recommendations would be shaped by their own religious beliefs and practices, however, threatens the core assumptions of conventional medical ethics.

Medical ethics as we know it today arose in the second half of the twentieth century, when theologians began to push back against scientists' pretenses to addressing the moral implications of scientific advances without regard to religious concerns (see Evans, 2012). Over the ensuing decades, a variety of stakeholders have contended with each other to establish jurisdiction over the domain of clinical medical ethics. This history is described in some depth by Evans (2012), but for our purposes it is enough to know that in the domain of medical ethics, theologians and other religious scholars have been largely displaced by other experts. Hailing from a variety of disciplinary backgrounds, these experts share in common a medical ethics framework that emphasizes patient autonomy and focuses on procedures for resolving disagreements. This conventional framework calls practitioners to facilitate clinical decisions that align with patients' wishes. It matters not whether those wishes are shaped by religious (or other) values and norms. As a corollary of emphasizing patient autonomy, however, conventional medical ethics opposes the undue influence of clinicians' so-called "personal values," and particularly their religious values. Physicians are expected to be scientific and evidence-based, neutral regarding religion, and steeled against the influence of their own moral convictions.

The fact that physicians' religious characteristics appear to strongly shape their clinical practices exposes the limits of conventional medical ethics. Differences in physicians' practices force us to look beneath the surface of clinical ethical disputes to examine the deeper disagreements that lead not only to arguments about which clinical interventions are ethical, but also to arguments about how one should *do* medical ethics in the face of such disagreements. As we will see, religious traditions call the assumptions and practices of conventional medical ethics into question particularly when they critique the broader culture of contemporary medicine.

Before proceeding further I make two stipulations. First, although this volume takes up the subjects of "religion and spirituality," I will focus on religion. That seems appropriate to the subject. When religion and spirituality are spoken of together, the term *spirituality* is typically used to mark off a domain of human experience that does not necessarily involve particular institutions, communities, teachings, and practices—which are seen as the stuff of religion. It is precisely those particular institutions, communities, teachings, and practices, however, that most influence medical ethics. As such, for simplicity I will not speak further here of spirituality, though to my knowledge nothing I say is contradicted by any operative understanding of that concept. Second, I will take "medical ethics" to refer to what might also be called *clinical ethics*—those questions that arise for clinicians and patients regarding what they ought to do with respect to the uses and practices of medicine. I will not address issues that are more peripheral to the clinical encounter, such as the ethics of embryonic stem cell research or health care financing or environmental ethics, even though these have obvious implications for health care and are typically included within the broader domain of *bioethics*.

PRACTICAL DISPUTES: HOW RELIGION "SHOWS UP" IN MEDICAL ETHICS

With respect to clinical medicine, religion shows up at precisely the point that medical ethics shows up: when a question emerges regarding what should be done. A patient wonders if the clinical options available are all morally permissible for him. A physician wonders if she can ethically provide the option the patient requests. A patient declines something her physician thinks she really needs, and the physician wonders what he should do in response. Religion becomes starkly visible one or both parties to a disagreement give a religious reason for their position. The patient may forego some assisted reproductive technology that her physician recommends, out of concern to honor the Roman Catholic Church's teaching regarding sexuality and marriage. A physician may refuse to hasten a patient's death out of concern to honor the requirements of Jewish law. A patient may decline the surgery his physician recommends, because, in the patient's view, the surgery requires too much "contrivance and fuss and . . . turns [the patient's life] into one long *provision for the flesh* (Rom. 13:14)" (Silvas, 2005, p. 266). His physician may wonder how she can "stand idly by the blood of [her] neighbor."[1] In these cases, religion comes dressed in vestments. In other cases, religion hides under the plain clothes of conventional moral language regarding beneficence and justice, burdens and benefits, autonomy and professional responsibility. Either way, religion shows up, because religions teach and form responses to clinical ethical questions.

In the United States, the great majority of patients *and* clinicians identify a religious affiliation, and most say they try hard to carry their religious beliefs over into all their other dealings in life (Curlin et al., 2005).[2] In a 2003 study, my colleagues and I found that 55% of US physicians agreed or strongly agreed that their religious beliefs influence their practices of medicine (Curlin et al., 2005). Over the ensuing years, we have sought to describe *how*, using data from six representative national studies of physicians and one of medical students, which together include more than 6,000 respondents. These studies help to fill in a virtual atlas of religion-associated differences in physicians' approaches to an array of ethically disputed clinical practices. To illustrate the ways religion shows up in clinical ethical disputes, I here provide a snapshot of our findings in three domains: (1) addressing religious concerns in the clinical encounter, (2) sexual and reproductive health care, and (3) care for patients at the end of life.

ADDRESSING RELIGIOUS CONCERNS IN THE CLINICAL ENCOUNTER

We found that physicians' religious characteristics largely account for differences in their judgments about whether and how physicians should address religious and spiritual concerns in the clinical encounter. Paralleling public and professional interest in the intersection of medicine and religion, medical and bioethical writing has supported a lively debate about whether and how clinicians should address religious concerns in the clinical encounter (Daniel Hall and I contributed to this debate: Curlin & Hall, 2005b). Critics have argued that clinicians who take on religious concerns in their interactions with patients thereby cross professional boundaries and threaten patient privacy and autonomy.

In our 2003 study, we found that physicians who were more religious or more spiritual were significantly more likely to report inquiring about religious and spiritual concerns, sharing their own religious/spiritual ideas and experiences, encouraging patients' religious/spiritual beliefs and practices, and praying with patients (see Curlin et al., 2006). In general, religiosity and spirituality interacted such that, at a given level of one, an increase in the other increased the likelihood of practicing the behavior and endorsing it as ethically appropriate. Differences persisted even after adjusting for differences in physicians' religious affiliations and an array of demographic and practice characteristics.

In a particularly telling finding, physicians of high religiosity and spirituality were three times as likely as those of low religiosity and spirituality to say they inquire about religion and spirituality (76% vs. 23%; adjusted odds ratio [AOR], 95% confidence interval [95% CI] = 6.6, 3.5–12.5), and they were almost three times as likely to say they *never* change the subject when religious and spiritual issues comes up (56% vs. 22%; AOR, 95% CI = 3.4, 1.9–6.1). Despite these findings, they were also more than three times as likely (63% vs. 18%, $P < 0.001$) to say they spend too little time discussing religion and spirituality with patients. In sum, it appears that differences in religious practice lie beneath the surface of arguments about whether it is ethical for physicians to engage with patients regarding religious and spiritual concerns. Those who are less religious tend to oppose practices that those who are more religious not only find unproblematic, but to which they aspire.[3]

SEXUAL AND REPRODUCTIVE HEALTH CARE

No domain of medicine has stirred more clinical ethical disputes than the domain of sexual and reproductive health care. In the winter of 2008-2009, we surveyed a nationally representative sample of obstetrician gynecologist physicians (Ob/Gyns). In that study, we found that Ob/Gyns' religious characteristics were strongly associated with their opinions and practices regarding an array of issues in sexual and reproductive health care.

Consider contraceptives. Although embraced by the large majority of American women, the use of different contraceptive technologies continues to be contested in some communities. In particular, the Roman Catholic Church still teaches that using contraceptives is immoral because it intentionally separates the "procreative" and "unitive" aspects of sexual intercourse. In other religious communities, concerns have been raised about contraceptives having an abortifacient effect, or about the widespread use of contraceptives leading to corruption in sexual mores. In our study (Lawrence et al., 2011b), we found that compared with doctors who attend religious services twice a year or less often, those who attend at least twice a month were much more likely to object to at least one of six contraceptive methods (9% vs. 1%; AOR, 95% CI = 7.4, 2.5–22), and they were also more likely to say they would refuse to provide one or more contraceptive methods (9% vs. 5%; AOR, 95% CI = 1.9, 1.0–3.7).

The advent of post-coital or "emergency" contraception (levonorgestrel, initially marketed as "Plan B") was attended by further debates both about contraception and about whether physicians have a professional ethical obligation to provide a technology that they may oppose on moral grounds. In 2004 the Food and Drug Administration (FDA) denied an application for over-the-counter sales, and in 2006 the FDA made the drug available without prescription for women 18 years and older, but kept it behind the pharmacy counter. Both decisions were criticized in the professional and lay media as being based on politics and ideology rather than on scientific data. This public criticism exposed the limits of science with respect to medical ethics (for our take on this, see Curlin & Hall, 2005a), a subject to which I will return below. In our study of Ob/Gyns (see Lawrence et al., 2011b), we found that those who attend religious services twice a month or more often were somewhat less likely to believe that using emergency contraception lowers rates of unintended pregnancy (84% vs. 95% of Ob/Gyns who never attend; AOR, 95% CI = 0.3, 0.1–0.7), and they were much more likely to believe that access to emergency contraception leads to more sexual partners (22% vs. 7%; AOR, 95% CI = 4.1, 1.9–9.1). Those who attend religious services frequently also were more likely to say they never offer emergency contraception or that they offer it only to victims of sexual assault (21% vs. 5%; AOR, 95% CI = 4.2, 1.6–11), whereas Ob/Gyns who never attend were more likely to offer emergency contraception to all women at risk of pregnancy (65% vs. 41%; AOR, 95% CI = 2.3, 1.4–3.6).

In the same study, we included a vignette in which a 17-year-old college freshman requests birth control pills and does not want her parents to know (see Lawrence et al., 2011a). Doctors with any religious affiliation (except Jewish) were more likely than unaffiliated doctors to encourage the young woman to abstain from sexual activity until she is older, with Evangelical Protestants most likely to encourage abstinence (76% vs. 31% of those with no affiliation; AOR, 95% CI = 7.0, 3.7–14). Similarly, doctors who attend services twice a month or more often were more likely to advise abstinence than doctors who never attend services (68% vs. 32%; AOR, 95% CI = 4.4, 2.7–7.2), and they were also more likely to encourage the young woman to talk to a parent (53% vs. 37%; AOR, 95% CI = 1.9, 1.2–3.1).

Some opposition to contraceptives stems from concerns that particular contraceptive technologies prevent nascent human embryos from implanting in the uterine wall, and thereby act as abortifacients (Chung et al., 2012).[4] Intrauterine devices are known to prevent implantation, and although hormonal contraceptives act primarily by blocking ovulation, debate persists about whether and how often they act secondarily by preventing implantation. These questions have fresh relevance in light of two recent policy changes. First, the FDA approved the "five-day pill" (ulipristal acetate), a prescription-only contraceptive that is effective when taken within 120 hours of unprotected sexual intercourse. Second, regulations from the Affordable Care Act require employers to pay for health insurance that includes coverage for all FDA-approved contraceptives (physicians' opinions about these regulations are described in Antiel et al., 2014). Challenges to that law have been raised by numerous religiously-affiliated institutions, particularly Roman Catholic and evangelical Protestant ones, that oppose contraceptive methods that may act by preventing implantation.

A common retort to concerns about contraceptives blocking implantation has been to note that pregnancy does not begin until implantation, and so loss of a fertilized ovum prior to implantation is not an interruption of pregnancy, and therefore not abortifacient. We asked US Ob/Gyns,

"Which of the following statements comes closest to your beliefs about when pregnancy begins?" and they were given the response options "at conception," "at implantation of the embryo," and "not sure." We found that fewer than one third (28%) believed pregnancy begins "at implantation of the embryo" (57% indicated at conception, 16% not sure), and this minority was disproportionately irreligious (46% of those for whom religion is not at all important, compared to 14% of those for whom religion is most important, $p < 0.01$). Catholics (21%) and evangelicals (17%) were less than half as likely as Jewish (52%), Muslim (47%), and unaffiliated (47%) physicians to believe pregnancy begins with implantation.

The public role of religion in contemporary medicine has been contested perhaps most strongly in relation to the subject of abortion (Kim et al., 2014).[5] We asked Ob/Gyns directly whether they objected to abortion in several clinical scenarios (see Harris et al., 2011). A large majority (82%) of Ob/Gyns objected to a woman seeking abortion because the fetus was female. Setting that scenario aside, compared to Ob/Gyns for whom religion is not very or not at all important, those for whom their religion is most important were much more likely to object to abortion (AOR, 95% CI = 16.9, 7.7–37.1) and they were less likely to be willing to help a patient obtain an abortion if asked (AOR, 95% CI = 0.4, 0.2–0.7). Even after adjusting for differences in religious importance, compared to those with no religious affiliation, Jewish physicians were less likely to object to abortion (AOR, 95% CI = 0.3, 0.1–0.7), whereas Muslim (3.4, 1.2–9.6), Catholic (2.7, 1.4–5.1), and Evangelical Protestant (3.7, 1.4–10.0) physicians were all more likely to object.

Only 14% of Ob/Gyns ever perform abortions (see Stulberg, Dude, Dahlquist, & Curlin, 2011). Compared to physicians reporting no religious affiliation, Jewish physicians were more likely (AOR, 95% CI = 3.3, 1.5–6.9), and Christian physicians were less likely (evangelicals, 0.1, 0.0–0.7; non-evangelical Protestants, 0.5, 0.2–0.9; and Catholics, 0.4, 0.2–0.9), to report performing abortions. Physicians for whom religion is not very or not at all important were significantly more likely to provide abortions (AOR, 95% CI = 2.7, 1.5–5.1, compared to those for whom religion is "most important").

CARE FOR PATIENTS AT THE END OF LIFE

Disputes about how to care for a patient with advanced illness and at the end of life are the most common cause for referrals to clinical ethics consultants. In the 2003 study, we asked, "Please note if you object to any of the following medical practices, and if so, whether your objection is for religious reasons, reasons unrelated to religion, or both." We included three practices relevant to end of life care: "Physician assisted suicide," "Sedation to unconsciousness in dying patients," and "Withdrawal of artificial life support" (see Curlin et al., 2008). Physicians who were more religious, however measured, were markedly more likely to report objections to physician-assisted suicide and to sedation to unconsciousness in dying patients. Hindu physicians were particularly likely (43%, compared to ~ 20% of Protestants, Catholics, and Muslims) to object to sedating dying patients to unconsciousness. This finding may reflect Hindu writings that have discouraged measures that unduly sedate or impair mental clarity at the time of death because of concern that individuals have sufficient opportunity to expunge Karma in preparation for the next life.

To probe further how religion shows up in care for patients at the end of life, in 2010 we surveyed a nationally representative sample of physicians likely to care for patients with advanced illness (see Putman et al., 2013). In that study we included a vignette:

> KD is a 62-year-old woman dying at home from metastatic lung cancer. Her pain has been treated with high-dose, long-acting narcotics. Her dyspnea has been treated with a combination of oxygen, narcotics, and intermittent nebulizer treatments. KD tells her physician that her pain and dyspnea are well-controlled, but she is distressed at the constant thought of her impending death. She says, "I know I am going to die; I just cannot tolerate lying here thinking about it day after day." KD asks her physician to sedate her to unconsciousness until she dies.

After the vignette, physicians were asked, "In your judgment, how appropriate would it be in this case for KD's physician to sedate her to unconsciousness until she dies?"

We found that 72% of physicians believed it would be *not very* or *not at all* appropriate to grant KD's request for sedation. In response to another item, 85% agreed that "Unconsciousness is an acceptable side effect of palliative sedation, but should not be directly intended." Hindu affiliation was inversely associated with believing that it would be appropriate to grant KD's request for sedation (20% vs. 38% *no religion*; AOR, 95% CI = 0.4, 0.1-0.9), and also inversely associated with believing that "doctors should sometimes treat the psychological and spiritual suffering of terminally ill patients by sedating the patient to unconsciousness" (20% vs. 41% *no religion*; AOR, 95% CI = 0.4, 0.2-0.9). Notably, physicians who were more religious were significantly more likely to oppose intentionally hastening a patient's death.

Religious convictions also generate clinical ethical disputes about tube feeding, also called "artificial nutrition and hydration" (for details regarding religion and tube feeding, see Wolenberg et al., 2013). US law and conventional medical ethics allow patients or their surrogates to withhold or withdraw tube feeding as they would any other medical intervention. Yet withholding and withdrawing tube feeding can be morally problematic in some Jewish, Christian, and Muslim communities. Within Judaism, questions focus on whether tube feeding is life-sustaining, and therefore obligatory, or merely death-prolonging, and therefore optional. Within Roman Catholicism, questions focus on whether tube feeding should be regarded as ordinary (obligatory) or extraordinary (optional) care, and recent church statements have indicated that patients, and their surrogates and clinicians, have a prima facie obligation to use tube feeding unless doing so will not effectively provide nutrition, or the patient is actively dying.[6] Debates within Islam have focused on whether tube feeding is basic care (obligatory) or medical treatment (sometimes optional).

In our study, we found that irreligious physicians (those with no religious affiliation, or for whom religion is not important/not applicable, or who never attend religious services) were significantly less likely than other physicians to object to withholding or withdrawing tube feeding. Moreover, compared to non-evangelical Protestant physicians, Jewish and Muslim physicians were both significantly more likely to oppose withholding tube feeding (AOR, 95% CI = 3.4, 1.9–6.2 and 2.7, 1.3–5.5, respectively), and Muslim physicians were also more likely to oppose withdrawing tube feeding (AOR, 95% CI = 2.8, 1.2–6.5).

Across these domains of continuing debate within the field of medical ethics, we did not merely find that religious characteristics matter. Rather, we found that religious characteristics typically account for more of the variation in physicians' responses than all other (measured) characteristics combined. Why would that be? It seems clinical ethical disputes are signals that deeper issues are at stake about which religions have important things to say. For example, differences regarding contraception and abortion reflect deeper disagreements about the meaning of human sexuality and about which human organisms deserve fundamental respect. Differences regarding palliative sedation and hastening death reflect deeper disagreements about what sorts of suffering one should try to alleviate and what one should hope for in the face of death. Answers to such questions depend on and emerge from particular frameworks of meaning, which in many cases are religious traditions. As such, religious concepts and traditions (and their secular analogues) appear to be implicit in the choices clinicians and patients make in deploying medical science.

DISCERNING HOW TO MOVE FORWARD: DIFFERENT IDEAS ABOUT WHAT MEDICAL ETHICS IS FOR AND ABOUT THE ROLES OF THOSE INVOLVED

Religious differences not only give rise to clinical ethical disputes; they also give rise to disagreements about how one should *do* medical ethics in the face of such disputes. Suppose a clinical disagreement arises. What should happen next? What is the clinician's role, ethically? What role should the ethics consultant play? These are questions about the purposes of medicine itself, as well as about the proper role and authority of both clinicians and medical ethicists. They are unsettled questions, but conventional medical ethics emphasizes respect for patient autonomy as the primary ethical imperative for both clinicians and ethics consultants. As a result, conventional medical ethics generally encourages physicians to be nondirective in their counsel to patients, particularly in the face of disagreement. In support of this emphasis, a familiar narrative tells of how the paternalistic medicine of past generations unjustly imposed physicians' values onto patients. To resist this injustice, the narrative continues, physicians are professionally obligated to adhere to *scientific* standards and to resist the undue influence of their *personal values*.

This conventional narrative, however, results in problems for the doctor-patient relationship. Indeed, physicians and ethicists who disagree about all sorts of substantive ethical questions do agree that in moving away from the problems of physician paternalism, the pendulum has swung too far toward an emphasis on patient autonomy in which, as Quill and Brody put it, "the physician as a person, with values and experience, has become an impediment to rather than a resource for decision-making" (Emanuel & Emanuel, 1992; Quill & Brody, 1996; Siegler, 1981; Thomasma, 1983). The judgment of the physician, in such a framework, is beside the point with respect to the physician's obligation to competently provide the health care services that the patient chooses. In different ways, each of these ethicists insists that the clinical encounter should be characterized less as a transaction between a consumer or client and his or her technician-provider, and more as an encounter in which the physician engages in negotiation, persuasion, and seeking a mutually acceptable accommodation, out of her genuine concern for the patient's good. In such a model, as Emanuel and Emanuel (1992) put it, "the physician acts as a teacher or friend, engaging the patient in dialogue on what course of action would be best. Not only knowing what the patient could do, but, knowing the patient, the physician indicates what the patient should do."

With respect to the debate about how directive or nondirective a physician should be in her counsel to patients, it is clear that religious physicians are more likely to come down on the side of being directive. In our study of US Ob-Gyns (Yoon et al., 2010), we found that physicians who believe one religious tradition is uniquely or comprehensively true were less likely to endorse nondirective counseling (measured as agreeing that, "physicians should provide all relevant facts without trying to influence the patient's decision one way or another"). This was true with respect both to typical medical decisions and to morally controversial medical decisions. In two subsequent studies of US primary care physicians (see Putman et al., 2014), we found that those who attended religious services more frequently, or for whom their religion is very important, were more likely to endorse directive counsel ("a physician should encourage the patient to make the decision that the physician believes is best") regarding typical medical decisions. Similarly, after reading a vignette describing a patient requesting palliative sedation, physicians who were more religious were more likely to endorse giving the patient directive counsel.

How physicians should proceed in the face of disagreements with patients comes to a head with regard to the subject of physician conscience, and, specifically, conscientious refusals to provide or participate in interventions to which physicians have moral objections. In a study of US primary care physicians (see Lawrence & Curlin, 2009), we found that those who were more religious were more likely to believe that physicians are never obligated to do what they believe is wrong (AOR, 95% CI = 2.9, 1.2–7.2 for high intrinsic religiosity vs. low). In our 2003 study of all US physicians, we asked physicians, "If a patient requests a legal medical procedure, but the patient's physician objects to the procedure for religious or moral reasons: (1) Would it be ethical for the physician to plainly describe to the patient why he or she objects to the requested procedure? (2) Does the physician have an obligation to present all possible options to the patient, including information about obtaining the requested procedure? (3) Does the physician have an obligation to refer the patient to someone who does not object to the requested procedure?" As we noted in a report from the study (see Curlin, Lawrence, Chin, & Lantos, 2007), "physicians who are more religious, measured either by attendance at religious services or intrinsic religiosity, are more likely to report that doctors may describe their objections to patients, and they are less likely to report that physicians must present all options [including information about how to obtain the requested procedure] and refer patients to someone who does not object to the requested procedure. Compared to those with no religious affiliation, Catholics and Protestants are more likely to report that physicians may describe their moral objections and less likely to report that physicians are obligated to refer."

Much of the debate about conscientious refusals revolves around the question of whether doctors are obligated at least to refer patients to another physician for those legal interventions that they are unwilling to provide personally. The bioethicist Dan Brock has argued they must (see Brock, 2008). Describing what he calls the "conventional compromise," Brock concedes that because physician integrity is important, individual physicians should not be compelled to provide every medical intervention. He argues, however, that the profession of medicine as a whole is obligated to make all legal interventions available, and therefore that every physician is obligated to at least refer patients for interventions that they are not willing to provide. Brock's "conventional compromise" raises the question: what about situations in which a physician believes that making a referral is itself immoral? We studied the opinions of US physicians (all specialties) about this issue in a 2009 study led by Tilburt (see Combs, Antiel, Tilburt, Mueller, & Curlin, 2011). There we found that physicians are divided: 57% agreed that, "Physicians have a professional obligation to refer patients for all legal medical services for which the patients are candidates, even if the physician believes that such a referral is immoral." Again, physicians who were more religious, by any of several measures, were less likely to believe physicians have this obligation.

That religious physicians are more likely to endorse being morally directive, and more likely to endorse physicians practicing according to conscience, indicates that to have an imagination shaped by an authoritative religious tradition is to come to see medicine as having purpose and meaning not determined simply by the wishes or desires of patients (or any other party). Indeed, religious traditions speak explicitly to the meaning and purpose of medicine. They give accounts of why and how we should respond to those who are sick, and they spell out an identity, a calling, that has meaning for physicians and others who are involved in the task of caring. It is not incidental, for example, that in Judaism saving someone's life takes precedence over all but three of the Torah's commandments. It is not incidental that the concept of a hospital began when Christian monastic communities enfolded the care of the sick into their lives of liturgy and prayer. Judaism, Christianity, Islam, and other religions often ground care for the sick in sacred and transcendent obligations to God and neighbor. Religious traditions thus give medical ethics a moral starting point.

ARRIVING AT THE LIMITS OF "MEDICAL ETHICS": HOW RELIGIOUS TRADITIONS CALL CONVENTIONAL MEDICAL ETHICS INTO QUESTION

By generating different conclusions about what is ethical in particular clinical cases, as well as different notions about the purposes of medicine and how to contend for what is ethical in light of disagreements, religious traditions expose the limits of "medical ethics." Consequently, religious accounts of medicine and medical ethics call into question the assumptions, practices, and categories that govern today's medicine and medical ethics.

By way of illustration, consider excerpts from two texts that address medical ethics from within content-full religious traditions. First, Orthodox Jewish scholar Avraham Steinberg, in the "Introduction" to his *Encyclopedia of Jewish Medical Ethics*, writes:

> This Encyclopedia is based upon the Jewish sources from the Bible to current responsa literature. It is, therefore, pertinent to summarize the fundamentals and the structure of Jewish Law: "*Halakhah*" is the generic term for the whole legal system of Judaism, embracing all the laws, practices, and observances. Orthodox Jews consider the *Halakhah*, in its traditional form, to be absolutely binding. The source of *Halakhah* is Divine revelation. To the basic corpus of biblical law were added rabbinic enactments and decrees. The sources of

authority in *Halakhah* are composed of two fundamental parts: (a) the Written Law, a composition of 613 positive and negative commandments of Sinaitic origin, which are included in the five books of the Pentateuch; (b) the Oral law, which includes the interpretation of the written law transmitted in its entirety with its details and minutiae at Sinai, as well as logical deductions, rabbinical decrees, customs, and positive and negative enactments. (Steinberg, 2003)

Second, Jean Claude Larchet, in his book titled, *The Theology of Illness*, writes:

> To consider illness strictly as a phenomenon unto itself is almost inevitably to see it in a negative, sterile light: and this only increases the physical suffering and moral pain which result from a sense of its absurdity. The consequence of such an attitude is generally to leave the way open to the activity of demons and to develop in the soul troubling passions, such as fear, anxiety, anger, weariness, revolt and despair . . . . The illness then serves no good at all, but it becomes for the ill person a source of spiritual deterioration which puts his soul in jeopardy perhaps more than it does his body. It is because of this very danger that the Fathers stress the point that 'it is not in vain, nor without reason, that we are subject to illnesses.' [quoting St. John Chrysostom] This is why they encourage us to be vigilant when illness strikes, and not to trouble ourselves first of all with their natural causes and means to cure them. Rather, our first concern should be to discern their meaning within the framework of our relationship to God, and to throw light on the positive function they can have in furthering our salvation. (Larchet, 2002)

These two excerpts manifestly transgress the norms of conventional medical ethics. Both ways of talking emerge in cultures other than the culture of medicine with which we are familiar. Both accounts seem odd to our ear. I dare say it would be hard to imagine someone using this kind of language in an ethics case conference in an American medical center. By contrasting so starkly with conventional ways of talking about medical ethics, these accounts call conventional medical ethics into question. If it is not self-evident that these religious accounts are false, then it is not self-evident that conventional accounts of medical ethics are true. By being so obviously different, these religious accounts call into question what we are up to even when we are doing medical ethics according to the best available conventional standards.

Religious accounts expose the limits of "medical ethics" particularly when they critique as false what the culture of medicine takes for granted as true. Whether advanced by Jewish, Christian, or Muslim scholars, religious accounts of medical ethics all seem to criticize conventional medical ethics for being captive to an imagination in which nothing beyond the immanent is morally significant (see, for example, Bleich, 1998b; Engelhardt, 2000; Padela, Malik, Curlin, & De Vries, 2015). Conventional medical ethics, that is, has largely given up asking what it means to be human and to live well in the face of suffering, illness, and death. Such questions are treated as unanswerable—or at least as outside the realm of professional consideration. The medical community has defaulted to human choice (autonomy) as the activity that gives moral sense to our actions. If an action is chosen by the authorized chooser, the action is ethical. If not, the action is not ethical. As a result, conventional medical ethics deals almost exclusively with procedural ethics aimed at getting conflicts resolved. The focus tends to be on questions about who makes decisions: substituted judgment, legal parameters, advance directives, and so on. Medical ethicists much less commonly consider questions of moral substance. They rarely ask what would be a good decision for the decision maker to make.

"EVIDENCE-BASED" RECOMMENDATIONS

In light of the inextricable relationship between religion and medical ethics, and the way religious accounts of medical ethics call conventional medical ethics and the broader culture of medicine into question, I offer two modest recommendations.[7] First, clinicians and clinical ethicists should gain some familiarity with the religious traditions and practices that shape the patients and clinicians who show up in their clinical contexts. If holistic medicine requires attention to patients' cultural contexts, then holistic medical ethics consultation requires attention to religious accounts of illness, suffering, and the role of medicine. At this most rudimentary level, clinicians and clinical ethicists should become cultural demographers and linguists—they should listen to and learn about the people they will serve, most of whom, at least in North America, will be committed religious believers. I recommend learning about different religions from and in the company of experts who are also practitioners of the traditions in question. Doing so mitigates the tendency to oversimplify and caricature religious ideas and practices.

More important than gaining abstract knowledge about religious doctrines and practices, clinicians and clinical ethicists should develop the habit of asking questions and listening so as to understand how those doctrines and practices might be at work in a particular ethical dispute. Take a common case. A patient lies in the intensive care unit suffering multiple organ system failure. Clinicians hold a family conference to discuss the patient's poor prognosis and to raise the possibility of discontinuing life-sustaining technology. Family members of the patient insist that God will heal the patient, and they ask that life-sustaining technology be continued, because God is the one who should decide if the patient lives or dies.

With respect to such a case, it is more helpful to have the habit of seeking to understand the family's reasoning than to know what Pope John Paul II or Rabbi Jakobovits said about how much we are obligated to keep a mortally ill person alive. Better to listen carefully for what is at stake theologically for those involved, rather than to attempt to see through and explain away what patients say. The clinician or clinical ethicist who has developed the requisite habits of listening will come to discern, with greater accuracy, when families are using religious language to express concerns that are not obviously related to particular religious beliefs or practices. For example, the family's statement that God should decide if the patient lives or dies may express the family's conviction that they do not have authority to make the decision themselves. Anyone who attempts to respectfully negotiate clinical ethical disagreements will benefit both from knowledge about different religious traditions and from the practice of asking patients about religious concerns.

My second recommendation is that clinicians and ethicists should acknowledge, and be open to the ways religious traditions address, the questions that lie under the surface of clinical ethical disputes and conventional medical ethics language. In part, this means respecting the limits of conventional medical ethics—the fact that "evidence-based" or "principle-based" rubrics often fail to address deeper ethical questions. Paying attention to these deeper questions requires courage, because the structures of modern medicine overwhelmingly emphasize empirical and instrumental modes of reasoning, treating deeper questions as appropriate only for synagogue or church or mosque, or the privacy of one's closet. Yet the courage to push deeper will be rewarded by greater clarity, integrity, and respect in one's interactions with patients and colleagues.

Moreover, teachers of medical ethics will find that many learners are hungry to grapple with these deeper questions. Many learners are deeply unsatisfied with the way conventional medical ethics detaches from questions about the good, about the nature of medicine, its purposes, and how to practice medicine well. Many are ready to go beyond procedural ethics in order to discern what good medicine entails in contemporary contexts. Religious traditions provide surprising resources for that task, and teachers might introduce students to the religious concepts and practices that form different imaginations, and therefore give rise to clinical ethical disagreements. That would mean reading explicitly theological accounts of relevant ethical questions. For example, with respect to the care of patients with advanced illness, students might read Jewish (Bleich, 1998a), Catholic (Pellegrino, Thomasma, & Miller, 1996), Protestant Reformed (Verhey, 2011), or Buddhist (Halifax, 2008) accounts. A sampling of such works will make plain that religious traditions are oceans to swim in. They contain vast intellectual and moral resources found in centuries of reasoning about and attending practically to human life, the body, suffering and illness, and death.

In summary, religion matters for medical ethics and for the broader culture of medicine. Religious traditions and communities form patients and clinicians to endorse some medical practices as morally praiseworthy, and to condemn other practices as morally corrupt. This influence of religion will show up in clinical ethical disputes. Beneath the surface of those disputes, religious traditions and their communities form the imaginations of patients and clinicians—giving them visions for the meaning and purposes of medicine within faithful lives. Religious traditions and communities shape clinicians' judgments about how to practice medicine, and about how to negotiate clinical ethical decisions in the face of disagreements that inevitably arise. By challenging the core assumptions of today's medical ethics, religious traditions also call the overall culture of medicine into question, particularly insofar as that culture reduces medicine and ethics to procedure and technique, ignoring the deeper moral purposes of our practices. By taking religion more seriously, clinicians and clinical ethicists can practice with appropriate humility, candor, and understanding.

NOTES

1. Leviticus 19:16. Tanakh. Jewish Publication Society of America Version, 1917. Accessed online at: http://www.mechon-mamre.org/e/et/et0.htm
2. For a long time conventional wisdom held that physicians were, on average, much less religious than their patients. This conventional wisdom was due in part to studies of scientists, which have found scientists tend to be much less religious than the general population, as well as to broader studies in which those with more education and higher incomes tend to be less religious. Yet we found that physicians, despite

being scientists of a sort and having far above average income and education, are more or less as religious as members of the general population.

3. Interestingly, Jewish physicians were significantly more likely to find these practices problematic. That finding and its implications are explored in Stern, Rasinski, & Curlin (2011).
4. Debate about this question, and the data that follow, are presented in Chung et al. (2012).
5. See Kim et al. (2014) for a history of the Committee on Medicine and Religion and the Department of Medicine and Religion at the American Medical Association. We argue that the demise of both in 1972 came about as the result of conflicts over abortion.
6. See Directive 58 in United States Conference of Catholic Bishops, 2009.

REFERENCES

Antiel, R. M., James, K. M., Hardt, J. J., Curlin, F. A., Tilburt, J. C. (2014). Physician opinion and the HHS contraceptive mandate. *AJOB Empirical Bioethics*, 5(1), 56–60.

Bleich, J. D. (1998a). *Bioethical dilemmas: a Jewish perspective*. Hoboken, NJ: KTAV Publishing House.

Bleich, J. D. (1998b). *Bioethical Dilemmas: A Jewish Perspective*. Hoboken, NJ: KTAV Publishing House.

Brock, D. W. (2008). Conscientious refusal by physicians and pharmacists: Who is obligated to do what, and why? *Theor Med Bioeth*, 29(3), 187–200. doi:10.1007/s11017-008-9076-y

Chung, G. S., Lawrence, R. E., Rasinski, K. A., Yoon, J. D., & Curlin, F. A. (2012). Obstetrician-gynecologists' beliefs about when pregnancy begins. *Am J Obstet Gynecol*, 206(2), 132 e131–137. doi:10.1016/j.ajog.2011.10.877

Combs, M. P., Antiel, R. M., Tilburt, J. C., Mueller, P. S., & Curlin, F. A. (2011). Conscientious refusals to refer: Findings from a national physician survey. *Journal Med Ethics*, 37(7), 397–401. doi:10.1136/jme.2010.041194

Curlin, F. A., Chin, M. H., Sellergren, S. A., Roach, C. J., & Lantos, J. D. (2006). The association of physicians' religious characteristics with their attitudes and self-reported behaviors regarding religion and spirituality in the clinical encounter. *Med Care*, 44(5), 446–453. Retrieved from http://www.ncbi.nlm.nih.gov/entrez/query.fcgi?cmd=Retrieve&db=PubMed&dopt=Citation&list_uids=16641663

Curlin, F. A., & Hall, D. E. (2005a). Regarding Plan B: Science and politics cannot be separated. *Obstet Gynecol*, 105(5 Pt 1), 1148–1150; author reply 1150–1141. doi:10.1097/01.AOG.0000162540.26907.43

Curlin, F. A., & Hall, D. E. (2005b). Strangers or friends? A proposal for a new spirituality-in-medicine ethic. *J Gen Intern Med*, 20(4), 370–374. Retrieved from http://www.ncbi.nlm.nih.gov/entrez/query.fcgi?cmd=Retrieve&db=PubMed&dopt=Citation&list_uids=15857497

Curlin, F. A., Lantos, J. D., Roach, C. J., Sellergren, S. A., & Chin, M. H. (2005). Religious characteristics of U.S. physicians: a national survey. *J Gen Intern Med*, 20(7), 629–634. Retrieved from http://www.ncbi.nlm.nih.gov/entrez/query.fcgi?cmd=Retrieve&db=PubMed&dopt=Citation&list_uids=16050858

Curlin, F. A., Lawrence, R. E., Chin, M. H., & Lantos, J. D. (2007). Religion, conscience, and controversial clinical practices. *N Engl J Med*, 356(6), 593–600. Retrieved from http://www.ncbi.nlm.nih.gov/entrez/query.fcgi?cmd=Retrieve&db=PubMed&dopt=Citation&list_uids=17287479

Curlin, F. A., Nwodim, C., Vance, J. L., Chin, M. H., & Lantos, J. D. (2008). To die, to sleep: US physicians' religious and other objections to physician-assisted suicide, terminal sedation, and withdrawal of life support. *Am J Hosp Palliat Care*, 25(2), 112–120. doi:10.1177/1049909107310141

Emanuel, E. J., & Emanuel, L. L. (1992). Four models of the physician-patient relationship. *JAMA*, 267(16), 2221–2226. Retrieved from http://www.ncbi.nlm.nih.gov/pubmed/1556799

Engelhardt, H. T. (2000). *The foundations of Christian bioethics*. Amsterdam, Netherlands: Swets & Zeitlinger Publishers.

Evans, J. H. (2012). *The history and future of bioethics: A sociological view*. New York, NY: Oxford University Press

Halifax, J. (2008). *Being with dying: Cultivating compassion and fearlessness in the presence of death* (1st ed.). Boston, MA: Shambhala.

Harris, L. H., Cooper, A., Rasinski, K. A., Curlin, F. A., & Lyerly, A. D. (2011). Obstetrician-gynecologists' objections to and willingness to help patients obtain an abortion. *Obstet Gynecol, 118*(4), 905–912. doi:10.1097/AOG.0b013e31822f12b7

Kim, D., Curlin, F., Wolenberg, K., & Sulmasy, D. (2014). Religion in organized medicine: The AMA's Committee and Department of Medicine and Religion, 1961–1974. *Perspect Biol Med, 57*(3), 393–414. doi:10.1353/pbm.2014.0025

Larchet, J.-C. (2002). *The theology of illness*. Crestwood, NY: St. Vladimir's Seminary Press.

Lawrence, R. E., & Curlin, F. A. (2009). Physicians' beliefs about conscience in medicine: a national survey. *Acad Med, 84*(9), 1276–1282. doi:10.1097/ACM.0b013e3181b18dc5

Lawrence, R. E., Rasinski, K. A., Yoon, J. D., & Curlin, F. A. (2011a). Adolescents, contraception and confidentiality: A national survey of obstetrician—gynecologists. *Contraception, 84*(3), 259–265. doi:10.1016/j.contraception.2010.12.002

Lawrence, R. E., Rasinski, K. A., Yoon, J. D., & Curlin, F. A. (2011b). Obstetrician-gynecologists' views on contraception and natural family planning: A national survey. *Am J Obstetr Gynecol, 204*(2), 124 e121–127. doi:10.1016/j.ajog.2010.08.051

Padela, A. I., Malik, A. Y., Curlin, F., & De Vries, R. (2015). [Re]considering respect for persons in a globalizing world. *Dev World Bioeth, 15*(2), 98–106. doi:10.1111/dewb.12045

Pellegrino, E. D., Thomasma, D. C., & Miller, D. G. (1996). *The Christian virtues in medical practice*. Washington, DC: Georgetown University Press.

Putman, M. S., Yoon, J. D., Rasinski, K. A., & Curlin, F. A. (2013). Intentional sedation to unconsciousness at the end of life: Findings from a national physician survey. *J Pain Symptom Manage, 46*(3), 326–334. doi:10.1016/j.jpainsymman.2012.09.007

Putman, M. S., Yoon, J. D., Rasinski, K. A., & Curlin, F. A. (2014). Directive counsel and morally controversial medical decision-making: Findings from two national surveys of primary care physicians. *J Gen Intern Med, 29*(2), 335–340. doi:10.1007/s11606-013-2653-4

Quill, T. E., & Brody, H. (1996). Physician recommendations and patient autonomy: Finding a balance between physician power and patient choice. *Ann Intern Med, 125*(9), 763–769. Retrieved from http://www.ncbi.nlm.nih.gov/pubmed/8929011

Siegler, M. (1981). Searching for moral certainty in medicine: A proposal for a new model of the doctor-patient encounter. *Bull NY Acad Med, 57*(1), 56–69. Retrieved from http://www.ncbi.nlm.nih.gov/pubmed/6937229

Silvas, A. (2005). *The Asketikon of St Basil the Great*. Oxford; New York: Oxford University Press.

Steinberg, A. (2003). Encyclopedia of Jewish medical ethics (F. Rosner, Trans.) (pp. lxxv). Jerusalem, Israel: Feldheim Publishers.

Stern, R. M., Rasinski, K. A., & Curlin, F. A. (2011). Jewish physicians' beliefs and practices regarding religion/spirituality in the clinical encounter. *J Relig Health*. doi:10.1007/s10943-011-9509-1

Stulberg, D. B., Dude, A. M., Dahlquist, I., & Curlin, F. A. (2011). Abortion provision among practicing obstetrician-gynecologists. *Obstet Gynecol, 118*(3), 609–614. doi:10.1097/AOG.0b013e31822ad973

Thomasma, D. C. (1983). Beyond medical paternalism and patient autonomy: A model of physician conscience for the physician-patient relationship. *Ann Intern Med, 98*(2), 243–248. Retrieved from http://www.ncbi.nlm.nih.gov/pubmed/6824259

United States Conference of Catholic Bishops. Ethical and religious directives for catholic health care services. 5th ed. 2009. Retrieved from: http://www.usccb.org/issues-and-action/human-life-and-dignity/health-care/upload/Ethical-Religious-Directives-Catholic-Health-Care-Services-fifth-edition-2009.pdf

Verhey, A. (2011). *The Christian art of dying: Learning from Jesus*. Grand Rapids, MI: William B. Eerdmans.

Wolenberg, K. M., Yoon, J. D., Rasinski, K. A., & Curlin, F. A. (2013). Religion and United States physicians' opinions and self-predicted practices concerning artificial nutrition and hydration. *J Relig Health*, *52*(4), 1051–1065. doi:10.1007/s10943-013-9740-z

Yoon, J. D., Rasinski, K. A., & Curlin, F. A. (2010). Moral controversy, directive counsel, and the doctor's role: Findings from a national survey of obstetrician-gynecologists. *Acad Med*, *85*(9), 1475–1481. doi:10.1097/ACM.0b013e3181eabacc

CHAPTER 13

RELIGION AND SPIRITUALITY IN MEDICAL EDUCATION

Marta Herschkopf, Najmeh Jafari, and Christina Puchalski

What is the place of spirituality and religion in medical education? Leaders of the spirituality in health movement have been addressing this issue for the past two decades. In ancient times, spirituality and medicine were closely entwined, but in modernity, this relationship had been largely overlooked until the end of the twentieth century. In 1995, three medical schools offered courses in spirituality and health. According to recent surveys, 75 to 90% of US medical schools have now incorporated teaching on spirituality and health, with a majority doing so as part of the required curriculum (Koenig et al., 2010; Puchalski et al., 2014). This chapter will describe the current state of spirituality in medical education, reviewing evidence in the literature to support specific educational practices, with an emphasis on undergraduate medical education in North America.

While this volume concerns itself with the place of religion and spirituality within various parts of medical culture, in the realm of medical education the discourse and scientific evidence has consciously centered itself around the comprehensive concept of spirituality. A conference convened by the Association of American Medical Colleges to start developing learning objectives in this area defined spirituality as follows:

> "Spirituality [. . .] is expressed in an individual's search for ultimate meaning through participation in religion and/or belief in God, family, naturalism, rationalism, humanism, and the arts. All of these factors can influence how patients and health care professionals perceive health and illness and how they interact with one another" (Association of American Medical Colleges, 1999).

This definition of spirituality subsumes religion as well as other systems of meaning, and makes a case for its relevance to the practice of medicine. This chapter will focus on this definition but will also discuss aspects of medical education focusing more deliberately on religion, including educational programs situated within particular religious traditions.

One aspect of medical education is to teach physicians to respect the spiritual beliefs, values, and practices of their patients and provide culturally competent care. Yet it has become increasingly evident that spiritually competent care is not simply a matter of deferring to the beliefs and attitudes of patients, but encompasses a mode of relating to patients and families, to one's colleagues, and to one's own identity as a clinician. Modern educational theory points to educational institutions as tools of socialization, and medical educators have become acutely aware of the "hidden curriculum" that influences the ethical and moral development of physicians-in-training (Hafferty & Franks, 1994). This has led to increased educational resources devoted to ethics and professionalism, and spirituality has played a part in this. A recent study investigating the relationship of spirituality and the hidden curriculum found that survey participants who self-identified as religious or spiritual often struggled with issues of personal identity and self-confidence, but also were more likely to resist the hidden curriculum and avoid relationship conflicts within the medical team, work-life imbalance, and emotional stress arising from patient encounters (Balboni et al., 2015). The most recent guidelines for core competencies in spirituality and health for medical education (Puchalski et al., 2014) emphasize not only asking about a patient's spiritual beliefs, but also respecting those beliefs, understanding the role of spirituality in health care, practicing nonjudgmental listening skills, navigating spiritual resources within health-care systems, and recognizing one's own spiritual needs.

This chapter focuses on how to impart these lessons to physicians-in-training. It begins with a brief historical background, followed by a review of the National Competencies on Spirituality and Health, a 2011 consensus statement of faculty from seven medical schools delineating competencies and behavioral objectives, as well as potential teaching (pedagogical) methods and performance assessments, for spirituality in medical education. The chapter will then elaborate on work published regarding these methods in both undergraduate and graduate medical education, and conclude with a discussion of implications and future directions.

HISTORICAL BACKGROUND: EDUCATIONAL INITIATIVES AND RESEARCH

The current structure of American medical school training, with undergraduate science prerequisites, two preclinical basic science years, and two clinical clerkship years, dates back to the reforms of Abraham Flexner in the early twentieth century. Flexner was chiefly concerned with countering a trend towards accrediting physicians with little to no formal training in science and clinical medicine. In the years since, as the corpus of medical knowledge has grown, and as practitioners have become increasingly specialized, standard medical education has come to include internship and residency, and even post-residency fellowships.

In the latter half of the twentieth century, medical educators became increasingly attentive not only to the medical knowledge being imparted, but also to the mores and culture of medicine. Concerned that the physician-patient relationship was suffering as students struggled to master an exponentially growing corpus of medical knowledge, several medical school faculties in the 1950s developed experimental educational programs to emphasize communication skills and preventative medicine (Kendall & Reader, 1988). In response to social pressure in the 1980s, medical educators began to emphasize values of professionalism and cultural competence. While religion and spirituality were not generally discussed explicitly, there was significant theoretical overlap in the early work on professionalism and current aspects of spiritual competence (Herschkopf, 2011; Puchalski, 2006; Puchalski et al., 2014).

In 1984, the Panel on the General Professional Education of the Physician and College Preparation for Medicine (GPEP), a subsidiary of the Association of American Medical Colleges (AAMC), published a report calling for "Medical faculties [to...] emphasize the acquisition and development of skills, values, and attitudes by students at least to the same extent that they do the acquisition of knowledge" (Association of American Medical Colleges, 1984). However, there was little guidance regarding what values and attitudes were to be acquired, nor on how to impart them, and as a result, few medical schools adjusted their curricula. In response, the AAMC launched the Medical Schools Objectives Project (MSOP) to delineate measurable learning objectives in various domains of medical education (Association of American Medical Colleges, 1999). The 1999 MSOP report focused on communication, and included a Report from a Task Force on Spirituality, Cultural Issues, and End of Life Care. The latter included a definition of spirituality and seven specific learning objectives regarding spirituality and cultural issues. These objectives were further refined in 2011 by the National Initiative to Develop Competencies in Spirituality for Medical Education (NIDCSME) (Puchalski et al., 2014) (Table 13.1)

As various governing medical bodies were calling for the integration of spirituality into curricula, educators were seeking support to implement these recommendations. Various educators were successfully integrating spirituality into their curricula, but there was little being published describing the content and evaluation of these courses. Part of the reason for a lack of literature is that spirituality is often integrated into other courses, such as ethics, practice of medicine, communication skills, palliative medicine, humanities, and those on complementary and alternative medicine (CAM). For example, a 2002 survey of medical schools found that 64.4% of the 53 respondents included spirituality/faith/prayer in their CAM curricula (Brokaw et al., 2002). Another part of the reason is a lack of publications of curricular details/assessments, which is not unique to spirituality courses, but has also been noted regarding curricula on resident research and evidence-based medicine (Fortin & Barnett, 2004). These methodological challenges likely account for some of the discrepancies in various surveys quantifying the presence of religion and spirituality in medical school curricula.

A 1998 review described common elements in spirituality courses offered by approximately 50 US medical schools (Puchalski & Larson, 1998). A 2004 review found 10 articles describing elements of curricula on spirituality in medicine (Fortin & Barnett, 2004). A 2012 comprehensive global literature review identified 38 articles on the topic of spirituality in undergraduate and graduate medical education (Lucchetti et al., 2012). Thirty-one of these articles came from the United States, but only 8 of them described specific educational initiatives in US medical schools. More recently, there has been a push from funding bodies to have recipients of awards publish their findings more generally. Internationally, of the 38 articles in the 2012 survey, only 4 came from countries outside of North America (Lucchetti et al., 2012). Nevertheless, those articles do suggest that spirituality is being integrated into curricula globally in select countries.

TABLE 13.1 The National Initiative to Develop Competencies in Spirituality for Medical Education

Competency		Behaviors
Health Care Systems: Apply knowledge of health care systems to advocate for spirituality in patient care	HCS1	Describe the importance of incorporating spiritual care into a health care system
	HCS2	Describe and evaluate spiritual resources in a health care system and a community
	HCS3	Compare and contrast spiritual resources in different health care systems
	HCS4	Discuss the ways in which health care systems may complicate spiritual care
	HCS5	Describe methods of reimbursement for spiritual care, including funding for other disciplines (e.g., nursing, chaplains, counseling)
	HCS6	Discuss how the legal, political and economic factors of health care influence spiritual care
	HCS7	Explain how effective spiritual care impacts the overall quality of and improvements to patient care
	HCS8	Describe how spiritual care is provided by interdisciplinary team members and community resources
	HCS9	Apply advocacy skills to spiritual care within health care systems (e.g., local, regional, national)
Knowledge: Acquire the foundational knowledge necessary to integrate spirituality in patient care	K1	Compare and contrast spirituality (broadly defined) and religion
	K2	Discuss the relationships between spirituality, religious beliefs, and cultural traditions
	K3	Describe how spirituality interrelates with complementary and alternative medicine
	K4	Discuss major religious traditions as they relate to patient care
	K5	Differentiate between a spiritual history, spiritual screening, and spiritual assessment
	K6	Describe common religious/spiritual problems that arise in clinical care
	K7	Compare and contrast sources of spiritual strength and spiritual distress
	K8	Differentiate between spirituality and psychological factors (e.g., grief, hope, meaning)
	K9	Describe boundary issues in providing spiritual care
	K10	Outline key findings of spirituality-health research
	K11	Locate and evaluate spiritual/religious information resources (online and hard copy)
	K12	Describe how a patient's spirituality may affect his/her context-specific clinical care

TABLE 13.1 Continued

Competency		Behaviors
Patient Care: Integrate spirituality into routine clinical practice	PC1	Appropriately use patients' spiritual network and supports
	PC2	Perform a detailed spiritual history at appropriate times (e.g., complete medical history, giving bad news)
	PC3	Perform spiritual screening at appropriate time
	PC4	Perform ongoing assessment of patient's spiritual distress
	PC5	Integrate patient's spiritual issues and resources into ongoing treatment and discharge plans
	PC6	Collaborate with staff, family, pastoral care and other members of health care team to address patient's spiritual care
	PC7	Invite patients to identify and explore their own spirituality or inner life
	PC8	Respond appropriately to verbal and nonverbal signs of spiritual distress
	PC9	Make timely referral to chaplain or spiritual counselor
	PC10	Respect patients' spiritual/religious belief systems
Compassionate Presence: Establish compassionate presence and action with patients, families, colleagues	CP1	Discuss why it is a privilege to serve the patient
	CP2	Describe personal and external factors that limit your ability to be fully "present" with a given patient
	CP3	Discuss why the illness experience of the patient is an essential element of the physician-patient relationship
	CP4	Discuss how you as a provider may be changed by your relationship with the patient
	CP5	Demonstrate the ability to be engaged and fully "present" with a patient
	CP6	Describe strategies to be more present with patients
Personal and Professional Development: Incorporate spirituality in professional and personal development	PPD1	Explain the reasons and motives that drew you to the medical profession
	PPD2	Explore the role that spirituality plays in your professional life
	PPD3	Reflect on signs of personal spiritual crisis & methods of intervening
	PPD4	Identify your sources of spiritual strengths
	PPD5	Describe how spirituality functions as a way of connecting with health care team, family, and patients
	PPD6	Identify your personal and professional support communities

(continued)

TABLE 13.1 Continued

Competency		Behaviors
Communications: Communicate with patients, families, and health care team about spiritual issues	C1	Practice deep listening—hearing what is being communicated through and between the words, the body language, and the emotions.
	C2	Practice curious inquiry—a non-judgmental practice of exploration without goals or expectations
	C3	Practice perceptive reflections—mirroring for the client what you hear or perceive, but always checking the "truth" of your reflection with the client.
	C4	Communicate professionally with spiritual care providers and other team members about the patient's spiritual distress or resources of strength
	C5	Use appropriate nonverbal behaviors to signal interest in the patient
	C6	Demonstrate the use of silence in patient communication

In the United Kingdom, 59% of schools who participated in a national questionnaire survey in 2008 stated that they integrated at least some topics on spirituality into their undergraduate medical curriculum, with 50% including compulsory teaching (Neely & Minford, 2008). A cross-sectional study from Brazil showed that 41% of Brazilian medical schools have courses or content on spirituality and health and 10% have dedicated spirituality courses (Lucchetti et al., 2012). This chapter will focus on North America given the more comprehensive scope of literature focusing on these curricula.

GUIDELINES AND CONSENSUS STATEMENTS

There have been a few published expert opinions and consensus statements on how to design and evaluate courses on spirituality and health (Koenig, 2013; Puchalski, 2006). Specific recommendations as to the form of courses have been based on anecdotal evidence and include the following:

- Using a broad definition of spirituality
- Incorporating spirituality into the required curriculum, and not relegating it to elective courses
- Integrating spirituality throughout medical school curricula, in both preclinical and clinical years, and in residencies
- Stepwise curricula with basic material in preclinical years followed by reinforcement, modeling, and the introduction of more refined material in clinical and residency years

- Interdisciplinary courses with students and/or professionals from other fields, including nursing, social work, or pastoral care
- Creative, multimedia teaching methods, such as personal reflection, use of art/literature, field trips, role-play, and meditation
- Incorporating evaluative components to reinforce lessons and assess outcomes

These consensus statements also included recommendations regarding the general content of these courses, including knowledge and skills. The *Oxford Textbook of Spirituality in Healthcare* includes a table outlining a model curriculum on Spirituality and Medicine developed by educators at George Washington University (Cobb, Puchalski, & Rumbold, 2012).

The National Initiative to Develop Competencies in Spirituality for Medical Education took a more systematic approach, delineating learning objectives and framing them in terms of 49 behavioral competencies comprising skills, knowledge, and attitudes (Puchalski et al., 2014) (Table 13.1). Medical schools applied competitively to be chosen to participate in a consensus conference to develop competencies in spirituality and health in medical education, with interdisciplinary educators from selected schools participating in this meeting. The members of this conference adapted preexisting competency domains from guidelines used by the Accreditation Council for Graduate Medical Education (ACGME), and added a newly defined competency of compassionate presence (CP). The other domains are health care systems (HCS), knowledge (K), patient care (PC), personal and professional development (PPD), and communications (C). These domains will be referred to in the remainder of the chapter using these abbreviations. The full report (not reproduced here) also lists 49 potential teaching (pedagogical) methods and 23 potential modes of performance assessments, and maps the most applicable ones onto each competency domain.

As part of the application process for the George Washington Institute for Spirituality and Health (GWish)–Templeton Reflection Rounds (GTRR) (discussed further later in this chapter), medical schools were asked to provide a description of National Competencies in Spirituality and Health for Medical Education which is currently embedded in their medical education curriculum. All 33 participating medical schools reported that they were teaching competency topics either as stand-alone elective courses or as part of required courses. Out of the 33 medical schools who submitted their applications, 11 schools (33%) teach more than 60% of competency behaviors; 10 medical schools (30%) teach 30–60% of competency behaviors; and 27% teach 30% or less of the competency behaviors. Collectively, these applications indicate that a majority of the competency behaviors in spirituality and health are offered in these schools with the highest prevalence in the compassionate presence domain (CP6: Describe strategies to be more present with patients). The least prevalent competency behavior was locating and evaluating spiritual/religious informational resources (online and hard copy). (Table 13.2)

Overall, however, while there is significant content in spirituality and health in many schools, evaluation of the curricula has been lagging. As mentioned previously, many of the spirituality topics are integrated into broader courses such as the humanities or in history taking, making evaluation more difficult. Similarly, it is difficult to develop quantitative evaluation methodology for topics in humanities and ethics. Finally, the hidden curriculum continues to emphasize the biomedical over the psychosocial and spiritual as students still are primarily evaluated on their technical and scientific expertise. According to a 2010

TABLE 13.2 National Competency Behaviors in Spirituality and Health for Medical Education Offered by Medical Schools as Reported in their GTRR Applications (*n* = 33)

Competency	Behaviors	# Offered in Medical Schools
CP6	Describe strategies to be more present with patients	67
K2	Discuss the relationships between spirituality, religious beliefs, and cultural traditions	59
PC3	Perform spiritual screening at appropriate time	51
PC1	Appropriately use patients' spiritual network and supports	50
C1	Practice deep listening—hearing what is being communicated through and between the words, the body language, and the emotions.	48
C2	Practice curious inquiry—a non-judgmental practice of exploration without goals or expectations	48
K12	Describe how a patient's spirituality may affect his/her context-specific clinical care	43
C3	Practice perceptive reflections—mirroring for the client what you hear or perceive, but always checking the "truth" of your reflection with the client.	43
C6	Demonstrate the use of silence in patient communication	43
C5	Use appropriate nonverbal behaviors to signal interest in the patient	42
PC2	Perform a detailed spiritual history at appropriate times (e.g., complete medical history, giving bad news)	39
PC4	Perform ongoing assessment of patient's spiritual distress	36
PC7	Invite patients to identify and explore their own spirituality or inner life	34
C4	Communicate professionally with spiritual care providers and other team members about the patient's spiritual distress or resources of strength	34
PPD1	Explain the reasons and motives that drew you to the medical profession	33
K1	Compare and contrast spirituality (broadly defined) and religion	32
PPD2	Explore the role that spirituality plays in your professional life	29
K8	Differentiate between spirituality and psychological factors (e.g., grief, hope, meaning)	28
HCS1	Describe the importance of incorporating spiritual care into a health care system	28
CP1	Discuss why it is a privilege to serve the patient	26
PPD5	Describe how spirituality functions as a way of connecting with health care team, family and patients	26
PPD6	Identify your personal and professional support communities	26
HCS2	Describe and evaluate spiritual resources in a health care system and a community	24
HCS4	Discuss the ways in which health care systems may complicate spiritual care	24
HCS7	Explain how effective spiritual care impacts the overall quality of and improvements to patient care	24

TABLE 13.2 Continued

Competency	Behaviors	# Offered in Medical Schools
K4	Discuss major religious traditions as they relate to patient care	24
K6	Describe common religious/spiritual problems that arise in clinical care	24
K9	Describe boundary issues in providing spiritual care	24
PC8	Respond appropriately to verbal and nonverbal signs of spiritual distress	23
K3	Describe how spirituality interrelates with complementary and alternative medicine	22
PC5	Integrate patient's spiritual issues and resources into ongoing treatment and discharge plans	21
PPD3	Reflect on signs of personal spiritual crisis & methods of intervening	21
CP2	Describe personal and external factors that limit your ability to be fully "present" with a given patient	20
CP4	Discuss how you as a provider may be changed by your relationship with the patient	20
CP5	Demonstrate the ability to be engaged and fully "present" with a patient	20
PPD4	Identify your sources of spiritual strengths	20
CP3	Discuss why the illness experience of the patient is an essential element of the physician-patient relationship	19
HCS8	Describe how spiritual care is provided by interdisciplinary team members and community resources	17
PC6	Collaborate with staff, family, pastoral care and other members of health care team to address patient's spiritual care	15
HCS9	Apply advocacy skills to spiritual care within health care systems (e.g., local, regional, national)	14
PC10	Respect patients' spiritual/religious belief systems	13
K7	Compare and contrast sources of spiritual strength and spiritual distress	12
PC9	Make timely referral to chaplain or spiritual counselor	12
HCS3	Compare and contrast spiritual resources in different health care systems	11
HCS6	Discuss how the legal, political and economic factors of health care influence spiritual care	10
K5	Differentiate between a spiritual history, spiritual screening, and spiritual assessment	9
K10	Outline key findings of spirituality-health research	9
HCS5	Describe methods of reimbursement for spiritual care, including funding for other disciplines (e.g., nursing, chaplains, counseling)	5
K11	Locate and evaluate spiritual/religious information resources (online and hard copy)	4

survey of medical school deans, while the majority did integrate spirituality in health into their required curricula (80%) and agreed that such content was valuable (64%), only 33% agreed that it was important to have spirituality and health content encouraged by AAMC guidelines, and only 30% agreed that it was important to develop methods of evaluation (Association of American Medical Colleges, 1999). The reasons for these attitudes are not covered in the survey but, anecdotally, are often related to concerns that other areas of the curriculum are more valuable and already given short shrift. Additionally, some surveys suggest that physicians' attitudes towards spirituality in the clinical encounter may be influenced by their own spiritual beliefs, encouraging speculation that the same may apply to educators' attitudes regarding teaching on this subject (McEvoy et al., 2014). A survey of primary care residents found that residents participating in organized religious activities or endorsing a higher level of personal spirituality were more likely to feel that they should play a role in their patients' spiritual or religious lives (Luckhaupt et al., 2005). Similarly, a survey of 2000 practicing US physicians found that physicians with high religiosity were more likely to report that patients mentioned religion/spirituality issues, to believe that religion/spirituality strongly influences health, and to interpret the influence of religion/spirituality in positive rather than negative ways (Curlin et al., 2007). Published surveys on the religious/spiritual demographics of medical educators are lacking, but could theoretically play a role. Thus, there remains a relative dearth of outcomes-based research in this field.

REVIEW OF THE LITERATURE: TEACHING (PEDAGOGICAL) METHODS AND PERFORMANCE ASSESSMENTS

As previously mentioned, currently there is not sufficient data to recommend particular evidence-based educational techniques. There is not space in this chapter to cover all areas described by the NIDCSME guidelines. Instead, selected interventions that have been described and evaluated in the literature with particular promise will be reviewed.

PERFORMANCE ASSESSMENTS AND INTERVENTION EVALUATIONS: CHALLENGES AND INNOVATIONS

How does one evaluate an educational intervention? The most obvious way is to test students to see whether they have acquired the skills and knowledge being imparted. Thus the development of performance assessments is integral to outcomes-research in this field. This review will use the term "performance assessments" to refer to interventions evaluating students for primarily pedagogical purposes, which can secondarily be used for research purposes. The term "intervention evaluations" will refer to evaluations used primarily for research purposes. It should be noted that some of the best performance assessments also serve a didactic role; for example, one learns to formulate a case by writing it up and receiving feedback.

Traditional medical education has relied upon examination questions, particularly of the multiple-choice format, to test knowledge acquisition, and this mode is appropriate to some spiritual competences. However, short-answer and essay formats are better suited to more conceptual knowledge. Case write-ups can also be used to evaluate acquisition of clinical concepts.

Skills and attitudes require other modes of assessment. Student self-report surveys can serve a role as performance assessments by asking students whether/how strongly they agree with statements that represent attitudes that educators wish to impart (e.g., "On a scale of 1 to 5, how strongly do you agree that spiritual factors play a role in health?"). However, no form of self-report survey necessarily reflects clinical practice (Adams et al., 1999), and all are thus limited in their ability to evaluate the behavioral competencies being advocated. Many research projects continue to use surveys and other self-report measures as intervention evaluations, for example, asking students whether they feel comfortable about their knowledge in a particular area, feel confident in their ability to accomplish a given skill, or think that a particular educational intervention was useful or enjoyable. Such measures are cost-effective and easily quantifiable, but remain limited in their ability to capture whether behaviors will indeed be practiced. There are few studies focusing on methods of assessment in this area: one study found that physician trainees' self-assessments of their communication skills regarding religion/spirituality correlated with patient ratings of the clinical encounter (Ford et al., 2014), although another found that self-assessments of spiritual history-taking did not correlate with performance in a standardized patient encounter (Musick et al., 2003).

Reflection essays and journals are didactic models that also are well-suited to performance assessment of compassionate presence and personal and professional development competencies. Many published studies incorporate written reflection into other interventions to both reinforce material and analyze themes that emerge in these writings for intervention evaluation purposes (Culliford, 2009; Kuczewski et al., 2014; McEvoy et al., 2014; Talley & Magie, 2014). Designed reflection essay prompts have asked specifically about NIDCSME domains (communications, compassionate presence, patient care, and personal and professional development). Ledford and colleagues (Ledford et al., 2014) developed an ordinal stages of change model coding scheme (pre-contemplation, contemplation, preparation, action, maintenance) for family medicine residents learning to interact with patients who bring up religious or spiritual concerns. The two authors who developed the scheme analyzed journal entries and interview transcripts according to it, with an eye towards progression between the stages. Inter-rater reliability was high (kappa = 0.937, $P < 0.001$). While this assessment method is likely better suited to the research setting, it could be the basis for less work-intensive rating tools. In the United Kingdom, an 8-week spirituality and health elective included reflections in which students described their own attitudes before and after the course (Culliford, 2009).

Direct observation of clinical practice remains the gold standard of performance assessments, but requires time, training, and staff. It is also subjective and can be difficult to quantify for research purposes. Many programs evaluate students using videotapes of standardized patient encounters (King et al., 2004) and objective structured clinical examinations, or OSCEs (discussed more later). In vivo supervision of spiritual competency behaviors in the clinical years of medical school has not been described in the literature, and would require extensive faculty training and buy-in. This would likely be best accomplished within a particular core clerkship rather than across all the various clinical departments. As a model, the University of South Carolina psychiatry residency describes successfully integrating 360-degree performance assessments of their residents: these included self-report, patient-satisfaction questionnaires, reports of individual supervisors, and peer chart-reviews to see if residents integrated spirituality into their documentation of history, formulation, and treatment planning (Campbell et al., 2012).

Another challenge for intervention evaluation is that performance assessments generally focus on short-term rather than long-term outcomes. This is one reason that it is important to integrate performance assessments into different levels of educational curricula. Long-term outcomes are difficult to evaluate without randomization, although some researchers have tried to retrospectively trace individual physician practice to different modes of spirituality education (Rasinski et al., 2011). Some promising data come from the Cambridge Health Alliance, which in 2004 piloted a longitudinal integrated clerkship for third-year Harvard Medical School students with clearly articulated goals of engendering patient-centered care and countering ethical erosion. While this is not a specifically spiritual intervention, it does demonstrate a comprehensive program aimed at enhancing professional development. Students in this program were contrasted with classmates who were randomized to complete their third-year clerkships at a different Harvard-affiliated hospital. Four to six years later, these students were surveyed and it was found that the outcomes measures of patient-centered attitudes immediately post-clerkship had persisted at statistically significant rates (Gaufberg et al., 2014).

SPECIFIC MATERIALS AND SPIRITUAL ASSESSMENT TOOLS

Most of the literature does not recommend specific textbooks or materials to include in didactic sessions. One report mentions having students watch a documentary about how a Muslim patient's religious beliefs affect his health care (McEvoy et al., 2014). Schonfeld and colleagues (Schonfeld et al., 2016) used two main texts supplemented with articles and other chapters: Harold Koenig's second edition of *Spirituality in Patient Care: Why, How, When, and What,* (Koenig, 2013) and Jerome Groopman's series of case portraits, *The Measure of Our Days* (Groopman, 1997). Koenig (2007) lists some of his favorite articles as resources. The *Oxford Textbook of Spirituality in Healthcare* (Cobb et al., 2012), which is designed to be a comprehensive textbook on this subject, has several chapters appropriate for didactic contexts.

Many curricula do mention specific spiritual history or assessment tools. Integral to patient care is the ability to talk to patients about their spiritual concerns. The NIDCSME guidelines differentiate between spiritual history, screening, and assessment (Puchalski et al., 2014), but broadly speaking, medical students must be given language with which to begin these conversations. One of the more influential innovations of spirituality and health has been the development of spiritual assessment scales, which define different domains of spirituality relevant to patient care and suggest questions to ask patients. The name of each assessment tool is an acronym to help remember these domains. Potential tools include the FICA (Puchalski & Romer, 2000), the HOPE questionnaire (Anandarajah & Hight, 2001), and the SPIRITual History (Maugans, 1996). Among these tools, FICA is a validated standard tool, serving as a guide for clinicians to incorporate open-ended questions regarding spirituality into the standard comprehensive history (Borneman et al., 2010; Lucchetti et al., 2013). This tool is a set of questions designed to invite patients to share their religious or spiritual beliefs based on four domains of spiritual assessment: the presence of Faith, belief, or meaning; the Importance of spirituality in an individual's life; the individual's spiritual Community; and interventions to Address spiritual needs (Puchalski & Romer, 2000). Tools are often taught in formal didactic sessions, but some programs reinforce this skill by having students read articles on the importance of eliciting a spiritual history, and/or role-playing history-taking in small-groups or with standardized patients (Barnett, 2004; Barnett & Fortin, 2006; Graves et al., 2002; King et al., 2004; Talley & Magie, 2014). The Kansas City University of Medicine and Biosciences went further and had students complete a spiritual self-assessment by applying the FICA to themselves (Talley & Magie, 2014), an innovative way to address competencies in the Personal and Professional Development domain.

OBJECTIVE STRUCTURED CLINICAL EXAMINATIONS (OSCES)

Objective Structured Clinical Examinations, or OSCEs, are useful as both evaluative and educational tools. These are scripted experiences involving a standardized patient (SP) meant to test particular clinical competences. Ledford and colleagues describe formulating an OSCE case in a family medicine residency to use as a "sensitizing practice," or what might be termed experiential-based learning. In other words, incorporating spiritual concerns into simulated clinical encounters without warning helps students integrate their knowledge and realize the need to respond to patient cues. The case in this report involved a 63-year-old woman visiting her primary care physician to follow-up a new diagnosis of hypertension. During the encounter, the woman mentions that her mother died at age 63 and that she is scared and has been praying to God that she not die. Immediately following the 10-minute interview were 10-minutes of written self-reflection, followed then by semi-structured reflective interviews and group reflection sessions 1–2 weeks later. These sessions were intended to reinforce the lessons from the encounter itself (Ledford et al., 2014).

Some medical schools have similarly begun to incorporate spiritual issues into OSCEs, *and OSCEs* which are well-suited to test competencies in several domains, including patient care (e.g., referring the SP to a chaplain, responding to SP signs of spiritual distress), compassionate presence (e.g., being engaged and fully present with a SP in distress), and communications (practicing deep, nonjudgmental listening). OSCEs can also be used to direct curriculum development. McEvoy and colleagues describe implementing a spiritual competency OSCE with third-year medical students, in which a 65-year-old man with acute chest pain who is now medically stable mentions that he is religious and has fears of dying. They found that while many students referred the SP to a chaplain, few engaged directly with the SP's spiritual distress. It should be noted that this case was one of eight in a larger evaluative experience, a setting which can reinforce it as a sensitizing practice: in this study, lessons were reinforced with a post-encounter written exercise with open-ended questions regarding the nature and treatment of the SP's distress (McEvoy et al., 2014).

SESSIONS INCLUDING SPIRITUAL CARE

Several published articles describe medical schools and residencies incorporating departments of spiritual care into their training. Such interventions can serve not only to familiarize students with the role of chaplains (health care systems domain), but also to have chaplains teach and model behaviors in the patient care, compassionate presence, personal and professional development, and communications domains. One common intervention is to have students shadow a chaplain, often followed by a reflection paper (Frazier et al., 2015; Perechocky et al., 2014; Schonfeld et al., 2016; Talley & Magie, 2014). Student surveys cited by these studies indicate that students find this a valuable experience.

Chaplains may also be incorporated into panel discussions, lectures, and other classroom-based experiences (Barnett, 2004; Barnett & Fortin, 2006; McEvoy et al., 2014; Stuck et al., 2012). Two examples of this approach follow. The University of South Carolina Psychiatry Residency piloted an interdisciplinary training program that included general psychiatry residents, child psychiatry residents, psychology interns, and seminary students. The workshops involved targeted teaching to each group, and small-group discussions incorporating members of all groups to help address preconceived biases and promote collaboration (Stuck et al., 2012). This is similar to the GWish-Templeton Reflection Rounds (GTRR), currently being implemented in 18 medical schools as part of an ongoing research effort, for third- and fourth-year clerkship students (GTRR website, 2014). GTRR is designed to nurture physicians' inner or spiritual growth through a unique reflection process facilitated by teams of specially trained physicians, chaplains, and counseling professionals. Through mentor and peer-facilitated reflection, participants consider how their encounters with patients affect them emotionally, spiritually, and formatively. Preliminary program evaluation data shows impact on student and faculty awareness of spirituality, on student ability to be present to others, and on student wellbeing. Faculty have also described the impact of these sessions on their own rekindling of joy and meaning in their profession.

Finally, some departments of spiritual care offer their own educational programs for health care providers. The Chaplaincy Department at Massachusetts General Hospital offers a five-month fellowship in spiritual care to health care providers from different disciplines focusing on the integration of religious and spiritual care into clinical practice. The course includes 100 hours of educational components and 300 hours of clinical components. Survey data from participants showed statistically significant increases in frequency of and confidence in providing such care, as well as increased prayer with patients (Zollfrank et al., 2015).

FIELD TRIPS

The literature reviewed on medical student spirituality courses does not specifically mention field trips, although this is a promising immersive intervention and is used in some psychiatry residencies (Kozak et al., 2010). Anecdotally, although not described much in the literature, it is becoming increasingly common for medical students and trainees to attend open meetings of Alcoholic Anonymous or Narcotics Anonymous, which present opportunities to learn about a successful spiritually-based health intervention (Stuck et al., 2012).

CEREMONIES, SERVICES, AND OATHS

Although they are rarely considered as part of the formal curriculum, formal ceremonies play an important part in undergraduate medical education and the imparting of spiritual and professional principles. Students are often initiated into their training with a White Coat Ceremony, a tradition designed by the Arnold P. Gold Foundation first held in 1993 at the Columbia University College of Physicians & Surgeons. According to the Gold Foundation website, currently 97% of AAMC-accredited US medical schools begin with a White Coat Ceremony or similar service (White Coat Ceremony, 2013). While these ceremonies may involve speakers and other elements, they are characterized by a "cloaking" of each student by a faculty member already part of the profession of medicine, who literally places the white coat on the student's shoulders as "a personally delivered gift of faith, confidence, and compassion" (White Coat Ceremony, 2013). The Gold Foundation is currently administering grants for schools and residency programs to develop other rituals to instill the values of humanism throughout medical training (Goldzweig et al., 2010).

Another increasingly common ceremony is a memorial service for human anatomy cadaver donors, conducted in the vast majority of the programs responding to a recent survey (Jones et al., 2014). These ceremonies generally include speeches as well as other modes of expression, such as music and art. In many cases, the family members of the cadaver donors play an active role. Furthermore, the ceremonies often have a religious/spiritual tone to them, with the majority referred to as "services," and with many having religious leaders be part of those organizing the event or be among those in attendance. However, there were some programs that did not include religious leaders due to objections raised in response to their attendance at prior ceremonies, and others that made a conscious effort not to include religious content that would seem to privilege one faith over another. These ceremonies are often considered part of the anatomy curriculum, although at one medical school the service of remembrance is a part of the required curriculum in spirituality and health; it is humanistic and inclusive of all beliefs, values and perspectives (Cobb, Puchalski, Rumbold, 2012). The focus of most of these programs is to allow the students to express gratitude for the gift of the cadaver donors to their education.

Another part of medical education where there is a potential intersection of spirituality and health care (though largely overlooked in the literature) is oath-taking. Oaths are often tied to one's call or reason to serve patients, or to the ethical responsibilities that the caregiving role entails. When first studied in the year 2000, all accredited US allopathic and osteopathic medical schools administered oaths, most of them variations on the Hippocratic Oath or the Declaration of Geneva, many involving students in writing them (Kao & Parsi, 2004). Some have begun to include oath-writing in courses on spirituality and health (Roseman, 2014). Oaths are often part of graduation ceremonies, but may also be integrated into White Coat ceremonies or other transition periods in medical education (Programs: Arnold P. Gold Foundation, 2013). The studies cited have surveyed the frequency and content of these various ceremonies, but there is little literature evaluating how they impact medical students and professionals. A 2009 survey of practicing US physicians found that while 79% of the 1,032 respondents recalled an oath-taking ceremony in medical school, only 26% identified such oaths as significantly influencing their professional practice, and were more likely to cite influences such as "personal sense of right and wrong" or "great moral teachers" (Antiel et al., 2011).

While this chapter has focused on programs in spirituality offered by non-denominational institutions, some scholars argue that the virtues of medical professionalism are based not the culture of medicine itself, but rather in a multiplicity of ethical and cultural traditions external to medical culture. Thus, teaching and training in medical professionalism should engage deeply with specific traditions with a spirit of "open pluralism" to help ground the virtues being taught (Kinghorn et al., 2007). Non-denominational programs often achieve this by incorporating departments of spiritual care (as described), or encouraging students to speak from their diverse cultural backgrounds in discussion sessions. Another approach is to include readings or lectures from health care providers speaking deliberately from within their own personal religious or spiritual traditions. A Harvard Medical School elective using this method published a collection with chapters authored by health care providers describing the intersection of different religious or spiritual traditions and medicine, often including personal reflections (Peteet & D'Ambra, 2011).

While not part of the formal curriculum, anecdotally many medical schools have a number of student organizations with religious affiliations that help connect students with other members of their religious communities for religious and cultural activities. For example, the Harvard Medical School website lists student groups for Catholics, Christians, and Jews (HMS/HSDM Student Council Web site., 2015), and there is also a branch of the university's Islamic Society at the medical school (Harvard Longwood Muslims, 2015). At times, programming includes lectures and discussions about the intersection of their particular religious traditions and medicine, serving as a forum for students to explore these relationships.

Finally, there are educational programs aimed at health care providers offered by a number of divinity schools and religiously affiliated universities that are situated within particular religious traditions. The Theology, Medicine, and Culture initiative at Duke Divinity School offers a fellowship program aimed at health care professionals that includes coursework toward a degree offered by the divinity school as well as seminars, retreats, and communal prayer (Duke Divinity School, 2015). Loyola University Chicago, a Jesuit institution, offers a four-year Physician's Vocation Program for medical students interested in exploring the intersection of their own faith and medical practice. The program includes educational components as well as community service, prayer, and retreats to foster a sense of spiritual community (The Physician's Vocation Program, 2015).

RESIDENCY, FELLOWSHIP, AND CONTINUING MEDICAL EDUCATION

The literature from residency and fellowship curricula will not be reviewed here, although some innovative educational approaches have been mentioned in the preceding section. Psychiatry is the specialty that appears to have the greatest amount of literature on this topic, including specialty-specific learning objectives and model curricula (Lucchetti et al., 2012). Other specialties with literature on this topic include primary care and family medicine (Ledford et al., 2014), oncology and palliative care (Otis-Green et al., 2012), and internal medicine (Lucchetti et al., 2012).

Continuing Medical Education Opportunities that are not specialty-specific are centered around several academic centers and institutes, including the Duke Center for Spirituality, Theology, and Health; the George Washington Institute for Spirituality and Health (GWish); the Institute for the Study of Health & Illness (ISHI); and the University of Chicago Program on Medicine and Religion, which sponsors an annual conference on medicine and religion. There are also many specific faith tradition-based academic and advocacy groups.

CONCLUSIONS AND FUTURE DIRECTIONS

This is a challenging but exciting time in medicine. While the scientific underpinnings of practice continue to advance at a rapid rate, physician burn-out and patient disaffection loom larger. As legislators, third-party payers, and other interests shape the culture of medicine, the role of medical educators in instilling values and safeguarding the place of ultimate meaning in health care delivery becomes all the more pressing. Fortunately, the conversation has been underway for some time.

While significant progress has been made in integrating spirituality into medicine generally, and into medical education in particular, there remains a great deal of work to be done. The relevance of spirituality to health and health care delivery remains an area of substantial controversy. While many clinicians, educators, and researchers continue to feel that spirituality does not have a place in their medical practice, there has been substantial progress in integrating spirituality into medical education over the last twenty years. Educational efforts can play a part in shifting cultural outlooks, but these efforts are hampered by a number of factors. For one, while there are clinical guidelines in some fields, such as palliative care, there is a lack of standardized clinical guidelines across all clinical areas that might inform and reinforce curricular content. The NIDCSME objectives provide a framework, but each clinical field must define its own best practices. As one example, the field of palliative care has formulated a consensus statement on delivering quality spiritual care as part of palliative care (Puchalski et al., 2009). Similar efforts in other clinical fields would streamline educational efforts and provide opportunities to evaluate those efforts. Furthermore, outcomes-based research on spiritual interventions could inform what clinical practices constitute evidence-based care. Many clinical initiatives have been driven by educators themselves, and we are just beginning to collect data from the courses developed in response to educational mandates. While we are starting to learn which kinds of educational efforts are successful in imparting particular knowledge and attitudes, the implications of those lessons remain an area for further study.

REFERENCES

Adams, A. S., Soumerai, S. B., Lomas, J., & Ross-Degnan, D. (1999). Evidence of self-report bias in assessing adherence to guidelines. *International Journal for Quality in Health Care: Journal of the International Society for Quality in Health Care / ISQua, 11*(3), 187–192.

Anandarajah, G., & Hight E. (2001). Spirituality and medical practice: Using the HOPE questions as a practical tool for spiritual assessment. *American Family Physician, 63*(1), 81–88.

Antiel, R. M., Curlin, F. A., Hook, C. C., & Tilburt, J. C. (2011). The impact of medical school oaths and other professional codes of ethics: Results of a national physician survey. *Archives of Internal Medicine, 171*(5), 469–471.

Association of American Medical Colleges. (1984). Physicians for the twenty-first century: The GPEP report (report of the project panel on the general and professional education of the physician and college preparation for medicine). *J Med Educ, 59.*

Balboni, T. (2015). Religion, spirituality, and the hidden curriculum: Medical student and faculty reflections. *Journal of Pain and Symptom Management, 50*(4), 507–515.

Barnett, K. G. (2004). Medical school curricula in spirituality and medicine. *JAMA: The Journal of the American Medical Association, 291*(23), 2883.

Barnett, K. G., & Fortin, A. H. (2006). Spirituality and medicine. *Journal of General Internal Medicine, 21*(5), 481–485.

Borneman, T., Ferrell, B., & Puchalski, C. M. (2010). Evaluation of the FICA tool for spiritual assessment. *Journal of Pain and Symptom Management, 40*(2), 163–173.

Brokaw, J. J., Tunnicliff, G., Raess, B. U., & Saxon, D. W. (2002). The teaching of complementary and alternative medicine in US medical schools: A survey of course directors. *Academic Medicine, 77*(9), 876–881.

Campbell, N., Stuck, C., & Frinks, L. (2012). Spirituality training in residency: Changing the culture of a program. *Academic Psychiatry, 36*(1), 56.

Cobb, M., Puchalski, C. M., & Rumbold, B. D. (2012). *Oxford textbook of spirituality in healthcare.* Oxford: Oxford University Press.

Culliford, L. (2009). Teaching spirituality and health care to third year medical students. *The Clinical Teacher, 6*(1), 22–27.

Curlin, F. A., Sellergren, S. A., Lantos, J. D., & Chin, M. H. (2007). Physicians' observations and interpretations of the influence of religion and spirituality on health. *Archives of Internal Medicine, 167*(7), 649–654.

Duke Divinity School:Theology, Medicine, and Culture. (2015). Retrieved from https://tmc.divinity.duke.edu/TMCprograms/#. Accessed December 20, 2015.

Ford, D. W., Downey, L., Engelberg, R., Back, A. L., & Curtis, J. R. (2014). Association between physician trainee self-assessments in discussing religion and spirituality and their patients' reports. *Journal of Palliative Medicine, 17*(4), 453–462.

Fortin, A. H., & Barnett, K. G. (2004). Medical school curricula in spirituality and medicine. *Jama, 291*(23), 2883.

Frazier, M., Schnell, K., Baillie, S., & Stuber, M. L. (2015). Chaplain rounds: A chance for medical students to reflect on spirituality in patient-centered care. *Academic Psychiatry, 39*(3), 320–323.

Gaufberg, E., Hirsh, D., Krupat, E., Ogur, B., Pelletier, S., Reiff, D., & Bor, D. (2014). Into the future: Patient centredness endures in longitudinal integrated clerkship graduates. *Medical Education, 48*(6), 572–582.

Goldzweig, G., Hasson-Ohayon, I., Meirovitz, A., Braun, M., Hubert, A., & Baider, L. (2010). Agents of support: Psychometric properties of the cancer perceived agents of social support (CPASS) questionnaire. *Psycho-Oncology, 19*(11), 1179–1186. doi:10.1002/pon.1668

Graves, D. L., Shue, C. K., & Arnold, L. (2002). The role of spirituality in patient care: Incorporating spirituality training into medical school curriculum. *Academic Medicine, 77*(11), 1167.

Groopman, J. (1997). *The measure of our days: New beginnings at life's end.* New York: Viking.

GTRR website - The Physician's Vocation Program. (2015). Retrieved from http://hsd.luc.edu/bioethics/content/physicianvocationprogram/

The GW institute for spirituality and health and the John Templeton foundation announce reflection rounds award winners. (2014). Retrieved from http://smhs.gwu.edu/news/gw-institute-spirituality-and-health-and-john-templeton-foundation-announce-reflection-rounds Accessed February 18, 2016.

Hafferty, F. W., & Franks, R. (1994). The hidden curriculum, ethics teaching, and the structure of medical education. *Academic Medicine, 69*(11), 861–871.

Harvard Longwood Muslims. (2015). Retrieved from http://www.hcs.harvard.edu/his/branches-2/harvard-longwoodmuslims. Accessed December 20, 2015.

Herschkopf, M. (2011). Teaching and learning at the medicine/spirituality interface. In J. R. Peteet, & M. N. D'Ambra (Eds.), *The soul of medicine: Spiritual perspectives and clinical practice* (pp. 237–255). Baltimore: Johns Hopkins University Press.

HMS/HSDM Student Council. (2015). Retrieved from http://studentcouncil.hms.harvard.edu/student-organizations/ Accessed December 20, 2015.

Jones, T. W., Lachman, N., & Pawlina, W. (2014). Honoring our donors: A survey of memorial ceremonies in united states anatomy programs. *Anatomical Sciences Education, 7*(3), 219–223.

Kao, A. C., & Parsi, K. P. (2004). Content analyses of oaths administered at US medical schools in 2000. *Academic Medicine, 79*(9), 882–887.

Kendall, P. L., & Reader, G. G. (1988). Innovations in medical education of the 1950s contrasted with those of the 1970s and 1980s. *Journal of Health and Social Behavior, 29*(4), 279–293.

King, D. E., Blue, A., Mallin, R., & Thiedke, C. (2004). Implementation and assessment of a spiritual history taking curriculum in the first year of medical school. *Teaching and Learning in Medicine, 16*(1), 64–68.

Kinghorn, W. A., McEvoy, M. D., Michel, A., & Balboni, M. (2007). Professionalism in modern medicine: Does the emperor have any clothes? *Academic Medicine: Journal of the Association of American Medical Colleges, 82*(1), 40–45.

Koenig, H. G. (2013). *Spirituality in patient care: Why, how, when, and what.* West Conshohocken: Templeton Foundation Press.

Koenig, H. G., Hooten, E. G., Lindsay-Calkins, E., & Meador, K. G. (2010). Spirituality in medical school curricula: Findings from a national survey. *International Journal of Psychiatry in Medicine, 40*(4), 391–398.

Kozak, L., Boynton, L., Bentley, J., & Bezy, E. (2010). Introducing spirituality, religion and culture curricula in the psychiatry residency programme. *Medical Humanities, 36*(1), 48–51.

Kuczewski, M. G., McCarthy, M. P., Michelfelder, A., Anderson, E. E., Wasson, K., & Hatchett, L. (2014). "I will never let that be ok again": Student reflections on competent spiritual care for dying patients. *Academic Medicine: Journal of the Association of American Medical Colleges, 89*(1), 54–59.

Ledford, C. J., Seehusen, D. A., Canzona, M. R., & Cafferty, L. A. (2014). Using a teaching OSCE to prompt learners to engage with patients who talk about religion and/or spirituality. *Academic Medicine: Journal of the Association of American Medical Colleges, 89*(1), 60–65.

Lucchetti, G., Bassi, R. M., & Lucchetti, A. L. G. (2013). Taking spiritual history in clinical practice: A systematic review of instruments. *Explore: The Journal of Science and Healing, 9*(3), 159–170.

Lucchetti, G., Lucchetti, A. L. G., Espinha, D. C. M., de Oliveira, L. R., Leite, J. R., & Koenig, H. G. (2012). Spirituality and health in the curricula of medical schools in Brazil. *BMC Medical Education, 12*(1), 1.

Lucchetti, G., Lucchetti, A. L. G., & Puchalski, C. M. (2012). Spirituality in medical education: Global reality? *Journal of Religion and Health, 51*(1), 3–19.

Luckhaupt, S. E., Michael, S. Y., Mueller, C. V., Mrus, J. M., Peterman, A. H., Puchalski, C. M., & Tsevat, J. (2005). Beliefs of primary care residents regarding spirituality and religion in clinical encounters with patients: A study at a midwestern US teaching institution. *Academic Medicine, 80*(6), 560–570.

Maugans, T. A. (1996). The spiritual history. *Archives of Family Medicine, 5*(1), 11–16.

McEvoy, M., Burton, W., & Milan, F. (2014). Spiritual versus religious identity: A necessary distinction in understanding clinicians' behavior and attitudes toward clinical practice and medical student teaching in this realm. *Journal of Religion and Health, 53*(4), 1249–1256.

McEvoy, M., Schlair, S., Sidlo, Z., Burton, W., & Milan, F. (2014). Assessing third-year medical students' ability to address a patient's spiritual distress using an OSCE case. *Academic Medicine: Journal of the Association of American Medical Colleges, 89*(1), 66–70.

Musick, D. W., Cheever, T. R., Quinlivan, M. S., & Nora, L. M. (2003). Spirituality in medicine: A comparison of medical students' attitudes and clinical performance. *Academic Psychiatry, 27*(2), 67–73.

Neely, D., & Minford, E. J. (2008). Current status of teaching on spirituality in UK medical schools. *Medical Education, 42*(2), 176–182.

Otis-Green, S., Ferrell, B., Borneman, T., Puchalski, C., Uman, G., & Garcia, A. (2012). Integrating spiritual care within palliative care: An overview of nine demonstration projects. *Journal of Palliative Medicine, 15*(2), 154–162.

Perechocky, A., DeLisser, H., Ciampa, R., Browning, J., Shea, J. A., & Corcoran, A. M. (2014). Piloting a medical student observational experience with hospital-based trauma chaplains. *Journal of Surgical Education, 71*(1), 91–95.

Peteet, J. R., & D'Ambra, M. N. (2011). *The soul of medicine: Spiritual perspectives and clinical practice.* Baltimore: Johns Hopkins University Press.

Programs: Arnold P. Gold Foundation. (2013). Retrieved from http://www.gold-foundation.org/programs/. Accessed April 18, 2015.

Puchalski, C. (2006). Spirituality and medicine: Curricula in medical education. *Journal of Cancer Education, 21*(1), 14–18.

Puchalski, C. M., & Larson, D. B. (1998). Developing curricula in spirituality and medicine. *Academic Medicine, 73*(9), 970–974.

Puchalski, C., Ferrell, B., Virani, R., Otis-Green, S., Baird, P., Bull, J., . . . Prince-Paul, M. (2009). Improving the quality of spiritual care as a dimension of palliative care: The report of the consensus conference. *Journal of Palliative Medicine, 12*(10), 885–904.

Puchalski, C., & Romer, A. L. (2000). Taking a spiritual history allows clinicians to understand patients more fully. *Journal of Palliative Medicine, 3*(1), 129–137.

Puchalski, C. M., Blatt, B., Kogan, M., & Butler, A. (2014). Spirituality and health: The development of a field. *Academic Medicine: Journal of the Association of American Medical Colleges, 89*(1), 10–16.

Rasinski, K. A., Kalad, Y. G., Yoon, J. D., & Curlin, F. A. (2011). An assessment of US physicians' training in religion, spirituality, and medicine. *Medical Teacher, 33*(11), 944–945.

Roseman, J. L. (2014). Honoring the medicine: Searching for the embodiment of spiritual commitment and philosophy for student physicians. *Advances in Mind-Body Medicine, 28*(2), 6–9.

Schonfeld, T. L., Schmid, K. K., & Boucher-Payne, D. (2016). Incorporating spirituality into health sciences education. *Journal of Religion and Health, 55*(1), 85–96.

Stuck, C., Campbell, N., Bragg, J., & Moran, R. (2012). Psychiatry in the deep south: A pilot study of integrated training for psychiatry residents and seminary students. *Academic Psychiatry, 36*(1), 51–55.

Talley, J. A., & Magie, R. (2014). The integration of the "spirituality in medicine" curriculum into the osteopathic communication curriculum at Kansas City University of Medicine and Biosciences. *Academic Medicine : Journal of the Association of American Medical Colleges, 89*(1), 43–47.

White Coat Ceremony. (2013). Retrieved from http://www.gold-foundation.org/programs/white-coat-ceremony/. Accessed April 18, 2015.

Zollfrank, A. A., Trevino, K. M., Cadge, W., Balboni, M. J., Thiel, M. M., Fitchett, G., . . . Balboni, T. A. (2015). Teaching health care providers to provide spiritual care: A pilot study. *Journal of Palliative Medicine, 18*(5), 408–414.

CHAPTER 14

RELIGION AND SPIRITUALITY IN NURSING

John Swinton and Lynne Vanderpot

As one reflects on the literature, it is clear that nurses have quite specific sensibilities around issues of religion and spirituality as these things relate to the practice of nursing (Pike, 2011). This evidence highlights the ways in which the profound intimacy that is an inexorable aspect of the nursing encounter lends itself to the mysterious and the personal. Such intimacy opens up those dimensions of human encounter that can easily be overlooked by those who perceive the nursing task as primarily technical and instrumental, having to do with standing back, observing, and limiting interactions with those who are sick. The beauty of the practice of nursing is that the distance between the nurse and the patient is never the point. It is the space between that matters. The space between is the place of meeting; it is a space that is not created by distance, but by a mutual movement towards one another in an attempt to create space for care that values, respects, and offers hospitality towards both participants. Those who are afraid to come close, to touch, to feel, to empathize, and to connect have probably misunderstood the relational nature of nursing as well as the complex and deeply personal narrative processes that shape and form both the experience of illness and the process and practices of medicine. In this chapter, we will try to tease out something of the nature of nursing-as-communion, and the ways in which a focus on spirituality and religion can move nurses to take seriously the sensuous and spiritual nature of nursing. We will briefly describe the nursing literature that focuses on religion and spirituality, before providing a conceptual framework that can allow nurses effectively to engage with the religious and spiritual needs of patients. In the final part of the chapter we will offer some examples of how nurses should engage patients at the level of the spiritual.

NURSING RESEARCH IN RELIGION AND SPIRITUALITY

The area of spirituality and nursing is growing exponentially. There is a good deal of evidence to suggest that while nurses may not always be confident about how to meet spiritual needs

(Lewinson et al., 2015), and in spite of the fact that there is some dispute about the rigor and validity of some of the studies that have been carried out thus far (Swinton, 2006; Paley, 2007, 2008), spirituality remains of deep significance for nurses. In terms of research, the field of spirituality-in-nursing is broad in its focus and intention. A good deal of the conversation to date has focused around conceptual and definitional issues: *what exactly is this "thing" we call spirituality?* This literature tends to focus around two issues:

1. The separation of religion from spirituality
2. The nature of generic, non-religious spirituality

It is clear from the literature, particularly that which emerges from Europe, Australia, and New Zealand, thatfor many nurses, spirituality is something to be understood apart from religion. Spirituality is considered to be a generic and often universal feature of human beings which may include, but is not defined by, religion (Torskenæs et al., 2015; Lopez et al., 2014; Reinert et al., 2013; Macleod et al., 2011). This generic spirituality is basically a form of self-actualization, defined in terms of a personal search for meaning, purpose, value, hope, love, and for some a sense of the holy. There is no commonly agreed-upon definition of this kind of spirituality, which has led some to suggest that it is so broad and diverse that it has become meaningless (Paley, 2008). However, others have pointed out that even without a commonly agreed-upon definition, a focus on meaning, purpose, hope, and so forth serves to raise the consciousness of nurses to issues that might otherwise be overlooked within a technologically-oriented healthcare system. Spirituality doesn't have to be "real" to be important (Swinton, 2014; Swinton & Pattison, 2010).

The literature overall leans toward this generic understanding of spirituality; as such, the primary methodological approach is often qualitative. Qualitative research is diverse, covering such things as nurses' awareness of spirituality and spiritual needs, education, end-of-life care, spiritual distress, and the experience of being cared for (McSherry & Jamieson, 2013; Roach, 2013; Taylor & Mamier, 2013; Cockell & McSherry, 2012; Skomakerstuen et al., 2015). This approach enables nurses to understand and respond to the deep and personal meanings of the spirituality of both nurses and patients. Such studies resonate very closely and clearly with the relational tasks of nursing.

There is a second strand within the research which adopts a more quantitatively-oriented approach. This strand seeks to apply the methods of the hard sciences to the spiritual practices of nursing. This research tends to focus specifically on religion and religious practices such as prayer, meditation, and religious observance (Koenig et al., 2012; Kim-Godwin, 2013; Spadaro & Hunker, 2016; Habibian et al., 2015). In this sense, implicitly and explicitly it aligns itself with the so-called "religion and health" movement which seeks to examine the ways in which practicing religion can be good for your health (Koenig et al., 2012). Although the focus is often on religion, the emphasis is on the *function* of religious beliefs as shapers of behaviors and responses, rather than on the content of specific belief systems. The growing evidence base that has emerged from this approach indicates that religious behavior can have a positive effect on physical and mental health. Such behavior has been shown to be beneficial on a number of levels and in relation to a wide variety of conditions. Health benefits include (Koenig et al., 2001)

- Extended life expectancy
- Lower blood pressure
- Lower rates of death from coronary artery disease
- Reduction in myocardial infarction
- Increased success in heart transplants
- Reduced serum cholesterol levels
- Reduced levels of pain in cancer sufferers
- Reduced mortality among those who attend church and worship services
- Increased longevity among the elderly
- Reduced mortality after cardiac surgery

Those working with this religiously-focused model do at times speak about the more general term "spirituality" (Koenig & Larson 2001). However, it is clear that the majority of the research done within this approach emphasizes religion and for the most part the Christian religion. Although nurses have touched on this approach, there is clearly a need for more of this kind of empirical research.

Both of these approaches hold value for nursing. The existentialist perspective opens up a humanistic spiritual space for practices that value the whole person. The more specifically religious approaches indicate that it may be possible to develop a convincing quantitative evidence base to underpin spiritual care and practice. Taken together, this body of literature serves to indicate and support the suggestion that spirituality is a vital aspect of nursing practice. With these provisional observations in mind, we would now like to develop a new framework that can help nurses to work in both the realm of the spiritual and the religious.

A CONCEPTUAL FRAMEWORK FOR NURSING CARE IN RELIGION AND SPIRITUALITY

ILLNESS AS NARRATIVE

The beginning point for what follows is a quite basic observation: illness is not simply a medical condition with symptoms that require to be treated. Rather, *illness is a narrative event with medical implications*. The experience of illness involves a subtle or major change in someone's narrative: a change that needs to be recognized and responded to in all of its fullness. We might think of it in this way. A person's personal identity is constituted by the various stories that we tell about ourselves and others tell about is. In a real sense, our perceptions of ourselves comprises an *autobiographical self* (Brockmeier, 2004). If I develop influenza, I might find myself saying something like "I am not feeling myself today." Not to "feel like one's self" has to do with the impact of a particular illness on the story that one uses to make sense of oneself. If a relatively minor viral infection such as influenza can bring about a change in someone's perception of who they are—a shift in their autobiographical self—how much more will a major diagnosis such as cancer, schizophrenia, or

Parkinson's disease alter the stories we tell about ourselves? Illness inevitably impacts upon the coherence of the fundamental narratives that comprise our identity.

ORIENTATION—DISORIENTATION—REORIENTATION

In drawing this point out, it will be helpful to reflect on the work of the biblical scholar Walter Brueggemann. In his exploration of the Psalms, Brueggemann points to the fact that the Psalms are intended to be form full of people's suffering (Brueggemann, 1995, 1977). What he means by this is that they are intended to shape and form our experiences of suffering. Suffering and distress are not things that occur outside of a particular context. The shape and form that the experience of suffering takes is deeply affected by where we experience our suffering. In one sense we are *taught* how to suffer. For example, the level of distress that we are able to express will depend on the response of those around us. If people are awkward in the presence of our suffering and respond in ways which indicate embarrassment or intolerance, we will more than probably limit the expression of our suffering in an attempt to prevent distress in the other or embarrassment in ourselves. The response of the other shapes our expression of suffering and determines our options for dealing with it.

Brueggemann suggests that the psalms are designed to provide a particular shape for people's suffering. Brueggemann focuses particularly on the Psalms of lament, that is, those psalms which give vent to deep suffering, pain, injustice, and anger:

How long, O LORD? Will you forget me forever? How long will you hide your face from me?
How long must I wrestle with my thoughts and every day have sorrow in my heart? How long will my enemy triumph over me?
Look on me and answer, O LORD my God. Give light to my eyes, or I will sleep in death;
my enemy will say, "I have overcome him," and my foes will rejoice when I fall.
But I trust in your unfailing love; my heart rejoices in your salvation.
I will sing to the LORD, for he has been good to me.
(Psalm 13)

The task of the psalms of lament, Brueggemann argues, was to teach the Hebrews a particular way in which to suffer and to give them a specific language to express such suffering. He points out that the psalms of lament are designed to take a person from a place of orientation to a place of disorientation and onwards towards a place of reorientation. *Orientation* occurs when life is presumed to be fundamentally good. In such times it is assumed that God is in control and that the world is a safe place. God is living peaceably in God's heaven. But then something goes wrong. People experience oppression, injustice, and suffering. They become *disoriented*. Everything seems to have gone wrong. The covenant appears to have been broken; loss and disorientation reign. But then, as the psalm moves on, the sufferer finds a new orientation: a *reorientation*. Here the psalmist finds himself in a new place where things may still make little sense, but where the Psalmist can nonetheless find an assurance that God still loves him, that he is safe and that God's unending *hesed* (love) has won the day. The shape of the psalm provides a structure and a language that enables people to work through this process and discover hope in the midst of what seems to be utter hopelessness. It is important to notice that the place of reorientation Brueggemann talks about is not a movement backwards towards a person's initial orientation. It is not an attempt to regain something that has been lost. Rather, it is a new state of being in the world which contains new possibilities. The original trauma is not taken from the psalmist. The trauma remains and the situation is still painful. The difference is that now, within the process of reorientation, he sees the trauma differently. He gives the situation a different meaning as he learns to trust in God's unfailing love.

THE DISORIENTATION OF ILLNESS

We can use this framework of orientation to disorientation to reorientation as a way of narrating the experience of illness. When we become ill, we enter into a new land of illness and disorientation. Susan Sontag describes this new land in this way:

> Illness is the night side of life, a more onerous citizenship. Everyone who is born holds dual citizenship, in the kingdom of the well and in the kingdom of the sick. Although we all prefer to use the good passport, sooner or later each of us is obliged, at least for a spell, to identify ourselves as citizens of that other place (Sontag, 1977, 47–48).

Within the kingdom of the sick, the old stories that we used to explain our lives and to make sense of the world simply don't fit. The old maps don't lead to the same places; the old methods of coping no longer enable us to cope. Our lives are filled with dissonance, unease, dis-ease, disorientation. It is here, within the tension between disorientation and reorientation that the spiritual inevitably rises to the surface: *Who am I? Where do I come from? Where am I going to? Why?*

We may well need medical treatment, but more than anything else, what we need is a new story; a story helps us to understand our "new selves" and which moves us to re-narrate our story and in so doing provide fresh possibilities to guide us as we struggle to negotiate the strange new world of illness. For the psalmist, the new story began with the recognition of God's unending love. This may be the case for people who are religious. However, for all patients, finding the centerpoint of meaning that can be the beginning place for the creation of a new re-orienting story is the key to effective spiritual care. Spiritual care is one way that nurses have of re-narrating the story of illness and reconstructing the shape of people's suffering.

In working through the meaning of reorientation in the context of illness and disability, the focus is not on cure or even necessarily on the eradication of any particular problem. The key thing for the psalmist is that nothing really changed. He simply looked at things differently in the light of his centerpoint of meaning: God's unending love. The focus is on the meaning of events for the individual. This means shifting our question around illness from "How can I help you; what can I do for you?"—a set of questions that tend to be perceived in terms of tasks to be done rather than people to become—to "What does this thing *mean* for you and your family?" "How do you see the future?" "Where is your source of hope and meaning in the midst of this situation?" Such questions form the core of our spirituality and demand not simply logical answers, but new stories;

stories that people can use to integrate their experience of illness within their autobiographical selves. The art of spiritual care is learning to listen to stories and to work with patients to create new stories that initiate spiritual reorientation.

UNDERSTANDING THE SPIRITUAL

Understood in this way, spirituality is perceived not as a "thing," like a table or a chair. Spirituality is a way of being in the world wherein we can learn to dwell within particular narratives that give us hope and provide meaning even in the midst of the most difficult of circumstances. Likewise, spiritual care is not a competence like giving medicine or changing beds. Spiritual care is the process of facilitating people's search for meaning as they journey towards their reoriented goals. Spiritual care has to do with discovering the diversity of ways in which nurses can learn to listen to, be with, and assist patients in finding satisfactory answers to the key questions that emerge from the experience of illness.

GENERIC SPIRITUALITY

This narrative perspective enables us to work creatively with the dichotomy within the nursing literature between religion and spirituality (Emblem, 1992; Swinton, 2001). There seems to be a general consensus that spirituality and religion should be separated into two related genres, one which applies to religious people and the other which has to do with *all* people. The broader definition of spirituality includes such things as a search for meaning, purpose, value, hope, love, relationships, and for some people, the sacred (again broadly defined; Weathers et al., 2015; Reinert & Koenig, 2013). Within this understanding *everyone* is presumed to have a spirituality and everyone has these basic existential needs. When illness impinges upon an individual and their sense of who they are begins to shift and change—Who am I? Where do I come from? Where am I going? Why?—the recognition of such existential needs opens up space for the creation of new stories of hope and reorientation. These stories may include, but do not necessitate, the presence of the divine. For example, imagine for a moment someone who has received a diagnosis that has changed his or her autobiographical self in profound ways. What kind of a story does a person require to cope effectively with such a change in status?

One of the authors remembers working alongside a woman who had terminal breast cancer. The doctor gave her three months to live. How was she to make sense of this new story? Where was her sense of identity and hope to come from? For this woman, her point of reorientation came in relation to her daughter's forthcoming wedding. She had promised her daughter that she would not only be at her wedding, but that she would make her wedding dress. So for the next few months that's what she did. She prepared, she sewed, and she put the dress together. Six months went by. In the end she attended her daughter's wedding and watched the gown she had so lovingly created do its work. Two weeks later she died.

Viktor Frankl has observed that if people have enough meaning in their lives they can survive even the most horrendous events (Frankl, 2004). For this woman, it was in the simplicity of preparing for her daughter's wedding that she discovered who she was, and the meaning of her life even though its ending was imminent. Her new story focused on how she could sustain her status as a mother who has things to do with and for her children while simultaneously facing the imminent loss of this central role. Spiritual care here related to supporting her as she struggled to re-narrate her maternal story in a way that brought hope, meaning, and fresh possibilities even if the end of the story remained tragic. Spirituality in this generic open mode enables people to find meaning, purpose, hope, and a new story within which they can reorient their experience.

RELIGIOUS CARE

As we have seen, while many nurse researchers frame spirituality as something that everyone in some sense has and participates in, other researchers highlight the importance of religion. Everyone has spirituality, it is argued, but only some people work it out via religion. Religion contains a particular story and a set of accompanying sub-narratives, a more or less fixed set of beliefs, and a set of formal rituals and practices such as worship, prayer, and Scripture reading. Religion helps individuals to narrate their experiences in quite particular ways. Put slightly differently in Brueggemann's terms, it provides a shape for people's suffering. People interpret and receive their illness experience in line with the narrative that underpins their religious beliefs—that is, that which provides their sense of identity and their sense of self in the world. So the change in story that is brought on by illness may be perceived by an "outsider" in quite a different way from the way in which an insider may perceive the story.

An example will help to highlight the significance of this point. A colleague of one of the authors recently preached a sermon on suffering and healing. The essence of his message was that the world is fallen and broken, pain and suffering do exist, but God doesn't will such suffering. In the end, God will wipe away every tear and end all human suffering. On the face of it, it sounded like a powerfully healing and compassionate way of framing the problem of suffering. However, after the service two elderly sisters approached the minister. They were very angry. One of them was in the latter stages of breast cancer. Both sisters were Christians and both sisters had always been involved with the church. However, they were unhappy with the minister's sermon. For them it was really important that God *had* done this to them. Why? Because if God had done this—had brought this affliction on them—it was under God's control. If God was in control, there was meaning, purpose, hope, and above all the certainty of life after death. Their current pain and suffering would be overcome in the long-term. The sisters were locating their tragic story within a bigger story that was filled with hope and new possibilities. They were using the big story to reorient their "small" story. Importantly, what looked like healing words actually took something profoundly hopeful away from them. Likewise, what, for some, might have looked like a pathological religious belief—God has done this to me—turned out to be the locus for healing and reorientation. Learning to listen to stories in the right way is the heart of spiritual care.

NARRATIVE COMPETENCY

If we put to one side the ongoing and probably insurmountable conceptual issues surrounding the definition of spirituality and religion and take seriously this narrative approach, we can see that both religion and spirituality have practical utility despite their lack of conceptual clarity. What nurses need to do is learn to be people who can listen to spiritual stories and work with others as they renegotiate these stories in the midst of the turmoil of illness. Nurses needs to develop what we might describe as *narrative competency*. In a post-modern context wherein a multiplicity of different forms of narratives may be considered spiritual, the expression of people's spiritual needs will be articulated in lots of different ways. The key for the nurse is to be spiritually attuned to the way in which she receives the story of the patient. Narrative competency relates to

- The assumption that a patient has the ability to tell his or her own story well
- The ability to listen and to hear beyond the obvious
- The ability to identify the spiritual in the midst of the ordinary

In a professional context within which the big stories of diagnosis and etiology can easily swallow up the smaller stories of transformation and reorientation, the task of the nurse as a spiritual carer is to facilitate the development of a setting wherein people's stories can be heard held, respected, and reoriented. The ability to hear the spiritual in the midst of the mundane is the beginning point for care of the spirit.

CASE STUDIES OF ILLNESS NARRATIVES

In order to further explore what some of these ideas might look like when applied to people living with illness, we will operationalize the framework outlined thus far within the context of two case studies. The narratives are taken from a larger qualitative study recently completed by one of the authors of this chapter (Lynne). The larger study looked at the interrelationship between spirituality and the use of psychiatric medication (Vanderpot, 2015). Central to that study was the crucial insight that the experience of mental health problems involves a change in someone's identity: his or her self-narrative. Spirituality was found to be central to the narrative reconstruction that follows the experience of severe mental health problems. In this section of our chapter, we will expand this observation and examine the ways in which *treatment* for an illness can also impact upon people's identity, and can be a disorienting agent that serves to occlude their sense of who they are and where they are going.

In the following cases, the framework of orientation—disorientation—reorientation will be used as a way of narrating the experience of illness in the context of the use of psychopharmacological medication. These cases will illustrate how the building blocks of spirituality's deep existential questions—*Who am I? Where do I come from? Where am I going? Why?*—helped guide the recovery process and reorient individuals by creating new stories of healing, hope, and a renewed sense of direction. The reader is asked to pay particular attention to the ways in which the proposed task of nurses as spiritual carers—facilitators of the conditions which allow such stories to be developed and heard—was fulfilled or denied by the professionals caring for Susan and Maria (not their real names).

SUSAN

Susan is a 53-year-old housewife from North West England whose illness narrative began with what her doctor called a psychotic episode, but what she perceived as a spiritual crisis brought on by several traumas she had endured earlier in life. Prior to her crisis, Susan's life was oriented in ways that were stable and good, and firmly centered on a settled life that included a quite clearly articulated spiritual life. She held (and still holds) the firm conviction that life is fundamentally a spiritual journey:

> We're spiritual beings having an experience in a human body, and not the other way 'round.'

Susan says she is blessed with the abilities of a psychic medium, and can receive spiritual messages from the transcendent, which are healing for her. For many years she was active in a Spiritualist church. The spirituality so central to her identity became lost in the disorienting experience of her illness and treatment. The spiritual crisis was both fearsome and entirely confusing. Without apology it appropriated her familiar place in the world:

> That's what I believe; I experienced, the negative side of spirituality . . . I was in a battle of good against evil. It's an opening up, but in a chaotic kind of way. It's very powerful, and it really overcomes you.

Susan's disorientation was compounded by the use of antipsychotic medication. Her already vulnerable sense of self bore further injury under the weight of her prescriptions. The medication blocked her ability to feel emotions, which she had always considered as the doorway to her spirituality:

> I find it hard to practice spirituality on medication. The medication blunts emotions. I don't cry. I don't feel the joy in living and the joy in being spiritual . . . It creates a different kind of thought pattern, which is kind of flattened.

Losing the capacity to feel her "spiritual feelings" was a devastating loss for Susan at the deepest level of how she sensed herself to be in the world.

An immense space emerged within which Susan desperately needed to find a way to navigate the strange new world of her illness. Instinctively, she seemed to know that her turmoil and hopelessness could be transformed if she were able to redraft her answers to those basic spiritual questions—who was she, where was she going, and why. With the loss of her old maps and explanations, Susan was faced with the need to create new understandings of her life; new stories that offered her a sense of hope and new direction. Part of this process involved finding meaning and purpose through learning more about her illness and subsequent prescriptions. The more she read, the more she felt she had at least some control over the situation. She started reading widely in the areas of psychiatry and psychology, and she attended conferences on spiritual crises and psychoses. Central to Susan's re-narration of her situation was her ability to place her new story within a spiritual frame that helped her to make sense of it. Over time, she came to view her experiences as a valuable part of her ongoing spiritual journey:

> I see it as part of my spiritual path. I wouldn't have gained such an understanding of it, unless it had happened. Maybe I was meant to follow this path in the hope that one day I'm off medication.

What we see here is the way in which Susan has managed to integrate her new experience into the ongoing narrative of her spiritual journey. She did not desire to have a mental health problem and she did not desire to take medication. However, she was able to make sense of the undesirability of her circumstances by re-writing her story in a way that enabled her to take ownership and some degree of control. It is important to be clear on this point. Making meaning out of her illness and medication use wasn't simply a therapeutic exercise. For Susan it was really a matter of survival:

> I have to find a meaning in it, to be able to live.

Finding space for illness and medication within her new spiritual narrative was not just helpful, it was absolutely necessary. Spiritual care for Susan was not an added extra, it was fundamental.

The process of reorientation for Susan meant that she had to reject the medical narrative put forth by professionals, a narrative that she felt was de-spiritualizing and forced upon her. The seemingly inflexible focus of the professionals on her neurochemistry as opposed to her personhood was incongruent with her spiritual need for deeper meanings:

> If I just went along with, "this is a chemical imbalance," and I went along with [their] pessimistic beliefs about me, I think I would go mad. I think that would drive me crazy.

In showing no interest in attuning to her story, or connecting with her in any kind of deep, personal way, the psychiatric staff treating Susan missed that which was central to her life and ultimately to her recovery. When she did attempt to share the importance of her spirituality, she felt that it was invalidated or ignored:

> You can't get your point across. I insisted that it was a spiritual experience, because that's what I recognized it as. One psychiatrist said, 'you'll have a hard job convincing me,' and the others just ignored what I was saying.

Communion with her carers was not possible for Susan. The powerful opportunity to forge a closer connection, and move the relationship beyond the confines of a medical encounter was not fulfilled. Without communion there can be no understanding; without understanding there can be no connection and without connection there can be no healing. In the end, in spite of a lack of supportive communion with her carers, Susan found her own way to create a reorienting narrative that offered hope and deeper meaning. The spiritual teachings of her many disorienting experiences became places where she came to recognize new things about her spirituality and discovered new aspects of what it might mean to recover from serious mental health problems.

Yet let us imagine for a moment what it would look like for nurses to engage with Susan's spiritual needs in a way that demonstrates the concept of nursing-as-communion. Illustrating practical ways in which nurses might respond will help us better understand what this model could look like in practice. Nurses might have started out by listening reflectively to Susan's perceptions of a spiritual crisis and by responding in a way that validates her experience: *"I'm hearing you say that you believe there is a spiritual basis for what brings you here. It sounds like you have deep insight into the connection between what's happening right now and some traumatic experiences from your past."* The nurse is affirming Susan's ability to tell her own story, and showing that in the midst of responding to Susan's symptoms, he/she is willing to hear the spiritual.

Once the nurse has validated Susan's narrative, the next step might be to communicate an intention of relationality, beyond the technical aspects of care: *"As your nurse, I will certainly be on hand to help you and perform the expected tasks related to your care. But beyond that, I want you to know that I'm here to support you, whatever that might look like, as you figure out what this illness means for you and your family, and how you want to go about things in the future. I'd like to suggest setting aside some time each day in which we can address what's most important to you."* By explicitly letting Susan know that he/she is open to deeper levels of connection, the nurse gives Susan the option for communion, something she likely would have chosen, given the opportunity.

MARIA

Susan's spirituality, although emerging from spiritualist roots, was quite free floating and not formally connected with any kind of religion. Maria on the other hand does have a religious faith, but her relationship with it is somewhat ambivalent. Maria is a 39-year-old Catholic nun living in the Midwest United States. She works as a chaplain in prisons and hospitals. Maria's illness narrative involves serious and persistent mental health issues:

> What was happening was some intense states of anxiety and emotion and then pretty constant self-harming thoughts and images. I had so many cutting thoughts I wasn't really able to function.

Maria is currently diagnosed with PTSD, anxiety disorder, and dissociative disorder non-specific. Maria's illness has caused powerful changes in her identity narrative. There are times when she can get really lost, and go to a place of extreme dysfunction. For the last eight years she has been in treatment involving a therapeutic milieu of medication, Dialectical Behavior Therapy (DBT), and the day-to-day discipline of self-care. Maria pays close attention to her eating, sleeping, and exercise habits.

Spirituality for Maria is not always positive. Indeed, it is a component of the disorienting aspect of her illness. She is so open to anomalous spiritual experiences that they can then overwhelm and flood her senses. When this happens she doesn't know how to turn it off. Psychiatric medication provides her with a much needed boundary from God. The mixture of Prozac, Ativan, and Risperdal she takes reduces her vulnerability to the omnipotent, fast moving lava that she imagines God to be:

> Like if God is like this waterfall or this stream, I often think of God as lava, I think that the meds and other supports keep me from being flooded.

Unlike Susan, Maria is still able to feel intense spiritual feelings on medication. It's the medication that helps her be more stable. This has deep implications for her spirituality in that it allows her to be functional and increases her ability to connect with others. Spirituality is a key part of Maria's reorientation. In spite of living with on-going and disabling bouts of mental illness, her spirituality, with its foundation of meaning and stability, holds and shapes the process of creating and sustaining her identity narrative in the midst of significant change.

What does reorientation look like for Maria?

> *There's so much broken relationship, and so much woundedness and injustice in our world that trying to live in right relationship with that is essential I think, to spirituality.*

Fundamentally, reorientation has to do with her spirituality, which relates to living in right relationship and honoring her commitment to stay within a certain range of functioning, which in turn, creates and sustains consistency and stability in her relationships. Maria's new sense of hope and direction emerges from the story of her dedication to her community of religious sisters and to the people whom she serves as a chaplain. Maria works closely with a nurse practitioner who provides her not only with effective medical treatment, but with a sense of healing communion as well:

> *She's accessible to me. I can contact her at any time. We communicate really regularly. Even though she just does my meds, I feel like she pays attention to me as a person, and the larger sense of my life.*

Maria's healthcare experience of being understood as a whole person provided crucial support during the process of working through her illness narrative and constructing a new identity narrative. It made it a lot easier for her to address the existential questions of who she was and where she was going with the feeling that her story mattered to someone, and had been genuinely valued by another. Maria talked about how helpful and healing she found working side-by-side with her caregiver on matters that went beyond the technical aspects of her prescriptions. The intimate accessibility of her practitioner and her practitioner's integrated approach to care offer a good example of one way that nurses can show spiritual attunement with patients. Maria's experiences illustrate what nursing-as-communion might look like in practice, and what some of the benefits can feel like to the patient.

To flesh out further the practical applications of this chapter's model of nursing-as-communion, let's imagine additional ways that Maria's nurse could engage with her religious needs around maintaining stability in relationships. The nurse might initiate regular discussions to review Maria's spiritual care needs, creating the opportunity for deeper relationality: *"Maria, I'm glad you've let me know that my paying attention to other aspects of you, besides your medication, has been helpful in your treatment. I believe that you said relationships are essential to your spirituality, and I've seen how prioritizing them has been so helpful in your recovery. I think that includes our relationship as well. If it interests you, I'd like to schedule occasional sessions not concerning medication, but to explore whatever's coming up for you that is impacting your ability to connect with the people in your life."* Maria has already indicated that such interactions with her nurse support her spiritual needs, so in this case the nurse is providing positive reinforcement for that, and searching for and expressing interest in deepened communion with her patient.

REFLECTIONS ON THE CASE STUDIES

What becomes clear from looking at the two cases of Susan and Maria is that, from the patient's perspective, the experience of illness is predominantly lived as a narrative event which appears to include a deep, spiritual need for others to bear witness to its disorienting power. Part of the inexorable intimacy of the nursing encounter is the role of witnessed significance (Fleischman, 1989, p. 7). Nursing-as-communion has to do with remaining present with whatever patients find most bewildering and lethal about their illness narrative, in a way that expresses faith in the patient's ability to create a new and healing story. This welcoming approach to the illness narrative is a spiritually supportive way to care for patients as they journey toward themselves, in their search to discover meaning and purpose within their experience of illness.

That both Susan and Maria were experiencing serious mental health conditions with considerable medical implications is neither contested nor criticized. Without medical treatment, Susan admits she may not have been capable of running a household and protecting the well-being of her 12-year-old daughter:

> *I take it for the family's sake. I'm considering my 12-year-old daughter mostly, I can get on with the normal things in life.*

Medicine is important, but it is not the only game in town! Susan's story informs us that it is a mistake to allow the medical narrative of diagnosis and evidence-based treatment to overpower the other important stories that surround and comprise mental health problems. The task of healthcare has not been fulfilled or exhausted when its technical duties have been effectively carried out. To think otherwise is to reveal an egregiously limited awareness of the spiritual and narrative dimensions that are inextricably intertwined within the illness experience. The case studies we have presented here reflect an increasing awareness of the importance of the personal and narrative aspects of recovery, and the significance of healing beyond the level of symptom reduction.

In each case presented, psychiatric medication played a significant role in the orientation-disorientation-reorientation model of narrating the spiritual experience of illness. For Maria, medication provided an important boundary to the spiritual world, which helped her maintain a level of functioning, and enabled her to create her new story around the spiritual pursuit of right relationship. The hindering effects of psychiatric medication on Susan's spirituality became the inspiration for the pursuit of higher learning, which offered great meaning and purpose to her story. In both cases, the process of reorientation involved new interpretations of the basic spiritual/existential questions. The role of spiritual care in Maria's case provided a good example of nursing-as-communion in practice, and highlights the healing power of intimacy within the nursing encounter. Maria's nurse created a caring space in which respect and validation were prioritized and valued as key components of treatment. The mutual hospitality held within the space embraced Maria's new orientation, and her spiritual need for *right relationship*. The manner in which Susan's experience was denied and invalidated by professionals is perhaps an extreme example of the cost of narrative incompetency, and the distance that can form in settings between nurses and patients when personal illness stories are undermined by a strictly medicalized perspective. Fortunately, Susan was able to find her own way toward a new story filled with hope and personal meaning.

The main argument of this chapter has suggested that identity narratives are a key component of the illness experience which requires nurses to respond not only with technical and instrumental competency, but with intimacy and relational skills as well. By its very nature, the space between nurses and patients lends itself to connection and to the intimate. Given the spiritual need for patients to heal by reorienting their experience toward new narratives of hope and meaning, the intimacy of the nursing encounter serves to shape and form a person's experience of illness and recovery. Similar to the ways in which the psalms provide the structure and language of suffering and a way for people to rediscover hope in the midst of suffering, nursing-as-communion provides a form-full way of understanding patient's experiences of illness and a way of creating what they perhaps need most: a new reorienting story. When nurses develop narrative competency and learn how to listen in the right ways, they teach their patients how to negotiate their way toward the creation of new narratives based on those things that bring patients deeper meaning and purpose.

Hearing stories in the right way—with narrative competency—fosters true spiritual care. Narrative competency is about presuming that the patient is highly capable of telling his or her own story. It's about narrative communion, and being able to listen to the people we work alongside in ways that move us beyond the surface of things and into the deeper aspects of what it means to be ill and to recover from illness. Given the multiplicity of spiritual narratives within post-modern pluralist societies, it is expected that people's narratives will take many forms and be expressed in many ways. Nurses should expect that some people will embrace a more generic spirituality, while others will tell narratives based on a particular religious perspective. Nursing-as-communion is about the movement toward one another that acknowledges, respects and values the healing power of relational intimacy. This is in part achieved by narrative competency, by bearing witness to the significance of patients' illness and spiritual narratives, and by providing the structure and space for new stories to be created and enacted.

REFERENCES

Brockmeier, J. (2004). "Identity, agency, and embodiment." In Hydén, Lars C., & Lindemann, Hilde, *Beyond loss: Dementia, identity, personhood.* New York: Oxford University Press.

Brueggemann, W. (1977). "The formfulness of grief." *Interpretation: A Journal of Bible and Theology,* 31(3), 263–275.

Brueggemann, W. (1995). *The psalms and the life of faith.* Minneapolis, MN: Fortress Press.

Cockell, N., & McSherry, W. (2012). "Spiritual care in nursing: An overview of published international research." *Journal of Nursing Management,* 20(8), 958–969.

Emblem, J. D. (1992). "Religion and Spirituality defined according to current use in nursing literature." *Journal of Professional Nursing,* 8, 41–47.

Fleischman, P. (1989). *The healing spirit.* London: SPCK.

Frankl, V. (2004). *Man's search for meaning. An introduction to logotherapy.* Boston: Beacon and Random House / London: Rider.

Habibian, N., Ahmadi, R., Vashian, A., Mortazavi, S. M., & Dadkhah-Tehrani, T. (2015). "Investigating the correlation between the life and religious attitudes with psychological well-being in nurses working in health

Centers at Qom Universities of Medical Sciences in 2014." *Mediterranean Journal of Social Sciences, 6*(6 S4), 168.

Kim-Godwin, Y. (2013). "Prayer in Clinical Practice: What does evidence support?" *Journal of Christian Nursing, 30*(4), 208–215.

Koenig, H., King, D., & Carson, V. B. (2012). *Handbook of religion and health.* Oxford University Press.

Lewinson, L. P., McSherry, W., & Kevern, P. (2015). "Spirituality in pre-registration nurse education and practice: A review of the literature." *Nurse Education Today, 35*(6), 806–814.

Lopez, V., Fischer, I., Leigh, M. C., Larkin, D., & Webster, S. (2014). "Spirituality, religiosity, and personal beliefs of Australian undergraduate nursing students." *Journal of Transcultural Nursing, 25*(4), 1–8.

McSherry, W., & Jamieson, S. (2013). "The qualitative findings from an online survey investigating nurses' perceptions of spirituality and spiritual care." *Journal of Clinical Nursing, 22*(21–22), 3170–3182.

Paley, J. (2008). "Spirituality and nursing: A reductionist approach." Nursing Philosophy, 9(1), 3–18.

Pike, J. (2011). "Spirituality in nursing: A systematic review of the literature from 2006–10." *British Journal of Nursing, 20*(12), 743–749.

Pullen, L., McGuire, S., Farmer, L., & Dodd, D. (2015). "The relevance of spirituality to nursing practice and education." *Mental Health Practice, 18*(5), 14–18.

Reinert, K. G., & Koenig, H. G. (2013). "Re-examining definitions of spirituality in nursing research." *Journal of Advanced Nursing, 69*(12), 2622–2634.

Roach, M. S. (2013). "Caring: The human mode of being." In Watson Caring Science Institute (Eds.) *Caring in nursing classics: An essential resource.* New York: Springer Publishing Company, 165–179.

Skomakerstuen Ødbehr, L., Kvigne, K., Hauge, S., & Danbolt, L. J. (2015). "A qualitative study of nurses' attitudes towards and accommodations of patients' expressions of religiosity and faith in dementia care." *Journal of advanced nursing, 71*(2), 359–369.

Sontag, S. 1977. *Illness as metaphor.* New York: Picador Publishing.

Spadaro, K. C., & Hunker, D. F. (2016). "Exploring the effects of an online asynchronous mindfulness meditation intervention with nursing students on stress, mood, and cognition: A descriptive study." *Nurse Education Today, 39*, 163–169.

Swinton, J. (2001) Spirituality in Mental Health care: Rediscovering a "forgotten" dimension. London: Jessica Kingsley Publishers.

Swinton, J. (2006). "Identity and resistance: Why spiritual care needs 'enemies.'" *Journal of Clinical Nursing, 15*(7), 918–928.

Swinton, J. (2014). "Spirituality-in-healthcare: Just because it may be 'made up' does not mean that it is not real and does not matter (Keynote 5)." *Journal for the Study of Spirituality, 4*(2), 162–173.

Swinton, J., & Pattison, S. (2010). "Moving beyond clarity: Towards a thin, vague, and useful understanding of spirituality in nursing care." *Nursing Philosophy, 11*(4), 226–237.Taylor, E. J., & Mamier, I. (2013). "Nurse responses to patient expressions of spiritual distress." *Holistic Nursing Practice, 27*(4), 217–224.

Torskenæs, K. B., Baldacchino, D. R., Kalfoss, M., Baldacchino, T., Borg, J., Falzon, M., & Grima, K. (2015). "Nurses' and caregivers' definition of spirituality from the Christian perspective: A comparative study between Malta and Norway." *Journal of Nursing Management, 23*(1), 39–53.

Vanderpot, L. (2015). *The interrelationship between spirituality and psychiatric medication: A hermeneutic phenomenological study.* PhD. Thesis, University of Aberdeen.

Weathers, E. McCarthy, G., & Coffey, A. (2015) "Concept analysis of spirituality: An evolutionary approach." *Nursing Forum/* Early online version: http://onlinelibrary.wiley.com/doi/10.1111/nuf.12128/full. Accessed 06/12/2015.

PART 2

SCHOLARLY DISCIPLINARY PERSPECTIVES

CHAPTER 15

MEDICINE, SPIRITUALITY, RELIGION, AND PSYCHOLOGY

Kelly M. Trevino and Kenneth I. Pargament

The intersection of religion/spirituality (R/S) and medicine is apparent from the societal to individual level of American culture (Cadge & Fair, 2010). In 2012, Hobby Lobby and Conestoga Wood Specialties, businesses run by Christian owners, sued the federal government for requiring them to provide health insurance coverage for birth control methods that violated their religious beliefs (Cohen et al., 2014). In 2013, a case in Ohio received national attention when Amish parents refused potentially life-saving chemotherapy for their daughter with leukemia, citing their daughter's suffering and their faith in "God's will" as reasons for their decision. While these cases may be extreme examples, over half of Americans report praying for their own health (Barnes et al., 2004; Mao et al., 2007) and over two-thirds want their medical providers to ask about their religious beliefs (Best et al., 2015). A growing body of research over the past 30 years has consistently documented relationships between R/S and health behaviors and outcomes (Koenig et al., 2012; Koenig, 2015). With the advent of care models such as patient-centered care (Institute of Medicine, 2001), the importance of R/S to medical care is increasingly, although not completely, recognized.

The relationship between R/S and medicine is complex and can be viewed from multiple perspectives, many of which are represented in this volume. The current chapter examines this relationship from a psychological perspective. The American Psychological Association defines psychology as the "study of the mind and behavior" (American Psychological Association, n.d.) in all aspects of the human experience. Certainly, for many people that experience includes illness and interactions with the health care system as patients, caregivers, and/or health care providers. In the following pages, we provide a theoretical framework for understanding the relationship between R/S and medicine and review research on this relationship in patients, informal caregivers, and health care providers. We conclude with a brief review of psycho-spiritual interventions in medical populations.

Of note, when discussing issues of religion and spirituality, clarifying definitions can be extremely important. We refer readers to chapter 1 of this volume for a discussion of the definitions of religion and spirituality. For the purposes of this chapter, we will refer to religion and spirituality together (R/S) while recognizing that this overlooks differences between religion and spirituality and oversimplifies complex constructs.

THEORETICAL LEVEL

Much of the research on the role of R/S in medicine has been informed by a religious coping perspective. According to this model, each individual has an orienting system or way of viewing and responding to the world that includes values, relationships, beliefs, and habits (Pargament, 2001). Individuals draw on this orienting system during difficult times. Orienting systems include helpful resources such as prior experience, self-efficacy, and social support and unhelpful burdens such as pessimism and personality problems (Pargament, 2001).

R/S is often one aspect of this general orienting system. Individuals whose R/S beliefs and practices are well integrated in their orienting systems may be more likely to access R/S resources in the face of a stressor like illness and to integrate R/S into their efforts to cope with illness (Pargament, 2001). For example, patients and caregivers for whom R/S is important may turn to their R/S beliefs to understand and make meaning of their illness. They may seek comfort through prayer or spending time with a religious community. Beliefs about the nature of God or a divine being can be another component of the spiritual orienting system. Religious attachment theory has identified three styles of attachment to God: secure, avoidant, and anxious/ambivalent (Granqvist & Kirkpatrick, 2013; Kirkpatrick, 1992, 1999). Securely attached individuals view God as a loving being who will protect and comfort them (Kirkpatrick, 1992). Individuals with an avoidant attachment view God or the divine as impersonal and distant while individuals with an anxious/ambivalent attachment experience God as inconsistent and unpredictable (Kirkpatrick, 1992). These attachment types appear to be differentially related to patients' response to illness. In a study of patients with cancer or renal impairment, a secure attachment to God was associated with adaptive coping responses while an insecure attachment to God was associated with hopelessness (Cassibba et al., 2014). Similarly, in a sample of bereaved individuals, a secure attachment to God was associated with lower levels of depression and grief and greater growth (Kelley & Chan, 2012).

Many aspects of the spiritual orienting system can be viewed from the perspective of positive psychology, a relatively new subfield of psychology that emphasizes strengths, virtues, and positive qualities and experiences rather than disorder and mental illness (Seligman & Csikszentmihalyi, 2000). While positive psychology extends beyond R/S, R/S constructs such as forgiveness, meaning, and spiritual experience fall within the framework of positive psychology (Seligman, 2012; Seligman & Csikszentmihalyi, 2000). From this perspective, R/S can be viewed as a component of positive psychology. Alternatively, R/S can be viewed as distinct from positive psychology and the relationship between R/S and positive psychology constructs can be examined (Barton & Miller, 2015). This perspective is reflected in much of the research on medical populations in which R/S is related to constructs such as well-being and growth. However, it is important to note that R/S is not always a positive force in individuals' response to illness. As discussed below, negative R/S appraisals and coping responses do occur and are associated with problematic outcomes across medical populations.

The religious coping model provides a framework for understanding the role of R/S in medicine. In the following sections, we review research on components of the spiritual orienting system and the relationship between these components and mental and physical health in patients, caregivers, and health care providers.

PATIENT LEVEL

Perhaps unsurprisingly, the role of R/S in medicine has been most studied at the patient level. R/S values and beliefs impact how many patients view and respond to illness and make treatment decisions (Ehman et al., 1999; Silvestri et al., 2003). In 2007, 49% of a national sample reported praying for their health, with higher rates in individuals with functional limitations and health changes (Wachholtz & Sambamoorthi, 2011). Patients rely on many aspects of their spiritual orienting systems. We will focus on R/S beliefs about illness and the role of R/S in coping with, understanding, and making meaning of illness.

Many patients have beliefs about God's role in illness. These beliefs vary and include that God is responsible for physical health, God works through the doctor, illness is God's will, only God can influence life and death, and divine intervention and miracles do occur (Johnson et al., 2005; Mansfield et al., 2002). In a sample of gynecologic cancer survivors, over one-third (39.2%) reported that God's will was a moderately to very important factor in the development of cancer. In addition, a majority of the sample reported that prayer (87.9%) and God's will (69.3%) were moderately to very important factors in the prevention of a cancer recurrence (Costanzo et al., 2005). Patients also vary in the degree to which they believe God can control their illness (Cattich & Knudson-Martin, 2009; Koffman et al., 2008; Johnston et al., 1999; Wallston et al., 1999), with some evidence to suggest that greater belief in God's control over illness is associated with worse psychological adjustment (Wallston et al., 1999). Negative beliefs about God's role in illness are less common though not rare. In a sample of community-dwelling older adults, approximately one-quarter of participants viewed illness as a punishment from God (Bearon & Koenig, 1990).

The prevalence of these beliefs demonstrates the relevance of R/S to medicine from the patient's perspective. However, beliefs about God's role in illness also have implications for patients' psychological well-being, health behaviors, treatment preferences, and physical health. Across medical illnesses, positive views of God are associated with better mental health, including greater happiness (Dezutter et al., 2010), better role and emotional function (Gall, 2004), and better psychological well-being and less distress (Schreiber, 2011). Conversely, negative beliefs about God such as believing God had abandoned the patient or that illness is a punishment from God are associated with greater concerns about death, worse pain, and poor physical and mental health (Edmondson et al., 2008; Jones et al., 2015; Kaldjian et al., 1998). Believing that illness is God's will is complex and has been associated with positive (Gall, 2003, 2004) and negative outcomes (Collin, 2012). In a study of ill older adults, viewing illness as God's will was associated with seeing the illness as an opportunity for growth (Gall, 2003). However, cancer patients who attribute their cancer and possible recurrence to God's will report greater worry about cancer recurrence (Costanzo et al., 2005).

The importance of R/S to patients' illness experience is also evident in how patients appraise or interpret their illness. R/S appraisals can be negative or positive and focus specifically on the implications of stressful events for values of deepest significance. Sacred loss and desecration are two negative R/S appraisals that have been studied in medical populations. Sacred loss is the perception that a sacred aspect of life, an aspect "perceived as having divine character and significance" has been lost (Pargament et al., 2005; Pargament & Mahoney, 2005, p. 183). In the context of medicine, this loss is due to illness or injury. Desecration is the perception that a sanctified aspect of life has been violated (Pargament et al., 2005). Benevolent religious appraisal is a positive R/S appraisal in which a stressor is redefined "through religion as benevolent and potentially beneficial" (Pargament et al., 2000, p. 522).

Positive religious appraisals tend to be more common than negative religious appraisals (Burker et al., 2004; Pargament et al., 2001, 2004). In a sample of patients admitted to an acute medical rehabilitation facility, 85.7% reported some degree of benevolent religious appraisal of their health, 71.4% some degree of sacred loss, and 42.9% some degree of desecration (Magyar-Russell et al., 2013). These appraisals are also relevant for patient's mental health. In longitudinal analyses of this medical rehabilitation sample, desecration at hospital admission predicted greater depression 7-8 weeks post-discharge, controlling for age, severity of the health event, global religiousness, and baseline depression levels. Sacred loss at admission was associated with greater growth at follow-up in controlled analyses. In a final model that compared the relative predictive power of sacred loss, desecration, and benevolent religious appraisal, desecration at baseline predicted greater depression at follow-up and sacred loss predicted greater growth (Magyar-Russell et al., 2013).

The R/S appraisals described can be part of the process of making meaning of an illness. According to the meaning-making model, stress occurs when appraisals of particular situations, such as illness or injury, are different from or violate patients' global meaning, the framework through which they view themselves and the world (Park, 2013a, 2013b). For example, myocardial infarction patients who felt their heart attack interfered with the divine purpose of their life reported feeling angry at God (Walton, 1999). Patients attempt to resolve the discrepancy between global and situational meaning by changing their appraisal of the situation or their global meaning (Park, 2013a, 2013b; Skaggs & Barron, 2006). Meaning can be made in both secular and R/S contexts. However, the role of R/S in the meaning-making process is apparent across medical populations including in patients with heart disease (Baldacchino, 2011; Walton, 1999), dementia (Agli et al., 2015), diabetes (Cattich & Knudson-Martin, 2009), and cancer (Adelstein et al., 2014; Farsi, 2015).

In the process of meaning-making, situational appraisals (or re-appraisals) can include viewing illness as an opportunity for spiritual growth (Cattich & Knudson-Martin, 2009) and greater connection with the self, family and friends, community, nature, and the divine (Walton, 1999). For example, a patient may initially interpret illness as a sacred loss but, over time, reappraise the illness as an opportunity to become closer to God. Rather than reappraise the situation, patients may also change their global meaning to account for their view of their illness. For example, patients may view God as less powerful, convert to a new religious tradition, abandon their R/S beliefs, seek a divine purpose, or identify a "personal calling or vocation" (Walton, 1999, p. 47) as a way of changing global meaning. Of course, finding meaning in serious illness can be difficult. A woman with newly diagnosed dementia struggled to understand her illness in the context of her religious beliefs: ". . .sometimes I think to myself, 'but my faith should be that whatever happens, God will look after me, and then sometimes my faith waivers, thinking 'who is looking after me?' you know" (Dalby et al., 2012, p. 82).

In addition to patients' beliefs and understanding of their illness, R/S is visible in how patients cope with illness. R/S can serve various functions in the coping process, including emotional regulation, gaining control, maintaining self-identity, anxiety reduction, and increasing social connectedness (Cummings & Pargament, 2010). R/S coping consists of positive and negative coping responses. Positive religious coping includes a sense of love, compassion, secure partnership with the divine, and a spiritual connection to others (Pargament et al., 1998). For example, a woman with breast cancer stated, "Before we left the house on the morning of my mastectomy, my husband took me in his arms and said, 'God will be with us today'. We both felt His presence on a very frightening day" (Schreiber, 2011, p. 615). Negative religious coping or spiritual struggle is characterized by spiritual conflicts, a strained relationship with the divine, and doubt in one's religious beliefs (Pargament et al., 2005; Pargament et al., 1998). For example the father of a child with cystic fibrosis stated, "At first when we got to know the diagnosis, I used to doubt my faith in God. . .I used to ask, "What did I do wrong in my life for this to happen to our child? . . . Why has this happened to us?" (Baldacchino et al., 2012, p. 838).

Positive religious coping is more common than negative religious coping across patient populations (Cotton et al., 2006; Hebert et al., 2009; McGee et al., 2013; Pedersen et al., 2013; Sherman et al., 2009; Zwingmann et al., 2006) but has shown mixed relationships with various types of psychological well-being (Gall et al., 2011; Hebert et al., 2009; Tarakeshwar et al., 2006; Zwingmann et al., 2006). Many studies suggest that positive religious coping is associated with better emotional, interpersonal, and global functioning (Agarwal et al., 2010; Ai et al., 2006; Cotton et al., 2006; Gall, 2004), better overall quality of life (Tarakeshwar et al., 2006), greater life satisfaction (Cotton et al., 2006), and greater growth (Allmon et al., 2013; Pargament et al., 2004; Urcuyo et al., 2005). These findings suggest that positive religious coping may help reduce patient distress. However, positive religious coping has also been associated with greater transplant concerns post-transplant in multiple myeloma patient (Sherman et al., 2009), more physical symptoms in advanced cancer patients (Tarakeshwar et al., 2006), and less HIV mastery and worse overall functioning in patients with HIV/AIDS (Cotton et al., 2006). These findings may reflect a religious coping mobilization effect in which religious resources are accessed in the context of stressful events (Cummings & Pargament, 2010). Further, other studies have found no relationship between positive religious coping and well-being (Hebert et al., 2009; McGee et al., 2013; Pedersen et al., 2013).

Conversely, negative religious coping, although endorsed at low levels, is consistently associated with greater psychological distress including higher levels of depression (Ai et al., 2007; Hebert et al., 2009; Sherman et al., 2009; Trevino et al., 2010) and anxiety (Ai et al., 2007; McGee et al., 2013; Sherman et al., 2009), lower levels of life satisfaction and quality of life (Hebert et al., 2009; Manning-Walsh, 2005; Pargament et al., 2004; Pedersen et al., 2013; Tarakeshwar et al., 2006; Trevino et al., 2010), and worse mental health (Cotton et al., 2006; Hebert et al., 2009; Pérez & Smith, 2015) and adjustment to illness (Exline et al., 2011; Trevino et al., 2010) across medical diagnoses (Ano & Vasconcelles, 2005; Koenig et al., 2012). In addition, there is evidence to suggest that the relationship between negative religious coping and distress may be stronger in people with a medical illness than those without (McConnell et al., 2006). Interestingly, negative religious coping has also been associated with higher rates of growth (Allmon et al., 2013; Pargament et al., 2006; Trevino et al., 2010). For example, in a sample of breast cancer patients, negative religious coping assessed prior to diagnosis and 6 months after surgery predicted greater growth at 12 months post-surgery (Gall et al., 2011). Findings such as these are consistent with psychological theories (e.g., Piaget, Erikson) that highlight the value of periods of struggle and challenge for development and maturation. Nevertheless, overall it appears that negative religious coping may be tied to both growth and decline. Researchers are now beginning to examine those factors that may determine the trajectory of change following periods of negative religious coping, including illness severity and chronicity, the individual's coping resources, and the strength of the individual's spiritual worldview (Pargament et al., 2006).

Fewer studies have examined R/S coping and physical health. As with mental health, research on positive religious coping and physical health is mixed. Positive religious coping has been associated with improvements in physical and cognitive function in elderly medical inpatients (Pargament et al., 2004), a lower rate of cognitive decline in dementia patients (Agli et al., 2015), and better post-operative global function in patients undergoing cardiac surgery (Ai et al., 2006). However, positive religious coping has also been associated with worse physical outcomes (Sherman et al., 2009; Tarakeshwar et al., 2006), which, as stated, may indicate that religious resources are mobilized in the context of more severe illnesses (Rippentrop et al., 2005; Koenig et al., 2012). Negative religious coping is consistently associated with worse physical heath. In a study of multiple myeloma patients undergoing transplant evaluation, negative religious coping was associated with poor physical health after controlling for demographic and medical variables and general religiousness, suggesting that NRC contributes uniquely to cancer patients' health (Sherman et al., 2009; Sherman et al., 2005). Negative religious coping in congestive heart failure patients was associated with more time spent hospitalized (Park et al., 2011). In patients with mild Alzheimer's disease, negative religious coping was associated with greater frequency and severity of neuropsychiatric symptoms of dementia (McGee et al., 2013). The chronicity of negative religious coping may be an important indicator patient health. Negative religious coping was associated with declines in functional status (Pargament et al., 2004) and increased mortality risk over two years in elderly medical inpatients (Pargament et al., 2001). However, only patients who endorsed negative religious coping at baseline and follow-up experienced greater declines in mental and physical health than patients who did not endorse negative religious coping at both time points (Pargament et al., 2004).

Negative religious coping has also been associated with physiological indicators of poor health. In a sample of patients with HIV/AIDS, negative religious coping predicted change in CD4 counts, an indicator of immune system function, after controlling for demographic variables and positive religious coping (Trevino et al., 2010). Patients with high negative religious coping scores experienced a decrease in CD4 counts indicating worsening immune function while patients low in negative religious coping experienced an increase in CD4 counts over time (Trevino et al., 2010). In a sample of patients undergoing cardiac surgery, negative religious coping was associated with higher levels of interleukin-6, an indicator of inflammatory stress, after controlling for medical and psychosocial correlates (Ai et al., 2009). These findings suggest that negative religious coping may impact disease directly through immune function and inflammatory processes.

Patients bring R/S to medicine through their beliefs, coping strategies, and attempts to understand their illness. These patients are not in the minority. Numerous studies suggest that the majority of patients rely on their spiritual orienting system in some way during their illness experience. Further, mounting research suggests that R/S is related to patient outcomes. However, research in this area is relatively young. Additional studies are needed to identify those factors that determine whether R/S leads to growth or decline following an illness. Yet, these findings highlight the importance of patient R/S to health care provision. Ignoring R/S in patient care risks overlooking a prevalent and prominent part of the patient experience and a potential resource for the promotion of health and well-being.

CAREGIVER LEVEL

Patients' informal or unpaid caregivers (who are often family members) play an important role in the care and support of individuals with illness. According to a national survey conducted by the National Alliance for Caregiving, 65.7 million people in the United States provided unpaid care to a family member or friend in 2009 (National Alliance for Caregiving, 2009). On average, caregivers served in this role for 4.6 years and over two-thirds (69%) of caregivers were caring for an individual with a long-term physical health condition (National Alliance for Caregiving, 2009). Caregivers spent an average of 20.4 hours per week providing care. Medical care is increasingly provided in an outpatient setting, increasing the number and complexity of tasks completed by informal caregivers (Pasacreta & McCorkle, 2000). Perhaps not surprising given the chronicity and complexity of caregiving, caregivers are at increased risk for negative psychological and physical outcomes including depression, anxiety, sleep disturbance, fatigue, cardiovascular disease, and mortality (Aoun et al., 2013; Applebaum & Breitbart, 2013; Bhimani, 2014; Girgis et al., 2013; Haines et al., 2015; Rofail et al., 2013; Seeher et al., 2013). Further, illness often impacts the patient and caregiver as a unit (Li & Loke, 2013; Murray et al., 2010). This mutuality is evident in rates of distress (Aoun et al., 2013; Northouse et al., 2012; Whittingham et al., 2013) and psychiatric diagnoses (Bambauer et al., 2006). For example, caregivers of advanced cancer patients who meet criteria for a psychiatric diagnosis are 7.9 times more likely to have a psychiatric diagnosis themselves (Bambauer et al., 2006). This mutuality is also apparent in the spiritual domain; there is a direct relationship between caregiver and patient spiritual well-being (Kim et al., 2011) and spiritual distress (Murray et al., 2010). Understanding the needs and experiences of the caregiver is likely to benefit both the patient and caregiver.

Like patients, many caregivers turn to their spiritual orienting systems to help them cope with the caregiving role (Mehrotra & Sukumar, 2007; Sheridan et al., 2014; Delgado-Guay et al., 2013; Leonardi et al., 2012; Thornton & Hopp, 2011). In a single site study of 150 cancer caregivers, 88.6% endorsed a religious affiliation, 81.3% reported attending religious services "occasionally" or "regularly," and 65.3% reported praying for their own health. These percentages were higher than those reported in national and state-wide surveys (Williams et al., 2014). In a multi-site study of dementia caregivers, 77% of participants reported praying daily, 70% described their R/S faith as important, and 42% attended religious services at least weekly (Hebert et al., 2007). There is also evidence of racial differences in caregivers' use of R/S to cope (McDonald et al., 1999). Much of this work comes from the Resources for Enhancing Alzheimer's Caregivers Health Study (Coon et al., 2004; Haley et al., 2004). This research suggests that Latina (Coon et al., 2004; Mausbach et al., 2003) and Black (Haley et al., 2004) dementia caregivers report higher levels of R/S coping than White caregivers, which may explain racial differences in caregiver mental health and perceived burden of caregiving (Hodge & Sun, 2012; Sun et al., 2010). Unfortunately, spiritual distress is also common in caregivers (Murray et al., 2010). In a study of caregivers of advanced cancer patients, 58% reported experiencing spiritual pain (Delgado-Guay et al., 2013). Caregivers experiencing spiritual pain reported higher levels of depression and anxiety, worse quality of life, and greater use of maladaptive coping strategies than those without spiritual pain (Delgado-Guay et al., 2013).

R/S is also associated with caregiver well-being. Affiliation with a religious denomination, a blunt indicator of R/S, is associated with positive caregiver outcomes including better quality of life (Leow et al., 2014) and greater perceived benefits of caregiving (Kang et al., 2013). More frequent engagement in R/S activities such as prayer and service attendance has been associated with lower levels of depression (Hebert et al., 2007; Lopez et al., 2012; Sun & Hodge, 2014), perceived caregiving burden (Barber, 2014; Herrera et al., 2009), and hopelessness (Kim et al., 2014; Mehrotra & Sukumar, 2007), better quality of life (Banthia et al., 2007), and more positive appraisals of the caregiving role (Mehrotra & Sukumar, 2007), such as greater perceived meaning in and benefits from caregiving (Barber, 2014; Hodge & Sun, 2012; Quinn et al., 2012). In a longitudinal study of dementia caregivers, greater frequency of religious service attendance and prayer and greater importance of R/S prior to the patient's death were associated with lower levels of depression after the patient's death. More frequent attendance at religious services prior to the death was also associated with fewer symptoms of complicated grief post-loss (Hebert et al., 2007).

In addition to R/S practices, caregiver self-report of degree of R/S has been associated with positive outcomes. Higher levels of caregiver R/S on these measures have been associated with better mental health (Yeh & Bull, 2009), including lower levels of depression (Fenix et al., 2006; Newberry et al., 2013; Roscoe et al., 2009; Williams et al., 2014) and anxiety (Newberry et al., 2013), better quality of life (Lo Coco et al., 2005; Tang, 2009), greater life satisfaction (Roscoe et al., 2009), and more perceived benefits of caregiving (Roscoe et al., 2009). In married couples caring for aging parents, higher levels of R/S were associated with greater marital satisfaction (Murphy et al., 2015). Greater intrinsic religiosity has been associated with lower perceived caregiver burden (Herrera et al., 2009) and less hopelessness (Kim et al., 2014). Research on the relationship between R/S and caregiver physical health is limited and has relied on self-report measures of caregiver physical health, often as a component of quality of life measures. However, there is some evidence to suggest that greater R/S is associated with better physical health (Roscoe et al., 2009). Notably, in a sample of cancer survivors and their caregivers, higher caregiver R/S was associated with better survivor physical health and higher survivor R/S predicted better caregiver physical health (Kim et al., 2011). These results demonstrate the potential importance of R/S to physical health and provide further evidence of the mutuality of patient and caregiver well-being.

However, to conclude that R/S is associated with better caregiver outcomes is an over-simplification of a complex relationship. While most studies report a positive relationship between R/S and caregiver outcomes, some studies have reported null (Herrera et al., 2009; Kapari et al., 2010; Leblanc et al., 2004; Meller, 2001) or negative findings. For example, private R/S practices, such as prayer, have been associated with worse caregiver mental health (Herrera et al., 2009), including higher levels of depression (Winter et al., 2015) and caregiver strain (Wakefield et al., 2012). In a sample of cancer caregivers, stronger faith was associated with caregiver self-report of poor physical health (Kim et al., 2011). As in research on patients, one explanation for these negative relationships is that R/S resources are mobilized in the context of more severe stressors, resulting in an association between R/S and poor mental and physical health.

Further, the relationship between R/S and caregiver outcomes may depend on the outcome assessed and the nature of the patient-caregiver relationship. In a study of cancer caregivers, the relationship between caregiver stress and poor mental health was weaker for caregivers with greater R/S, suggesting a stress-buffering effect of R/S (Colgrove et al., 2007). However, the relationship between caregiver stress and poor physical function was only significant in caregivers with higher R/S levels, indicating a "stress-aggravating effect" of R/S (Colgrove et al., 2007, p. 95). Regarding the patient-caregiver relationship, differences have emerged between spouse and adult child caregivers. In a sample of caregivers of older adults, stronger faith was associated with greater stress and worse self-reported physical health in spousal caregivers (Meller, 2001). Opposite relationships emerged in adult child caregivers in which stronger faith was associated with less stress, greater life satisfaction, better physical health, and greater social connection (Meller, 2001). In a separate study of caregivers of disabled older adults, higher levels of R/S were associated with low levels of depression in spouses while the reverse relationship emerged in adult child caregivers (Zunzunegui et al., 1999). Variation in results across studies may be due to differences in the samples and assessments used and require additional study. However, these findings demonstrate the complex relationship between caregiver R/S and well-being. Additional research is needed to understand the nuances of these relationships.

As previously stated, many caregivers report using R/S to cope with caregiving responsibilities. Similar to R/S coping in patients, relationships between positive religious coping and caregiver outcomes are mixed (Heo & Koeske, 2013; Kinney et al., 2003). For example, in a sample of caregivers of advanced cancer patients, greater use of positive religious coping strategies was associated with more caregiver burden and greater satisfaction with the caregiving role after controlling for demographic characteristics (Pearce et al., 2006). However, negative religious coping is consistently associated with problematic outcomes including greater depression (Herrera et al., 2009; Shah et al., 2001), worse quality of life (Khanjari et al., 2012), less growth (Thombre et al., 2010), and greater perceived caregiving burden (Shah et al., 2001). In the same sample of cancer caregivers, greater use of negative religious coping was associated with worse quality of life, greater burden, lower satisfaction with caregiving, and increased risk for major depressive disorder and an anxiety disorder (Pearce et al., 2006). Although research is limited, R/S coping has also been associated with indicators of physical health. In a study of Latina and White dementia caregivers, negative religious coping was associated with greater cumulative health risk, assessed with a measure of engagement in health behaviors. Positive religious coping was associated with reduced health risk but only in Latina caregivers (Rabinowitz et al., 2010). However, in dementia caregivers, greater use of positive religious coping has been associated with worse diurnal salivary cortisol patterns (Merritt & McCallum, 2013) and worse self-reported health (Mausbach et al., 2003).

Many caregivers turn to their spiritual orienting systems to cope with the stresses of caregiving and much of the research suggests that R/S is associated with positive outcomes. However, research on caregiver R/S has focused primarily on R/S behaviors and degree of R/S assessed with self-report measures. Research on more specific R/S indicators such as R/S appraisals of the caregiving role and the role of R/S in making meaning of the patient's illness would provide a more comprehensive view of the role and impact of caregiver R/S. Further, caregivers are at increased risk for poor physical health but research on caregiver R/S and physical health is limited. Additional research on this relationship would determine whether R/S is a protective factor that can be accessed to protect and improve caregiver health.

CARE TEAM LEVEL

For the purposes of this chapter, the care team includes the health care providers who treat the patient. These teams are often interdisciplinary but vary in their inclusion of R/S care providers such as health care chaplains. Research on R/S in medicine has focused primarily on the nature and outcomes of patients' R/S beliefs and practices. However, like patients and caregivers, many health care providers bring their own R/S attitudes, beliefs, and practices to clinical care (Ramondetta et al., 2011). In addition, the majority of providers believe that patient R/S is an important component of patients' illness experience (Chibnall & Brooks, 2001; Curlin et al., 2007; McCauley et al., 2005; Taylor et al., 1994) and that addressing R/S issues is part of the role of a health care provider (Balboni et al., 2013; Luckhaupt et al., 2005; McCauley et al., 2005; Neeleman & King, 1993; Rodin et al., 2015), particularly when providing end-of-life care (Balboni et al., 2014; Berg et al., 2013; Ramondetta et al., 2011; Sheppe et al., 2013; Siegel et al., 2002). These attitudes are consistent with patients' preferences. Across studies, the majority of patients (median 70.5%) report wanting their health care provider to inquire about R/S needs (Best et al., 2015). As expected, patients who endorse higher levels of religiosity are more likely to want physicians to inquire about their R/S (Best et al., 2015; Daaleman & Nease Jr, 1994; Ehman et al., 1999; Phelps et al., 2012). However, up to half of patients with low levels of religiosity would like some degree of integration of spiritual care into medical care (Best et al., 2015; Daaleman & Nease Jr, 1994; Ehman et al., 1999), particularly in the context of severe illness (MacLean et al., 2003).

While some research suggests that physicians have lower R/S levels than the general population (Neeleman & King, 1993), there is also evidence that rates of R/S in physicians are similar to those in the general population (Cheever et al., 2005; Curlin et al., 2005). Up to three-quarters of physicians describe themselves as religious or spiritual (Curlin et al., 2005; Peckham, 2015; Voltmer et al., 2014), over half regularly attend religious services (Curlin et al., 2005; Peckham, 2015), and more than half state that their religious beliefs influence their medical practice (Catlin et al., 2008; Cheever et al., 2005; Curlin et al., 2005; Peteet & Balboni, 2013). Further, physicians' R/S beliefs are related to their beliefs about patient care. For example, more religious physicians are less likely to believe in withdrawing life-sustaining treatment, approve of prescribing needed pain medications that will hasten death, agree with euthanasia, and be willing to perform an abortion (Aiyer et al., 1999; Christakis & Asch, 1995; Curlin et al., 2008; Wenger & Carmel, 2004). Providers with strong personal R/S beliefs also have more positive attitudes about R/S and spiritual care (Curlin et al., 2007; Luckhaupt et al., 2005; Musgrave & McFarlane, 2004). They are more likely to believe that providers should discuss R/S with patients and that patients desire these discussions, that R/S beliefs play a role in healing, that the doctor-patient relationship is strengthened by discussing R/S, and that R/S providers should be integrated into patient care (Berg et al., 2013; Curlin et al., 2006; Curlin et al., 2007; Sheppe et al., 2013; Siegel et al., 2002). Providers' R/S may also impact their conceptualization of patients' problems. In a study of primary care providers and psychiatrists, physicians with higher self-reported R/S were more likely to interpret medically unexplained symptoms as reflecting a spiritual problem and to recommend that the patient attend to spiritual issues (Shin et al., 2013). Finally, providers' R/S beliefs are also related to patient care. Providers with higher self-reported R/S are more likely to address R/S with patients (Grossoehme et al., 2007; Johnston Taylor et al., 1994; Voltmer et al., 2014), make referrals to religious leaders (Neeleman & King, 1993), and disclose their R/S beliefs to patients (Al-Yousefi, 2012; Neeleman & King, 1993).

R/S may also help care team members cope with the challenges of patient care (Ayele et al., 1999; Pawlikowski et al., 2012; Ramondetta et al., 2011). In medical residents, higher levels of R/S were associated with less emotional exhaustion and patient depersonalization, and a greater sense of personal accomplishment (Doolittle et al., 2013). Like patients, providers can experience R/S changes, particularly growth, as a result of their interactions with patients (Penderell & Brazil, 2010). The patient-provider encounter may also be experienced in R/S terms. In a sample of mental health providers, over half (55.5%) stated that an important moment in treatment was sacred or had qualities associated with the divine or higher powers (Pargament et al., 2014). Higher levels of provider perceptions of sacred qualities were associated with provider report of greater improvements in client and provider outcomes (e.g., gaining new insight), a stronger patient-provider relationship, and higher levels of providers' motivation in their work (Pargament et al., 2014). Additional research is needed in this area. However, these findings suggest that R/S is evident, not just in patients and providers individually, but in the interaction between patients and providers.

Despite the preferences of patients and providers, rates of spiritual care provision are low (Chibnall & Brooks, 2001; Phelps et al., 2012; Ramondetta et al., 2011; Voltmer et al., 2014) and less than providers' enthusiasm for this type of care (Balboni et al., 2014; Kalish, 2012). In a sample of cancer patients, only 6% reported that their spiritual needs were assessed by a member of their health care team (Astrow et al., 2007). Similarly, the large majority of advanced cancer patients reported receiving no spiritual care from the medical team (13% received spiritual care from nurses and 6% from physicians; Balboni et al., 2013). This gap in care is felt by providers as well as patients. Approximately one-third of oncology nurses and physicians provide spiritual care less often than they would like to provide such care (Balboni et al., 2014). Addressing patients' R/S needs is important for comprehensive patient care and is relevant to patient outcomes. Unmet spiritual needs are associated with lower patient ratings of care quality (Astrow et al., 2007; Winkelman et al., 2011) and satisfaction with care (Astrow et al., 2007; Balboni et al., 2013), and higher medical costs at the end of life, particularly among minority patients and those who use rely on R/S to cope (Balboni et al., 2011). However, advanced cancer patients whose spiritual needs were supported by the health care system received more hospice care and had better quality of life at the end of life than patients whose spiritual needs were not supported (Balboni et al., 2011; Balboni et al., 2010).

Understanding the barriers to provision of spiritual care may help reduce rates of unmet spiritual care needs and avoid the negative outcomes associated with these needs. Barriers identified by providers include lack of time (Balboni et al., 2014; Daaleman et al., 2008; Keall et al., 2014; McCauley et al., 2005; Rassouli et al., 2015; Vermandere et al., 2012), inadequate training (Keall et al., 2014; McCauley et al., 2005; Rassouli et al., 2015; Vermandere et al., 2012), provider discomfort and concern about professional boundaries (Keall et al., 2014; Phelps et al., 2012; Rassouli et al., 2015; Vermandere et al., 2012), lack of privacy during patient appointments (Daaleman et al., 2008; Keall et al., 2014; Rassouli et al., 2015), and differences in patients' and providers' beliefs (Daaleman et al., 2008; Gallison et al., 2013; Keall et al., 2014). However, in a sample of oncology nurses and physicians, the only barrier significantly associated with rates of spiritual care provision was lack of training in spiritual care (Balboni et al., 2014).

There is increasing recognition of the inadequacy of provider training in spiritual care and the need to incorporate spiritual care training into medical school curricula (Lucchetti et al., 2012; Puchalski, 2006; Talley & Magie, 2014) and provider education (Harbinson & Bell, 2015; Lewinson et al., 2015; Schonfeld et al., 2014; Timmins et al., 2015). Programs that train health care providers in the provision of spiritual care are available (Lovanio & Wallace, 2007; Mitchell et al., 2006; Todres et al., 2005; Wasner et al., 2005; Zollfrank et al., 2015), although research on their efficacy is quite limited. Further, providers with stronger R/S beliefs may be more likely to seek such training and allocate the time required to benefit from it (Balboni et al., 2014; Rasinski et al., 2011). Developing programs that are efficacious and feasible for busy clinicians may improve provider access to training and increase the number of providers trained in spiritual care.

In addition to spiritual care training, clinical resources are available to help providers address patients' R/S issues. Numerous assessment tools have been developed for use in clinical care (Anandarajah & Hight, 2001; Borneman et al., 2010; Lucchetti et al., 2013; Sessanna et al., 2011). However, evaluation of the reliability and validity of these tools is limited (Draper, 2012; Lucchetti et al., 2013). In addition, R/S assessments are often too complex to integrate into routine clinical care (Lunder et al., 2011; Timmins & Kelly, 2008) and are not culturally sensitive (Lewis, 2008; Lunder et al., 2011). Yet preliminary research suggests that integrating R/S assessment into clinical care is feasible and effective (Borneman et al., 2010; Puchalski & Romer, 2000). The Oncologist Assisted Spirituality Intervention Study (OASIS) evaluated the feasibility, acceptability, and patient impact of a physician initiated assessment of spiritual concerns (Kristeller et al., 2005). Patients and oncologists in the intervention condition were comfortable with the intervention and found it to be helpful. The average length of the intervention was six minutes per oncologist report and was associated with only a 1.7 minute increase in the length of the session. In addition, the intervention was associated with improved patient mood and quality of life immediately following the intervention and three weeks later.

The importance of R/S in medicine is not restricted to the patient and caregiver experience. Like patients, providers turn to their spiritual orienting systems in ways that likely impact patient care. Notably, most providers believe that addressing patients' R/S issues is part of their professional role. However, many barriers to greater provision of R/S care exist. Removing these barriers may improve comprehensive patient-centered care, reduce problems associated with unmet R/S needs, and perhaps improve providers' satisfaction with the care they provide.

PSYCHO-SPIRITUAL INTERVENTIONS

Research on psycho-spiritual interventions in medical populations is limited and focuses primarily on patients. However, evidence suggests that psycho-spiritual interventions may be beneficial and are an important addition to secular psychotherapies (Pargament, 2007).

MINDFULNESS-BASED THERAPIES

Mindfulness is based on Buddhist spiritual practices and focuses on experiencing the present moment without judging or trying to change it (Bishop et al., 2004; Kabat-Zinn, 2013; Marchand, 2012). Experiencing the present is achieved by being aware of external (e.g., auditory and visual) and internal (e.g., pain, thoughts, emotions) stimuli without becoming attached to or overly influenced by them. Mindfulness has been integrated into two psychotherapeutic techniques: mindfulness-based stress reduction (MBSR; Kabat-Zinn, 2013) and mindfulness-based cognitive therapy (MBCT; Marchand, 2012; Segal et al., 2002). Mindfulness in MBSR includes meditation, a focus on bodily sensations, and hatha yoga. MBSR also includes education on stress, training in assertiveness and effective coping, and cultivation of acceptance of the present moment. MBSR has been evaluated in various medical populations including patients with cancer (Johns et al., 2015; Piet et al., 2012; Zainal et al., 2013), multiple sclerosis (Simpson et al., 2014), fibromyalgia (Cash et al., 2015; Lauche et al., 2013), chronic insomnia (Lauche et al., 2013), pain (Reiner et al., 2013), and vascular disease (Abbott et al., 2014). MBSR has also been evaluated in non-patient populations including caregivers of dementia patients (Hoppes et al., 2012) and health care professionals (Beddoe, 2004; Irving et al., 2009; Martín-Asuero & García-Banda, 2010). Across studies, MBSR has been associated with improvements in anxiety (Simpson et al., 2014; Zainal et al., 2013), depression (Johns et al., 2015; Simpson et al., 2014; Zainal et al., 2013), stress (Cash et al., 2015; Zainal et al., 2013), quality of life (Lauche et al., 2013; Simpson et al., 2014), pain (Lauche et al., 2013; Reiner et al., 2013; Simpson et al., 2014), weight loss (Olson & Emery, 2015), and fatigue and sleep disturbance (Cash et al., 2015; Johns et al., 2015).

MBCT was originally developed to prevent relapse of depression by combining mindfulness and cognitive therapy. MBCT teaches patients to recognize changes in mood and disengage from patterns of negative thinking that contribute to relapse. MCBT has been tested in various medical populations including patients with diabetes (Tovote et al., 2014; Tovote et al., 2015; van Son et al., 2014), cancer (Brotto et al., 2012; Stafford et al., 2013; van der Lee & Garssen, 2012), fertility problems (Sherratt & Lunn, 2013), chronic fatigue syndrome (Rimes & Wingrove, 2013), tinnitus (Philippot et al., 2012), pain (Day et al., 2014; Dowd et al., 2015; Peilot et al., 2014), HIV (Gonzalez-Garcia et al., 2013; Yang, Liu, Zhang, & Liu, 2015), psoriasis (Fordham et al., 2015), and traumatic brain injury (Bedard et al., 2014; Bedard et al., 2012). While fewer studies have been conducted on MBCT than MBSR in medical populations, the results are promising. MBCT has been associated with improvements in stress (Tovote et al., 2014; van Son et al., 2014), anxiety (Gonzalez-Garcia et al., 2013; Tovote et al., 2014; van Son et al., 2014), depression (Bedard et al., 2014; Gonzalez-Garcia et al., 2013; Rimes & Wingrove, 2013; Tovote et al., 2014; van Son et al., 2014), fatigue (Rimes & Wingrove, 2013; van der Lee & Garssen, 2012), well-being (Tovote et al., 2014; van der Lee & Garssen, 2012), quality of life (Gonzalez-Garcia et al., 2013; Stafford et al., 2013), and sexual function (Brotto et al., 2012). In a randomized controlled trial of MBCT compared to treatment as usual in patients with HIV, patients in the MCBT condition had significant increases in CD4 counts over a six-month follow-up (Gonzalez-Garcia et al., 2013).

MEANING-CENTERED PSYCHOTHERAPY

Meaning-centered group psychotherapy (MCGP) is an eight-session manualized treatment for patients with advanced cancer. The goal of MCGP is to enhance patients' spiritual well-being and sense of meaning, peace, and purpose by exploring sources of meaning, the impact of cancer on meaning and identity, and the historical and personal contexts of patients' lives (Breitbart et al., 2010; Breitbart et al., 2015). In a recent randomized controlled trial, patients were randomized to eight sessions of MCGP or supportive group psychotherapy (SGP; Breitbart et al., 2015). An analysis of patients who completed at least three sessions of the intervention found significant improvements over time for MCGP in quality of life, spiritual well-being, depression, hopelessness, desire for hastened death, and physical symptom distress relative to SGP. In intent-to-treat analyses, treatment effects were reduced but remained significant for spiritual well-being, quality of life, depression, hopelessness, and desire for hastened death (Breitbart et al., 2015). Notably, only 52% of patients randomized to MCGP and 48% randomized to SGP completed post-treatment assessments. Attrition did not differ across groups and was due primarily to worsening health and scheduling conflicts. These attrition rates highlight the challenges associated with designing and evaluating interventions for advanced cancer patients and should be taken into consideration when interpreting these results. MCGP is currently being evaluated in cancer caregivers (Applebaum et al., 2015) and cancer survivors (van der Spek et al., 2014).

DIGNITY THERAPY

Dignity therapy addresses psychosocial and existential distress in patients with terminal illness by fostering patients' sense of meaning and purpose (Chochinov et al., 2005). A framework of questions based on the dignity-conserving model of care is used by clinicians to guide patients through an individualized discussion of what matters most to the patient and how they want to be remembered (Chochinov, 2002; Chochinov et al., 2011). The dignity-conserving model includes three areas that influence patients' dignity: illness-related concerns (e.g., symptom distress, level of independence), dignity-conserving repertoire (e.g., generativity, maintaining normalcy), and the social dignity inventory (e.g., social support, concern about burdening others; Chochinov, 2002). Sessions are audiotaped, transcribed, and formatted into a narrative. The narrative is read aloud to the patient who can edit the document. The final narrative is given to the patient to share or leave with loved ones (Chochinov et al., 2005, 2011).

A randomized controlled trial by the intervention developers compared dignity therapy to supportive psychotherapy and standard palliative care (Chochinov et al., 2011). Change over time in spiritual well-being, dignity, anxiety, depression, and quality of life did not differ across groups. However, patients in the dignity therapy group were more likely to find the study helpful and report that it improved their quality of life and sense of dignity. These findings were mirrored in a recent systematic review of research on dignity therapy which found high levels of patient acceptability and satisfaction but few differences in psychological and spiritual outcomes when compared to control conditions. Further, as with MCGP, many studies suffered from study recruitment and retention issues (Fitchett et al., 2015).

ADDITIONAL PSYCHO-SPIRITUAL INTERVENTIONS

Additional psycho-spiritual interventions have been developed in medical populations. These interventions have less empirical support than those discussed but represent promising areas for ongoing research. For example, a randomized controlled trial compared a 6-week spiritual reminiscence group therapy to a control condition in patients with mild to moderate dementia (Wu & Koo, 2015). Treatment was based on the spiritual model of dementia (MacKinlay & Trevitt, 2012) and addressed life meaning, relationships, hopes and fears, transcendence, and R/S beliefs and practices. Patients in the treatment condition reported improvements in hope, life satisfaction, spiritual well-being, and cognitive function while patients in the control condition experienced declines on all outcomes.

A recent study compared religiously integrated cognitive behavioral therapy (RCBT) to traditional cognitive behavioral therapy (CBT) for depression in patients with chronic medical illness (Koenig et al., 2015). RCBT uses resources from patients' religious traditions to replace cognitive distortions and increase adaptive behaviors. For example, RCBT incorporates scripture verses and prayers to provide a context for the cognitive and behavioral strategies of CBT. Manuals were created for the five major world religions: Christianity, Judaism, Islam, Buddhism, and Hinduism (Pearce et al., 2015). In a pilot randomized controlled trial, patients were assigned to 10 sessions of telephone administered RCBT or CBT. The groups did not differ in changes in depression (Koenig et al., 2015), generosity (Pearce et al., 2015), or optimism (Koenig et al., 2015) over time although there was some evidence to suggest that RCBT was more effective in more religious patients (Koenig et al., 2015).

Finally, a pre-post within group evaluation of a spiritual coping intervention for patients with HIV resulted in significant increases in patients' self-rated religiosity and decreases in negative spiritual coping and depression (Tarakeshwar et al., 2005). The 8-session group intervention addressed issues such as body image, stigma and guilt, relationships, control, mental and physical health, and personal goals from a religious coping framework.

Research on psycho-spiritual interventions in medical populations is limited and based on small sample sizes in largely Christian samples collected from academic medical institutions. In addition, heterogeneity across study designs, assessments, and the content and duration of interventions preclude conclusive statements regarding optimal intervention design and intervention efficacy (Kruizinga et al., 2015). However, preliminary findings are promising and suggest that psycho-spiritual interventions are worthy of continuing evaluation.

CONCLUSION

In this chapter, we discussed the relationship between R/S and medicine from a religious coping perspective in patients, caregivers, and health care providers. A large body of research demonstrates the important role of R/S in how patients and caregivers understand and cope with illness. Similarly, many health care providers view illness and their clinical care through a R/S lens and believe that attending to patients' spiritual needs is part of their professional role. This research has led to preliminary work on psycho-spiritual interventions for medical populations. However, additional work is needed to translate findings from observational studies to clinical care. Yet available research suggests that failing to integrate R/S into the care of patients and caregivers overlooks an important aspect of patients' and caregivers' experiences, with negative implications for patient and caregiver mental and physical well-being.

REFERENCES

Abbott, R. A., Whear, R., Rodgers, L. R., Bethel, A., Coon, J. T., Kuyken, W., . . . Dickens, C. (2014). Effectiveness of mindfulness-based stress reduction and mindfulness based cognitive therapy in vascular disease: A systematic review and meta-analysis of randomised controlled trials. *J Psychosom Res, 76*(5), 341–351. doi: 10.1016/j.jpsychores.2014.02.012

Adelstein, K. E., Anderson, J. G., & Taylor, A. G. (2014). Importance of meaning-making for patients undergoing hematopoietic stem cell transplantation. *Oncol Nurs Forum, 41*(2), E172–184. doi: 10.1188/14.onf.e172-e184

Agarwal, M., Hamilton, J. B., Crandell, J. L., & Moore, C. E. (2010). Coping strategies of African American head and neck cancer survivors. *Journal of Psychosocial Oncology, 28*(5), 526–538.

Agli, O., Bailly, N., & Ferrand, C. (2015). Spirituality and religion in older adults with dementia: A systematic review. *International Psychogeriatrics, 27*(5), 715–725. doi: 10.1017/S1041610214001665

Ai, A. L., Park, C. L., Huang, B., Rodgers, W., & Tice, T. N. (2007). Psychosocial mediation of religious coping styles: A study of short-term psychological distress following cardiac surgery. *Pers Soc Psychol Bull, 33*(6), 867–882. doi: 10.1177/0146167207301008

Ai, A. L., Peterson, C., Bolling, S. F., & Rodgers, W. (2006). Depression, faith-based coping, and short-term postoperative global functioning in adult and older patients undergoing cardiac surgery. *J Psychosom Res, 60*(1), 21–28. doi: 10.1016/j.jpsychores.2005.06.082

Ai, A. L., Seymour, E. M., Tice, T. N., Kronfol, Z., & Bolling, S. F. (2009). Spiritual struggle related to plasma interleukin-6 prior to cardiac surgery. *Psychology of Religion and Spirituality, 1*(2), 112–128. doi: 10.1037/a0015775

Aiyer, A. N., Ruiz, G., Steinman, A., & Ho, G. Y. (1999). Influence of physician attitudes on willingness to perform abortion. *Obstet Gynecol, 93*(4), 576–580.

Al-Yousefi, N. A. (2012). Observations of Muslim physicians regarding the influence of religion on health and their clinical approach. *J Relig Health, 51*(2), 269–280. doi: 10.1007/s10943-012-9567-z

Allmon, A. L., Tallman, B. A., & Altmaier, E. M. (2013). Spiritual growth and decline among patients with cancer. *Oncology Nursing Forum, 40*(6), 559–565. doi: 10.1188/13.ONF.559–565

American Psychological Association. (n.d.). Psychological Science. Retrieved from http://www.apa.org/research/

Anandarajah, G., & Hight, E. (2001). Spirituality and medical practice: Using the HOPE questions as a practical tool for spiritual assessment. *Am Fam Physician, 63*(1), 81–89.

Ano, G. G., & Vasconcelles, E. B. (2005). Religious coping and psychological adjustment to stress: A meta-analysis. *J Clin Psychol, 61*(4), 461–480. doi: 10.1002/jclp.20049

Aoun, S. M., Bentley, B., Funk, L., Toye, C., Grande, G., & Stajduhar, K. J. (2013). A 10-year literature review of family caregiving for motor neurone disease: Moving from caregiver burden studies to palliative care interventions. *Palliat Med, 27*(5), 437–446. doi: 10.1177/0269216312455729

Applebaum, A. J., & Breitbart, W. (2013). Care for the cancer caregiver: A systematic review. *Palliat Support Care, 11*(3), 231–252. doi: 10.1017/s1478951512000594

Applebaum, A. J., Kulikowski, J. R., & Breitbart, W. (2015). Meaning-Centered Psychotherapy for Cancer Caregivers (MCP-C): Rationale and overview. *Palliat Support Care*, 1–11. doi: 10.1017/s1478951515000450

Astrow, A. B., Wexler, A., Texeira, K., He, M. K., & Sulmasy, D. P. (2007). Is failure to meet spiritual needs associated with cancer patients' perceptions of quality of care and their satisfaction with care? *J Clin Oncol, 25*(36), 5753–5757. doi: 10.1200/jco.2007.12.4362

Ayele, H., Mulligan, T., Gheorghiu, S., & Reyes-Ortiz, C. (1999). Religious activity improves life satisfaction for some physicians and older patients. *J Am Geriatr Soc, 47*(4), 453–455.

Balboni, M. J., Sullivan, A., Amobi, A., Phelps, A. C., Gorman, D. P., Zollfrank, A., . . . Balboni, T. A. (2013). Why is spiritual care infrequent at the end of life? Spiritual care perceptions among patients, nurses, and physicians and the role of training. *J Clin Oncol, 31*(4), 461–467. doi: 10.1200/jco.2012.44.6443

Balboni, M. J., Sullivan, A., Enzinger, A. C., Epstein-Peterson, Z. D., Tseng, Y. D., Mitchell, C., . . . Balboni, T. A. (2014). Nurse and physician barriers to spiritual care provision at the end of life. *J Pain Symptom Manage, 48*(3), 400–410. doi: 10.1016/j.jpainsymman.2013.09.020

Balboni, T. A., Balboni, M., Enzinger, A. C., Gallivan, K., Paulk, M. E., Wright, A., . . . Prigerson, H. G. (2013). Provision of spiritual support to patients with advanced cancer by religious communities and associations with medical care at the end of life. *JAMA Intern Med, 173*(12), 1109–1117. doi: 10.1001/jamainternmed.2013.903

Balboni, T., Balboni, M., Paulk, M. E., Phelps, A., Wright, A., Peteet, J., . . . Prigerson, H. (2011). Support of cancer patients' spiritual needs and associations with medical care costs at the end of life. *Cancer, 117*(23), 5383–5391. doi: 10.1002/cncr.26221

Balboni, T. A., Paulk, M. E., Balboni, M. J., Phelps, A. C., Loggers, E. T., Wright, A. A., . . . Prigerson, H. G. (2010). Provision of spiritual care to patients with advanced cancer: Associations with medical care and quality of life near death. *J Clin Oncol, 28*(3), 445–452. doi: 10.1200/jco.2009.24.8005

Baldacchino, D. (2011). Myocardial infarction: A turning point in meaning in life over time. *Br J Nurs, 20*(2), 107–114. doi: 10.12968/bjon.2011.20.2.107

Baldacchino, D. R., Borg, J., Muscat, C., & Sturgeon, C. (2012). Psychology and theology meet: Illness appraisal and spiritual coping. *Western J NursRes, 34*(6), 818–847. doi: 10.1177/0193945912441265

Bambauer, K. Z., Zhang, B., Maciejewski, P. K., Sahay, N., Pirl, W. F., Block, S. D., & Prigerson, H. G. (2006). Mutuality and specificity of mental disorders in advanced cancer patients and caregivers. *Soc Psychiatry Psychiatr Epidemiol, 41*(10), 819–824. doi: 10.1007/s00127-006-0103-x

Banthia, R., Moskowitz, J. T., Acree, M., & Folkman, S. (2007). Socioeconomic differences in the effects of prayer on physical symptoms and quality of life. *J Health Psychol, 12*(2), 249–260. doi: 10.1177/1359105307074251

Barber, C. E. (2014). Is religiosity a protective factor for Mexican-American filial caregivers? *Journal of Religion, Spirituality & Aging, 26*(2-3), 245–258. doi: 10.1080/15528030.2013.867422

Barnes, P. M., Powell-Griner, E., McFann, K., & Nahin, R. L. (2004). Complementary and alternative medicine use among adults: United States, 2002. *Adv Data, May 27*(343), 1–19.

Barton, Y. A., & Miller, L. (2015). Spirituality and positive psychology go hand in hand: An investigation of multiple empirically derived profiles and related protective benefits. *J Relig Health, 54*(3), 829–843. doi: 10.1007/s10943-015-0045-2

Bearon, L. B., & Koenig, H. G. (1990). Religious cognitions and use of prayer in health and illness. *The Gerontologist, 30*(2), 249–253. doi: 10.1093/geront/30.2.249

Bedard, M., Felteau, M., Marshall, S., Cullen, N., Gibbons, C., Dubois, S., … Moustgaard, A. (2014). Mindfulness-based cognitive therapy reduces symptoms of depression in people with a traumatic brain injury: Results from a randomized controlled trial. *J Head Trauma Rehabil, 29*(4), E13–22. doi: 10.1097/HTR.0b013e3182a615a0

Bedard, M., Felteau, M., Marshall, S., Dubois, S., Gibbons, C., Klein, R., & Weaver, B. (2012). Mindfulness-based cognitive therapy: Benefits in reducing depression following a traumatic brain injury. *Adv Mind Body Med, 26*(1), 14–20.

Beddoe, A. E. (2004). Does mindfulness decrease stress and foster empathy among nursing students? *Journal of Nursing Education, 43*(7), 305.

Berg, G. M., Crowe, R. E., Budke, G., Norman, J., Swick, V., Nyberg, S., & Lee, F. (2013). Kansas physician assistants' attitudes and beliefs regarding spirituality and religiosity in patient care. *J Relig Health, 52*(3), 864–876. doi: 10.1007/s10943-011-9532-2

Best, M., Butow, P., & Olver, I. (2015). Do patients want doctors to talk about spirituality? A systematic literature review. *Patient Educ Couns.* doi: 10.1016/j.pec.2015.04.017

Bhimani, R. (2014). Understanding the Burden on Caregivers of People with Parkinson's: A Scoping Review of the Literature. *Rehabil Res Pract, 2014*, 1–8. doi: 10.1155/2014/718527

Bishop, S. R., Lau, M., Shapiro, S., Carlson, L., Anderson, N. D., Carmody, J., … Velting, D. (2004). Mindfulness: A proposed operational definition. *Clinical psychology: Science and Practice, 11*(3), 230–241.

Borneman, T., Ferrell, B., & Puchalski, C. M. (2010). Evaluation of the FICA Tool for Spiritual Assessment. *J Pain Symptom Manage, 40*(2), 163–173. doi: 10.1016/j.jpainsymman.2009.12.019

Breitbart, W., Rosenfeld, B., Gibson, C., Pessin, H., Poppito, S., Nelson, C., … Olden, M. (2010). Meaning-centered group psychotherapy for patients with advanced cancer: A pilot randomized controlled trial. *Psycho-Oncology, 19*(1), 21–28. doi: 10.1002/pon.1556

Breitbart, W., Rosenfeld, B., Pessin, H., Applebaum, A., Kulikowski, J., & Lichtenthal, W. G. (2015). Meaning-centered group psychotherapy: An effective intervention for improving psychological well-being in patients with advanced cancer. *J Clin Oncol, 33*(7), 749–754. doi: 10.1200/jco.2014.57.2198

Brotto, L. A., Erskine, Y., Carey, M., Ehlen, T., Finlayson, S., Heywood, M., … Miller, D. (2012). A brief mindfulness-based cognitive behavioral intervention improves sexual functioning versus wait-list control in women treated for gynecologic cancer. *Gynecol Oncol, 125*(2), 320–325. doi: 10.1016/j.ygyno.2012.01.035

Burker, E. J., Evon, D. M., Sedway, J. A., & Egan, T. (2004). Religious coping, psychological distress and disability among patients with end-stage pulmonary disease. *J Clin Psychol Med Settings, 11*(3), 179–193.

Cadge, W., & Fair, B. (2010). Religion, spirituality, health, and medicine: Sociological intersections. In C. E. Bird, P. Conrad, A. M. Fremont & S. Timmermans (Eds.), *Handbook of medical sociology* (pp. 341–362). Nashville, TN: Vanderbilt University Press.

Cash, E., Salmon, P., Weissbecker, I., Rebholz, W. N., Bayley-Veloso, R., Zimmaro, L. A., … Sephton, S. E. (2015). Mindfulness meditation alleviates fibromyalgia symptoms in women: Results of a randomized clinical trial. *Ann Behav Med, 49*(3), 319–330. doi: 10.1007/s12160-014-9665-0

Cassibba, R., Papagna, S., Calabrese, M. T., Costantino, E., Paterno, A., & Granqvist, P. (2014). The role of attachment to God in secular and religious/spiritual ways of coping with a serious disease. *Mental Health, Religion & Culture, 17*(3), 252–261. doi: 10.1080/13674676.2013.795138

Catlin, E. A., Cadge, W., Ecklund, E. H., Gage, E. A., & Zollfrank, A. A. (2008). The spiritual and religious identities, beliefs, and practices of academic pediatricians in the United States. *Acad Med, 83*(12), 1146–1152. doi: 10.1097/ACM.0b013e31818c64a5

Cattich, J., & Knudson-Martin, C. (2009). Spirituality and relationship: A holistic analysis of how couples cope with diabetes. *J Marital Fam Ther, 35*(1), 111–124. doi: 10.1111/j.1752–0606.2008.00105.x

Cheever, K. H., Jubilan, B., Dailey, T., Ehrhardt, K., Blumenstein, R., Morin, C. J., & Lewis, C. (2005). Surgeons and the spirit: A study on the relationship of religiosity to clinical practice. *J Relig Health, 44*(1), 67–80.

Chibnall, J. T., & Brooks, C. A. (2001). Religion in the clinic: The role of physician beliefs. *South Med J, 94*(4), 374–379.

Chochinov, H. M. (2002). Dignity-conserving care—a new model for palliative care: Helping the patient feel valued. *JAMA, 287*(17), 2253–2260.

Chochinov, H. M., Hack, T., Hassard, T., Kristjanson, L. J., McClement, S., & Harlos, M. (2005). Dignity therapy: A novel psychotherapeutic intervention for patients near the end of life. *Journal of clinical oncology, 23*(24), 5520–5525.

Chochinov, H. M., Kristjanson, L. J., Breitbart, W., McClement, S., Hack, T. F., Hassard, T., & Harlos, M. (2011). Effect of dignity therapy on distress and end-of-life experience in terminally ill patients: A randomised controlled trial. *Lancet Oncol, 12*(8), 753–762. doi: 10.1016/s1470-2045(11)70153-x

Christakis, N. A., & Asch, D. A. (1995). Physician characteristics associated with decisions to withdraw life support. *Am J Public Health, 85*(3), 367–372.

Cohen, I. G., Lynch, H. F., & Curfman, G. D. (2014). When religious freedom clashes with access to care. *The New England Journal of Medicine, 371*(7), 596–599. doi: 10.1056/NEJMp1407965

Colgrove, L. A., Kim, Y., & Thompson, N. (2007). The effect of spirituality and gender on the quality of life of spousal caregivers of cancer survivors. *Ann Behav Med, 33*(1), 90–98. doi: 10.1207/s15324796abm3301_10

Collin, M. (2012). The search for a higher power among terminally ill people with no previous religion or belief. *Int J Palliat Nurs, 18*(8), 384–389. doi: 10.12968/ijpn.2012.18.8.384

Coon, D. W., Rubert, M., Solano, N., Mausbach, B., Kraemer, H., Arguelles, T., . . . Gallagher-Thompson, D. (2004). Well-being, appraisal, and coping in Latina and Caucasian female dementia caregivers: findings from the REACH study. *Aging Ment Health, 8*(4), 330–345. doi: 10.1080/13607860410001709683

Costanzo, E. S., Lutgendorf, S. K., Bradley, S. L., Rose, S. L., & Anderson, B. (2005). Cancer attributions, distress, and health practices among gynecologic cancer survivors. *Psychosomatic Medicine, 67*(6), 972–980. doi: 10.1097/01.psy.0000188402.95398.c0

Cotton, S., Puchalski, C. M., Sherman, S. N., Mrus, J. M., Peterman, A. H., Feinberg, J., . . . Tsevat, J. (2006). Spirituality and religion in patients with HIV/AIDS. *J Gen Int Med, 21*(S5), S5–S13. doi: 10.1111/j.1525-1497.2006.00642.x

Cummings, J. P., & Pargament, K. I. (2010). Medicine for the spirit: Religious coping in individuals with medical conditions. *Religions, 1*(1), 28–53.

Curlin, F. A., Chin, M. H., Sellergren, S. A., Roach, C. J., & Lantos, J. D. (2006). The association of physicians' religious characteristics with their attitudes and self-reported behaviors regarding religion and spirituality in the clinical encounter. *Med Care, 44*(5), 446–453. doi: 10.1097/01.mlr.0000207434.12450.ef

Curlin, F. A., Lantos, J. D., Roach, C. J., Sellergren, S. A., & Chin, M. H. (2005). Religious characteristics of U.S. physicians: A national survey. *J Gen Intern Med, 20*(7), 629–634. doi: 10.1111/j.1525-1497.2005.0119.x

Curlin, F. A., Nwodim, C., Vance, J. L., Chin, M. H., & Lantos, J. D. (2008). To die, to sleep: US physicians' religious and other objections to physician-assisted suicide, terminal sedation, and withdrawal of life support. *Am J Hosp Palliat Care, 25*(2), 112–120. doi: 10.1177/1049909107310141

Curlin, F. A., Sellergren, S. A., Lantos, J. D., & Chin, M. H. (2007). Physicians' observations and interpretations of the influence of religion and spirituality on health. *Arch Intern Med, 167*(7), 649–654. doi: 10.1001/archinte.167.7.649

Daaleman, T. P., & Nease Jr., D. E. (1994). Patient attitudes regarding physician inquiry into spiritual and religious issues. *J Fam Pract, 39*(6), 564–568.

Daaleman, T. P., Usher, B. M., Williams, S. W., Rawlings, J., & Hanson, L. C. (2008). An exploratory study of spiritual care at the end of life. *Ann Fam Med, 6*(5), 406–411. doi: 10.1370/afm.883

Dalby, P., Sperlinger, D. J., & Boddington, S. (2012). The lived experience of spirituality and dementia in older people living with mild to moderate dementia. *Dementia, 11*(1), 75–94.

Day, M. A., Thorn, B. E., Ward, L. C., Rubin, N., Hickman, S. D., Scogin, F., & Kilgo, G. R. (2014). Mindfulness-based cognitive therapy for the treatment of headache pain: A pilot study. *Clin J Pain, 30*(2), 152–161. doi: 10.1097/AJP.0b013e318287a1dc

Delgado-Guay, M. O., Parsons, H. A., Hui, D., De la Cruz, M. G., Thorney, S., & Bruera, E. (2013). Spirituality, religiosity, and spiritual pain among caregivers of patients with advanced cancer. *American Journal of Hospice & Palliative Medicine, 30*(5), 455–461. doi: 10.1177/1049909112458030

Dezutter, J., Luyckx, K., Schaap-Jonker, H., Bussing, A., Corveleyn, J., & Hutsebaut, D. (2010). God image and happiness in chronic pain patients: The mediating role of disease interpretation. *Pain Med, 11*(5), 765–773. doi: 10.1111/j.1526-4637.2010.00827.x

Doolittle, B. R., Windish, D. M., & Seelig, C. B. (2013). Burnout, coping, and spirituality among internal medicine resident physicians. *J Grad Med Educ, 5*(2), 257–261. doi: 10.4300/jgme-d-12-00136.1

Dowd, H., Hogan, M. J., McGuire, B. E., Davis, M. C., Sarma, K. M., Fish, R. A., & Zautra, A. J. (2015). Comparison of an Online Mindfulness-Based Cognitive Therapy Intervention With Online Pain Management Psychoeducation: A randomized controlled study. *Clin J Pain, 31*(6), 517–527. doi: 10.1097/ajp.0000000000000201

Draper, P. (2012). An integrative review of spiritual assessment: implications for nursing management. *J Nurs Manag, 20*(8), 970–980. doi: 10.1111/jonm.12005

Edmondson, D., Park, C. L., Chaudoir, S. R., & Wortmann, J. H. (2008). Death without God: Religious struggle, death concerns, and depression in the terminally ill. *Psychol Sci, 19*(8), 754–758. doi: 10.1111/j.1467-9280.2008.02152.x

Ehman, J. W., Ott, B. B., Short, T. H., Ciampa, R. C., & Hansen-Flaschen, J. (1999). Do patients want physicians to inquire about their spiritual or religious beliefs if they become gravely ill? *Archives of Internal Medicine, 159*(15), 1803–1806. doi: 10.1001/archinte.159.15.1803

Exline, J. J., Park, C. L., Smyth, J. M., & Carey, M. P. (2011). Anger toward God: Social-cognitive predictors, prevalence, and links with adjustment to bereavement and cancer. *J Pers Soc Psychol, 100*(1), 129–148. doi: 10.1037/a0021716

Farsi, Z. (2015). The meaning of disease and spiritual responses to stressors in adults with acute leukemia undergoing hematopoietic stem cell transplantation. *Journal of Nursing Research, Publish Ahead of Print*. doi: 10.1097/jnr.0000000000000088

Fenix, J. B., Cherlin, E. J., Prigerson, H. G., Johnson-Hurzeler, R., Kasl, S. V., & Bradley, E. H. (2006). Religiousness and major depression among bereaved family caregivers: A 13-month follow-up study. *J Palliat Care, 22*(4), 286–292.

Fitchett, G., Emanuel, L., Handzo, G., Boyken, L., & Wilkie, D. J. (2015). Care of the human spirit and the role of dignity therapy: A systematic review of dignity therapy research. *BMC Palliat Care, 14*, 8. doi: 10.1186/s12904-015-0007-1

Fordham, B., Griffiths, C. E., & Bundy, C. (2015). A pilot study examining mindfulness-based cognitive therapy in psoriasis. *Psychol Health Med, 20*(1), 121–127. doi: 10.1080/13548506.2014.902483

Gall, T. L. (2003). The role of religious resources for older adults coping with illness. *J Pastoral Care Counsel, 57*(2), 211–224.

Gall, T. L. (2004). Relationship with God and the quality of life of prostate cancer survivors. *Qual Life Res,* *13*(8), 1357–1368.

Gall, T. L., Charbonneau, C., & Florack, P. (2011). The relationship between religious/spiritual factors and perceived growth following a diagnosis of breast cancer. *Psychology & Health, 26*(3), 287-305. doi: 10.1080/08870440903411013

Gallison, B. S., Xu, Y., Jurgens, C. Y., & Boyle, S. M. (2013). Acute care nurses' spiritual care practices. *J Holist Nurs, 31*(2), 95–103. doi: 10.1177/0898010112464121

Girgis, A., Lambert, S., Johnson, C., Waller, A., & Currow, D. (2013). Physical, psychosocial, relationship, and economic burden of caring for people with cancer: a review. *J Oncol Pract, 9*(4), 197–202. doi: 10.1200/jop.2012.000690

Gonzalez-Garcia, M., Ferrer, M. J., Borras, X., Munoz-Moreno, J. A., Miranda, C., Puig, J., . . . Fumaz, C. R. (2013). Effectiveness of mindfulness-based cognitive therapy on the quality of life, emotional status, and CD4 cell count of patients aging with HIV infection. *AIDS Behav.* doi: 10.1007/s10461-013-0612-z

Granqvist, P., & Kirkpatrick, L. A. (2013). Religion, spirituality, and attachment. In K. I. Pargament, J. J. Exline, J. W. Jones (Eds.), *APA handbook of psychology, religion, and spirituality (Vol 1): Context, theory, and research* (pp. 139–155). Washington, DC: American Psychological Association.

Grossoehme, D. H., Ragsdale, J. R., McHenry, C. L., Thurston, C., DeWitt, T., & VandeCreek, L. (2007). Pediatrician characteristics associated with attention to spirituality and religion in clinical practice. *Pediatrics, 119*(1), e117–123. doi: 10.1542/peds.2006-0642

Haines, K. J., Denehy, L., Skinner, E. H., Warrillow, S., & Berney, S. (2015). Psychosocial outcomes in informal caregivers of the critically ill: A systematic review. *Crit Care Med, 43*(5), 1112–1120. doi: 10.1097/ccm.0000000000000865

Haley, W. E., Gitlin, L. N., Wisniewski, S. R., Mahoney, D. F., Coon, D. W., Winter, L., . . . Ory, M. (2004). Well-being, appraisal, and coping in African-American and Caucasian dementia caregivers: Findings from the REACH study. *Aging Ment Health, 8*(4), 316–329. doi: 10.1080/13607860410001728998

Harbinson, M. T., & Bell, D. (2015). How should teaching on whole person medicine, including spiritual issues, be delivered in the undergraduate medical curriculum in the United Kingdom? *BMC Med Educ, 15*(1), 96. doi: 10.1186/s12909-015-0378-2

Hebert, R. S., Dang, Q., & Schulz, R. (2007). Religious beliefs and practices are associated with better mental health in family caregivers of patients with dementia: Findings from the REACH study. *Am J Geriatr Psychiatry, 15*(4), 292–300. doi: 10.1097/01.JGP.0000247160.11769.ab

Hebert, R., Zdaniuk, B., Schulz, R., & Scheier, M. (2009). Positive and negative religious coping and well-being in women with breast cancer. *J Palliat Med, 12*(6), 537–545. doi: 10.1089/jpm.2008.0250

Heo, G. J., & Koeske, G. (2013). The role of religious coping and race in Alzheimer's disease caregiving. *Journal of Applied Gerontology, 32*(5), 582–604.

Herrera, A. P., Lee, J. W., Nanyonjo, R. D., Laufman, L. E., & Torres-Vigil, I. (2009). Religious coping and caregiver well-being in Mexican-American families. *Aging Ment Health, 13*(1), 84–91. doi: 10.1080/13607860802154507

Hodge, D. R., & Sun, F. (2012). Positive feelings of caregiving among Latino Alzheimer's family caregivers: Understanding the role of spirituality. *Aging Ment Health, 16*(6), 689–698. doi: 10.1080/13607863.2012.678481

Hoppes, S., Bryce, H., Hellman, C., & Finlay, E. (2012). The effects of brief mindfulness training on caregivers' well-being. *Activities, Adaptation & Aging, 36*(2), 147–166. doi: 10.1080/01924788.2012.673154

Institute of Medicine. (2001). *Crossing the quality chasm.* Washington, DC: National Academy Press.

Irving, J. A., Dobkin, P. L., & Park, J. (2009). Cultivating mindfulness in health care professionals: A review of empirical studies of mindfulness-based stress reduction (MBSR). *Compl Ther Clinical Practice, 15*(2), 61–66.

Johns, S. A., Brown, L. F., Beck-Coon, K., Monahan, P. O., Tong, Y., & Kroenke, K. (2015). Randomized controlled pilot study of mindfulness-based stress reduction for persistently fatigued cancer survivors. *Psycho-Oncol, 24*(8), 885–893. doi: 10.1002/pon.3648

Johnson, K. S., Elbert-Avila, K. I., & Tulsky, J. A. (2005). The influence of spiritual beliefs and practices on the treatment preferences of African Americans: A review of the literature. *J Am Geriatr Soc, 53*(4), 711–719. doi: 10.1111/j.1532-5415.2005.53224.x

Johnston Taylor, E., Highfield, M., & Amenta, M. (1994). Attitudes and beliefs regarding spiritual care. A survey of cancer nurses. *Cancer Nurs, 17*(6), 479–487.

Johnston Taylor, E., Outlaw, F. H., Bernardo, T. R., & Roy, A. (1999). Spiritual conflicts associated with praying about cancer. *Psycho-Oncology, 8*(5), 386–394.

Jones, A., Cohen, D., Johnstone, B., Yoon, D. P., Schopp, L. H., McCormack, G., & Campbell, J. (2015). Relationships between negative spiritual beliefs and health outcomes for individuals with heterogeneous medical conditions. *J Spirit Ment Health, 17*(2), 135–152. doi: 10.1080/19349637.2015.1023679

Kabat-Zinn, J. (2013). *Full catastrophe living: Using the wisdom of your body and mind to face stress, pain, and illness.* New York, NY: Bantam Books.

Kaldjian, L. C., Jekel, J. F., & Friedland, G. (1998). End-of-life decisions in HIV-positive patients: The role of spiritual beliefs. *AIDS, 12*(1), 103–107.

Kalish, N. (2012). Evidence-based spiritual care: A literature review. *Curr Opin Support Palliat Care, 6*(2), 242–246. doi: 10.1097/SPC.0b013e328353811c

Kang, J., Shin, D. W., Choi, J. E., Sanjo, M., Yoon, S. J., Kim, H. K., . . . Yoon, W. H. (2013). Factors associated with positive consequences of serving as a family caregiver for a terminal cancer patient. *Psycho-Oncol, 22*(3), 564–571.

Kapari, M., Addington-Hall, J., & Hotopf, M. (2010). Risk factors for common mental disorder in caregiving and bereavement. *J Pain Symptom Manage, 40*(6), 844–856. doi: 10.1016/j.jpainsymman.2010.03.014

Keall, R., Clayton, J. M., & Butow, P. (2014). How do Australian palliative care nurses address existential and spiritual concerns? Facilitators, barriers and strategies. *J Clin Nurs, 23*(21-22), 3197–3205.

Kelley, M. M., & Chan, K. T. (2012). Assessing the role of attachment to God, meaning, and religious coping as mediators in the grief experience. *Death Stud, 36*(3), 199–227.

Khanjari, S., Oskouie, F., & Langius-Eklöf, A. (2012). Lower sense of coherence, negative religious coping, and disease severity as indicators of a decrease in quality of life in Iranian family caregivers of relatives with breast cancer during the first 6 months after diagnosis. *Cancer Nurs, 35*(2), 148–156. doi: 10.1097/NCC.0b013e31821f1dda

Kim, S. S., Reed, P. G., Hayward, R. D., Kang, Y., & Koenig, H. G. (2011). Spirituality and psychological well-being: Testing a theory of family interdependence among family caregivers and their elders. *Res Nurs Health, 34*(2), 103–115. doi: 10.1002/nur.20425

Kim, S. Y., Kim, J. M., Kim, S. W., Kang, H. J., Shin, I. S., Shim, H. J., . . . Yoon, J. S. (2014). Determinants of a hopeful attitude among family caregivers in a palliative care setting. *Gen Hosp Psychiatry, 36*(2), 165–171. doi: 10.1016/j.genhosppsych.2013.10.020

Kim, Y., Carver, C. S., Spillers, R. L., Crammer, C., & Zhou, E. S. (2011). Individual and dyadic relations between spiritual well-being and quality of life among cancer survivors and their spousal caregivers. *Psychooncology, 20*(7), 762–770. doi: 10.1002/pon.1778

Kinney, J. M., Ishler, K. J., Pargament, K. I., & Cavanaugh, J. C. (2003). Coping with the uncontrollable: The use of general and religious coping by caregivers to spouses with dementia. *Journal of Religious Gerontology, 14*(2-3), 171–188. doi: 10.1300/J078v14n02_06

Kirkpatrick, L. A. (1992). An attachment-theory approach to the psychology of religion. *International Journal for the Psychology of Religion, 2*(1), 3–28. doi: 10.1207/s15327582ijpr0201_2

Kirkpatrick, L. A. (1999). Attachment and religious representations and behavior. In J. Cassidy & P. R. Shaver, (Eds.), *Handbook of attachment: Theory, research, and clinical applications.* (pp. 803–822). New York, NY: Guilford Press.

Koenig, H. G. (2015). Religion, spirituality, and health: A review and update. *Adv Mind Body Med, 29*(3), 19–26.

Koenig, H., King, D., & Carson, V. B. (2012). *Handbook of religion and health.* New York, NY: Oxford University Press.

Koenig, H. G., Pearce, M. J., Nelson, B., & Daher, N. (2015). Effects of religious versus standard cognitive-behavioral therapy on optimism in persons with major depression and chronic medical illness. *Depress Anxiety.* doi: 10.1002/da.22398

Koenig, H. G., Pearce, M. J., Nelson, B., Shaw, S. F., Robins, C. J., Daher, N. S., . . . King, M. B. (2015). Religious vs. conventional cognitive behavioral therapy for major depression in persons with chronic medical illness: A pilot randomized trial. *Journal of Nervous and Mental Disease, 203*(4), 243–251. doi: 10.1097/NMD.0000000000000273

Koffman, J., Morgan, M., Edmonds, P., Speck, P., & Higginson, I. J. (2008). "I know he controls cancer": The meanings of religion among Black Caribbean and White British patients with advanced cancer. *Soc Sci Med, 67*(5), 780–789. doi: 10.1016/j.socscimed.2008.05.004

Kristeller, J. L., Rhodes, M., Cripe, L. D., & Sheets, V. (2005). Oncologist assisted spiritual intervention study (OASIS): Patient acceptability and initial evidence of effects. *Int J Psychiatry Med, 35*(4), 329–347.

Kruizinga, R., Hartog, I. D., Jacobs, M., Daams, J. G., Scherer-Rath, M., Schilderman, J. B. A. M., . . . Van Laarhoven, H. W. M. (2015). The effect of spiritual interventions addressing existential themes using a narrative approach on quality of life of cancer patients: A systematic review and meta-analysis. *Psycho-Oncol.* doi: 10.1002/pon.3910

Lauche, R., Cramer, H., Dobos, G., Langhorst, J., & Schmidt, S. (2013). A systematic review and meta-analysis of mindfulness-based stress reduction for the fibromyalgia syndrome. *J Psychosom Res, 75*(6), 500–510. doi: 10.1016/j.jpsychores.2013.10.010

Leblanc, A. J., Driscoll, A. K., & Pearlin, L. I. (2004). Religiosity and the expansion of caregiver stress. *Aging Ment Health, 8*(5), 410–421. doi: 10.1080/13607860410001724992

Leonardi, M., Giovannetti, A. M., Pagani, M., Raggi, A., & Sattin, D. (2012). Burden and needs of 487 caregivers of patients in vegetative state and in minimally conscious state: Results from a national study. *Brain Inj, 26*(10), 1201–1210. doi: 10.3109/02699052.2012.667589

Leow, M. Q. H., Chan, M.-F., & Chan, S. W. C. (2014). Predictors of change in quality of life of family caregivers of patients near the end of life with advanced cancer. *Cancer Nurs, 37*(5), 391–400.

Lewinson, L. P., McSherry, W., & Kevern, P. (2015). Spirituality in pre-registration nurse education and practice: A review of the literature. *Nurse Educ Today, 35*(6), 806–814. doi: 10.1016/j.nedt.2015.01.011

Lewis, L. M. (2008). Spiritual assessment in African-Americans: A review of measures of spirituality used in health research. *J Relig Health, 47*(4), 458–475.

Li, Q., & Loke, A. Y. (2013). A literature review on the mutual impact of the spousal caregiver-cancer patients dyads: 'Communication', 'reciprocal influence', and 'caregiver-patient congruence'. *Eur J Oncol Nurs.* doi: 10.1016/j.ejon.2013.09.003

Lo Coco, G., Lo Coco, D., Cicero, V., Oliveri, A., Lo Verso, G., Piccoli, F., & La Bella, V. (2005). Individual and health-related quality of life assessment in amyotrophic lateral sclerosis patients and their caregivers. *J Neurol Sci, 238*(1-2), 11–17. doi: 10.1016/j.jns.2005.05.018

Lopez, J., Romero-Moreno, R., Marquez-González, M., & Losada, A. (2012). Spirituality and self-efficacy in dementia family caregiving: Trust in God and yourself. *International Psychogeriatrics, 24*(12), 1943–1952. doi: 10.1017/S1041610212001287

Lovanio, K., & Wallace, M. (2007). Promoting spiritual knowledge and attitudes: A student nurse education project. *Holist Nurs Pract, 21*(1), 42–47.

Lucchetti, G., Bassi, R. M., & Lucchetti, A. L. (2013). Taking spiritual history in clinical practice: A systematic review of instruments. *Explore (NY)*, 9(3), 159–170. doi: 10.1016/j.explore.2013.02.004

Lucchetti, G., Lucchetti, A. L., & Puchalski, C. M. (2012). Spirituality in medical education: Global reality? *J Relig Health*, 51(1), 3–19. doi: 10.1007/s10943-011-9557-6

Luckhaupt, S. E., Yi, M. S., Mueller, C. V., Mrus, J. M., Peterman, A. H., Puchalski, C. M., & Tsevat, J. (2005). Beliefs of primary care residents regarding spirituality and religion in clinical encounters with patients: A study at a midwestern U.S. teaching institution. *Acad Med*, 80(6), 560–570.

Lunder, U., Furlan, M., & Simonic, A. (2011). Spiritual needs assessments and measurements. *Curr Opin Support Palliat Care*, 5(3), 273–278. doi: 10.1097/SPC.0b013e3283499b20

MacKinlay, E., & Trevitt, C. (2012). *Finding meaning in the experience of dementia. The place of spiritual reminiscence work.* London: Jessica Kingsley.

MacLean, C. D., Susi, B., Phifer, N., Schultz, L., Bynum, D., Franco, M., . . . Cykert, S. (2003). Patient preference for physician discussion and practice of spirituality. *J Gen Intern Med*, 18(1), 38–43.

Magyar-Russell, G., Pargament, K.I., Trevino, K.M., Sherman, J.E. (2013). Religious and spiritual appraisals and coping strategies among patients in medical rehabilitation. *Research in the Social Scientific Study of Religion*, 24, 93–131.

Manning-Walsh, J. (2005). Spiritual struggle: effect on quality of life and life satisfaction in women with breast cancer. *J Holist Nurs*, 23(2), 120–140. doi: 10.1177/0898010104272019

Mansfield, C. J., Mitchell, J., & King, D. E. (2002). The doctor as God's mechanic? Beliefs in the Southeastern United States. *Social Science & Medicine*, 54(3), 399–409. doi: http://dx.doi.org/10.1016/S0277-9536(01)00038-7

Mao, J. J., Farrar, J. T., Xie, S. X., Bowman, M. A., & Armstrong, K. (2007). Use of complementary and alternative medicine and prayer among a national sample of cancer survivors compared to other populations without cancer. *Complement Ther Med*, 15(1), 21–29. doi: 10.1016/j.ctim.2006.07.006

Marchand, W. R. (2012). Mindfulness-based stress reduction, mindfulness-based cognitive therapy, and Zen mediation for depression, anxiety, pain, and psychological distress. *Journal of Psychiatric Practice*, 18(4), 233–252. doi: 10.1097/01.pra.0000416014.53215.86

Martín-Asuero, A., & García-Banda, G. (2010). The mindfulness-based stress reduction program (MBSR) reduces stress-related psychological distress in healthcare professionals. *The Spanish journal of psychology*, 13(02), 897–905.

Mausbach, B. T., Coon, D. W., Cardenas, V., & Thompson, L. W. (2003). Religious coping among Caucasian and Latina dementia caregivers. *Journal of Mental Health and Aging*, 9(2), 97–110.

McCauley, J., Jenckes, M. W., Tarpley, M. J., Koenig, H. G., Yanek, L. R., & Becker, D. M. (2005). Spiritual beliefs and barriers among managed care practitioners. *J Relig Health*, 44(2), 137–146.

McConnell, K. M., Pargament, K. I., Ellison, C. G., & Flannelly, K. J. (2006). Examining the links between spiritual struggles and symptoms of psychopathology in a national sample. *Journal of Clinical Psychology*, 62(12), 1469–1484. doi: 10.1002/jclp.20325

McDonald, P. E., Fink, S. V., & Wykle, M. L. (1999). Self-reported health-promoting behaviors of black and white caregivers. *West J Nurs Res*, 21(4), 538–548.

McGee, J. S., Myers, D. R., Carlson, H., Funai, A. P., & Barclay, P. A. (2013). Spirituality, faith, and mild Alzheimer's Disease. *Research in the Social Scientific Study of Religion*, 24, 221–257.

Mehrotra, S., & Sukumar, P. (2007). Sources of strength perceived by females caring for relatives diagnosed with cancer: An exploratory study from India. *Support Care Cancer*, 15(12), 1357–1366. doi: 10.1007/s00520-007-0256-5

Meller, S. (2001). A comparison of the well-being of family caregivers of elderly patients hospitalized with physical impairments versus the caregivers of patients hospitalized with dementia. *J Am Med Dir Assoc*, 2(2), 60–65.

Merritt, M. M., & McCallum, T. (2013). Too much of a good thing?: Positive religious coping predicts worse diurnal salivary cortisol patterns for overwhelmed African American female dementia family caregivers. *The American Journal of Geriatric Psychiatry, 21*(1), 46–56.

Mitchell, D. L., Bennett, M. J., & Manfrin-Ledet, L. (2006). Spiritual development of nursing students: Developing competence to provide spiritual care to patients at the end of life. *J Nurs Educ, 45*(9), 365–370.

Murphy, J. S., Nalbone, D. P., Wetchler, J. L., & Edwards, A. B. (2015). Caring for aging parents: The influence of family coping, spirituality/religiosity, and hope on the marital satisfaction of family caregivers. *Am J Family Ther, 43*(3), 238–250. doi: 10.1080/01926187.2015.1034636

Murray, S. A., Kendall, M., Boyd, K., Grant, L., Highet, G., & Sheikh, A. (2010). Archetypal trajectories of social, psychological, and spiritual wellbeing and distress in family care givers of patients with lung cancer: Secondary analysis of serial qualitative interviews. *BMJ, 340*, c2581. doi: 10.1136/bmj.c2581

Musgrave, C. F., & McFarlane, E. A. (2004). Israeli oncology nurses' religiosity, spiritual well-being, and attitudes toward spiritual care: A path analysis. *Oncol Nurs Forum, 31*(2), 321–327. doi: 10.1188/04.onf.321-327

National Alliance in Caregiving. (2009). Caregiving in the U.S.: Executive summary. Retreived from http://www.caregiving.org/pdf/research/CaregivingUSAllAgesExecSum.pdf

Neeleman, J., & King, M. B. (1993). Psychiatrists' religious attitudes in relation to their clinical practice: A survey of 231 psychiatrists. *Acta Psychiatr Scand, 88*(6), 420–424.

Newberry, A. G., Choi, C. W., Donovan, H. S., Schulz, R., Bender, C., Given, B., & Sherwood, P. (2013). Exploring spirituality in family caregivers of patients with primary malignant brain tumors across the disease trajectory. *Oncol Nurs Forum, 40*(3), E119–125. doi: 10.1188/13.onf.e119-e125

Northouse, L. L., Katapodi, M. C., Schafenacker, A. M., & Weiss, D. (2012). The impact of caregiving on the psychological well-being of family caregivers and cancer patients. *Semin Oncol Nurs, 28*(4), 236–245. doi: 10.1016/j.soncn.2012.09.006

Olson, K. L., & Emery, C. F. (2015). Mindfulness and weight loss: A systematic review. *Psychosomatic Med, 77*(1), 59–67. doi: 10.1097/PSY.0000000000000127

Pargament, K. I. (2001). *The psychology of religion and coping: Theory, research, practice.* New York, NY: Guilford Press.

Pargament, K. I. (2007). *Spiritually integrated psychotherapy: Understand and addressing the sacred.* New York, NY: Guilford Press.

Pargament, K. I., Desai, K. M., McConnell, K. M. (2006). Spirituality: A pathway to posttraumatic growth or decline. In L. Calhoun & R. Tedeschi (Eds.), *Handbook of posttraumatic growth: Research and practice* (121–137). New York, NY: Lawrence Erlbaum Associates, Inc.

Pargament, K. I., Koenig, H. G., & Perez, L. M. (2000). The many methods of religious coping: Development and initial validation of the RCOPE. *J Clin Psychol, 56*(4), 519–543.

Pargament, K. I., Koenig, H. G., Tarakeshwar, N., & Hahn, J. (2001). Religious struggle as a predictor of mortality among medically ill elderly patients: A 2-year longitudinal study. *Arch Int Med, 161*(15), 1881–1885.

Pargament, K. I., Koenig, H. G., Tarakeshwar, N., & Hahn, J. (2004). Religious coping methods as predictors of psychological, physical and spiritual outcomes among medically ill elderly patients: A two-year longitudinal study. *J Health Psychol, 9*(6), 713–730.

Pargament, K. I., Lomax, J. W., McGee, J. S., & Fang, Q. (2014). Sacred moments in psychotherapy from the perspectives of mental health providers and clients: Prevalence, predictors, and consequences. *Spirit Clin Pract, 1*(4), 248–262.

Pargament, K. I., Magyar, G. M., Benore, E., & Mahoney, A. (2005). Sacrilege: A study of sacred loss and desecration and their implications for health and well-being in a community sample. *J Sci Study Religion, 44*(1), 59–78.

Pargament, K. I., & Mahoney, A. (2005). Sacred matters: Sanctification as a vital topic for the psychology of religion. *Int J Psychol Religion*, 15(3), 179–198.

Pargament, K. I., Murray-Swank, N. A., Magyar, G. M., & Ano, G. G. (2005). Spiritual struggle: A phenomenon of interest to psychology and religion. In W. R. Miller & H. D. Delaney (Eds.), *Judeo-Christian perspectives on psychology: Human nature, motivation, and change* (pp. 245–268). Washington, DC: American Psychological Association.

Pargament, K. I., Smith, B. W., Koenig, H. G., & Perez, L. (1998). Patterns of positive and negative religious coping with major life stressors. *J Sci Study Religion*, 37(4), 710–724.

Park, C. L. (2013a). Positive psychology perspectives across the cancer continuum: Meaning, spirituality, and growth. In B. I Carr and J. Steel (Eds.), *Psychological aspects of cancer* (pp. 101–117). New York, NY: Springer.

Park, C. L. (2013b). Religion and meaning. In R. F. Paloutzian & C. L. Park (Eds.), *Handbook of the psychology of religion and spirituality* (pp. 357–379), New York, NY: Guilford Press.

Park, C. L., Wortmann, J. H., & Edmondson, D. (2011). Religious struggle as a predictor of subsequent mental and physical well-being in advanced heart failure patients. *J Behav Med*, 34(6), 426–436. doi: 10.1007/s10865-011-9315-y

Pasacreta, J. V., & McCorkle, R. (2000). Cancer care: Impact of interventions on caregiver outcomes. *Annu Rev Nurs Res*, 18, 127–148.

Pawlikowski, J., Sak, J. J., & Marczewski, K. (2012). Physicians' religiosity and attitudes towards patients. *Ann Agric Environ Med*, 19(3), 503–507.

Pearce, M. J., Koenig, H. G., Robins, C. J., Daher, N., Shaw, S. F., Nelson, B., . . . King, M. B. (2015). Effects of religious versus conventional cognitive-behavioral therapy on generosity in major depression and chronic medical illness: A randomized clinical trial. *Spirit Clin Pract*, 2(3), 202–215. doi: 10.1037/scp0000076

Pearce, M. J., Koenig, H. G., Robins, C. J., Nelson, B., Shaw, S. F., Cohen, H. J., & King, M. B. (2015). Religiously integrated cognitive behavioral therapy: A new method of treatment for major depression in patients with chronic medical illness. *Psychotherapy*, 52(1), 56–66. doi: 10.1037/a0036448

Pearce, M. J., Singer, J. L., & Prigerson, H. G. (2006). Religious coping among caregivers of terminally ill cancer patients: main effects and psychosocial mediators. *J Health Psychol*, 11(5), 743–759. doi: 10.1177/1359105306066629

Peckham, C. (2015). Medscape physician lifestyle report 2015. Retrieved from http://www.medscape.com/features/slideshow/lifestyle/2015/public/overview#20

Pedersen, H. F., Pedersen, C. G., Pargament, K. I., & Zachariae, R. (2013). Coping without religion? Religious coping, quality of life, and existential well-being among lung disease patients and matched Controls in a secular society. *Res Soc Sci Study Religion*, 24, 163–192.

Peilot, B., Andrell, P., Samuelsson, A., Mannheimer, C., Frodi, A., & Sundler, A. J. (2014). Time to gain trust and change—experiences of attachment and mindfulness-based cognitive therapy among patients with chronic pain and psychiatric co-morbidity. *Int J Qual Stud Health Well-being*, 9, 24420. doi: 10.3402/qhw.v9.24420

Penderell, A., & Brazil, K. (2010). The spirit of palliative practice: A qualitative inquiry into the spiritual journey of palliative care physicians. *Palliat Support Care*, 8(4), 415–420. doi: 10.4300/jgme-d-12-00136.110.1017/s1478951510000271

Pérez, J. E., & Smith, A. R. (2015). Intrinsic religiousness and well-being among cancer patients: The mediating role of control-related religious coping and self-efficacy for coping with cancer. *J Behav Med*, 38(2), 183–193. doi: 10.1007/s10865-014-9593-2

Peteet, J. R., & Balboni, M. J. (2013). Spirituality and religion in oncology. *CA Cancer J Clin*, 63(4), 280–289. doi: 10.3322/caac.21187

Phelps, A. C., Lauderdale, K. E., Alcorn, S., Dillinger, J., Balboni, M. T., Van Wert, M., . . . Balboni, T. A. (2012). Addressing spirituality within the care of patients at the end of life: Perspectives of patients with advanced cancer, oncologists, and oncology nurses. *J Clin Oncol*, 30(20), 2538–2544. doi: 10.1200/jco.2011.40.3766

Philippot, P., Nef, F., Clauw, L., de Romree, M., & Segal, Z. (2012). A randomized controlled trial of mindfulness-based cognitive therapy for treating tinnitus. *Clin Psychol Psychother, 19*(5), 411–419. doi: 10.1002/cpp.756

Piet, J., Wurtzen, H., & Zachariae, R. (2012). The effect of mindfulness-based therapy on symptoms of anxiety and depression in adult cancer patients and survivors: A systematic review and meta-analysis. *J Consult Clin Psychol, 80*(6), 1007–1020. doi: 10.1037/a0028329

Puchalski, C. M. (2006). Spirituality and medicine: Curricula in medical education. *J Cancer Educ, 21*(1), 14–18. doi: 10.1207/s15430154jce2101_6

Puchalski, C., & Romer, A. L. (2000). Taking a spiritual history allows clinicians to understand patients more fully. *J Palliat Med, 3*(1), 129–137. doi: 10.1089/jpm.2000.3.129

Quinn, C., Clare, L., & Woods, R. T. (2012). What predicts whether caregivers of people with dementia find meaning in their role? *Int J Geriatr Psychiatry, 27*(11), 1195–1202.

Rabinowitz, Y. G., Hartlaub, M. G., Saenz, E. C., Thompson, L. W., & Gallagher-Thompson, D. (2010). Is religious coping associated with cumulative health risk? An examination of religious coping styles and health behavior patterns in Alzheimer's dementia caregivers. *J Religion Health, 49*(4), 498–512.

Ramondetta, L., Brown, A., Richardson, G., Urbauer, D., Thaker, P. H., Koenig, H. G., . . . Sun, C. (2011). Religious and spiritual beliefs of gynecologic oncologists may influence medical decision making. *Int J Gynecol Cancer, 21*(3), 573–581. doi: 10.1097/IGC.0b013e31820ba507

Rasinski, K. A., Kalad, Y. G., Yoon, J. D., & Curlin, F. A. (2011). An assessment of US physicians' training in religion, spirituality, and medicine. *Med Teach, 33*(11), 944–945. doi: 10.3109/0142159x.2011.588976

Rassouli, M., Zamanzadeh, V., Ghahramanian, A., Abbaszadeh, A., Alavi-Majd, H., & Nikanfar, A. (2015). Experiences of patients with cancer and their nurses on the conditions of spiritual care and spiritual interventions in oncology units. *Iran J Nurs Midwifery Res, 20*(1), 25–33.

Reiner, K., Tibi, L., & Lipsitz, J. D. (2013). Do mindfulness-based interventions reduce pain intensity? A critical review of the literature. *Pain Medicine, 14*(2), 230–242. doi: 10.1111/pme.12006

Rimes, K. A., & Wingrove, J. (2013). Mindfulness-based cognitive therapy for people with chronic fatigue syndrome still experiencing excessive fatigue after cognitive behaviour therapy: A pilot randomized study. *Clin Psychol Psychother, 20*(2), 107–117. doi: 10.1002/cpp.793

Rippentrop, E. A., Altmaier, E. M., Chen, J. J., Found, E. M., & Keffala, V. J. (2005). The relationship between religion/spirituality and physical health, mental health, and pain in a chronic pain population. *Pain, 116*(3), 311–321. doi: http://dx.doi.org/10.1016/j.pain.2005.05.008

Rodin, D., Balboni, M., Mitchell, C., Smith, P. T., VanderWeele, T. J., & Balboni, T. A. (2015). Whose role? Oncology practitioners' perceptions of their role in providing spiritual care to advanced cancer patients. *Support Care Cancer, 23*(9), 2543–2550. doi: 10.1007/s00520-015-2611-2

Rofail, D., Maguire, L., Kissner, M., Colligs, A., & Abetz-Webb, L. (2013). A review of the social, psychological, and economic burdens experienced by people with spina bifida and their caregivers. *Neurol Ther, 2*(1-2), 1–12. doi: 10.1007/s40120-013-0007-0

Roscoe, L. A., Corsentino, E., Watkins, S., McCall, M., & Sanchez-Ramos, J. (2009). Well-being of family caregivers of persons with late-stage Huntington's disease: Lessons in stress and coping. *Health Communication, 24*(3), 239–248. doi: 10.1080/10410230902804133

Schonfeld, T. L., Schmid, K. K., & Boucher-Payne, D. (2014). Incorporating spirituality into health sciences education. *J Relig Health*. doi: 10.1007/s10943-014-9972-6

Schreiber, J. A. (2011). Image of God: Effect on coping and psychospiritual outcomes in early breast cancer survivors. *Oncol Nurs Forum, 38*(3), 293–301. doi: 10.1188/11.onf.293-301

Seeher, K., Low, L. F., Reppermund, S., & Brodaty, H. (2013). Predictors and outcomes for caregivers of people with mild cognitive impairment: A systematic literature review. *Alzheimers Dement, 9*(3), 346–355. doi: 10.1016/j.jalz.2012.01.012

Segal, Z.V., Williams, J.M.G., & Teasdale, J.D. (2002). *Mindfulness-based cognitive therapy for depression: A new approach to preventing relapse.* New York, NY: Guilford Press.

Seligman, M. E. (2012). *Flourish: A visionary new understanding of happiness and well-being*: New York, NY: Simon and Schuster.

Seligman, M. E., & Csikszentmihalyi, M. (2000). Positive psychology. An introduction. *Am Psychol, 55*(1), 5–14.

Sessanna, L., Finnell, D. S., Underhill, M., Chang, Y. P., & Peng, H. L. (2011). Measures assessing spirituality as more than religiosity: A methodological review of nursing and health-related literature. *J Adv Nurs, 67*(8), 1677–1694. doi: 10.1111/j.1365-2648.2010.05596.x

Shah, A. A., Snow, A. L., & Kunik, M. E. (2001). Spiritual and religious coping in caregivers of patients with Alzheimer's disease. *Clin Gerontol: J Aging Mental Health, 24*(3-4), 127–136. doi: 10.1300/J018v24n03_11

Sheppe, A. H., Nicholson, R. F., 3rd, Rasinski, K. A., Yoon, J. D., & Curlin, F. A. (2013). Providing guidance to patients: Physicians' views about the relative responsibilities of doctors and religious communities. *South Med J, 106*(7), 399–406. doi: 10.1097/SMJ.0b013e31829ba64f

Sheridan, M. J., Burley, J., Hendricks, D. E., & Rose, T. (2014). 'Caring for one's own': Variation in the lived experience of African-American caregivers of elders. *J Ethnic CultDiversity Soc Work: Innov Theory Res Pract, 23*(1), 1–19. doi: 10.1080/15313204.2013.849642

Sherman, A. C., Plante, T. G., Simonton, S., Latif, U., & Anaissie, E. J. (2009). Prospective study of religious coping among patients undergoing autologous stem cell transplantation. *J Behav Med, 32*(1), 118–128. doi: 10.1007/s10865-008-9179-y

Sherman, A. C., Simonton, S., Latif, U., Spohn, R., & Tricot, G. (2005). Religious struggle and religious comfort in response to illness: Health outcomes among stem cell transplant patients. *J Behav Med, 28*(4), 359–367. doi: 10.1007/s10865-005-9006-7

Sherratt, K. A., & Lunn, S. (2013). Evaluation of a group programme of mindfulness-based cognitive therapy for women with fertility problems. *J Obstet Gynaecol, 33*(5), 499–501. doi: 10.3109/01443615.2013.786031

Shin, J. H., Yoon, J. D., Rasinski, K. A., Koenig, H. G., Meador, K. G., & Curlin, F. A. (2013). A spiritual problem? Primary care physicians' and psychiatrists' interpretations of medically unexplained symptoms. *J Gen Intern Med, 28*(3), 392–398. doi: 10.1007/s11606-012-2224-0

Siegel, B., Tenenbaum, A. J., Jamanka, A., Barnes, L., Hubbard, C., & Zuckerman, B. (2002). Faculty and resident attitudes about spirituality and religion in the provision of pediatric health care. *Ambul Pediatr, 2*(1), 5–10.

Silvestri, G. A., Knittig, S., Zoller, J. S., & Nietert, P. J. (2003). Importance of faith on medical decisions regarding cancer care. *J Clin Oncol, 21*(7), 1379–1382.

Simpson, R., Booth, J., Lawrence, M., Byrne, S., Mair, F., & Mercer, S. (2014). Mindfulness based interventions in multiple sclerosis—A systematic review. *BMC Neurol, 14*. doi: 10.1186/1471-2377-14-15

Skaggs, B. G., & Barron, C. R. (2006). Searching for meaning in negative events: Concept analysis. *J Adv Nurs, 53*(5), 559–570. doi: 10.1111/j.1365-2648.2006.03761.x

Stafford, L., Foley, E., Judd, F., Gibson, P., Kiropoulos, L., & Couper, J. (2013). Mindfulness-based cognitive group therapy for women with breast and gynecologic cancer: A pilot study to determine effectiveness and feasibility. *Support Care Cancer, 21*(11), 3009–3019. doi: 10.1007/s00520-013-1880-x

Sun, F., & Hodge, D. R. (2014). Latino Alzheimer's disease caregivers and depression: Using the stress coping model to examine the effects of spirituality and religion. *Journal of Applied Gerontology, 33*(3), 291–315. doi: 10.1177/0733464812444462

Sun, F., Kosberg, J. I., Leeper, J., Kaufman, A. V., & Burgio, L. (2010). Racial differences in perceived burden of rural dementia caregivers: The mediating effect of religiosity. *J Appl Gerontol, 29*(3), 290–307. doi: 10.1177/0733464809343205

Talley, J. A., & Magie, R. (2014). The integration of the "spirituality in medicine" curriculum into the osteopathic communication curriculum at Kansas City University of Medicine and Biosciences. *Acad Med, 89*(1), 43–47. doi: 10.1097/acm.0000000000000078

Tang, W. R. (2009). Hospice family caregivers' quality of life. *J Clin Nurs, 18*(18), 2563–2572. doi: 10.1111/j.1365-2702.2008.02753.x

Tarakeshwar, N., Pearce, M. J., & Sikkema, K. J. (2005). Development and implementation of a spiritual coping group intervention for adults living with HIV/AIDS: A pilot study. *Ment Health, Religion Culture, 8*(3), 179–190. doi: 10.1080/13694670500138908

Tarakeshwar, N., Vanderwerker, L. C., Paulk, E., Pearce, M. J., Kasl, S. V., & Prigerson, H. G. (2006). Religious coping is associated with the quality of life of patients with advanced cancer. *J Palliat Med, 9*(3), 646–657. doi: 10.1089/jpm.2006.9.646

Thombre, A., Sherman, A. C., & Simonton, S. (2010). Religious coping and posttraumatic growth among family caregivers of cancer patients in India. *J Psychosoc Oncol, 28*(2), 173–188. doi: 10.1080/07347330903570537

Thornton, N., & Hopp, F. P. (2011). 'So I just took over': African American daughters' caregiving for parents with heart failure. *Families Soc, 92*(2), 211–217.

Timmins, F., & Kelly, J. (2008). Spiritual assessment in intensive and cardiac care nursing. *Nurs Crit Care, 13*(3), 124–131. doi: 10.1111/j.1478-5153.2008.00276.x

Timmins, F., Neill, F., Murphy, M., Begley, T., & Sheaf, G. (2015). Spiritual care competence for contemporary nursing practice: A quantitative exploration of the guidance provided by fundamental nursing textbooks. *Nurse Educ Pract.* doi: 10.1016/j.nepr.2015.02.007

Todres, I. D., Catlin, E. A., & Thiel, M. M. (2005). The intensivist in a spiritual care training program adapted for clinicians. *Crit Care Med, 33*(12), 2733–2736.

Tovote, K. A., Fleer, J., Snippe, E., Peeters, A. C., Emmelkamp, P. M., Sanderman, R., . . . Schroevers, M. J. (2014). Individual mindfulness-based cognitive therapy and cognitive behavior therapy for treating depressive symptoms in patients with diabetes: Results of a randomized controlled trial. *Diabetes Care, 37*(9), 2427–2434. doi: 10.2337/dc13-2918

Tovote, K. A., Schroevers, M. J., Snippe, E., Sanderman, R., Links, T. P., Emmelkamp, P. M., & Fleer, J. (2015). Long-term effects of individual mindfulness-based cognitive therapy and cognitive behavior therapy for depressive symptoms in patients with diabetes: A randomized trial. *Psychother Psychosom, 84*(3), 186–187. doi: 10.1159/000375453

Trevino, K. M., Pargament, K. I., Cotton, S., Leonard, A. C., Hahn, J., Caprini-Faigin, C. A., & Tsevat, J. (2010). Religious coping and physiological, psychological, social, and spiritual outcomes in patients with HIV/AIDS: Cross-sectional and longitudinal findings. *AIDS and Behavior, 14*(2), 379–389. doi: 10.1007/s10461-007-9332-6

Urcuyo, K. R., Boyers, A. E., Carver, C. S., & Antoni, M. H. (2005). Finding benefit in breast cancer: Relations with personality, coping, and concurrent well-being. *Psychol Health, 20*(2), 175–192. doi: 10.1080/08870440512331317634

van der Lee, M. L., & Garssen, B. (2012). Mindfulness-based cognitive therapy reduces chronic cancer-related fatigue: A treatment study. *Psychooncology, 21*(3), 264–272. doi: 10.1002/pon.1890

van der Spek, N., van Uden-Kraan, C. F., Vos, J., Breitbart, W., Tollenaar, R. A. E. M., van Asperen, C. J., . . . Verdonck-de Leeuw, I. M. (2014). Meaning-centered group psychotherapy in cancer survivors: A feasibility study. *Psycho-Oncology, 23*(7), 827–831. doi: 10.1002/pon.3497

van Son, J., Nyklicek, I., Pop, V. J., Blonk, M. C., Erdtsieck, R. J., & Pouwer, F. (2014). Mindfulness-based cognitive therapy for people with diabetes and emotional problems: Long-term follow-up findings from the DiaMind randomized controlled trial. *J Psychosom Res, 77*(1), 81–84. doi: 10.1016/j.jpsychores.2014.03.013

Vermandere, M., Choi, Y. N., De Brabandere, H., Decouttere, R., De Meyere, E., Gheysens, E., . . . Aertgeerts, B. (2012). GPs' views concerning spirituality and the use of the FICA tool in palliative care in Flanders: A qualitative study. *Br J Gen Pract, 62*(603), e718–725. doi: 10.3399/bjgp12X656865

Voltmer, E., Bussing, A., Koenig, H. G., & Al Zaben, F. (2014). Religiosity/spirituality of German doctors in private practice and likelihood of addressing R/S issues with patients. *J Relig Health, 53*(6), 1741–1752. doi: 10.1007/s10943-013-9776-0

Wachholtz, A., & Sambamoorthi, U. (2011). National trends in prayer use as a coping mechanism for health concerns: Changes from 2002 to 2007. *Psychol Religion Spiritual, 3*(2), 67–77. doi: 10.1037/a0021598

Wakefield, B. J., Hayes, J., Boren, S. A., Pak, Y., & Davis, J. W. (2012). Strain and satisfaction in caregivers of veterans with chronic illness. *Res Nurs Health*, 35(1), 55–69.

Wallston, K., Malcarne, V., Flores, L., Hansdottir, I., Smith, C., Stein, M., . . . Clements, P. (1999). Does God determine your health? The God Locus of Health control scale. *Cogne Ther Res*, 23(2), 131–142. doi: 10.1023/A:1018723010685

Walton, J. (1999). Spirituality of patients recovering from an acute myocardial infarction: A grounded theory study. *J Holist Nurs*, 17(1), 34–53.

Wasner, M., Longaker, C., Fegg, M. J., & Borasio, G. D. (2005). Effects of spiritual care training for palliative care professionals. *Palliat Med*, 19(2), 99–104.

Wenger, N. S., & Carmel, S. (2004). Physicians' religiosity and end-of-life care attitudes and behaviors. *Mt Sinai J Med*, 71(5), 335–343.

Whittingham, K., Barnes, S., & Gardiner, C. (2013). Tools to measure quality of life and carer burden in informal carers of heart failure patients: A narrative review. *Palliat Med*, 27(7), 596–607. doi: 10.1177/0269216313477179

Williams, A. L., Dixon, J., Feinn, R., & McCorkle, R. (2015). Cancer family caregiver depression: Are religion-related variables important? *Psycho-Oncol*, 24(7):825–831. doi: 10.1002/pon.3647.

Winkelman, W. D., Lauderdale, K., Balboni, M. J., Phelps, A. C., Peteet, J. R., Block, S. D., . . . Balboni, T. A. (2011). The relationship of spiritual concerns to the quality of life of advanced cancer patients: preliminary findings. *J Palliat Med*, 14(9), 1022–1028. doi: 10.1089/jpm.2010.0536

Winter, L., Moriarty, H. J., Atte, F., & Gitlin, L. N. (2015). Depressed affect and dimensions of religiosity in family caregivers of individuals with dementia. *J Relig Health*, 54(4), 1490–1502. doi: 10.1007/s10943-015-0033-6

Wu, L. F., & Koo, M. (2015). Randomized controlled trial of a six-week spiritual reminiscence intervention on hope, life satisfaction, and spiritual well-being in elderly with mild and moderate dementia. *Int J Geriatr Psychiatry*. doi: 10.1002/gps.4300

Yang, Y., Liu, Y.-H., Zhang, H.-F., & Liu, J.Y. (2015). Effectiveness of mindfulness-based stress reduction and mindfulness-based cognitive therapies on people living with HIV: A systematic review and meta-analysis. *Int J Nurs Sci*. doi: http://dx.doi.org/10.1016/j.ijnss.2015.07.003

Yeh, P. M., & Bull, M. (2009). Influences of spiritual well-being and coping on mental health of family caregivers for elders. *Res Gerontol Nurs*, 2(3), 173–181. doi: 10.3928/19404921-20090421-08

Zainal, N. Z., Booth, S., & Huppert, F. A. (2013). The efficacy of mindfulness-based stress reduction on mental health of breast cancer patients: A meta-analysis. *Psycho-Oncol*, 22(7), 1457–1465. doi: 10.1002/pon.3171

Zollfrank, A. A., Trevino, K. M., Cadge, W., Balboni, M. J., Thiel, M. M., Fitchett, G., . . . Balboni, T. A. (2015). Teaching health care providers to provide spiritual care: A pilot study. *J Palliat Med*, 18(5), 408–414. doi: 10.1089/jpm.2014.0306

Zunzunegui, M. V., Beland, F., Llacer, A., & Keller, I. (1999). Family, religion, and depressive symptoms in caregivers of disabled elderly. *J Epidemiol Commun Health*, 53(6), 364–369.

Zwingmann, C., Wirtz, M., Muller, C., Korber, J., & Murken, S. (2006). Positive and negative religious coping in German breast cancer patients. *J Behav Med*, 29(6), 533–547. doi: 10.1007/s10865-006-9074-3

CHAPTER 16

SPIRITUALITY, RESISTANCE, AND MODERN MEDICINE: A SOCIOLOGICAL PERSPECTIVE

Jonathan B. Imber

Social science has not been an especially enthusiastic partner with the profession of medicine. Nineteenth-century reports of a nascent social-scientific (understood today as social-epidemiological and preventative) perspective described the emerging tensions between the observations and treatments of disease at the clinical level and at the broader societal level (i.e., public health). Competing observations would lead twentieth-century social scientists, economists in particular, to hold the medical profession culpable for what George Bernard Shaw famously concluded was a conspiracy against the laity. This characterization has endured until very recently and was also advanced in specific ways by several generations of sociologists. The latest controversies about "evidence-based" medicine, personalized medicine, and precision medicine are further illustrations of the abiding tensions concerning physician judgment, scientific knowledge, and patient trust.

This chapter offers an account of the enduring nature of these tensions between patient-centered and social, now global, analyses that at different times have reflected the principal interests of sociologists in medicine and the health care professions. System-wide critiques made by sociologists have generally received the greatest public attention, for example, in the Pulitzer Prize winning work of Paul Starr, *The Social Transformation of American Medicine*, first published in 1982. Around the same time, patient-focused accounts of physician-patient interactions led, in particular, by feminist sociologists offered new ways to account for problems of communication in the medical encounter (West, 1984; Fisher, 1986; Ong et al., 1995). The system-wide critiques have increased over the decades, and the systemic reform of health care has become among the most politically controversial subjects in American life. But these debates conceal more than they reveal about transformations in the ways that the clinical encounter has been scrutinized and challenged by a focus on how patients experience illness and how doctors and nurses recognize their responsibilities toward culturally and religiously diverse populations. Even as major social forces - economic, political, and scientific - have engulfed the clinical encounter, the sociological response in its various perspectives has provided a kind of spiritual resistance to the widespread pessimism about the nature and future of that encounter.

SOCIOLOGICAL ACCOUNTS OF THE MEDICAL SYSTEM

It is worth recalling that sociological interest in the medical profession had substantial roots in the work of Harvard University sociologist Talcott Parsons (1902–1979). Parsons was influenced by the work of Lawrence J. Henderson (1878–1942), a Harvard biochemist who wrote "Physician and Patient as a Social System" (Henderson, 1935) in the *New England Journal of Medicine*, and who introduced the writings of the Italian sociologist, Vilfredo Pareto, to America (Imber, 2008:87f; Bloom, 2002:83–90). In the tenth chapter of *The Social System* (1951), Parsons presented his formulation of the doctor-patient relationship, deeply indebted to Freudian thought and framed exclusively in terms of the doctor's and the patient's different but nevertheless converging social roles. "Role theory," as it was called a half century ago, was a way to categorize social or normative definitions of what was expected of people in their various life capacities. Parsons' approach is useful to recount here at the outset.

The "sick role," as Parsons named it, defined expectations on both sides of the doctor-patient relationship. From the patient's side, one was not expected to be held responsible for being ill. The ill person was exempted from social obligations and expected *not* to fulfill them. The patient was expected to follow the doctor's orders in order to get well and to consult with designated helpers. The sick role was defined as a contingent and temporary role. It could easily encompass more than the patient alone, including family members and others. Its temporary character was based on what in 1950 was the dominant view of endemic disease. With the prevalence of polio, childhood diseases, and other infectious diseases, the age of chronic illness—which might be regarded as starting in 1964 with the first Surgeon General's report on smoking—had yet to gain public acknowledgment by way of professional organizations and the media.

From the physician's side, Parsons noted that doctors were required to be trained in their occupation, their status being achieved rather than ascribed. Their profession was defined by a specificity of function: that is, as science improved, specialization increased. Both training and function were part of the evolution of the system of medicine. Parsons also emphasized the "character" of the physician. Doctors were to emulate an "affective neutrality," responding first and foremost to the medical condition of the patient. This neutrality was intended to radically limit judgments that criticized or condemned how that medical condition might be linked to a patient's behavior. Such behavior (e.g., continuing to smoke, not eating well, etc.) was never to be the basis of a physician's willingness to treat a patient. Finally, unlike other occupations (e.g., business and law), the medical vocation was expected to suppress the profit motive, directing the physician away from a self-orientation toward a commitment to the collectivity (Parsons, 1951:428–79).

Sixty-five years later, the focus on system-wide attributes has been overwhelming and at times relentless, resulting in what sociologists have defined as multiple social processes that have diminished the physician's taken-for-granted authority, the pinnacle of which one historian described as "American medicine's golden age" (Burnham, 1982, Imber, 1991, and Brandt and Gardner, 2000). A host of observations have been made about the various social processes that transformed both internal and external expectations about medical and professional responsibility. The jargon used to define these processes has included deprofessionalization, proletarianization, corporatization, commodification, medicalization, demedicalization, technologification, and bureaucratization. Taken as critiques of the medical system almost exclusively, each one incorporates a view of change in that system that is viewed by some as positive, by others as inevitable, and by still others as lamentable. Nevertheless, however conceived, they represent both resistances to change and concerns about that change (Freidson, 1970, 1994).

Deprofessionalization and its consequences have been challenged *and* endorsed, depending on how competence, cost and coordination of care are viewed. The increase in gate- keeping responsibilities by nurse-practitioners follows in the wake of increased specialization in medicine during the past half century. At the same time, these forces internal to medicine have coincided with external developments, including a greater number of better informed patients by way of self-help movements, the internet, and more publicized accounts of medical-scientific uncertainty. Proletarianization derived its perspective from Marxist theory that broadened the system-wide analysis to the larger-scale social processes of capitalism and class interests. From one perspective, doctors were pawns in rapidly emerging for-profit developments led by corporate and insurance interests. Concerns about cost-containment which led to the formation of health-maintenance organizations in the 1980s created not only a much larger workforce of medical care providers as "paid-wage laborers" but also opened the way to dramatically increased opportunities for physicians and others to determine their hours of work. Preceding these developments, doctors were either in solo or group practices, working in private offices, called to the hospital at all times of the day and night. One unforeseen consequence of the proletarianization of medical work was opening the way for much greater numbers of women to enter the profession because of the greater control they could achieve over their work circumstances. This is perhaps one of the least acknowledged changes that grew out of a social process that also served the interests of corporate managers who have sought to increase revenue while controlling costs (Larson, 1977).

The commodification of medicine is directly related to the simultaneous processes of medicialization and demedicalization. The concept originated also in Marxist theory, but it has acquired more general applications raising questions about the limits of the market in organizing and promoting medical care. The provision of such care beyond the norms defined by Parsons has extended the boundaries of what is offered under the dispensation of allopathic medicine. Once upon a time, the claims by those neither trained in medicine nor subject to its norms of licensure were typically regarded as quackery, that is, medical fraudulence that capitalized on a patient's anxious search for treatments and cures not available within medicine. The major chronic illnesses (e.g., cancer, diabetes, neurological disorders) have intensified interest in treatments that show little prospect for cure but that nevertheless are promoted even by some celebrity physicians. The appeal to scientific proof is largely ignored or so limited in scope as to be irrelevant. Government and public concerns typically arise when some of these treatments are shown to cause harm.

Commodification goes hand-in-hand with medicalization which is the process by which a condition that normally develops (for example, aging) becomes subject to medical intervention. Pharmaceutical interventions that have been made as a result of a diagnosis of attention deficit disorder are also consistent with the medicalizing of normally observed behavior at young ages.

Demedicalization, that is the deauthorizing of medical attention to and involvement in various conditions, is as much a cultural and political process as a medical one; for example, requests for abortion in the United States do not require medical justification as they once did, and homosexuality is no longer described medically as it once was. At particular moments in time, the surveillance that is part of the jurisdiction of doctors is believed to be too extensive and at other times not extensive enough. Opportunities for greater commodification result from both processes (Fox, 1977; Halfmann, 2012).

Technologification and bureaucratization have been addressed by both the "disappearance" of the doctor dependent upon technology in the form of machine generated knowledge (Reiser, 2014) as well as by the "disappearance" of the patient in a health bureaucracy that makes coordinated care ever more difficult to achieve. Recognition of such problems was already evident forty years ago (Mechanic, 1977). What is now called patient "literacy" determines how well any patient is able to navigate the complicated systems of contacts, referrals, and insurance. In some areas of the country, "concierge" medicine has appeared, providing increased access to doctors and to greater coordinated care for those willing to pay a premium.

The social processes reviewed here illustrate numerous ways in which the critiques of the medical system at particular points in time have been described. Sociologists in general have argued that these processes are the most important elements in understanding not only how the medical system is organized and how it functions but also how it fails to provide adequate care to all in need of it. The focus on system-wide factors found its political apotheosis in the work of Paul Starr (cited earlier). Many other sociologists of an earlier generation were already aware of the political and economic forces at work in the nature of all professions, but Starr's work established a public credibility for holding the medical system to a higher standard, reflected today, for example, in the burgeoning research on health disparities.

In April 1976, the National Institutes of Health held a conference on *The Doctor-Patient Relationship in the Changing Health Scene* over three days with more than seventy participants serving as presenters and discussants. A volume of the proceedings included prescient themes such as "The Orientation of the Professional," "The Orientation of the Consumer," and "Technological Medicine." The substitution of "consumer" for "patient" signaled already a decade before Paul Starr's work an underlying tension whose political manifestations would become more explicit in the years that followed. At the same time, an account of "Migration, Manpower, and the Doctor-Patient Relationship" by John Z. Bowers, President of the Josiah Macy, Jr. Foundation, concluded that "The restless mobility of the American people lessens the strength and the durability of the doctor-patient relationship." And, "The soaring numbers of women entering medicine should have a beneficial effect on the doctor-patient relationship" (Gallagher, 1976:411).

FROM SYSTEM TO PERSON

Talcott Parsons was unable to attend the 1976 conference, but he was invited to write an Epilogue to the volume of proceedings, thus giving him a fuller opportunity to respond to many of its themes. His chief concern was expressed in terms that address the abiding tension, greater today than forty years ago, between policy-making and clinical practice. The sociological perspective recounted in the various types of major social processes had implications for policy *and* clinical practice, but Parsons' prescience was obvious:

> From the social science point of view it is conspicuous that the main preoccupation of the conference was with what we call macrosocial problems. These touched the nature of the social organization in which health care functions are carried out and even the setting of these organizations in the larger society. Of course there was also considerable concern with trends of change in such organizations. I think it important though to emphasize that while varying enormously in nature and degree of severity, illness or the threat of it is an extremely intimate personal concern of human individuals. Health care personnel, notably physicians, must penetrate into areas which are ordinarily treated as areas of intimacy such as access to the body and confidential information. Furthermore, illness is a primary focus of anxiety. It often involves disability and pain as well as various other deprivations such as highly restrictive diets. For reasons such as these the relational system in which health care takes place seems to have a markedly different character from those relational systems in which other functions are performed, such as the manufacture and sale of goods or the organization of administrative functions like tax collection. In many respects, the relational nexus which generally becomes involved in health care resembles that of the family, with the physician or other agent of care playing a quasi-parental role which emphasizes the adequate handling of the patient, and the latter playing a quasichild role. Certainly affects and emotions can be aroused in the context of health care in a way which has no parallel in tax collection or the sale of goods. At the same time, modern health care draws importantly upon science and upon technologies based on scientific knowledge. Scientific research and the teaching and technological application of advanced knowledge are sometimes characterized as universalistic and impersonal, which gives them a very different sociological character from activities which involve high degrees of personal intimacy (Parsons, 1976: 445–446).

The "relational system" of the medical encounter that Parsons described, largely by contrasting it to other relational systems "such as the manufacture and sale of goods or the organization of administrative functions like tax collection," took for granted a kind of trust that was more parental in nature than dependent on *caveat emptor* with its assumption that the personal trust of another person alone was not necessarily sufficient to make the best informed decisions. When Parsons wrote, the "second opinion" still rankled an older generation of medical practitioners who might refer a patient to a specialist but not to a similarly trained colleague.

Continuing his assessment of the conference, Parsons noted that

> In the preoccupation of the participants with macrosocial problems there was a strong tendency to emphasize models of social organization which are considerably at variance with those which have historically been predominant in the health care field. I should like to make a comment briefly on three of them. The first is the *market* model which regards the patient as a "consumer" with the implications that the health care agent, notably the physician, should be regarded as the seller of a service, and that the basis of the relationship is primarily economic. The second model is that of *bureaucratic organization* which would be

appropriate to predominantly administrative functions as in the tax collection agency I have mentioned. Closely related to the bureaucratic model is the notion of the proletarianization of the medical profession. The third model, which appears on a more implicit level, is that of, the doctor-patient relationship as a *democratic association*. While each of these models has a range of applicability, each also has serious limitations (Parsons, 1976:446).

Parsons identified two models: the patient as consumer (i.e., a market model) and the physician as employee (i.e., a bureaucratic model), which a half-century later have their advocates and critics. But he was not arguing empirically against the reality in which "health care is a service and must be financed in some way or other" and in which consumerism and proletarianization would be the new and dominant forces. Quite the contrary, he was lamenting his colleagues' assessments that such a reality and the shape it was taking were inevitable or should be further pursued or advocated. He sought to acknowledge physicians' asymmetric power by placing it in a larger context of their necessary and inevitable authority that could not be bought and could not be defined by bureaucratic fiat.

SPIRITUALITY AS RESISTANCE

The implications of Talcott Parsons' acknowledgment of the sociologically dominant approach to the medical system in general, and the medical encounter in particular, were not lost on subsequent generations of sociologists. They recognized that the "social transformation of American medicine" (as the title of Starr's book described it) had both macro- and micro-contexts which led them to explore medical advance and patient experience in a variety of ways that were characteristically Parsonian in expectation. In other words, the concerns about medical power and authority represented by such macro-social processes as consumerism and proletarianization served in some cases as forms of resistance to both their disempowering and unintended consequences. Yet what Parsons had recognized long before others was that this resistance had micro-social implications which belonged to the very nature and meaning of the medical encounter. The authority of the doctor and the vulnerabilities of the patient endured regardless of the macro-social processes at work at any given moment in time.

The sociological study of the role that religion and spirituality have played in health and well-being runs along typically conventional quantitative and qualitative lines, reflecting sometimes conflicting and sometimes mutual interests among these different types of research. Ellen L. Idler, for example, has pursued a thirty-year career addressing the social epidemiological perspective on religion, spirituality and health. Her research has provided sophisticated empirical measures of this relationship (Idler, 1987; Idler et al., 2003; Idler, 2015). The social epidemiological perspective has been taken up by researchers far beyond the discipline of sociology (Idler, 2014; Christakis, 1999). The focus of and support for this research has long been for the purpose of shaping public health policy, thus emulating precisely what Parsons acknowledged was necessary but not sufficient for a full understanding of health and the provision of medical care.

Sociologists have also engaged in research from the other end of the methodological spectrum, using qualitative and ethnographic approaches to the clinical encounter, revealing what may be taken as a different set of priorities toward "policy" concerns. Among the most original and influential works in this tradition of research is Renée C. Fox's *Experiment Perilous*, first published in 1959. In her memoir published in 2011, Fox wrote,

> There are those who regard *Experiment Perilous* as a precursor to bioethics, a field that had its genesis in the United States in the 1960s. James Gustafson, a distinguished theologian who was a major teacher of a core group of first-generation bioethicists, has described the book as one that "combines rigorous sociological research methods with perceptive moral sensitivity in a way that opens both the complexity and the poignancy of decisions in medical research and care" (Fox, 2011:92; see also Fox, 1996).[1]

The significance of the rise of bioethics for sociological research from an ethnographic and qualitative perspective is beyond the scope of this essay, but its ascendency in various spheres of intellectual and public life remains an important development in what rapidly became a new alliance between bureaucracy and ethics embodied in the institutional review board and between the medical profession and the government (Rothman, 1991; Evans, 2002; Stark, 2012).

James Gustafson's use of words such as "sensitivity," "complexity" and "poignancy" suggests an awareness of not only the role of the ethnographer but of the less examined and less often addressed characterological and patient-centered responsibilities of the practitioner. Medical schools have begun to emphasize less the rules of ethical thinking and more the examples of engaged empathy as health care providers confront a diverse and both better- and less-informed patient population. The terms of such engagement (illustrated in the words used by Gustafson in his praise of Fox) are embedded deeply in the sociological outlook that has examined the age-old anxieties of sickness and death which remain as powerful as ever whatever scientific and technical progress has been made toward their relief and delay (see, for example, Bosk, 1992, 2008; Anspach, 1993; Chambliss, 1996).

The work of the sociologist Arthur W. Frank provides a conceptual basis to a renewed focus on the lived encounter between physician and patient in contrast to a theoretical account of ethical responsibility.[2] Frank called for a multivocal clinical ethic. Scrutiny of the physician-patient encounter served in his estimation as a form of witnessing, drawing from religious and "spiritual" ideas of personal transformation (Frank, 1991, 1995, 2009). His focus would be on the situation and experience of the patient for whom the system of the medical encounter was preceded by the anxiety and suffering of the body. This represented a new way to conceptualize the sick role which was derived from a sense of mission or purpose when possible.

Frank's ambition to empower patienthood with a sensibility of mission was intentionally nonconfrontational in contrast to other ways in which the critique of medical practice was mounted. Rather than depict doctors or the normative expectations of the community as inevitably shaping and defining how illness should be understood, Frank called for a defiance of conventional expectations altogether. The idea of a narrative—a story or account of illness—was an antidote to the overly technological and role-specific aspects of caring about and for an ill person (Frank, 2004).

---

1. *Experiment Perilous* was reissued with a new Epilogue in 1997 by Transaction Publishers. James Gustafson's statement was part of an endorsement for an earlier reissue published by the University of Pennsylvania Press in 1974.

2. What follows is drawn directly from my previous work in Imber, 2008:122–26.

Suffering was not simply an experience; it was the basis for a special communication of experience, if only those suffering less would listen. The problem was that the specific narrative of illness, that is, the specific worldview about the perception that the ill had of illness, could limit how well such communication was accomplished. Frank portrayed three such worldviews: restitution, chaos, and quest.

In the restitution narrative, illness is not memorable, because its duration is short and the ill person follows the doctor's orders and gets well. Frank is impressed with the power of this kind of narrative, empirically the most common of all: "The restitution narrative has its proper sphere: images of health can model behavior that many people can adopt and adapt. The problem arises when the ill person does not find restitution, or when someone who can only tell restitution stories encounters another whose health will not be restored" (Frank, 1995:92).

Restitution narratives symbolize the achievement of modern life. In Frank's assessment. They are the proof of medical progress, though he laments that the costs of treatment for certain illnesses may preclude access. This has always been the case to some extent, and Frank seeks to indict the objectivity of progress for its complicity in the inequalities it inevitably creates. The restitution narrative had particular relevance to the historical moment when Talcott Parsons first formulated the sick role, at the tail end of widespread infectious disease and the beginning of a concerted effort to address chronic illness. Frank makes an important point that the restitution narrative does not account for all who are ill, a point that shifts attention away from the structure of modern society and its narrative of recovery and survival to the more intimate realities of illness among others. He concludes, "The tragedy is not death, but having the self-story end before the life is over" (Frank, 1995:96).

A second narrative, the opposite of restitution, describes the abyss of illness as it spreads chaos in the normal ordering of life. The loss of control is paramount, until some semblance of control returns, whether or not illness is defeated, and the possibility of reporting the "chaos narrative" in such a state is limited, if not impossible. Frank's determination to describe how such a narrative of the sheer experience of pain and the disorientation of illness is beyond reporting lead him to explore narratives of the Holocaust as a basis of comparison. He cannot be begrudged his recognition of the powerful resonance between the specificity of historical experience and the universality of human pain and despair beyond speech. But he pushes this recognition to an image of total chaos in which many reasonable human responses such as defiance or the acceptance of help from others are deemed extraneous, even irrelevant. That the implications of the chaos of the Holocaust did not end for those who survived it marks something greater, of course, than the "discovery" of the many clinical realities of post-traumatic syndromes. What Frank proposes, as a kind of postmodern understanding of illness, is how the experience of chaos informs a middle ground—the quest narrative—between itself and routine restitution, one that may become the basis for a new ethic of human encounter. It is a remarkable ambition for narrative accounts, with broad public attraction, allowing as it does for the entry of less often heard voices in the drama of illness.

Because the restitution narrative accounts for the routine triumphs of medicine and because the chaos narrative is beyond communication, Frank introduces the quest narrative, which accepts illness and seeks "to use it" (Frank, 1995:115). As he observes, "involvement in patient advocacy is one enactment of a quest story; making significant vocational and personal changes in one's life following illness is another" (Frank, 1995:116). Citing Joseph Campbell's *The Hero with a Thousand Faces*, Frank carefully remarks, "If the idea of 'journey' has become a New Age spice sprinkled indiscriminately to season almost any experience, pop psychology could have done worse. The journey may be a fad, but it nevertheless represents a form of reflexive monitoring" (Frank, 1995:117)

"Reflexive monitoring" in an older rendition is what might have been called coming to terms, that is, finding a way to express intellectually and emotionally the meaning of one's situation or condition. The postmodern vocation of patienthood derives much of its contemporary force precisely in the mutual reinforcement that self-expression gives to the authentication of experience. At the same time, self-help is not at all an individual or lonely quest.

The possibility of finding others with similar conditions to whom one can turn for support is something that was, in fact, initially created by the conditions of medical research itself. When Renée Fox described how physicians and patients "came to terms" with their mutual ignorance about disease and its treatment, she took for granted that reflexive monitoring arose in the shared reality of physician and patient. Frank did not. Instead he believed that, in many instances, "medical care becomes the health care industry" (Frank, 1995:175; see also Frank, 2015).

The quest narrative is not exclusively about the physician-patient encounter. Illness itself is not only existential in that sense; it is also authentic beyond the terms of any therapeutic intervention. This suggests the broader role played by a host of concerned people in the care of the ill and dying. That concern has in the recent past been taken up by the sociologist, Wendy Cadge, in her work on hospital chaplaincy and the role that spirituality plays in health care (Cadge, 2009, 2012a, 2014, 2015). Cadge, in particular, has demonstrated an elective affinity between the research interests of those committed to addressing the spiritual well-being of patients and providers and the use of ethnographic and participant observation methods in social science.

One example illustrates the longstanding continuity between the initial reflections made by Talcott Parsons sixty-five years ago, maintained and furthered by his student, Renée Fox, and embodied in the work of Wendy Cadge. In *Experiment Perilous*, Fox introduced the concept of "detached concern" (Fox, 1959:86). Wendy Cadge and Clare Hammonds (2012) reported in a study of 37 intensive-care nurses that the history of the uses of "detached concern" focused more on detachment than concern. Their effort to understand how nurses in particular negotiated detachment and concern, not as dichotomies but as dualities, shows how concern, rather than being viewed as a failure to cope with patients' suffering, acknowledges the person who *is* the patient. This, in turn, does not ignore or diminish how system-wide factors affect this concern but directs attention to and recognition of the spiritual lives of all concerned.

FUTURE AGENDAS

The work of contemporary sociologists as it pertains to the growing "spirituality and health field" in and around medicine is clearly reflected in the quantitative and qualitative work of such people as Ellen Idler, Arthur Frank, and Wendy Cadge, whose various interests seek to make sense of the role that religion and spirituality play in the medical enterprise. In certain respects the "protest movement" in their work which assumes a central importance about the existential status of the person who is at times also a patient, runs parallel with sociological work that continues to hammer at the profession in the much longer tradition exemplified in Paul Starr's and Eliot Freidson's work, among others. More recent work in that more conventional tradition of protest in sociology has focused increasingly on the limits of biomedicine, a perspective that coincides with critiques of the costs of medical care and the concerns about justice claims in its provision (see Davis and González, 2016).

At the same time, although not the focus of this essay, the emergence of a "spirituality and health field" itself is indicative of a form of protest in developments in the focus and direction of medical care that has been led by what should be described as practitioners in the trenches who are very often trained and practicing physicians. Until relatively recently, such efforts to communicate the interests and findings of such early leaders in this field such as David B. Larson (Levin and Koenig, 2005) have been limited by the broader conventional silos of research and contact that define both medicine and social science. In the past few years, a variety of public conferences have been organized that have addressed the broad mandate of how spirituality relates to medicine and medical care (for example, the Program on Medicine and Religion [http://www.medicineandreligion.com/] and The American Association of Medicine and the Person [http://www.medconference.org/] have virtually no connection to the traditional protests in sociology, but they have embodied a fascinating evolution of the spirit of those protests, less committed to critiques of broad systems per se, and more inclined to offer powerful statements on the cultures and religious traditions at work in the medical encounter (Lazenby et al., 2014). A more pointed spirit of protest that has emerged from within the medical profession is exemplified in debates over some of the most contentious issues facing practitioners in real time. A statement on physician assisted suicide in *JAMA* captures that protest (Yang and Curlin, 2016). What distinguishes this kind of statement from others is its focus on the physician's vocation as distinct from the often arcane and politically directed arguments that define much of contemporary bioethical discourse. And the growing interest in how faith traditions relate to the practice of medicine is an important social development and promises to influence discussions about medicine in the years to come.

REFERENCES

Anspach, Renee R. (1993) *Deciding Who Lives: Fateful Choices in the Intensive-Care Nursery*. Berkeley: University of California Press.

Bloom, Samuel W. (2002) *The Word as Scalpel: A History of Medical Sociology*. New York: Oxford University Press.

Bosk, Charles (1992) *All God's Mistakes: Genetic Counseling in a Pediatric Hospital*. Chicago: University of Chicago Press.

Bosk, Charles (2008) *What Would You Do? Juggling Bioethics and Ethnography*. Chicago: University of Chicago Press.

Brandt, Allan M., and Martha Gardner (2000) "The Golden Age of Medicine?" In *Medicine in the 20th Century*, ed. Roger Cooter and John Pickstone. Amsterdam: Harwood Academic Publishers, pp. 21–37.

Burnham, John C. (1982) "American Medicine's Golden Age: What Happened to It? *Science* 215:1474–1479.

Cadge, Wendy (2012) *Paging God: Religion in the Hall of Medicine*. Chicago: University of Chicago Press.

Cadge, Wendy, and Clare Hammonds (2012) "Reconsidering Detached Concern: The Case of Intensive-Care Nurses." *Perspectives in Biology and Medicine* (55)2:266–82.

Cadge, Wendy et al. (2015) "Teaching Healthcare Providers How to Provide Spiritual Care: A Pilot Study." *Journal of Palliative Medicine* 18(5):408–414.

Cadge, Wendy, and Mary Ellen Konieczny (2014) "Making 'Invisible Religion' Visible: The Significance of Religion and Spirituality in Secular Organizations." *Sociology of Religion* 75(4):551–563.

Cadge, Wendy, Elaine Howard Ecklund, and Nicholas Short (2009) "Religion and Spirituality: A Barrier and a Bridge in the Everyday Professional Work of Pediatric Physicians." *Social Problems* 56(4): 702–721.

Chambliss, Daniel F. (1996) *Beyond Caring: Hospitals, Nurses, and the Social Organization of Ethics.* Chicago: University of Chicago Press.

Christakis, Nicholas A. (1999) *Death Foretold: Prophecy and Prognosis in Medical Care.* Chicago: University of Chicago Press.

Davis, Joseph E., and Ana Marta González (2016) *To Fix or To Heal: Patient Care, Public Health, and the Limits of Biomedicine.* New York: New York University Press.

Evans, John H. (2002) *Playing God? Human Genetic Engineering and the Rationalization of Public Bioethical Debate.* Chicago: University of Chicago Press.

Fisher, Sue (1986) *In the Patient's Best Interest: Women and the Politics of Medical Decisions.* New Brunswick, NJ: Rutgers University Press.

Fox, Renée C. (1977) "The Medicalization and Demedicalization of American Society." *Daedalus,* Winter: 9–22.

Fox, Renée C. (1996) *"Experiment Perilous*: Forty-Five Years as a Participant Observer of Patient-Oriented Clinical Research." *Perspectives in Biology and Medicine,* 39(2):206–226.

Fox, Renée C. (2011) *In the Field: A Sociologist's Journey.* New Brunswick, NJ: Transaction Publishers.

Frank, Arthur W. (1991) *At the Will of the Body: Reflections on Illness.* Boston: Houghton Mifflin.

Frank, Arthur W. (1995) *The Wounded Storyteller: Body, Illness, and Ethics.* Chicago: University of Chicago Press.

Frank, Arthur W. (2004) "Asking the Right Question about Pain: Narrative and Phronesis." *Literature and Medicine* 23(2):209–225.

Frank, Arthur W. (2009) "Why I wrote ... *The Wounded Storyteller*: A Recollection of Life and Ethics." *Clinical Ethics,* 4:106–108.

Frank, Arthur W. (2015) "The Angel and IV Pump." *Society* 52:(5):469–474.

Freidson, Eliot [1970] (1988) *Profession of Medicine: A Study of the Sociology of Applied Knowledge.* Chicago: University of Chicago Press.

Freidson, Eliot (1994) *Professionalism Reborn: Theory, Prophecy and Policy.* Chicago: University of Chicago Press.

Gallagher, Eugene B., ed. (1976) *The Doctor-Patient Relationship in the Changing Health Scene* (Washington, D.C.: U.S. Department of Health, Education, and Welfare, DHEW Publication No. (NIH) 78-183).

Halfmann, Drew (2012) "Recognizing Medicalization and Demedicalization: Discourses, Practices, and Identities." *Health* (London) March (16)2:186–207.

Henderson, Lawrence J. (1935) "Physician and Patient as a Social System." *New England Journal of Medicine,* 212:819–823.

Idler, Ellen L. (1987) "Religious Involvement and the Health of the Elderly: Some Hypotheses and an Initial Test." *Social Forces,* 66:226–238.

Idler, Ellen L., ed.. (2014) *Religion as a Social Determinant of Public Health.* New York: Oxford University Press.

Idler, Ellen L. (2015) "Religion and Health: Sociological Considerations." In James D. Wright, ed., *International Encyclopedia of the Social & Behavioral Sciences,* 2nd edition, Vol 20. Oxford: Elsevier, pp. 269–272.

Idler, Ellen L. et al. (2003) "Measuring Multiple Dimensions of Religion and Spirituality for Health Research: Conceptual Background and Findings from the 1998 General Social Survey." *Research on Aging,* 25:327–365.

Imber, Jonathan B. (1991) "Doctor No Longer Knows Best: Changing Attitudes toward Medicine and Health." Chapter 14 in *America at Century's End,* ed. by Alan Wolfe. Berkeley, CA: University of California Press, pp. 298–317.

Imber, Jonathan B. (2008) *Trusting Doctors: The Decline of Moral Authority in American Medicine.* Princeton, NJ: Princeton University Press.

Larson, Magali Sarfatti (1977) *The Rise of Professionalism: A Sociological Analysis*. Berkeley, CA: University of California Press.

Lazenby, Mark, Ruth McCorkle, and Daniel P. Sulmasy (2014) *Safe Passage: A Global Spiritual Sourcebook for Care at the End of Life*. New York: Oxford University Press.

Levin, Jeff, and Harold C. Koenig, eds. (2005) *Faith, Medicine, and Science: A Festschrift in Honor of Dr. David B. Larson*. New York: The Haworth Pastoral Press.

Mechanic, David (1977) "The Growth of Medical Technology and Bureaucracy: Implications for Medical Care." *The Milbank Memorial Fund Quarterly. Health and Society*. 55(1) (Winter):61–78.

Ong L.M.L., et al. (1995) "Doctor-Patient Communication: A Review of the Literature," *Social Science and Medicine*, 40:903–918.

Parsons, Talcott (1951) *The Social System*. New York: Free Press.

Parsons, Talcott (1976) "Epilogue." In Eugene B. Gallagher, ed. *The Doctor-Patient Relationship in the Changing Health Scene* (Washington, D.C.: U.S. Department of Health, Education, and Welfare, DHEW Publication No. (NIH) 78-183). 445–455.

Reiser, Stanley Joel (2014) *Technological Medicine: The Changing World of Doctor and Patient*. New York: Cambridge University Press.

Rothman, David J. (1991) *Strangers at the Bedside: A History of How Law and Bioethics Transformed Medical Decision Making*. New York: Basic Books.

Stark, Laura (2012) *Behind Closed Doors: IRBS and the Making of Ethical Research*. Chicago: University of Chicago Press.

West, Candace (1984) *Routine Complications: Troubles with Talk between Doctors and Patients*. Bloomington: Indiana University Press.

Yang, V. Tony, and Farr A. Curlin (2016) "Why Physicians Should Oppose Assisted Suicide." *Journal of the American Medical Association*, 315, (3):247–248.

CHAPTER 17

ANTHROPOLOGIES OF MEDICINE, RELIGION, AND SPIRITUALITY AND THEIR APPLICATION TO CLINICAL PRACTICE

Linda L. Barnes and Lance D. Laird

Medical Anthropology emerged as a discipline in the 1960s, and coalesced during the mid-1970s, addressing topics related to "medicine and health." Early researchers came from cultural anthropology, public health, medical sociology, and ethnomedicine. Their work resulted in the formulation of key concepts, with the goal of determining ways to interpret, analyze, and compare different dimensions of the world's therapeutic traditions. At the time, it seemed a given that "medicine" referred to the clinical practices rooted in the biological sciences as these had developed in European-descended settings. Medical Anthropology reclassified this tradition as "biomedicine," one tradition among many, each with its own history, cultural roots, distinctive characteristics, and claims to truth.

Following the Immigration and Nationality Act of 1965, the entry into the United States of immigrants from a growing number of non-European countries gradually changed the demographics of the United States. Particularly in urban areas, more Americans had occasion for greater engagement with groups from other parts of the world who had brought with them other cultural, religious, and therapeutic traditions. These encounters contributed to a new and more direct awareness of both therapeutic and religious pluralism throughout the country. What would come to be known as the "New Age" tapped these influences, along with self-help movements, transpersonal psychology, and a comprehensive application of the term "holism." A pivotal part of this movement lay in its attention to non-biomedical orientations to sickness, suffering, and healing, resulting in the grassroots popularization of "unconventional" therapies or what would be called "alternative medicine," "complementary medicine," "complementary and alternative medicine" or "CAM," and eventually "integrative medicine."

Just as the term "medicine" became more nuanced, so did the term "religion." Although generations of Americans had learned to think of the United States as a Christian (and primarily Protestant) nation—and therefore of "religion" as synonymous with Christianity—the new realities of pluralism challenged such assumptions. As it became possible to interact more directly with other traditions, Americans redefined their understandings of religious identity, with some rejecting the category of "religion" altogether in favor of the more amorphous category of "spirituality." The appeal of "spirituality" as opposed to "religion" grew out of a sense that something deeper and unified existed beneath the different religions. This orientation carried over into therapeutic traditions linked to religious and spiritual traditions. As new generations of clinicians grew up in the midst of these cultural changes, boundaries between categories that had once seemed clear now blurred, particularly as some of these clinicians looked for ways to introduce their individual commitments into biomedical settings.

Efforts to integrate religiosity into clinical settings represent a longstanding American tradition. Such syntheses generally privileged the theologies and religious worldviews of Protestant Christian denominations. They assumed the primacy of biomedicine and, often, the givenness of Christian practice, and dated back to ministers like John Wesley (1703–1791), who authored *Primitive Physick: An Easy and Natural Method of Curing Most Diseases* (Wesley, 2003 [1747]) for a lay audience. However, such assumptions gradually lost their apparent inevitability, giving way to religiously grounded non-biomedical therapies like meditation, yoga, acupuncture, and other interventions deriving from Hindu, Buddhist, Daoist, and other traditions.

These variables filtered into anthropological perspectives on medicine, religion, and spirituality. This chapter will first review how medical anthropology has characterized and interpreted biomedicine as a cultural system in its own right. Because so much of the field has attended to how practitioners and patients *experience* their engagement in biomedicine and other systems of healing, we will introduce related dimensions. Some medical anthropologists have also drawn from what is known as the Anthropology of Religion, as a way of exploring religious traditions related to healing. Their work adds useful dimensions to the topic at hand. Finally, we address applied implications that include how the emphasis on particular kinds of evidence, combined with the bureaucratization of biomedicine, affects how biomedical professionals can introduce issues related to religion/spirituality in their clinical work.

ANTHROPOLOGY OF BIOMEDICINE: CULTURES OF BIOMEDICINE

Medical anthropologists, following sociologists in the 1970s, turned their gaze toward biomedicine itself as the product of particular cultural assumptions and relations of power. Alternately designated with terms such as Western medicine, cosmopolitan medicine, or scientific medicine, these scholars locate biomedicine as one among many "ethnomedicines." Charles Leslie, for instance, characterized "cosmopolitan medicine" among the "great traditions" of medicine, alongside Ayurvedic and Chinese medical traditions that compete for explanatory and therapeutic power in Asian societies, and often merge in hybrid, complementary forms (Leslie, 1976). Other scholars developed cross-cultural categories for ethnomedical systems and mapped patients' varied pathways to health through interaction with popular, folk/traditional, and professional healers (Chrisman, 1977; Fabrega, 1979; Kleinman, 1978).

Lorna Rhodes (Rhodes, 1996) characterizes one stream of medical anthropological scholarship as investigating the "historical, social and linguistic contexts" in which biomedical "facts" about the human body and disease emerged. Exploring territory opened up by Michel Foucault's analysis of the "clinical gaze" and the "disciplinary power" of public health systems, medical and psychiatric institutions, such scholars have investigated the influence of cultural values on the development of clinical categories and treatment regimens for "diseases and disorders" such as drapetomania, hysteria, alcoholism, homosexuality, menopause (Lock, 1993), and PTSD (Hinton and Good, 2015; Young, 1995), among others. Deborah Gordon, for instance, points to the epistemological assumptions in biomedicine, including a naturalist cosmology that divides the material and biological from the spiritual and supernatural; a positivist and atomistic universalism that reduces the human to biological animals with secondary qualitative differences like rationality, culture and belief; and a concept of the autonomous individual as a rational agent, responsible to work on the health of the body as a project (Gordon, 1988).

Other medical anthropologists of biomedicine, Rhodes explains, take the clinic and hospital environment for granted and have applied their energies to improving patient care. Arthur Kleinman's "eight questions" for eliciting a patient's explanatory model of an illness episode, for instance, have become a mainstay of what some call "culturally competent care" (Kleinman et al., 1978); and the *Illness Narratives* influenced a field that Byron Good calls "meaning-centered analysis," an interpretive phenomenological approach to illness experience that may enable clinicians to understand what is at stake for their patients (Good, 1994). Along these lines, Byron Good and Mary Jo Delvecchio-Good have explored the cultural formation of physicians through the practice of "narrating patients":

> Students enter the world of medicine by learning how to constitute disease through a set of distinctive narrative practices. They gain competence as they learn to tell stories that accurately represent physiological reality and provide a basis for effective interventions. Maturing as physicians involves early experiences of naive realism, periods of disillusionment and a sense of the arbitrariness of the claims of medicine, periods of a sense of the absolute power of medicine, and, for many, an increasingly complex understanding about the relations among medical narratives, the human body, and the experiences of their patients. (1994, 65–66)

Critical medical anthropologists have approached biomedicine from a third perspective, as a product and reflection of relations of power within larger political, economic and social systems (Baer et al., 2003, Lock and Nguyen, 2010). Drawing on theories developed by Marx and Foucault, these scholars draw attention to "larger (macro) social problems such as class and gender inequality, corporate domination and the health-destroying features of capitalism" (Rhodes, 1996). Critical medical anthropologists define health broadly as "access to and control over the basic material and non-material resources that sustain and promote life at a high level of satisfaction" (Baer et al., 1986). These anthropologists examine the economic forces that introduce a market logic into health care management and public health, and frequently produce health disparities (Shaw, 2012). Others have explored the globalizing moral economies that undergird organ transplant programs (Scheper-Hughes and Wacquant, 2002) and promote medical and sex tourism (Edmonds, 2010; Padilla, 2007). Still others employ this critical lens to understand the emergence of infectious disease epidemics (Farmer, 2005) and the health effects of global pharmaceutical experimentation (Petryna, 2002).

ANTHROPOLOGY OF EXPERIENCE

Phenomenological inquiry has played a central role in anthropological investigations of religion, healing, and medicine. While North American sociologists have recently turned their attention to "lived religion" or "everyday religion," rather than normative and institutional practices (Ammerman, 2007; Hall, 1997; Orsi, 2005), anthropologists have historically paid more attention to contextualized ritual practices and embodied experiences and perceptions of the world. Phenomenological anthropologists contend that healing processes, religious practices, and moral formation arise from the "concrete engagements, concerns, and experiences of particular social actors acting in particular places and spaces in particular times" (Throop and Desjarlais, 2011). Key examples include Csordas's studies of "embodiment" in charismatic experiences of anointing, "words of knowledge," casting out of demons, and other healing practices (Csordas, 1990, 1993). He draws on examples from charismatic Catholicism, Puerto Rican espiritismo, and Navajo healing to challenge middle-class Protestant models of religious experience and expression. Other medical anthropologists have demonstrated the relevance of spirit possession, attack, and assistance in a variety of global settings, including immigrant and refugee communities in the West (Hinton et al., 2010).

Csordas and Kleinman also call on clinical medicine to attend to "therapeutic processes" of healing modalities (Csordas and Kleinman, 1996) rather than simply to focus on "clinical outcome." Phenomenological anthropologists situate the practices of medicine and religious healing in specific encounters between the lifeworlds of patients and healers: their individual or shared everyday experiences of being a self in the world. Likewise, Kleinman calls for attention to "local moral worlds" and "what really matters" in the formation of "caregiving" physicians and families (Kleinman, 2006). In this, he echoes insights by his colleague Byron Good into the often divergent and shifting social and existential worlds of chronic pain sufferers, medical students, and physicians (Good, 1994). While less often explicitly addressing spirituality and religion, phenomenological studies call attention to how different healing practices often carry implicit moralities or assume culturally constructed realities (physical, social, psychological, spiritual). Such attention is imperative for a nuanced, contextualized study of religion and spirituality in the cultures and spaces of medical practice.

While phenomenologists have alternatively emphasized hermeneutic/interpretive approaches, cultural/lifeworld approaches, and existential approaches to human experience, others have sought a "critical phenomenology" that "convincingly link[s] modalities of sensation, perception, and subjectivity to pervasive political arrangements and forms of economic production and consumption," (Willen, 2007; Desjarlais, 1997, p. 25). In other words, we need studies of religion, spirituality and medicine that link the experiences of being-in-the-world (with diverse "others"), in bodies suffering and bodies healing, with the larger discourses (e.g., of race, gender, class and individual responsibility) and power structures (e.g., health system, unemployment, insurance or immigration policies) that are implicated in such suffering and healing.

MEDICAL ANTHROPOLOGY & ANTHROPOLOGY OF RELIGION

Just as medical anthropologists have complicated the process of defining "medicine," so have anthropologists of religion and religious studies scholars done with "religion." Philosopher Charles Taylor cites anthropologist Fiona Bowie's argument that "the phenomena that scholars often approach as 'religious' (whether in religious studies or in anthropology, sociology, or psychology), are so diverse and shifting in their meanings, that we do well not to settle for one all-encompassing definition" (Taylor, 2004).

Both the anthropology of religion and medical anthropology address religious practices that include understandings of order, disorder, suffering, affliction, and pain. Both examine and analyze etiological, diagnostic, therapeutic, and evaluative practices, such as non-natural etiological factors and influences, divination, pulse reading, possession and trance, shamanism, ritual, the interaction with spirits, witchcraft and sorcery, magic, sent sickness, and communities of support. Therefore, it can be difficult to differentiate between these domains, or to separate out medical anthropology from the field of Religious Studies. The works of anthropologists like Clifford Geertz (1993) and Victor Turner (1967, 1995; Turner and Turner, 2011), among others, serve researchers in each of these fields.

However, one of the medical anthropologists who has worked most assiduously to integrate medical anthropology, the anthropology of religion, religious studies, and phenomenology is Thomas Csordas. His work encompasses the experience of Charismatic Catholics (Csordas, 1988, 1997) and of the Navajo people (Csordas and Lewton, 1998; Csordas, 1999, 2004), as well as theories of embodiment (Csordas, 1990, 1994). These intersections address the lived, embodied experience of groups who conceptualize illness and healing as inseparable from their religious identities.

THE BIOMEDICALIZING OF THE RELIGIOUS

A different interdisciplinary intersection occurs when biomedical researchers and groups approach the study of religiosity in relation to clinical settings, practices, practitioners, and patients. The methods employed within biomedical research are grounded in the evolving expectation that practice be based on specific forms of evidence, the most reliable of which is considered to be generated by the randomized, double (and sometimes triple-) blind, placebo-controlled clinical trials, or RCT. This approach draws on an epidemiological method— that is, one that examines phenomena at the level of larger groups or populations. It entails, among other things, testing for the effectiveness of a particular intervention either against a placebo or an existing therapy. Study participants are randomly assigned to the group receiving the intervention being tested and to a control group either not getting the treatment or getting a placebo. The objective is to eliminate the effects of chance and of bias. Even as the discussion of religion and healing unfolded in other disciplinary areas, some physicians were drawn to examine its potential ramifications—and beneficial effects—for biomedicine. However, to have any chance of persuading others in the biomedical community, this process requires the application of the RCT.

Four biomedical physicians in particular focused a significant part of their research, writing, and teaching on identifying and studying intersections between biomedicine and religion: cardiologist Herbert Benson (b. 1935), internist Larry Dossey (b. 1940), psychiatrist David Larson (1947–2002), and psychiatrist and gerontologist Harold Koenig (b. 1951–). At the time they began to do so, there was little overlap between the domains of the physician and the clergyman. Indeed, through the 1960s and into the 1970s, media attention to the issue of religion and healing focused largely on reporting about faith healers. Opinions were divided, with both warnings and support issuing from some of the mainline Christian denominations. Tragic stories of child deaths—due to parents' refusal of biomedical care on religious grounds and their reliance on a faith healer instead—contributed to a pervasive sense that faith, when mixed with illness, could harm the innocent. Such reports most frequently singled out Christian Scientists and Jehovah's Witnesses (see, for example, Swan, 1983; Merrick, 1994; Sheldon, 1996).

By the 1970s and into the 1980s, however, other kinds of healers had come to the public's attention, ranging from Native American medicine men to practitioners of Tibetan medicine. Discussions of the mind's influence over the body gained ground as well, with the word "biofeedback" being coined in 1969. Probably the single best-known figure was the Maharishi Mahesh Yogi (1914–2008), who made his first global tour in 1958. His practice of Transcendental Meditation came to the attention of Herbert Benson because its self-assigned secularity presented a lower threshold to cross than, say, the Hare Krishna movement might have. Although it had become something of a commonplace to refer to "mind-body medicine" when Benson published *The Relaxation Response* (Benson 1975), arguing that meditative techniques had certain features in common, the book marked a major milestone in the emerging field of alternative medicine. Like the Maharishi, he insisted that the Relaxation Response did not involve religious practice. He argued that one could divorce the process from religiosity or a particular tradition altogether—a position he largely maintained over time.

In contrast, Larry Dossey has advocated openly for the inclusion of prayer and other religious devotional practices in relation to medical care, arguing that both are associated with positive health outcomes. The consistent thread running through all of Dossey's work has been that prayer, which he defines as an attitude of the heart, can heal, effecting change from the cellular level to the level of disease. He therefore refers to it as a medicine that can be used in tandem with biomedical and other interventions. The premise upon which he bases this assertion is that the mind is not limited by time or by space. Instead, he argues, something in each person is infinite, eternal, and omnipresent.

Dossey characterizes this feature as an indefinable Absolute. Dossey traces the lineage of this idea to R. M. Bucke, Ralph Waldo Emerson, Arthur Lovejoy, and Carl Jung, among others, suggesting that they share the conviction that consciousness is larger than the individual mind. He asserts that prayer, which is not exclusive to any particular tradition, can take an infinite number of forms.

David Larson takes a different approach. Having served with the US Public Health Service Commissioned Corps, the NIH, the Department of Health and Human Services, and the National Institute of Mental Health, Larson developed a quantitative research method, systematic review, that facilitated comprehensive literature reviews. He applied this method to analyze the extent and ways in which religiosity was addressed in different branches of the psychiatric and biomedical literatures. These searches addressed, as well, the extent to which the literature appeared to suggest that religiosity contributed to both mental and physical health outcomes. As a psychiatrist, he was particularly interested in the topics of coping and mental illness. Identifying also as a Christian psychiatrist, he brought an added dedication to exploring integrations of faith with clinical work.

Koenig argues that there must be some mechanism through which religiosity can affect one's physical health, particularly through connections between religion, physical health, and mortality. He traces his interest in these questions to clinical experience as a psychiatrist, when patients talked with him about the importance of their religious lives in the face of their health challenges. Much of his work combines to build a case for the intentional inclusion of such discussions in clinical care. He does so by developing measures, gathering data related to the importance to patients of integrating religion and medicine, related health outcomes, and tools for actual practice, which he also tests.

From a number of medical anthropological perspectives, these works share the common feature of working with a relatively reductionist perspective. For example, Benson tends to represent the Relaxation Response as the generic underpinning of all meditative practices. The significance of religious and cultural differences, as well as the therapeutic specifics of each practice are, from this perspective, irrelevant and even disposable. Dossey's Absolute corresponds roughly to Ralph Waldo Emerson's Over-Soul (Emerson, 1865), a concept that Emerson synthesized from Unitarian, Transcendentalist, Hindu and other influences. A second parallel also appears, in Emerson's prescription that others "Make your own Bible. Select & Collect all those words & sentences that in all your reading have been to you like the blast of [a] trumpet out of Shakspear [sic], Seneca, Moses, John, and Paul" (Emerson, 1965, p. 186). If, he thought, one could intuit the Over-Soul in oneself, in Nature, and in others, then one could certainly discern its expression in all kinds of other sources, including religious texts and materials from all traditions. The starting point was oneself; the resulting "Bible" a composite fashioned after the image of one's personal understanding and experience of the Over-Soul. The claim was to have connected with a universal force that transcended the particulars of the individual religions.

On the surface, this claim to universalism appears to resolve potential tensions between the many traditions. In actuality, however, it also suggests that traditions themselves can be dispensed with, in favor of a highly personalized particularism—what religion scholar Huston Smith has characterized as "cafeteria spirituality" (Snell, 1997). The result is largely in the image of the compiler, with none of the communal commitments and disciplines provided by the traditions, or what Smith also refers to as "institutionalized spirituality" (Snell, 1997). While this orientation can hold great meaning for the individual, it can also lead to a disregard for the meaning that religious particularities may hold for patients and their families, or to a subtle assumption that they are narrow in their understanding.

Some medical anthropologists have adopted an approach known as "biocultural anthropology," which attempts to explore relationships between human culture and biology, and to synthesize the contributions of sociocultural and biological anthropology. (Others view the two as distinct subdisciplines, without pursuing an exchange between them.) In contrast, the research models that examine the effects of religiosity on health generally do not factor in sociocultural influences and an integral dimension. Moreover, the religiosity measures—although they have become relatively more nuanced over time—still often reflect an underlying Protestant Christian orientation that cannot, in itself, be considered a universal foundation.

APPLICATIONS TO CLINICAL PRACTICE

The question underlying this discussion as a whole involves what role, if any, clinicians should play in the spiritual and religious lives of their patients, and what contributions medical anthropology as a field might make in addressing this question. As Arthur Kleinman (1988) has observed, the very training of doctors—particularly through the "problem-oriented patient presentation"—emphasizes the translation of a meaning-centered narrative into a clinical case through strategies like the SOAP Note (**S**ubjective, **O**bjective, **A**ssessment, and **P**lan; Holmes and Ponte, 2011, p. 165).

Beginning in medical school, physicians-in-training receive the contradictory and persistent instruction to build an alliance with the patient on the one hand, while on the other hand, distilling the patient's experience into the case report. Medical students are corrected and sometimes reprimanded when their case presentations include what is construed as extraneous detail, instead of what is considered most relevant to arriving at a clear differential diagnosis. Although this training enables the learner to arrive at a more focused and precise analysis of the medical issues, it also discourages lingering on other details. As a result, it can be more difficult to persuade clinicians to fit yet another question into the clinic visit, especially when so many pressing issues inform patient health (e.g., the use of complementary/alternative therapies, the need to screen for depression, domestic violence, drug use, etc.).

In contrast, a fundamental component in the training of an anthropologist entails the process known as participant observation—an immersion in another culture, in the hope of moving from the vantage point of a complete outsider (*etic*) to that of a quasi-insider (*emic*). The development of an emic perspective involves learning to suspend—provisionally, and as much as possible— one's own categories, explanations, and interpretations of the world, and to engage in those of the other group. Ideally, it takes place over an extended period of time, in order to develop an in-depth relational familiarity with the diverse members of that group in their own setting. As a method, it relies on a complex synthesis of active engagement in the life of the group, ongoing observation, inquiry, and an ongoing reflection on the meanings assigned to different dimensions of life by the different kinds of stakeholders in the group. Most importantly, the purpose of anthropological inquiry is not to introduce one's own worldview when asking questions of research participants. The occasion may arise when a participant asks about the researcher's own culture, but that is not the focus of one's work.

Researchers who have advocated for the inclusion of "Spiritual History Taking" during clinical visits have intended a tool that is both neutral and inclusive (see, for example, Maugans, 2005; (Anandarajah and Hight, 2001; Culliford, 2002; LaRocca-Pitts, 2009). Perhaps the best known and most widely used example is the FICA (**F**aith and Belief, **I**mportance, **C**ommunity, **A**ddress in Care) assessment tool developed at the George Washington University Institute for Spirituality & Health, under the direction of its founder, physician Christina M. Puchalski. The related website suggests that spiritual histories can be "taken as part of the regular history during an annual exam or new patient visit, but can also be taken as part of follow-up visits, as appropriate. The FICA tool serves as a guide for conversations in the clinical setting" (George Washington University Institute of Spirituality and Health, 1996.).

The tools themselves cannot guarantee, however, that clinicians aim for a truly emic perspective. There is always the risk of the inadvertent imposition of the clinician's own presuppositions, even when he or she has received chaplaincy training. This is all the more likely when tools are presented as universally applicable. What may be missing is a personal, reflective process, to examine how one's own attitudes may shape one's understanding of the questions and of the responses. For example, the GWISH group provides a self-assessment tool intended to help providers take their own spiritual history, but this is not the same thing as reflecting on the ways in which one's own history may have created unexamined and unintended biases. We suggest that, without such awareness, biases are more likely to infuse discussions with patients. Sam Killerman's "30+ Examples of Christian Privilege" provides a particularly useful resource with which to detect and address these kinds of biases (Killerman, 2014; see Table 17.1).

They are not an attempt to criticize those who identify as Christian, but rather to help identify experiences that one learns not to notice. Particularly when working with patients whose religious/spiritual orientation may differ from one's own, these examples can facilitate an emic orientation.

In more recent work, Harold Koenig has joined with Daniel Hall, Keith Meador, and others to flag the influence of an Enlightenment paradigm in the study of religiosity, the "objectivity" of which has become "problematic, if not untenable." Perhaps the single most important insight deriving from this work is that

> If there is no objective frame of reference from which to measure religiousness, then the study of religion and health is fundamentally contingent on the specific languages and contexts in which particular religions find expression. While applying this cultural-linguistic approach to religion would require significant changes in the existing methods for studying religion and health, such changes may generate a deeper understanding of this relationship (Meador et al., 2004).

Hall, Koenig, and Meador note elsewhere that measures like "intrinsic" and "extrinsic" religiosity draw from, and are most applicable to, American Protestant religions (Hall et al., 2008), which makes them problematic when applied to other branches of Christianity and even more so when used with non-Christian traditions. We agree with their critique of the standard, "context-free" approach, and with their advocacy of developing tools that "measure religiousness in specific, theologically relevant contexts" (Hall et al., 2008). A case in point is their formulation of an Episcopal measure of faith (Hall et al., 2010).

TABLE 1 30+ Examples of Christian Privilege-Sam Killerman

1. You can expect to have time off work to celebrate religious holidays.
2. Music and television programs pertaining to your religion's holidays are readily accessible.
3. It is easy to find stores that carry items that enable you to practice your faith and celebrate religious holidays.
4. You aren't pressured to celebrate holidays from another faith that may conflict with your religious values.
5. Holidays celebrating your faith are so widely supported you can often forget they are limited to your faith (e.g., wish someone a "Merry Christmas" or "Happy Easter without considering their faith).
6. You can worship freely, without fear of violence or threats.
7. A bumper sticker supporting your religion won't likely lead to your car being vandalized.
8. You can practice your religious customs without being questioned, mocked, or inhibited.
9. If you are being tried in court, you can assume that the jury of "your peers" will share your faith and not hold that against you in weighing decisions.
10. When swearing an oath, you will place your hand on a religious scripture pertaining to your faith.
11. Positive references to your faith are seen dozens of times a day by everyone, regardless of their faith.
12. Politicians responsible for your governance are probably members of your faith.
13. Politicians can make decisions citing your faith without being labeled as heretics or extremists.
14. It is easy for you to find your faith accurately depicted in television, movies, books, and other media.
15. You can reasonably assume that anyone you encounter will have a decent understanding of your beliefs.
16. You will not be penalized (socially or otherwise) for not knowing other people's religious customs.
17. Your faith is accepted/supported at your workplace.
18. You can go into any career you want without it being associated with or explained by your faith.
19. You can travel to any part of the country and know your religion will be accepted, safe, and you will have access to religious spaces to practice your faith.
20. Your faith can be an aspect of your identity without being a defining aspect (e.g., people won't think of you as their "Christian" friend)
21. You can be polite, gentle, or peaceful, and not be considered an "exception" to those practicing your faith.
22. Fundraising to support congregations of your faith will not be investigated as potentially threatening or terrorist behavior.
23. Construction of spaces of worship will not likely be halted due to your faith.
24. You are never asked to speak on behalf of all the members of your faith.
25. You can go anywhere and assume you will be surrounded by members of your faith.
26. Without special effort, your children will have a multitude of teachers who share your faith.
27. It is easily accessible for you or your children to be educated from kindergarten through post-grad at institutions of your faith.
28. Disclosing your faith to an adoption agency will not likely prevent you from being able to adopt children.
29. In the event of a divorce, the judge won't immediately grant custody of your children to your ex because of your faith.
30. Your faith is taught or offered as a course at most public institutions.
31. You can complain about your religion being under attack without it being perceived as an attack on another religion.
32. You can dismiss the idea that identifying with your faith bears certain privileges.

Killerman, Sam. 2014. 30+ Examples of Christian Privilege. http://itspronouncedmetrosexual.com/2012/05/list-of-examplesof-christian-orivileo/ (Accessed April 12, 2016).

In 2005, Curlin and Hall reviewed the apprehensions and critiques related to including spiritual and/or religious issues in the clinical encounter: concerns for insufficient physician training or expertise; threats to patient autonomy and the apparent imposition of the clinician's agenda; tensions between religious and scientific inquiries; and the potential violation of professional boundaries. Their greatest concern involves the treatment of religion as a "therapeutic technique" rather than a life orientation. They advocate for clinicians to undertake related discussions "in an ethic of friendship, marked by wisdom, candor, and respect. Whether a particular conversation is ethical will depend on the character of those involved and the context of their engagement" (Curlin and Hall, 2005). The recommendation is admirable. At the same time, this final caveat leaves us with misgivings, insofar as the very concerns raised by critics who address religious questions as therapeutic techniques may just as readily arise even when clinicians believe themselves to be operating with an ethic of friendship.

Above all, we favor an orientation informed by "cultural humility," an approach developed by Melanie Tervalon and Jann Murray-Garcia. Cultural humility "incorporates a life-long commitment to self-evaluation and self-critique, to redressing the power imbalances in the patient-physician dynamic, and to developing mutually beneficial and nonpaternalistic clinical and advocacy partnerships with communities on behalf of individuals and defined populations" (Tervalon and Murray-Garcia, 1998) p. 117). The striking thing about this model is its emphasis on a reflective practice, in which clinicians lead with the things they do *not* know, and are slow to make assumptions about the things they imagine they do know. Melanie Tervalon and Jann Murray-Garcia, who coined the term, advocate for "patient-focused interviewing. . .that signals to the patient that the practitioner values what the patient's agenda and perspectives are, both biomedical and nonbiomedical" (Tervalon and Murray-Garcia, 1998) The model has been applied to the education of family medicine residents (Hook et al., 2013), and its effectiveness assessed for strengthening the working alliance between a client and a therapist (Juarez et al., 2006). Moreover, the approach has inspired analogous models like the *QIAN* 謙 (Humbleness) curriculum, which Chang et al. based on the works of Chinese philosophers and religious thinkers and the experience of Chinese immigrants. It encompasses "the importance of self-Questioning and critique, bi-directional cultural Immersion, mutually Active-listening, and the flexibility of Negotiation" (Chang et al., 2012, p. 269).

We illustrate this approach with two cases. The first (see Case I) involves Asha, a Somali Muslim woman, who developed severe headaches during childbirth. If a nurse or physician had asked Asha the FICA questions, she might have responded:

1. **F—Faith and Belief: "Do you consider yourself spiritual or religious?"** Yes, I am a Muslim. I know that I must bear patiently whatever suffering that God allows, and that God is the One who cures. God knows best, and I praise Him and thank Him for all His mercies. I will pray and listen to the Qur'an when I am in pain.

2. **I—Importance: "What importance does your spirituality have in your life?"** Spirituality is very important to me, and I pray several times a day. The Prophet Muhammad, peace be upon him, told us that we must be patient, but that we should also seek the cure, for God Almighty has created a cure for every disease.

3. **C—Community: "Are you part of a spiritual community?":** I usually pray at home, and sometimes I go to a Qur'an class at the masjid. Sometimes I get together with some other Somali women. Everyone comes to visit, but I'm too tired to see them.

4. **A—Address in Care: How would you like me, your health care provider, to address these issues in your health care?"**: I don't really need you to address anything. My family understands what I need, and they are here to help me.

Let us assume that the provider asked the FICA questions with sincerity, candor, and respect, and that Asha heard and responded to them in kind. Nevertheless, the assumption that spirituality or religiosity can be articulated as a faith in something, a set of beliefs and priorities, involvement in

---

CASE 1

Asha was a 27-year-old Somali woman who gave birth to her first child. During childbirth, she developed severe headaches, which caused her to be bedridden. In constant pain, she was unable to care for her child or to engage in daily activities. After a series of tests, her PCP referred her to a neurologist. Asha developed what looked like seizures, so her doctor decided to hospitalize her until she was stabilized and the specialists determined the cause.

Her mother and other family members became very angry and insisted on taking her home and caring for her themselves. The doctors asked a community advocate to explain to Asha and her family the need for hospitalization and medication. The advocate sat down with the family and asked them what they understood to be causing Asha's problem and why they refused further medical tests.

Asha's mother explained that this was something that she herself experienced as a young mother, as had her own mother. It was not a medical problem, but rather a family *wadaado* (a type of spirit affliction), which they—and not the doctors—knew how to cure.

The community advocate asked the family if they felt that medical care was interfering with the ritual for appeasing the *wadaacio*. They explained that the medication did not interfere, but by keeping her hospitalized, the doctors were preventing her from receiving the proper traditional treatment.

The advocate asked, "What if I allowed you to do the ritual in the hospital?" The family said that they would then agree to let her stay in the hospital and would allow her to receive the 'Western medicine.' The advocate arranged for the ritual to take place in the room, and the family accepted the treatment. Within a few days, the patient's "seizures" stopped, and she was released.

Ultimately, the advocate explained, "I told the family it did not matter what helped the patient: Western medicine or traditional healing. What mattered was that the patient was better"

Source: Saida Abdi, MSW, "Composite Case," Personal communication, April 27, 2016

community, and a coping strategy—while important—does not get at the many ways in which understandings and explanations of affliction derive from culturally informed religious models. It does not, for example, get at the ways in which certain spiritual forces can cause suffering.

In this case, the providers adopted an admirable stance of not-knowing—one dimension of cultural humility—turning instead to a community advocate to convey the team's concerns. Doing so created an opening for the family to explain their broader understanding of the problem, and of what needed to be done to address it. Note that they did not oppose the use of biomedical therapies. The second expression of cultural humility manifested itself in the team's willingness to accept the performance of a healing ritual, even though we suspect that, for some of them, it may have seemed merely a matter of humoring the family. (The more interesting question, which probably did not get asked, would be how we know that the family wasn't actually right in its assessment of the causal factor.) Although it is never a given that an advocate will necessarily be sympathetic to the views of another community member—a reminder of the internal variations and even disputes within a given cultural group—there is at least likely to be a higher level of understanding. Here, the advocate was able to broker an effective compromise.

In Case 2, the attending was able to teach the team about cultural underpinnings behind the rejection of surgery (we would guess that at least some of them had read Ann Fadiman's well-known book *The Spirit Catches You and You Fall Down* (Fadiman, 2012).

CASE 2

Npaim, a married, forty-seven-year-old Hmong mother of eight arrived at an emergency room complaining of severe right-upper-quadrant pain, fever, nausea, and vomiting. Ultrasound evaluation demonstrated significant gallbladder disease, with signs of advanced infection.

She was intubated and underwent an emergency Endoscopic Retrograde Cholangiopancreatography (ERCP) to drain pus from her gallbladder. Blood cultures quickly grew three strains of bacteria. Her blood pressure dropped and she was taken to the intensive care unit with a diagnosis of acute cholecystitis, ascending cholangitis and bacterial sepsis. The preferred treatment for this possibly fatal condition was emergency surgery.

The family refused and the surgical and medical residents were stunned. The case immediately raised two issues. First, who makes the decision in such a case; and second, what constitutes a legitimate decision? At stake was the question of competency.

The residents wanted to involve the legal system, to force a ruling. In this situation, however, the attending physician argued that the family's choice was reasonable, and that they were acting according to their values and presumably, as competent surrogates, by the woman's own wishes. "They have no reason to want her to die," she said, "and we'll respect them by abiding by their wishes."

The woman remained in intensive care and was treated aggressively with high-dose antibiotics and supportive care, but her condition grew progressively worse. The family became increasingly distressed, and finally asked the medical team to turn off the ventilator. Without it, the staff believed the patient would die. They also believed her case to be futile without surgery. They knew that the family had every right to decline an invasive or burdensome intervention, even if it resulted in death. However, several members of the medical team disagreed with the withdrawal of support from a young mother of eight with a reversible disease, and they tried to persuade the family to continue ventilator support.

What was unclear to the medical team was that the family wanted the patient to live. In the family's understanding of disease, "wind" brings and induces illness. The ventilator—as a wind machine—was bringing the patient wind that was responsible for her critical condition. Their request to turn off the ventilator was not a wish for a peaceful death in a situation of medical futility. Rather, it arose from their wish to protect her and to do everything in their power to keep her alive. They had brought her to the hospital with the expectation that, while certain courses of action might not be acceptable to them, others would be available that could still save her life.

To the medical staff's surprise, the antibiotic treatment proved successful and the woman walked out of the hospital one week after her admission (adapted from Barnes and Plotnikoff, 2001).

The medical team was then able to respond within a cultural framework. Yet as Barnes and Plotnikoff observe (Barnes and Plotnikoff, 2001), they continued to view "culture" as a set of "beliefs" about surgery, and did not explore the convergence of factors in other aspects of the case. "Wind" grows out of a larger cosmological life world that cannot be split between the cultural and the religious. Barnes and Plotnikoff note that, as a result, the team assumed that their own values were at work in the family's request to turn off the ventilator. This understandable and unintended blind spot almost resulted in their shutting down the case prematurely.

Medical anthropologists, like anyone doing comparative work, face the regular need to safeguard against the assumption that resemblance equals equivalence. Here, for example, the apparent resemblance masked what, in reality, were two radically different decisions. It can be one's own normative understandings that get in the way of even thinking to question such conclusions. In other words, we are all vulnerable to the perils of the blind spot.

As medical anthropologists, we support the commitment to exploring and challenging one's unconscious and unintended complicity in perpetuating power disparities. In the biomedical literature, one ordinarily one finds this particular commitment under the rubric of "cultural competence." We propose, however, a synthesis of the strengths of religious studies, medical anthropology, refined tools of spiritual inquiry that reflect the particularities of the different traditions, and a stance of cultural humility.

REFERENCES

Ammerman, Nancy Tatom. 2007. *Everyday religion: observing modern religious lives*. Oxford; New York: Oxford University Press.

Anandarajah, Gowri, and Ellen Hight. 2001. "Spirituality and Medical Practice: Using the HOPE Questions as a Practical Tool for Spiritual Assessment." *American Family Physician* 63 (1):81.

Baer, Hans A., Merrill Singer, and John H. Johnsen. 1986. "Toward a critical medical anthropology." *Social Science & Medicine* 23 (2):95–98.

Baer, Hans A., Merrill Singer, and Ida Susser. 2003. *Medical anthropology and the world system*. 2nd ed. Westport, CT: Praeger.

Barnes, Linda L., and Gregory A. Plotnikoff. 2001. "Fadiman and Beyond: The Dangers of Extrapolation." *Bioethics Forum* 17:32–40.

Benson, Herbert. 1975. *The relaxation response*. New York: William Morrow & Co.

Chang, E-shien, Melissa Simon, and XinQi Dong. 2012. "Integrating cultural humility into health care professional education and training." *Advances in Health Sciences Education* 17 (2):269–278.

Chrisman, Noel J. 1977. "The health seeking process: An approach to the natural history of illness." *Culture, Medicine, and Psychiatry* 1 (4):351–377.

Csordas, Thomas J. 1988. "Elements of charismatic persuasion and healing." *Medical Anthropology Quarterly* 2 (2):121–142.

Csordas, Thomas J. 1994. *Embodiment and experience: The existential ground of culture and self*. Vol. 2: Cambridge University Press.

Csordas, Thomas J. 1997. *The sacred self: A cultural phenomenology of charismatic healing*: Univ of California Press.

Csordas, Thomas J. 1999. "Ritual healing and the politics of identity in contemporary Navajo society." *American Ethnologist* 26 (1):3–23.

Csordas, Thomas J. 2004. "Healing and the human condition: scenes from the present moment in Navajoland." *Culture, medicine and psychiatry* 28 (1):1–14.

Csordas, Thomas J, and Elizabeth Lewton. 1998. "Practice, performance, and experience in ritual healing." *Transcultural Psychiatry* 35 (4):435–512.

Csordas, Thomas J. 1990. "Embodiment as a Paradigm for Anthropology." *Ethos* 18 (1):5–47.

Csordas, Thomas J. 1993. "Somatic Modes of Attention." *Cultural Anthropology* 8 (2):135–156.

Csordas, Thomas, and Arthur Kleinman. 1996. "The Therapeutic Process." In *Medical anthropology: contemporary theory and method*, edited by Carolyn Fishel Sargent and Thomas M. Johnson, 3–20. Westport, Conn.: Praeger.

Culliford, Larry. 2002. "Spiritual care and psychiatric treatment: an introduction." *Advances in Psychiatric Treatment* 8 (4):249–258.

Curlin, Farr A, and Daniel E Hall. 2005. "Strangers or friends?" *Journal of general internal medicine* 20 (4):370–374.

Desjarlais, Robert R. 1997. *Shelter blues: sanity and selfhood among the homeless, Contemporary ethnography*. Philadelphia, Pa.: University of Pennsylvania Press.

Edmonds, Alexander. 2010. *Pretty modern: beauty, sex, and plastic surgery in Brazil*. Durham, N.C: Duke University Press.

Emerson, Ralph Waldo. 1865. "Over-soul." In *Essays: First Series*, 213–235. Boston: Houghton, Mifflin and Company.

Emerson, Ralph Waldo. 1965. *Journals and Miscellaneous Notebooks of Ralph Waldo Emerson, Volume V: 1835-1838*. Vol. 4: Harvard University Press.

Fabrega, H., Jr. 1979. "Elementary systems of medicine." *Cult Med Psychiatry* 3 (2):167–98.

Fadiman, Anne. 2012. *The spirit catches you and you fall down: A Hmong child, her American doctors, and the collision of two cultures*: Macmillan.

Farmer, Paul. 2005. *Pathologies of power: health, human rights, and the new war on the poor: with a new preface by the author.* [2005 ed, *California series in public anthropology;.* Berkeley: University of California Press.

Geertz, Clifford. 1993. "Religion as a Cultural System." In *The interpretation of cultures: selected essays*, edited by Clifford Geertz, 87–125. Waukegan IL: Fontanta Press.

George Washington University Institute of Spirituality and Health. N.d. "Clinical." Accessed April 12. https://smhs.gwu.edu/gwish/clinical.

Good, Byron. 1994. *Medicine, rationality, and experience: an anthropological perspective, The Lewis Henry Morgan lectures; 1990.* Cambridge; New York: Cambridge University Press.

Gordon, Deborah. 1988. "Tenacious assumptions in Western medicine." In *Biomedicine examined*, edited by Margaret M. Lock and Deborah Gordon, 19–56. Dordrecht; Boston: Kluwer Academic Publishers.

Hall, Daniel E, Harold G Koenig, and Keith G Meador. 2008. "Hitting the target: why existing measures of 'religiousness' are really reverse-scored measures of 'secularism.'" *Explore: The Journal of Science and Healing* 4 (6):368–373.

Hall, Daniel E, Harold G Koenig, and Keith G Meador. 2010. "Episcopal measure of faith tradition: A context-specific approach to measuring religiousness." *Journal of religion and health* 49 (2):164–178.

Hall, Daniel E, Keith G Meador, and Harold G Koenig. 2008. "Measuring religiousness in health research: Review and critique." *Journal of religion and health* 47 (2):134–163.

Hall, David D. 1997. *Lived religion in America: toward a history of practice.* Princeton, N.J.: Princeton University Press.

Hinton, Devon E., and Byron Good. 2015. *Culture and PTSD: trauma in global and historical perspective, The ethnography of political violence.* Philadelphia: University of Pennsylvania Press.

Hinton, Devon E., Vuth Pich, Luana Marques, Angela Nickerson, and Mark H. Pollack. 2010. "Khyâl Attacks: A Key Idiom of Distress Among Traumatized Cambodia Refugees." *Culture, Medicine, and Psychiatry* 34 (2):244–278. doi: 10.1007/s11013-010-9174-y.

Holmes, Seth M, and Maya Ponte. 2011. "En-case-ing the patient: Disciplining uncertainty in medical student patient presentations." *Culture, Medicine, and Psychiatry* 35 (2):163–182.

Hook, Joshua N, Don E Davis, Jesse Owen, Everett L Worthington Jr, and Shawn O Utsey. 2013. "Cultural humility: Measuring openness to culturally diverse clients." *Journal of Counseling Psychology* 60 (3):353.

Juarez, Jennifer Anderson, Kim Marvel, Kristen L Brezinski, Cherie Glazner, Michael M Towbin, and Susan Lawton. 2006. "Bridging the gap: A curriculum to teach residents cultural humility." *FAMILY MEDICINE-KANSAS CITY-* 38 (2):97.

Killerman, Sam. 2014. "30+ Examples of Christian Privilege." Accessed April 12. http://itspronouncedmetrosexual.com/2012/05/list-of-examples-of-christian-privileg/.

Kleinman, A. 1978. "Concepts and a model for the comparison of medical systems as cultural systems." *Social Science & Medicine* 12 (2B):85–95.

Kleinman, Arthur. 1988. *The illness narratives: suffering, healing, and the human condition.* New York: Basic Books.

Kleinman, Arthur. 2006. *What really matters: living a moral life amidst uncertainty and danger.* New York: Oxford University Press.

Kleinman, Arthur, Leon Eisenberg, and Byron Good. 1978. "Culture, illness, and care: clinical lessons from anthropologic and cross-cultural research." *Annals of internal medicine* 88 (2):251–258.

LaRocca-Pitts, Mark A. 2009. "FACT: Taking a spiritual history in a clinical setting." *Journal of health care chaplaincy* 15 (1):1–12.

Leslie, Charles M. 1976. *Asian medical systems: a comparative study.* Berkeley: University of California Press.

Lock, Margaret M. 1993. *Encounters with aging: mythologies of menopause in Japan and North America*. Berkeley: University of California Press.

Lock, Margaret M., and Vinh-Kim Nguyen. 2010. *An anthropology of biomedicine*. Chichester, West Sussex; Malden, MA: Wiley-Blackwell.

Maugans, Todd A. 2005. "The SPIRITual History." *Archives of Family Medicine* 5:11–16.

Meador, Keith G, Daniel E Hall, and Harold George Koenig. 2004. "Conceptualizing" religion": how language shapes and constrains knowledge in the study of religion and health." *Perspectives in Biology and Medicine* 47 (3):386–401.

Merrick, Janna C. 1994. "Christian Science healing of minor children: spiritual exemption statutes, first amendment rights, and fair notice." *Issues L. & Med.* 10:321.

Orsi, Robert A. 2005. *Between heaven and earth: the religious worlds people make and the scholars who study them*. Princeton, N.J.: Princeton University Press.

Padilla, Mark. 2007. *Caribbean pleasure industry: tourism, sexuality, and AIDS in the Dominican Republic, Worlds of desire*. Chicago: The University of Chicago Press.

Petryna, Adriana. 2002. *Life exposed: biological citizens after Chernobyl, In-formation series*. Princeton, N.J.: Princeton University Press.

Rhodes, Lorna. 1996. "Studying Biomedicine as a Cultural System." In *Medical anthropology: contemporary theory and method*, edited by Carolyn Fishel Sargent and Thomas M. Johnson, 165–180. Westport, Conn.: Praeger.

Scheper-Hughes, Nancy, and Loïc J. D. Wacquant. 2002. *Commodifying bodies*. London; Thousand Oaks, Calif.: Sage Publications.

Shaw, Susan J. 2012. *Governing how we care: contesting community and defining difference in U.S. public health programs*. Philadelphia, Pa: Temple University Press.

Sheldon, Mark. 1996. "Ethical issues in the forced transfusion of Jehovah's Witness children." *The Journal of emergency medicine* 14 (2):251–257.

Snell, Marilyn. 1997. "The world of religion according to Huston Smith." *Mother Jones* 22 (6):40–43.

Swan, Rita. 1983. "Faith healing, Christian Science, and the medical care of children." *New England Journal of Medicine* 309 (26):1639–1641.

Taylor, Mark. 2004. "At the Crossroads of religion and medical anthropology." Conference of the Nordic Society of Medical Anthropologists, University of Helsinki, Mekrijarvie, Finland, March.

Tervalon, Melanie, and Jann Murray-Garcia. 1998. "Cultural humility versus cultural competence: a critical distinction in defining physician training outcomes in multicultural education." *Journal of health care for the poor and underserved* 9 (2):117–125.

Throop, C. Jason, and Robert Desjarlais. 2011. "Phenomenological Approaches in Anthropology." *Annual Review of Anthropology* 40:87–102. doi: 10.1146/annurev-anthro-092010-153345.

Turner, Victor Witter. 1967. *The forest of symbols: Aspects of Ndembu ritual*. Vol. 101: Cornell University Press.

Turner, Victor Witter. 1995. *The ritual process: Structure and anti-structure*: Transaction Publishers.

Turner, Victor Witter, and Edith LB Turner. 2011. *Image and pilgrimage in Christian culture*: Columbia University Press.

Wesley, John. 2003 (1747). *Primitive physic: An easy and natural method of curing most diseases*: Wipf and Stock Publishers.

Willen, S. S. 2007. "Toward a critical phenomenology of "illegality": State power, criminalization, and abjectivity among undocumented migrant workers in Tel Aviv, Israel." *International Migration* 45 (3):8–38. doi: DOI 10.1111/j.1468-2435.2007.00409.x.

Young, Allan. 1995. *The harmony of illusions: inventing post-traumatic stress disorder*. Princeton, N.J.: Princeton University Press.

CHAPTER 18

LAW, RELIGION, AND THE PHYSICIAN-PATIENT RELATIONSHIP

O. Carter Snead and Michael P. Moreland

The topic of religion and spirituality in the practice of medicine as it pertains to the law is a broad one, and it is also a topic that has generated a great deal of debate over the past several years. In particular, a debate about the role of a physician's religious or moral beliefs in objecting to certain medical procedures has become part of the larger debate about the place of religious freedom in contemporary American law and culture.

This essay will explore a range of legal and moral issues regarding the role of conscience in medicine, though out of necessity we will touch only briefly on important topics. Our discussion of these issues will proceed in three parts. In Part One, we will survey some of the leading recent contributions to the debate over physician conscience, both those arguing against such claims of conscience by physicians and those arguing for a broad protection for a physician's refusal to participate in or perform certain procedures. Second, we will address the legal issues surrounding claims based on a physician's conscientious objection or other forms of religious expression in medical practice. Such claims are at the intersection of two lines of cases, statutes, and regulations in current law: informed consent in medicine and freedom of religion. In the final part of this essay, we will briefly argue for a broad space for a physician's religious or moral beliefs in the clinical setting by drawing on the work of Alasdair MacIntyre on moral fragmentation.

The issue at the center of our discussion of these issues is what degree of autonomy rests with *physicians* during the medical decision making process, for there is already a vast literature on the topic of patient autonomy.[1] Specifically, we will explore questions about whether physicians should employ religious, spiritual, or moral concerns when carrying out their professional role. Such questions could arise in several ways, including (1) persuading patients to make certain decisions, (2) withholding medical information from patients, (3) refusing to provide certain medical treatments, or (4) religious expression by a physician. The following discussion outlines the pertinent literature about a physician's right to employ these concerns.

CONTEMPORARY CONTRIBUTIONS
TO THE DEBATE

The literature in support of a physician's ability to raise religious or moral concerns focuses primarily on the tradition of viewing physicians as moral agents. The historical practice behind this idea is—but need not be dependent on—a commitment to physician paternalism. Such paternalism is, broadly speaking, the idea that physicians know what is best for patients—not only medically, but also morally—and so a physician's subjective opinions should be allowed significant weight. But notwithstanding the views of critics, even this literature does not advocate for the unimpeded ability of physicians to determine the medical care of a patient based on such subjective factors (Wicclair, 2008).

Most of the literature in this area seeks to strike a balance between patients and physicians. Since the historical practice was to give more weight to a physician's beliefs, many have argued for more autonomy to be given to patients when making medical decisions. A popular recent argument has been that subjective beliefs of physicians should play no role because the medical profession already has ethical guidelines (Berke Fogel & Rivera, 2004; Ketler, 2001; Savulescu, 2006; Swartz, 2006). These commentators generally believe that physicians should be held to purportedly objective professional standards that require religious and spiritual beliefs to be left out, though some allow that so long as another physician is available to provide treatment, then physicians can refuse treatment. Others advocate for religion and spirituality to play some role without limiting patient's options, because such moral concerns may be valuable (Orr & Genesen, 1997; Pelligrino, 1993). Studies have shown that religion and spirituality do play a role in the habits of many physicians, and that some are more likely to refuse treatments based on their beliefs than others. But ultimately most doctors, even those with strong religious commitments, do not endorse changing medical treatments because of their beliefs (Curlin et al., 2007; Lawrence & Curlin, 2009).

There is additional literature on religion's role in the medical field generally, which looks primarily at health care providers and hospitals. These commentators discuss whether institutions should be able to employ the same standards as physicians. Most advocate for providers and hospitals that have religious affiliations to be able to abstain from providing certain treatments, such as physician-assisted suicide and abortion (Boozang, 1995; Doerflinger, 1995; Rizzo, 1996). Some commentators argue against this on account of a commitment to a constitutional right to abortion or physician-assisted suicide, though this is a minority position in the literature (Mitchell, 2006; Stacy, 1994).

Mark Wicclair offers one of the more robust and sophisticated defenses of physician conscientious refusal in his argument against a complete deference to patient autonomy (Wicclair, 2008). Specifically, Wicclair argues against what he terms the "incompatibility thesis," which holds that physicians who refuse legally permitted medical care on religious or moral grounds are neglecting their professional duty. Instead, Wicclair favors a limited right to conscientious objection. He critiques philosophical theories that are purported to support the incompatibility thesis, including a range of general ethical theories (consequentialism, contractarianism, and rights-based theories), internal morality (essentialist and non-essentialist conceptions), reciprocal justice, social contract, and promising.

Wicclair argues that consequentialism cannot support the incompatibility thesis because empirical evidence would support or deny the thesis, as the well-being of patients cannot be predicted in every situation. Contractarianism is problematic as well because there is reason to believe that equal value for the rights of both patients and of doctors would be preferred in a "veil of ignorance" scenario, rather than placing higher value on one side or the other. With regard to accounts based on internal morality, he rejects the view that the essential purpose of medicine, which is healing, is achieved by all possible treatments (essentialist), nor can it be said that the developing or traditional goals of medicine prohibit conscientious objection (non-essentialist). Reciprocity theory does not support the thesis because it would be unreasonable to require a professional physician to abandon moral grounds just because they are part of an asserted professional responsibility. Social contract theory provides little support because a policy favoring the incompatibility thesis would be unlikely to result from the political process—physicians have some discretion under current law, particularly in such deeply contested areas as abortion. Finally, there is no solid evidence that all physicians are required to promise, by choosing to become a medical professional, to provide all medical services without any accommodation for their personal religious beliefs. Wicclair's ultimate objective is a negative one—to demonstrate the weakness of the incompatibility thesis by arguing for how the range of plausible moral theories fails to prove it unequivocally.

Edmund Pellegrino provides a further step in a defense of conscientious objection by showing why physicians deserve a measure of autonomy in the first place (Pellegrino, 1993). Pellegrino argues that the moral beliefs of patients and physicians should both be considered in creating a policy on decision-making, and just because both parties have some degree of autonomy does not entail that they are pitted against each other in a non-beneficial way. Pellegrino certainly values the autonomy of patients, which historically has been neglected in medical practice and bioethics. He also, however, wants to see physician autonomy remain as part of the modern discussion of medical ethics, notwithstanding its recent neglect.

Pellegrino points out that there is always variation in medical cases and so it would be disingenuous to require an objective standard for different patients with unique situations. Likewise, individual physicians deserve autonomy as professionals who are burdened with a significant moral responsibility. Pellegrino calls us to remember that physicians are professionals who have an important duty of care but are also granted discretion in their exercise of that duty, and we should not strip physicians of that discretion but rather remain respectful of that autonomy. This will result in better medical care because medical decisions will be the product of input and deliberation from both parties (physician and patient). The best treatment for each individual patient can be achieved, Pellegrino argues, while also respecting the integrity of medical professionals.

A study by Lawrence and Curlin sheds light on Pellegrino's model in action (Lawrence & Curlin, 2009). It found that patient autonomy is the leading concern for most physicians who responded to their survey, but other concerns are prevalent and sometimes equal to patient autonomy. These concerns were largely moral, religious, or spiritual views about what was best for the patient. Though this runs contrary to much of the modern, patient-autonomy-centered literature in medical ethics, it supports the arguments of those such as Pellegrino who advocate for a balance between patient and physician autonomy. It also demonstrates that physicians do not control medical decisions entirely, and are usually interested only in exercising the discretion given them as professionals, as detailed by Pellegrino.

Katherine White provides some policy suggestions for balancing physician and patient autonomy (White, 1999). She explores and recommends support for three current policies: subscriber notification, continuity of care mandates, and open and direct access laws. Subscriber notifications alert patients when different physicians exercise conscientious refusal based on religious beliefs, in order that patients can choose physicians who are willing to provide certain medical services. This policy has been somewhat effective in states such as New York and Oregon, yet has not been widely adopted. Some concerns are raised that many people do not understand the basics of their medical care plan in the first place. Continuity of care mandates would require medical institutions to provide timely care or make a timely referral. In such instances, if a physician or institution refuses to perform a certain procedure, the patient will receive a quick referral to another provider. White and others, however, raise the concern that the original physician or institution may reject referring as well, because it is contributing to a procedure to which they object. Finally, open and direct access laws allow patients to seek medical care without referrals to work around institutions or physicians who object to making a referral. This too has been successful in New York; however there may still be issues if a patient is in a plan that is within a religious care network. Despite these and other challenges, though, White argues that these policies will allow patients to obtain the treatment they desire, while physicians can retain a measure of autonomy in their rights of refusal.

Elizabeth Sepper expands on that debate by discussing how decision making is affected by the Affordable Care Act (Sepper, 2012, 2013, 2014a, 2014b, 2015). In her works, she discusses the concept of corporate conscience and how the exemption from the contraceptive mandate under regulations implementing the Affordable Care Act has, in her view, expanded the rights of corporations too far. Sepper argues that expanding the constitutional rights of corporations by accepting the premise that corporations have a religious conscience is detrimental to employees in general—but to women in particular—as it will restrict the constitutional rights of those employees. Recent articles by Sepper focus on how the *Hobby Lobby* decision—in which the Supreme Court affirmed a right of exemption by such corporations—has confirmed her concerns, though we believe she vastly overstates the case.

PHYSICIAN CONSCIENCE, SPIRITUAL CARE, AND THE LAW

In order to illustrate the legal issues that arise in the context of physician conscience, consider a straightforward case of a pro-life obstetrician (perhaps practicing at a Catholic hospital, though the institutional setting is a distinct issue). Facing certain cases of maternal-fetal conflict in which some obstetricians might readily perform a therapeutic abortion, this physician would refuse to do so.[2] In such a case, what are the relevant legal questions and applicable statutes and case law?

Or consider a case in which a physician overtly expresses her religious beliefs in the patient care setting. Say a physician prays aloud with a patient after receiving the patient's consent, but other medical staff later complain to hospital administrators saying that the physician overstepped her professional role. The physician's supervisor reprimands the physician, and issues a warning in writing from the physician practice group that future violations will result in termination from the practice. Could a hospital suspend the physician from practicing in the institution, could a practice group fire the physician, or could a state licensing board suspend or remove the physician's license?

Questions about the scope of physicians' rights of conscience are relatively new in bioethics and the law, and this is for at least two reasons. First, patient autonomy became one of the governing principles of bioethics in the 1960s and 1970s, supplanting physician paternalism. Broadly stated, the period prior to such cases as *Canterbury v. Spence* in 1972 was one in which claims alleging that a physician had failed to inform a patient adequately before obtaining the patient's consent to a procedure were decided based on a reasonable professional standard. That is, courts looked to what a reasonable physician similarly situated to the physician in the case would have disclosed by way of the risks and benefits of a procedure. As summarized by the New Jersey Supreme Court:

> The "professional" standard rests on the belief that a physician, and only a physician, can effectively estimate both the psychological and physical consequences that a risk inherent in a medical procedure might produce in a patient. The burden imposed on the physician under this standard is to "consider the state of the patient's health, and whether the risks involved are mere remote possibilities or real hazards which occur with appreciable regularity. . . ." A second basic justification offered in support of the "professional" standard is that "a general standard of care, as required under the prudent patient rule, would require a physician to waste unnecessary time in reviewing with the patient every possible risk, thereby interfering with the flexibility a physician needs in deciding what form of treatment is best for the patient" (*Largey v. Rothman* (1998)).

In a series of cases such as *Canterbury* and *Largey*, courts replaced the "reasonable professional" standard with one centered on the prudent or reasonable patient. This trend was part of a larger movement in bioethics during the 1960s and 1970s that emphasized autonomy in contexts such as experiments on human subjects and informed consent. Again, as articulated by the New Jersey Supreme Court in *Largey*:

> The breadth of the disclosure of the risks legally to be required is measured, under *Canterbury*, by a standard whose scope is "not subjective as to either the physician or the patient," rather, "it remains objective with due regard for the patient's informational needs and with suitable leeway for the physician's situation." A risk would be deemed "material" when a reasonable patient, in what the physician knows or should know to be the patient's position, would be "likely to attach significance to the risk or cluster of risks" in deciding whether to forego the proposed therapy or to submit to it.[3]

Second, technological advances and liberalization of restrictions on such matters as abortion and assisted suicide have also brought new and sometimes morally controversial medical procedures into the practice of medicine, giving rise to a range of potential conflicts between a physician's religious or moral commitments and his or her medical practice. This has resulted in the past several years in a heated debate over a physician's right to refuse to participate in such procedures.

Such conflicts over a physician's right to refuse for religious reasons in performing certain procedures or engaging in religious expression in the clinical setting are also and interestingly part of a debate about religious freedom in American law. The conventional story of the recent history of free exercise claims is that from the time of the Supreme Court's decision in *Sherbert v. Verner* (1963) until *Employment Division v. Smith* (1990),[4] such claims were subject to strict scrutiny. [5] That is, a sincere religious believer claiming that a law imposed a substantial burden on the practice of his or her religion was entitled to an exemption unless the government could show that the law was narrowly tailored to advance a compelling government interest.[6] In practice, such claims were rarely successful, and the strict scrutiny applied was "strict in theory but futile in fact." An Air Force officer claiming an exemption to wear a yarmulke (*Goldman v. Weinberger* (1986)) and a challenge to the location of road next to a Native American burial ground (*Lyng v. Northwest Indian Cemetery Protective Association* (1988))[7] are just two examples of the many unsuccessful claims during that period. In fact, the only successful claims were either in cases similar to *Sherbert* insofar as they involved individually assessed claims for a government benefit[8] or in a challenge to a mandatory school attendance requirement brought by the Old Order Amish in *Wisconsin v. Yoder* (1972).

Employment Division v. Smith was the Supreme Court's effort to bring some predictability and coherence to the entire field. In *Smith*, the Court characterized its free exercise cases as "consistently [holding] that the right of free exercise does not relieve an individual of the obligation to comply with a valid and neutral law of general applicability on the ground that the law proscribes (or prescribes) conduct that his religion prescribes (or proscribes)"(*Employment Division v. Smith* (1990)). But notwithstanding *Smith's* holding that there is no right of constitutional exemption from a neutral law that is generally applicable, later cases, most notably *Church of the Lukumi Babalu Aye v. City of Hialeah*, demonstrate that there can be failures of neutrality or general applicability where religion is singled out for discriminatory treatment or is not treated on an equal basis with similar secular activities. As summarized by Douglas Laycock, "*Smith* changed free exercise from a substantive liberty—a rebuttable guarantee of freedom to act within the domain of religiously motivated behavior—to a comparative right, in which the constitutionally required treatment of religious practices depends on the treatment of some comparable set of secular practices" (Laycock, 2004).[9] Though there continues to be a debate about whether *Smith* was rightly decided, it forecloses most constitutional claims alleging an incidental burden on religious free exercise.[10] [11]

In the wake of *Smith*, Congress enacted the Religious Freedom Restoration Act (RFRA) in 1993, which sought to restore the strict scrutiny approach to free exercise claims. Though RFRA was held unconstitutional as applied to the states and local governments in 1997 (*Boerne v. Flores* (1997)), it remains in force as to programs administered by the federal government. In a series of cases and most notably in the *Burwell v. Hobby Lobby* decision in 2014, the Supreme Court has affirmed the rights of religious free exercise claimants.[12]

Beyond RFRA, there are other statutory protections for conscience and religious expression. Conscience provisions for abortion-related services date to 1973, when Congress enacted the Church Amendment providing that individuals and institutions receiving funds from certain federal programs may not be required to perform abortions if it "would be contrary to the [individual's or institution's] religious beliefs or moral convictions"(Church Amendment, 1973). Many states followed course by enacting similar abortion-related conscience protection statutes.[13] The Danforth Amendment to the 1988 Civil Rights Restoration Act (Danforth Amendment to the Civil Rights Restoration Act, 1988) provided that Title IX may not be used to prohibit or require an individual or institution to perform or pay for abortions. In 1997, Congress extended the federal abortion conscience clause protection to include refusals by Medicaid or Medicare managed care programs to provide referrals or counseling for abortion, and an annual rider on the HHS funding bill—the Weldon Amendment—has, since 2005, required that all HHS funding recipients not discriminate on the basis of refusals to provide, pay for, or refer for abortion (Weldon Amendment, 2005).

There remains a question about how to assess the proper *scope* of exemptions for conscience in particular cases. In recent years, Catholic hospitals have faced the issue of whether to administer Plan B contraception to sexual assault victims in emergency rooms.[14] Principles of cooperation might permit compliance with such requirements.[15] For example, Catholic hospitals have complied with the mandated administration of Plan B contraception for victims of sexual assault in emergency rooms (Sulmasy, 2006).

As to our earlier example about a physician who prays with a patient or otherwise engages in religious expression, protections under the law are more difficult to characterize. Discrimination in employment based on religion is prohibited (as to employers with more than 15 employees) under Title VII of the Civil Rights Act of 1964, which includes adverse employment decisions or harassment based on an employee's religious beliefs or expression. An employer (such as a hospital or physician practice group) must accommodate an employee's religious beliefs or expression so long as the accommodation does not impose an undue hardship on the employer.[16] Whether a physician engaging in this form of religious expression could be protected from adverse employment action would turn on whether permitting such expression is an unreasonable accommodation for the employer.

OVERCOMING MORAL FRAGMENTATION

In this brief concluding section, we wish to gesture toward a neglected aspect of the debate over physician conscientious refusal or religious expression in contemporary law and bioethics. Much of that debate proceeds as if physicians face a dilemma when dealing with cases in which they have a religious objection or wish to engage in religious expression: either conform to one's professional duty or act according to one's conscience. But perhaps this way of framing the entire debate—which much of the literature surveyed in Part I takes for granted—is itself rooted in a mistake.

How should we think about an understanding of medicine and the physician's role in which physicians would frequently believe themselves to be facing incommensurable moral demands? Here we incorporate the arguments of Alasdair MacIntyre on social structures and their threats to moral agency (MacIntyre, 1999). According to MacIntyre, such conflicts of conscience reflect a measure of compartmentalization and fragmentation in the moral life. As MacIntyre argues, we have good reasons—primarily from Aristotle—for believing that

> [B]oth rational enquiry in politics and ethics and rationality in action require membership in a community which shares allegiance to some tolerably specific overall conception of the ultimate human good. . . .What such a shared understanding provides is precisely the kind of standard independent of, not only individual desires, preferences, and wills, but also of the interests of particular groups within the community, by appeal to which rational debate on practical questions can be carried on" (MacIntyre, 1991).

In an essay addressing moral agency and social structures, Alasdair MacIntyre argues that

> [T]o have confidence in our deliberations and judgments we need social relationships of a certain kind, forms of social association in and through which our deliberations and practical judgments are subjected to extended and systematic critical questioning that will teach us how to make judgments in which both we and others may have confidence (MacIntyre, 1999).

What would result were such a shared conception of the human good obscured? First, MacIntyre argues, the "loss of a shared belief in the nature of the good would deprive the participants in debates over particular moral or evaluative issues of a common standard of judgment." [17] Where there is no standard for judgment, more and more conflict will result. Second, such a loss would "strengthen tendencies to construe appeals to principle as nothing more than disguised expressions of desire, preference, and will, whether recognized or not recognized as such by those making these appeals."[18] Finally, and most importantly for purposes of understanding the role of arguments from conscience in our culture, "a new need would arise for norms whose central purpose would be protective: to defend each person from becoming merely an instrument for the achievement of someone else's desires, preference, and will."[19] Appeals to individual conscience that seem to pose a conflict between a physician's religious views and his or her professional responsibilities are, then, the result of a deterioration of the common good.

The heated debate in contemporary bioethics over physician conscientious refusal is, in our view, just one among many such manifestations of a deterioration of the common good and the moral significance of medicine. As the literature on this debate that we surveyed in Part I shows, those who reject a physician's right of conscience in the practice of medicine could benefit from attention to the ways in which posing such dilemmas is itself a question-begging means of imposing their views on the ends of medicine.

NOTES

1. For differing perspectives on the importance of patient autonomy as a norm in bioethics, see Carl E. Schneider, *The Practice of Autonomy: Patients, Doctors, and Medical Decisions* (1998). Oxford: Oxford University Press. and T. E. Quill and H. Brody, "Physician Recommendations and Patient Autonomy: Finding a Balance Between Physician Power and Patient Choice," *Annals Intern Med* (1996) 125,763–769.

2. Much would turn, of course, on the nature of the underlying condition giving rise to a case of maternal-fetal conflict. The *Ethical and Religious Directives* contemplate some cases (a cancerous uterus is commonly cited as an example) where a procedure may be performed with the foresight (though not the intention) that an unborn child will die as a result. *See Ethical and Religious Directives for Catholic Health Care Services, 5th Edition* (2009). Washington, D.C.: United States Conference of Catholic Bishops. ¶ 47:

   > Operations, treatments, and medications that have as their direct purpose the cure of a proportionately serious pathological condition of a pregnant woman are permitted when they cannot be safely postponed until the unborn child is viable, even if they will result in the death of the unborn child.

3. Id.

4. Characterizing the Court's free exercise cases as "consistently [holding] that the right of free exercise does not relieve an individual of the obligation to comply with a valid and neutral law of general applicability on the ground that the law proscribes (or prescribes) conduct that his religion prescribes (or proscribes)."

5. For the most comprehensive and detailed survey of the free exercise exemption cases, see Kent Greenawalt, *Religion and the Constitution: Volume I: Free Exercise and Fairness* (2006).

6. Such strict scrutiny is still available in cases brought under federal or state religious freedom restoration acts (RFRAs), which I will leave to our discussion of available statutory accommodations of institutional conscience. See *Gonzales v. O Centro Espirita Beneficente Uniao do Vegetal*, 546 U.S. 418, 430–431 (2006) ("RFRA requires the Government to demonstrate that the compelling interest test is satisfied through application of the challenged law "to the person"-the particular claimant whose sincere exercise of religion is being substantially burdened. RFRA expressly adopted the compelling interest test as set forth in *Sherbert v. Verner* and *Wisconsin v. Yoder*.")

7. In *Lyng*, part of the reason for the Court's rejection of the free exercise claim was that such claims should not affect how the government conducts its own programs. *See also Bowen v. Roy*, 476 U.S. 693 (1986).

8. See *Frazee v. Ill. Dept. of Employment Sec.*, 489 U.S. 829 (1989); *Hobbie v. Unemployment Appeals Comm'n of Fla.*, 480 U.S. 136 (1987); and *Thomas v. Review Bd. of Ind. Employment Sec. Div.*, 450 U.S. 707 (1981).

9. Note that this does not necessarily require a showing of bad motive or discriminatory intent. See id. at 210:

   The persistent effort to read a bad motive requirement into the *Smith-Lukumi* rules distorts the structure of those rules. Bad motive may be one way to prove a violation, but first and foremost, *Smith-Lukumi* is about objectively unequal treatment of religion and analogous secular activities. The protection for religious liberty under the *Smith-Lukumi* rules lies in their effect on the political process. Legislatures can impose on religious minorities only those laws that they are willing to impose on all their constituents. . . . Even narrow secular exceptions rapidly undermine this interest. If the legislature can exempt those secular groups with the greatest motivation or ability to resist a proposed law, then the effective secular opposition would be left with no reason to continue its opposition, and the religious minority would be left without political protection in the legislature. And if these secular exceptions do not trigger strict scrutiny under *Smith-Lukumi*, the religious minority would also be left without the protection of judicial review. The focus on secular exceptions is thus an integral part of the *Smith-Lukumi* rules.

10. *See* Michael McConnell, *The Origins and Historical Understanding of Free Exercise of Religion*, 103 HARV. L. REV. 1409 (1990) and Philip A. Hamburger, *A Constitutional Right of Religious Exemption: An Historical Perspective*, 60 GEO. WASH. L. REV. 915 (1992).

11. Even accepting *Smith* as settled doctrine, several leading scholars have sought to avoid overly broad interpretations of *Smith* and to limit its effect on such doctrines as church autonomy. See, e.g., Douglas Laycock, *Theology Scholarships, the Pledge of Allegiance, and Religious Liberty: Avoiding the Extremes but Missing the Liberty*, 118 HARV. L. REV. 155 (2004) and Kathleen A. Brady, *Religious Organizations and Free Exercise: The Surprising Lessons of Smith*, 2004 B.Y.U. L. REV. 1633 (2004).

12. See *Burwell v. Hobby Lobby*, 134 S. Ct. 2751 (2014); *Gonzales v. O Centro Espirita Beneficente Uniao do Vegetal*, 546 U.S. 418 (2006).

13. See Robin Fretwell Wilson, *The Limits of Conscience: Moral Clashes over Deeply Divisive Healthcare Procedures*, 34 AM. J. L. & MEDICINE 41, 51 (2008) (discussing state statutes).

14. See, e.g., MASS. GEN. LAWS ch. 111, § 70E(o) (requiring all covered facilities to provide to female rape victims of childbearing age "accurate written information about emergency contraception from any facility, including any private or state run hospital, to be promptly offered the same, and to be provided with emergency contraception upon request").

15. *See* COOPERATION, COMPLICITY, AND CONSCIENCE: PROBLEMS IN HEALTHCARE, SCIENCE, LAW AND PUBLIC POLICY (Helen Watt, ed., 2005) and 1 HENRY DAVIS, S.J., MORAL AND PASTORAL THEOLOGY 341-52 (1949).

16. *See* Ansonia Board of Education v. Philbrook, 479 US 60 (1986) and Trans World Airlines Inc. v. Hardison 432 U.S. 63 (1977).

17. Id. at 100.
18. Id. at 101.
19. Id.

REFERENCES

Berke Fogel, S., & Rivera, L. (2004). Saving *Roe* Is Not Enough: When Religion Controls Healthcare. *Fordham Urb. L.J.*, 725, 728.

Boerne v. Flores, 521 U.S. 507 (1997).

Boozang, K. (1995). Deciding the Fate of Religious Hospitals in the Emerging Health Care Market. *Hous L. Rev*, 31, 1429, 1430.

Church Amendment, 42 U.S.C. § 300a—7(b) (1973).

Curlin, F., Lawrence, R., Chin, M., & Lantos, J. (2007). Religion, Conscience, and Controversial Clinical Practices. *N Engl J Med 2007*, 356, 593–600.

Danforth Amendment to the Civil Rights Restoration Act, 20 U.S.C. § 1688 (1988).

Doerflinger, R. (1995). The Good Samaritan and the 'Good Death': Catholic Reflections on Euthanasia. *Issues L. & Med*, 11, 149, 158.

Employment Division v. Smith, 494 U.S. 872 (1990a).

Goldman v. Weinberger, 475 U.S. 503 (1986).

Katherine, A. (1999). Crisis of Conscience: Reconciling Religious Health Care Providers' Beliefs and Patients' Rights. *Stan L. Rev.*, 51, 1703.

Ketler, S. (2001). The Rebirth of Informed Consent: A Cultural Analysis of the Informed Consent Doctrine after *Schreiber v. Physicians Insurance Co. of Wisconsin. NW. U. L. Rev.*, 95, 1029, 1034.

Largey v. Rothman, 540 A.2d 504 (N.J. 1998).

Lawrence, R., & Curlin, F. (2009). Autonomy, Religion, and Clinical Decisions: Findings from a National Physician Survey. *Journal of Medical Ethics*, 35.4, 214–218.

Laycock, D. (2004). Theology Scholarships, the Pledge of Allegiance, and Religious Liberty: Avoiding the Exremes but Missing the Liberty. *Harv. L. Rev*, 118, 155, 202.

Lyng v. Northwest Indian Cemetery Protective Association, 485 U.S. 439 (1988).

MacIntyre, A. (1991). Community, Law, and the Idiom and Rhetoric of Rights. *Listening: Journal of Religion and Culture*, 26, 99.

MacIntyre, A. (1999). Social Structures and Their Threats to Moral Agency. *Philosophy*, 74, 311, 316.

Mitchell, J. (2006). My Father, John Locke, and Assisted Suicide: The Real Constitutional Right. *Ind. Health L. Rev.*, 3, 45, 49.

Orr, R., & Genesen, L. (1997). Requests for 'Inappropriate' Treatment Based on Religious Beliefs. *Journal of Medical Ethics*, 23(3), 124, 142–147.

Pelligrino, E. (1993). Patient and Physician Autonomy: Conflicting Rights and Obligations in the Physician-Patient Relationship. *J. Contemp. Health L. & Pol'y*, 10, 47.

Rizzo, P. (1996). Religion-Based Arguments in the Public Arena: A Catholic Perspective on Euthanasia, *Compassion in Dying v. State of Washington* and *Quill v. Vacco. DePaul J. Health Care L*, 1, 243, 245.

Savulescu, J. (2006). Conscientious Objection in Medicine. *British Medical Journal*, 332, 294–297.

Sepper, E. (2012). Taking Conscience Seriously. *Va. L. Rev.*, 98, 1501.

Sepper, E. (2013). Not Only the Doctor's Dilemma: The Complexity of Conscience in Medicine. *Faulkner L. Rev.*, 4, 385.

Sepper, E. (2014a). Contraception and the Birth of Corporate Conscience. *Am. U.J. of Gender, Soc, Pol'y & L,* 22, 303.

Sepper, E. (2014b). Reports of Accommodation's Death Have Been Greatly Exaggerated. *Harv. L. Rev., Forum* 24 (invited response to Paul Horwitz (2014), "The Hobby Lobby Moment," 128 *Harv. L. Rev.* 154).

Sepper, E. (2015). Gendering Corporate Conscience. *Harv. J. Gender, 38,* 193.

Sherbert v. Verner, 374 U.S. 398 (1963).

Stacy, T. (1994). Euthanasia and the Supreme Court's Competing Conception of Religious Liberty. *Issues L. & Med, 10,* 55.

Sulmasy, D. (2006). Emergency Contraception for Women Who Have Been Raped: Must Catholics Test for Ovulation, or Is Testing for Pregnancy Morally Sufficient? *Kennedy Institute of Ethics J, 16,* 305.

Swartz, M. (2006). 'Conscience Clauses' or 'Unconscionable Clauses': Personal Beliefs Versus Professional Responsibilities *Yale J. Health Pol'y, L. & Ethics, 6*(269), 277–278.

Weldon Amendment, 108 P.L. 447 (2005).

Wicclair, M. (2008). Is conscientious objection incompatible with a physician's professional obligations? *Theor Med Bioeth, 29,* 171–185.

Wisconsin v. Yoder, 406 U.S. 205 (1972).

CHAPTER 19

MEDICINE AND SPIRITUALITY: A HISTORICAL PERSPECTIVE

Gary B. Ferngren

The intersection of medicine and spirituality is as old as recorded history. It is found in every human culture, ancient and modern. Widely regarded in our own time as an anachronism that is incompatible with modern biomedicine, religion nevertheless plays many of the same roles today that it did in times past, most often in the context of personal relationships. In the last century overt religion has been eliminated from every scientific discipline and every branch of medicine. Modern Western society has undergone a rapid process of desacralization in which religion has been required to limit or compromise its public nurturing and compassionate role in the face of several factors. How the modern world has seen the traditional roles of religion eliminated by medical professionalism, institutionalism, economic systems, and technology is the subject of this chapter. But we shall have to go back in human history more than two millennia to understand how the elements of medicine developed in order to understand how traditional medical care took shape and how religion came to play a supporting role in healing before it gave way to cultural challenges. In the last two centuries, these cultural challenges have divorced healing from medicine and in so doing have unintentionally transformed the healing process into something that our ancestors of a century ago would hardly have recognized.

ACCOUNTING FOR THE MEANING OF ILLNESS

In every culture societies have attempted to account for suffering in general and sickness in particular. We term these attempts *theodicies*. In the ancient world the most common explanation for suffering was that misfortune was retributive. When the gods were angry they sent plague, drought, famine, flood, defeat in battle, or some other calamity, which could only be removed by sacrifice or purificatory rites that would propitiate the gods or spirits by appeasing their anger (Garland

1995, 59–61). Homer's *Iliad* (Bk. 1, lines 43 ff.) provides a well-known example. The epic begins by describing a plague that has afflicted the Greek forces besieging Troy. The Greeks attribute the calamity to Apollo, who has for nine days been aiming pestilence-carrying arrows at his victims, with the result that piles of corpses are being burnt. On the tenth day a seer is consulted to determine why the god is angry. Once the seer discovers the cause, Apollo is propitiated and the plague ends. Throughout antiquity devastating natural disasters, such as plague, stimulated not only popular religious fervor, but also the tendency to look for scapegoats. Thus natural disasters evoked persecution of early Christians on the grounds that toleration of these "atheists" had provoked the wrath of the gods.

The tendency to moralize sickness by rendering its victims sinners in need of repentance was a late development in Egyptian and Mesopotamian religion, but it came to be almost universally held in antiquity that the sick were suffering deservedly because their disease was retributive. A sick person was not necessarily viewed compassionately, but rather as the recipient of deserved punishment. One finds this attitude everywhere in the ancient Near East, including the Old Testament. One does not pity the sick but encourages the afflicted person to repent. This is the attitude of Bildad the Shuhite in the biblical book of Job, who warns Job that Yahweh acts justly. Job and his sons have sinned against him, but if he repents and remains upright in his behavior, Yahweh will prosper him (Job 8:1–10). Bildad's attitude transcends cultural boundaries, and one finds it everywhere in the ancient world (Sigerist 1977, p. 39). So deeply rooted was this cultural prejudice that it hindered the establishment of any charitable concern for the sick.

THE ORIGINS OF PROFESSIONAL MEDICINE IN GREECE

Like so much of Western culture, professional medicine began with the Greeks. (For an extended treatment of much that follows, see Nutton, 2004.) Greek religion was polytheistic and diverse, focused on both personal and public rituals that united each city-state (*polis*) in a spiritual web. It had no defined creed or dogma, and religious belief was a matter of personal choice. With so many gods, syncretism was common and new gods from foreign cultures were easily assimilated to Greek deities and incorporated into the Greek pantheon. In the Archaic Age (c. 750–500 B.C.) the Greeks believed that the gods were active in all areas of life, including the sending of sickness and disease. Alongside religious explanations of disease as retributive punishment that required propitiation, there existed as early as Homer's time a naturalistic method of healing. Empirics, called *demiourgoi*, were members of a medical craft who relied on their accumulated experience to treat wounds and minor illnesses (*Iliad* 11.514 ff.; cf. Odyssey 17.382–386).

In the fifth century B.C. Greek medicine developed from an empirical craft into a profession. Medicine became both rational and empirical in the sense that in place of traditional methods of healing by merely treating symptoms it came to be explicitly based on medical theory, which physicians borrowed from Pre-Socratic philosophers, who had formulated it (Jouanna, 1999, pp. 181–209). One sees this development in the Hippocratic Corpus, a collection of some sixty treatises that were attributed in antiquity to the fifth-century B.C. physician Hippocrates (c. 460–380 B.C.) but in fact are anonymous, most of them written in the fifth or fourth century B.C. Some were written by physicians, others by laymen, but they consistently reject magical or religious categories in explaining disease, for which they employ natural explanations. One theory, which was to become widely influential in medicine, was that of the four humors, which was initially developed by the philosopher and physician Empedocles. The transition from a belief in divine to natural causation of disease can be seen in the Hippocratic treatise *On the Sacred Disease*, in which the anonymous author argues that epilepsy, which was called "sacred" because it was attributed to divine possession, is no more sacred than any other disease, but is the result of natural causes (van der Eijk, 2005, pp. 67–68). Most Hippocratic writers do not so much reject divine etiology of disease as they assume natural explanations and recommend healing by natural means.

Religious healing in Greek temples played an important subsidiary role in Greek life, but it was the birth of professional medicine that constituted a decisive break with religious and magical medicine. No other ancient culture viewed the physician as a distinctive medical professional who stood apart in his medical practice from the world of religion. It is true that Greek physicians claimed the god Asklepios as their divine patron and protector. But the practice of Greek medicine was a secular one, which constituted a different model from that of theocratic societies, such as those of Mesopotamia and Egypt. Medicine and religion were functionally separate. Physicians came to understand disease as the result of natural causes and they employed natural and empirical methods of healing. Along with creating a new professional class, the Greeks developed the first professional medical ethics, which are found in the deontological treatises of the Hippocratic Corpus, such as *Precepts, Decorum*, and *Law* (Jones, 1923–31). Though these works pay lip service to the gods, they are secular in defining the role of the physician, describing such elements as bedside manner, collegial relationships, and the payment of fees. The best-known of these ethical texts is the so-called Hippocratic Oath. Although it is first mentioned by the Latin writer Scribonius Largus in the first century A.D., it probably dates from several centuries earlier. It was, to our knowledge, not sworn by physicians upon entering their profession and it differs in some respects from the ordinary standards of Greek medical ethics by its prohibition of abortion, euthanasia, and surgery. But it constitutes a high standard for the ethical behavior of the physician and has been widely appealed to in Western medicine as providing an ethical basis for the practice of medicine (von Staden, 1996).

Greek medicine developed rapidly after the fifth century B.C. In the Hellenistic period (323–30 B.C.) that followed the death of Alexander the Great it spread throughout the Mediterranean world. The Romans had no native medical tradition of their own, but relied largely on folk remedies and magical and religious incantations. In the third century B.C. Greek physicians began to migrate to Rome, where there was a demand for the services of professionally trained physicians, and they quickly came to dominate Roman medical practice. By the first century A.D. most physicians who practiced in the Western Roman Empire were Greek, usually either freedmen or slaves (Nutton, 1993). Greek medicine-which was based on a humoral theory, as it came to be defined by Galen (A.D. c. 129–216), that viewed health as a balance of bodily fluids, or humors, and disease as the result of the lack of balance of these humors-became the model of Western medicine for more than 1,500 years. It outlasted the fall of the Roman Empire and hardly any systematic alternative was developed until Paracelsus (1493–1541) introduced a chemical one in the sixteenth century. And Hippocratic medical ethics was to influence Western medical ethics down to the latter half of the twentieth century (Jonsen, 2000). But although the Hippocratic treatises created the ideal of the physician as a wise and caring practitioner, it was a non-religious ideal that generally lacked religious or moral elements. Those elements would be added by Christianity.

MEDICINE IN EARLY CHRISTIANITY

Early Christians formulated a view of the human condition in which suffering assumed a positive role that it had previously lacked. They believed that rather than bringing shame and disapproval, disease and sickness gave to the sufferer a favored status that invited sympathy and compassionate care (Sigerist, 1943, pp. 69–70). In the classical world neither philosophy nor religion encouraged a compassionate response to human suffering. Greco-Roman values had no religious impulse for charity that involved personal concern for those who required help. Classical philanthropy excluded pity as a motive for medical treatment. It was influenced by the Stoic conception of *apatheia* (insensibility to suffering) and a spirit of quietism that thought it impossible to improve the world. Hence there existed in the Roman world no virtue or ideal of compassion that was urged on physicians (Ferngren, 2009, pp. 87–97). As a result there were no pre-Christian hospitals that served the purpose that hospitals were created to serve, namely, the offering of charitable aid, particularly health care, to those in need. During times of plague the sick and dying were abandoned, and corpses were sometimes left unburied in order to prevent the spread of contagion (Ferngren, 2009, pp. 116–118). This may be seen in a contemporary account by Dionysius, Patriarch of Alexandria, of the Plague of Cyprian in the mid-third century A.D.

> The heathen behaved in the very opposite way. At the first onset of the disease, they pushed the sufferers away and fled from their dearest, throwing them into the roads before they were dead, and treating unburied corpses as dirt, hoping thereby to avert the spread and contagion of the fatal disease; but do what they might, they found it difficult to escape (Eusebius, 1965, 7:22).

This description can be paralleled by several passages, beginning with Thucydides (Thucydides, 1974, 2.47.1–54), that describe popular reaction to plague in the classical world.

The Christians viewed suffering as an opportunity to provide care for the sick and dying, while at the same time they saw in it an opportunity for personal self-examination that could bring spiritual illumination. While Christians believed that suffering might be seen as God's chastisement for sin, they did not posit a simple correlation between sin and suffering. Rather they viewed it as a means of grace for the spiritual benefit of the sufferer. So universal, however, has been the connection between moral failing and sickness that it has remained a dominant theodicy in many societies, including our own. "To fall prey to a motor neuron disease," wrote the late historian Tony Judt regarding the diagnosis of his fatal ALS, "is surely to have offended the Gods at some point, and there is nothing more to be said" (Judt, 2010, pp. 13–14).

The distinctive Christian contribution to healing was the element of compassionate care of the suffering, which focused on the sick, particularly on the sick poor. The early church established congregational forms of organized assistance for the sick. Each congregation (*ecclesia*) maintained a clergy of presbyters (priests) and deacons, who cooperated in the direction of the church's ministry of mercy. The relief of physical want and suffering was assigned to deacons, who regularly visited those who were sick, while presbyters had charge of the administration of funds. Once each week, alms were collected and distributed among the sick and poor. The Christian church created the only organization in the Roman world that systematically cared for its sick (Ferngren, 2009, pp. 113–115; 120–122). Although infirmaries (*valetudinaria*) existed to treat Roman soldiers or slaves, there were no general or charitable hospitals or facilities to care for the sick in the ancient world before the founding of the first hospitals (*xenodocheia*) by Christians in the fourth century. The Basileias, founded by Basil in Caesarea, Cappadocia (in modern Turkey), c. A.D. 372, was the earliest, and thereafter hospitals spread quickly, first throughout the eastern Roman Empire and then to Rome, where the first hospital was founded by Fabiola, a Christian noblewoman. Hospitals offered care and sometimes (in the eastern Empire) medical treatment for the sick poor, while most who could afford it were cared for in their own homes. But hospitals especially cared for the terminally ill, who had no other place to go (Ferngren, 2009, pp. 124–130). In the practice of ancient medicine physicians refused to treat cases in which death seemed certain. Once a doctor's prognosis indicated that his treatment was unlikely to prevent death, he felt ethically free to refuse to treat (Amundsen, 1996, pp. 30–49). It was then possible for the sick to go to a temple whose god or goddess might heal miraculously. But the healing temples of Asklepios and other gods and goddesses that offered healing denied entrance to the dying, whose death was believed to pollute the sacred space. Only hospitals provided refuge and care.

Given the wide range of specialized early Christian charitable institutions that went by the name of *xenodocheia* (they included hospices, orphanages, leprosaria, and institutions for the elderly), not all cared for the sick, and only a minority of them had the resources to employ physicians. Peregrine Horden estimates that in the pre-1204 period some 23–25 Byzantine hospitals employed physicians. More common were *hypourgoi*, assistants who had no special medical training. It would be an anachronism to speak of a professional hospital "staff." It is for the most part in hospitals in Byzantium (the name given to the eastern Roman Empire after A.D. 476) that one finds physicians at all; in western Europe, except in Italy, there were few physicians in hospitals until the end of the Middle Ages (Horden, 2006, pp. 45–74).

THE MIDDLE AGES

In the late fifth century A.D., after more than two centuries of attacks by barbarian invaders along Rome's northern border (the Rhine and Danube Rivers), the western Roman Empire collapsed in A.D. 493. Its land mass was divided into several loosely governed kingdoms under the rule of Germanic tribes, a nomadic, pastoral people who were constantly moving and seeking new lands on which to settle. The result was chaos and disorder in Europe that lasted for the next five hundred years. Paved roads became impassible, trade disappeared, agriculture declined, and cities were deserted as their populations moved to large rural estates, called manors, to seek protection from marauding bands of barbarians. Roman government disappeared and with it education and most civic institutions. Nearly the entire population became illiterate and Roman cultural institutions were preserved only in monasteries, where monks kept precious Latin manuscripts and maintained a tradition of learning. Medicine, like all other elements of classical society, deteriorated under illiterate Germanic rulers, who were superstitious and introduced into European society folk medicines, magical incantations, and sorcery, which largely replaced medicine based on a Greek humoral model outside monasteries. The Germanic invaders were also attracted to miracles; and miraculous healing, sought at the tombs of saints and other sacred sites, became a common element of the Middle Ages (Amundsen, pp. 65–107, in Numbers and Amundsen 1986).

Greco-Roman medicine was transmitted in a synthesis that was created by Galen. His enormous body of works, written in Greek, was partially translated into Latin, as were some of the Hippocratic treatises, since the ability to read Greek had disappeared in the West. While some physicians could be found who received their training by apprenticeship, the tradition of learned medicine all but disappeared. Learned physicians were literate and educated men who had acquired their medical knowledge from reading books written by Galen, Hippocrates, and other standard classical (Greek and Roman) medical authors. Most were monks. They practiced classical medicine in the Galenic tradition, but also sometimes employed religious healing or even magic. Learned medicine was based on knowledge of humoral medical theory and limited to monasteries or to those trained in monasteries (Amundsen, 1996, pp. 65–107).

Most hospitals in the Middle Ages began as an outgrowth of monasteries. Their purpose was not chiefly medical but compassionate. Hospitals represented the most significant institutional outworking of Jesus' parable of the Good Samaritan in Christian cultures (Lk. 10:25–7). Hospitals were directed to the sick poor, who had no other place to go for medical care. They were often places in which to die. They had chaplains and nursing attendants, who were usually monks. Hospitals differed from place to place. While cleanliness and good care were emphasized in the best hospitals, in some, perhaps many, the care was poor and the cleanliness left much to be desired. The medicine administered was at a low level, given the limited facilities available. But hospitals cared for the soul as well as the body. The attention given to the healing of the soul in later, Western medieval hospitals, which was based on an understanding of the healthy soul's contribution to the health of the body, has been described as an early form of psychosomatic medicine. In the tradition of *Christus medicus* ("the Great Physician"), administering spiritual medicine was the first duty of medieval hospitals. Caregivers were aware of the importance of rest, diet, and nursing care, but they recognized that the "passions of the soul" encouraged cheerfulness (what we would call "a positive outlook" today). Hence Basil considered psalmody important in soothing the soul (Horden, 2007).

Little if any medical training existed in the West. Learned medicine was based on a knowledge of medical theory, which was studied in monasteries. Manuscripts before the invention of printing (c. 1447) were hand-copied. Treatises of Hippocrates, Galen, and other Greek and Roman medical writers were the source of this knowledge. But physicians also studied (in translation) the ethical treatises of the Hippocratic Corpus and integrated it into their own practice within the context of Christian ideals of medical philanthropy and the compassionate ideal of Christian medicine. Even the Hippocratic Oath was adapted to Christian (and later Jewish and Muslim) practice by replacing the names of the Greek gods with those appropriate to each faith tradition (Jones, 1924, pp. 17–27).

The medieval church was concerned with the moral implications of various occupations, including medicine, which were addressed in the confessional literature that are termed *Summae confessorum*. Several *summae* stressed the responsibility not to practice medicine unless the practitioner was competent. One *summa* asserted that physicians must be expert in the art by accepted standards and that simply having a doctorate was not sufficient. Practicing without the necessary competence, even if one were licensed, was a sin. If a physician harmed a patient from ignorance, whether by omission or commission, he sinned. Harming a patient by negligence was also defined as a sin, as was experimenting on patients, particularly on the poor or religious (monks or nuns). Keeping abreast of medical literature and techniques was a physician's responsibility, as was consulting with colleagues when in doubt. Rash treatment was condemned. Physicians in doubt about the effects of a particular medicine were expected to leave the patient in God's hands rather than expose him or her to the danger of an untried medicine. Surgeons in doubt about the need for an operation or about their own ability to perform it were supposed to leave the patient in God's hands. The physician sinned who intentionally neglected to administer an effective medicine that cured quickly merely to prolong the illness and collect additional fees. In the modern world these provisions became enshrined in codes of professional ethics. In the medieval world, which lacked such professional codes, they were given moral force by the church, which attempted to protect patients receiving medical care (Amundsen, 1996, pp. 222–288).

ARABIC MEDICINE

Islam, like Christianity, but unlike classical paganism, emphasized the community's responsibility to those who needed help. The earliest Arabic hospitals were founded in the lands of Arab conquest, modeled on the institutions founded by Nestorian Christians, and based on charitable giving. While they were not as widespread in the Islamic world as in the West, thirty-four hospitals are known to have existed in an area that stretched from Spain to India. The most famous was in Baghdad, the capital of the Muslim world and a hub of scientific activity and scholarship. It was founded in the tenth century by Ibn Zakariyya al-Razi (Latin Rhazes, c. 854–925), a polymath who was notable as a physician, philosopher, alchemist, and musician. The *bimaristan* (literally, "sick place") in Baghdad employed twenty-five staff physicians, who were mostly Christian or Jewish and who gave instruction in medicine. The story of al-Razi's establishment of the earliest Arabic hospital is well known. He was commissioned by the Caliph, al-Muktafi, to select a new site for a hospital. To find the most healthy locale, where the air was clear and pure, he ordered fresh meat to be hung in several districts of the city. Several days later he examined the meat and chose the site of the least rotten pieces for the building of the hospital. It was followed by several other hospitals in Baghdad, the largest of which, al-Bimaristan al-Muqtadiri, became famous for its amenities. Charitable endowments called *waqf* were established within Islamic law, making possible the rapid expansion of hospitals in large cities, such as Cordoba and Cairo. These hospitals were characterized by a high level of medical and administrative skill. Hospital physicians were required to sit for an examination and to swear an Arabic version of the Hippocratic Oath. They were expected to follow ethical standards described in Ishaq bin Ali al-Rahawi's *The Conduct of a Physician (Adab al-Tabib)*, the earliest treatise in Arabic devoted to medical ethics. Arab hospitals included specialized wards, including those for women and for the mentally deranged. While it is anachronistic to call them "psychiatric wards," there were separate sections that treated patients with mental conditions, and they were pioneered by Muslims. Al-Razi was in charge of the mental ward in the Baghdad hospital and later came to oversee several hospitals in the city.

Arabic learned medicine was based on Galenic and other medical texts that had been translated into Arabic. Al-Razi was an outstanding practicing clinician who incorporated his own notes alongside the Greek medical treatises in his celebrated and comprehensive medical text (*Kitab al-Hawi*). The work is not a formal medical encyclopedia but rather a compilation of his notebooks, to which he added commentaries on ancient texts and records of his own clinical experience. It includes his monograph on measles and smallpox, *Kitab al-Judari wal-Hasba,* the earliest treatise on the subject. The *al-Hawi* was translated into Latin as *Liber continens* in 1279 and became one of the most frequently cited medical textbooks in Europe for several centuries (al-Khalili, 2010, pp. 143–151; Ebrahimnejad, 2011, pp. 169–189).

There existed no schools for medical training in Western Europe until one was created at Salerno, south of Naples, in the ninth century, where a *civitas Hippocratica* or community of physicians had settled. The school employed Greek and Latin Christians as well as Jews and Arabs as masters. It accepted all students, irrespective of nationality, and women as well as men. Its students studied a medical course that took five years and was followed by a sixth year of apprenticeship. Its graduates practiced medicine throughout Europe. Students had access to a number of short Byzantine Greek medical texts that had been translated into Latin. In the late eleventh century, Constantine the African (c. 1020–1087), a merchant who had become a monk, brought twenty Arabic texts of Galen and Hippocrates to Salerno. He translated them into Latin, first at Salerno and later at the nearby monastery of Monte Cassino, thereby facilitating the transmission of Hippocratic and Galenic medicine into Europe. In doing so he redressed the impoverishment of medical knowledge in the Latin West (Green, 2001, pp. 3–14).

Before Constantine Latin texts of Arabic works were short and lacked physiological theory. His translations were later adopted by Salerno and the new universities (with an introduction or *Isagoge* by Constantine) as the basic texts of the medical curriculum. Constantine created the first comprehensive encyclopedia of medicine in Latin, called *Pantegni,* a rendering of an Arabic text by Majusi—who was known as Haly Abbas in Europe—with ten books each on theory and practice. The *Pantegni* gave the West its first view of Greek medicine as a whole. It was not until the late twelfth century, however, that the majority of Arabic medical texts were translated. Gerard of Cremona, working in Toledo in Spain, translated some twenty-one medical works from Arabic into Latin, including the *Canon* of Avicenna (Ibn Sina, c. 980–1037), which became a standard text in European medical faculties until the late seventeenth century. As a result of the translation movement, learned medicine in the Middle Ages became increasingly based on a Greek and Arab tradition, since the Arabs had access to more ancient medical texts than did Western Europeans.

MEDICINE AS A LIBERAL ART

In the eleventh century Europe began to emerge from the damage inflicted by the ninth- and tenth-century barbarian invasions of Vikings, Arabs, and Magyars that had caused much destruction for the past two centuries. The resumption of trade with the eastern Mediterranean in the eleventh century opened Europe to the influence of Arabic and Byzantine culture. As new towns sprang up along trade routes, Europe became re-urbanized and education shifted from rural monasteries to urban cathedrals. Cathedral schools developed a broader educational curriculum based on Greek writers that were translated into Latin, which was the lingua franca of educated persons of Western Europe. By 1600 some 60 universities had been created, which offered advanced study and higher degrees in three subjects: theology, medicine, and law.

Medicine and the liberal arts were taught alongside each other. University students first completed an arts degree before proceeding to advanced studies in medicine. From the late Middle

Ages to the seventeenth century medicine was taught as a humanistic subject, largely from texts. Students read Greek and Latin medical classics. University-trained doctors shared a background in the liberal arts in a tradition that had begun with Cicero and extended to Petrarch in the fourteenth century. In the fifteenth century refugee scholars from Constantinople brought Greek texts to Italy and began to teach Greek in Italian universities. Virtually the whole corpus of Galen's works, as well as those of many other Greek medical writers, were introduced to Western Europeans for the first time, and the invention of the printing press by Gutenberg made it possible for medical students and physicians to acquire them. But medicine remained what it had become in late classical antiquity: an art that was taught largely from ancient medical texts. It was not a scientific subject and there was little difference in the way medicine and other humanistic subjects were taught and practiced. Universities produced a large number of learned physicians, who based their knowledge of the body and medicine on the study of the medical classics but who also studied astrology, which was intended to help in prognosis; and they learned their anatomy from Galen.

Many new hospitals were founded in the late Middle Ages. Some of them became among the best-known in Europe, such as the Hotel-Dieu in Paris (founded according to tradition in 651, but probably centuries later), St. Bartholomew's (Barts) in London (1123), and St. Thomas's in London (1170). All were Christian foundations, established by monks (especially Augustinians) to care for both body and soul. They were examples of Christian medical philanthropy. "Receive the patients as you would Christ himself," was the rule of the Hotel-Dieu. "Treat each patient as if he were the master of the place" (Siraisi, 1990).

MEDICINE BECOMES A SCIENCE

It was not until the late seventeenth and eighteenth centuries that scientific medicine began to be studied and conceptualized. Indeed the word "science" (from Latin *scientia*, "knowledge") was of nineteenth-century coinage. In 1543 the Flemish anatomist Andreas Vesalius published his *De humani corporis fabrica* (*On the Fabric of the Human Body*), with fine woodcuts based on his personal dissection of cadavers. The *Fabrica* revolutionized the study of anatomy throughout Europe by replacing Galen's outdated works. Every faculty of medicine had an anatomical theater constructed in which physicians and medical students, as well as the public (who paid a fee), could watch the professor of anatomy perform dissections. But in spite of the fact that the dissection of animals was begun in the twelfth century at Salerno (Siraisi, 1990, pp. 86–91), dissection was not practiced by ordinary physicians, most of whom continued to gain their anatomical knowledge from books. It did, however, change the relative positions of doctor and patient in the iconography of the Renaissance. In the way medicine was depicted in Renaissance art the physician replaced the patient as the focal point. A famous example is Rembrandt's *The Anatomy Lesson of Dr. Nicolaes Tulp*, painted in 1632. Doctors rather than their suffering patients became central to medical iconography; the patients were subordinated to accessories. Although dissection marked a new chapter in the professionalization of the doctor, it was some time before physicians were encouraged to experiment and dissect cadavers themselves.

As dissection became a basic part of physicians' practice, clinical detachment came to be recommended in the place of a doctor's sympathy for his patients. One sees this in the career of the eighteenth-century physician John Hunter. The Hunter brothers, William and John, were both prominent Scottish physicians. William Hunter (1718–1783) was an old-fashioned doctor who took an arts degree. He studied the history of medicine, gave lectures on anatomy, read medical texts in Greek and Latin, and amassed a large collection of coins. His study of the humanities shaped his identity as a gentleman physician. His brother, John Hunter (1728–1793), was a new kind of doctor: a scientific physician, surgeon, and anatomist who did not place himself in the humane tradition of classical letters. He did not take an arts degree, did not read Greek or Latin, and by highly devious means gained cadavers for dissection, including the corpse of Charles O'Brien, the "Irish Giant," which he got for dissection against the latter's wishes by bribing an undertaker 500 pounds to deliver it. Dissection created a moral dilemma for John Hunter, who recognized that it appears brutal and that it dehumanizes the surgeon. He called it a "necessary inhumanity." Even more repugnant to his critics was his use of transplanted teeth taken from poor children for his upper-class clientele. Yet in nineteenth-century Scotland John Hunter was celebrated as the first scientific physician. The tradition of the arts-trained physician gradually declined and the birth of the clinic in France in the early nineteenth century helped to complete the transformation of the doctor into a scientific physician (Richardson, 2000, p. 105).

In spite of a growing secularization of medicine in seventeenth- and eighteenth-century Europe, religion and medicine retained a close connection. This is illustrated by two vignettes, one Catholic, the other Protestant, which demonstrate a similar approach to the spiritual care at the deathbed but with differences that reflect the particular characteristics of each faith tradition. The most famous hospital in Europe, Santa Maria Nuova in Florence, still enjoyed a superior reputation in the eighteenth century. Even with the secularization of hospitals during the Renaissance, which followed the Protestant Reformation, the care of the soul retained its primary importance. In Catholic practice the presence of the priest at the deathbed was crucial in administering the viaticum and extreme unction as the soul was prepared to meet his God. Catholic liturgical practice on the death of a patient was set forth in the hospital's statutes, where the medical and religious staff joined in solemn last rites that emphasized the care for both body and soul.

> When a patient is close to death, we place before him an image of Christ on the cross, and a nurse watches over him, never leaving his side and reading him the Creed, the Lord's Passion, and other holy texts. When he is dead, the head nurse comes with assistants; they take the dead man from the bed, clothe him in linen, and place him on a bier in the middle of the ward, where the chapel is, with a consecrated candle at his head and a lamp at his feet. At the appointed time a bell rings, and the priest comes with a cross. Two lay brothers light torches and the others take the body and bear it to the church, where the funeral service is sung (Henderson, 2001, p. 216).

In Protestant practice the role of the minister at the deathbed was not liturgically defined but was still important, with physician and minister playing different but complementary roles.

> Mistress Smith died a good death, attended by the parson, who ensured that she died on good terms with God and the Anglican Church. The minister managed the deathbed. The doctor, whose profession was, it has been argued, to gain importance at the deathbed later in the century, played only a subordinate role, retiring from the scene two days earlier.

Family and friends were present as supporting players. Because this was the death of a gentlewoman, it may not have been typical of those of the common people. Politics and personal links combined to give the clergy a more central role than may have been typical. . . .[But] Mrs. Smith's death represented a more intense variant of a pattern that prevailed widely. In the homes of ordinary villagers friends and neighbours managed deathbeds. Yet, although the role of the clergy was circumscribed, they nevertheless had an important role to play (Spaeth, 2000, p. 215).

The role of the clergyman at the bedside, whether Catholic or Protestant, not merely brought comfort to the bereaved, but also provided a spiritual framework for understanding the place of illness and death: the knowledge that the time and circumstances of one's leaving the world, like those of one's coming into it, were in God's hands. In spite of the many changes in custom, religion, ideology, and class that marked the period between the Protestant Reformation and the eighteenth-century Enlightenment (Houlbrooke, 1989, pp. 1–24; Porter, 1989), the spiritual framework was still present.

THE PROFESSIONALIZATION OF MEDICINE IN THE NINETEENTH CENTURY

For much of the eighteenth century hospitals remained what they had been since they were founded: houses for the poor that were operated by members of religious orders. Between 1770 and 1830 European hospitals became secularized, particularly in France after the French Revolution, with religious charitable care giving way to secular approaches that included the creation of pathology as a science and with an emphasis on hygiene, experimentation, and the application of statistical measurement to mortality rates. The French clinic, based on empiricist principles, featured external diagnosis, the introduction of widespread autopsy, and the use of auscultation in place of reliance on case histories. Paris became the center of a new movement that saw the hospital as an institution for research, teaching, and medical treatment, and it became the model for hospitals for the next century, and indeed down to the modern era. The result was the gradual abandonment of Galenic humoralism, which was replaced by the theory that disease was a localized phenomenon that could be traced to specific organs. A period of accelerated experimental research followed in the nineteenth century that produced the cellular theory of disease and in the 1870s and 1880s the germ theory that led to the field of bacteriology. The discovery of antisepsis made possible the rapid development of surgery (Jackson, 2011, pp. 91–93; Ludmerer, 1999, pp. 8–9).

Even more than the great advances in experimental medicine, evolutionary theory after the publication of Darwin's *Origin of Species* (1859) undercut the religious basis of Western societies. While Darwin's theory did not make a significant contribution to clinical medicine, many physicians became advocates of evolutionary naturalism, which abandoned belief in God or divine interaction with nature. The widespread adoption by physicians of evolutionary naturalism as a worldview was a factor in divorcing medicine from traditional religious ideas and in creating a new image of medicine as a scientific enterprise. Perhaps its greatest influence on medicine, however, was that it professionalized science and recast society as privileging scientific enquiry over religion (Numbers, 1998).

The professionalization of medicine in the late nineteenth century followed that of other scientific disciplines, such as geology and biology, which had begun earlier in the century. In geology, for example, non-clerical practitioners of the discipline sought to displace clerical naturalists who held many of the university positions in the field. In doing so they dropped all theological references, such as those relating to natural theology (knowledge of God derived from nature rather than from revelation), from their published work in a professionalizing strategy that was designed to allow them to replace "amateur" clerical geologists in the field (Turner, 1993). The new strategy encouraged in the scientific professions a spirit of secularism and a weakening of the long-standing close relationship between science and religion, especially in the expression of natural theology. The medical profession gradually became secularized as well. With the growing dominance of positivistic science in the latter half of the nineteenth century, medicine became even more a science and less an art. In 1910 the Flexner Report, commissioned by the Carnegie Foundation, recommended that American medical schools raise their standards of admission and graduation and that they include additional science in the curriculum. As a result of the Report most small proprietary medical schools were closed and the science curriculum of those remaining was strengthened. As medical schools began to demand of their students a rigorous training in science and devoted their attention increasingly to research, medicine came to insist on autonomy and to distance itself from Christian motives of compassion and calling. Practitioners without formal medical training, including clergymen, who had for centuries undertaken medical care in towns and villages that lacked physicians (Watson, 1991), were excluded altogether from the practice of medicine. As a result of the professionalization of medicine, the traditional Christian framework in Protestant (especially Anglo-Saxon) countries diminished in influence with every succeeding generation of physicians (Harrison et al., 2011).

THE REORGANIZATION OF THE HOSPITAL

Until the last three decades of the nineteenth century the medical care that one could receive from a physician in the home was considered superior to that received in a hospital. Advances in medicine and medical technology rapidly made the hospital a medical necessity, not merely for the indigent but for all seriously ill persons. The hospital lost its association with poverty and charity and became instead the center of medical care. The professionalization of nursing and the introduction of antiseptic surgery during the late nineteenth century led to a vast improvement in the environmental sanitation of hospitals, while the building of public hospitals vastly increased their number. As late as 1873 the United States had only 178 hospitals, including mental institutions, with fewer than 50,000 beds. By 1909 the number had jumped to 4,359 with 421,065 beds; and by 1939 to 6,991 hospitals with 1,186,262 beds. Increasingly reorganized on a public rather than a charitable model, they were governed no longer for the most part by nursing orders and religious authorities but by professional administrators and physicians. As the focus came to be on scientific medicine administered under a public model, the model of compassionate and spiritual care that had historically been the chief focus of hospitals was diminished over time. But it was not until the latter half of the twentieth century that even religiously based institutions were forced to lessen the overt connection between their religious and moral values and the care of patients. Nurses and other medical personnel were hired for their professional and medical qualifications without regard to their religious background (Starr, 1982, pp. 145–179).

THE DESACRALIZATION OF MEDICAL CARE

The alleged impersonality in health care that is often complained of by patients today is the result of many factors: large institutions, such as hospitals and nursing homes, which too often seem impersonal; technology, which promises accurate diagnosis and aid in healing, but is often little understood by patients who benefit from it and who regard it as mystifying, since it is controlled by technicians who operate in a different world of understanding; health care providers whose complex financial statements are difficult to decipher; health insurance providers and government agencies that operate through layers of bureaucracy that sometimes seem impenetrable; and governments that demand greater degrees of standardization and legislate ever more requirements. As many hospitals in the latter half of the twentieth century became corporate entities, often as part of large health care systems, decisions have seemed increasingly to be driven by economic considerations. Delays in scheduling laboratory examinations, constraints on hospital stays, the growth of out-patient care (including even post-operative care following surgery), limits on how much time physicians should spend on their patients—all have seemed to place profits over human concerns. Indeed they are often criticized as factors that dehumanize medicine, as patients complain of the perceived deficiencies of their health care.

In the sphere of public religion the "Protestant empire" that had dominated Anglo-Saxon values for some two centuries no longer retained its unchallenged influence in the formulation of widely accepted societal values. In the latter third of the twentieth century it appeared that religion was being pushed to the margins of society. Increasingly divorced from public life, it seemed to be largely confined to the private sphere as the structures of society reflected the pervasive cultural motifs of pluralism and diversity (Fessenden, 2007; Numbers, 2007, p. 129). As the link between hospitals and the religious communities that had initially founded many of them disappeared, procedures and health care adopted a non-religious model. What had previously been taken as commonalities of mission, symbolism, and compassionate care were now seen as sectarian, and were gradually withdrawn. Catholic and Protestant hospitals quietly placed religious symbols in storage. Hospital chapels were often closed or made non-sectarian (bare and without altars, crosses, or other religious symbols) for the sake of inclusivity or (in many cases) to avoid offending those without religious values. This was true of theologically derived moral values that informed medicine, such as Catholic opposition to abortion and contraceptives. Catholic institutions were sometimes required by municipal or federal officials to abandon their prohibition of practices that they found repugnant. Opposition to the dominance of one theological tradition in Western culture led to the desire to reflect the religious heterogeneity of communities. In Queensland, Australia, patients who were admitted to State public hospitals were invited on admission to indicate their religious preference, which until a generation ago had three options: "Anglican," "Roman

Catholic," "Other." These admittedly limited choices were replaced by a list of what are currently 92 religious and non-religious options. But the cultural opposition to the dominance of a single religious tradition has resulted not so much in creating a syncretistic approach that is inclusive of all faith traditions as it has in eliminating them all. Secular or more vaguely spiritual values have replaced religious ones. Indeed "spiritual" has replaced "religious" in the vocabulary of medicine and religion.

ALTERNATIVE MEDICINE

Concurrent with the growth of secularism in American public life has been the widespread following accorded New Age spirituality that developed in the latter half of the twentieth century (Sutcliffe, 2003, pp. 174–194). The movement drew on Eastern pantheistic religions and metaphysical traditions, as well as naturopathy, spiritualism, anthroposophy, and theosophy, which appealed to the now-fashionable motifs of religious inclusivism and pluralism. It claimed to merge science (which sometimes appeared to outsiders to be pseudoscience) with an alternative spirituality that sought to create an approach to healing that was holistic, based on natural substances, and vitalistic (the view that the body is animated by a life force (Smuts, 1926)).

New Age spirituality became popular in the 1970s and continues to attract widespread interest, even if in a diffused and attenuated fashion. Indeed it has become a component of the spirit of the age (Bivins 2007; Baruman et al. 1981) and has such as been mainstreamed. Because it rejects defined theology and creedal formulations in favor of pantheistic or non-particularized views, it has coalesced easily with modern secularism and has influenced education and the professions, including medicine. Complementary and alternative medicine (CAM) is very much an element of New Age belief, which rejects biomedical ethnocentrism and allopathic medicine in favor of self-healing and self-realization (the two are often intertwined) that are intended to create a harmony of body, mind, and spirit. CAM includes elements of traditional Chinese medicine (TCM), such as T'ai Chi, acupuncture, and herbal remedies, as well as naturopathy, reflexology, aromatherapy, Ayurveda, and various forms of psychic healing. While some of these practices remain marginal, others (such as yoga and acupuncture) have been incorporated into routine medical practice and mainstream medicine (Inglis, 1979).

A growing number of medical clinics offer integrative medicine that combines alternative medicine with orthodox practice, while a high proportion of American medical schools now offer courses in alternative therapies. There is a strong spiritual component in much of CAM, sometimes derived from Hindu or Tibetan roots, sometimes from Native American or European pagan backgrounds. But it more commonly appears as an amorphous patchwork of folk-healing practices drawn from a wide variety of spiritual sources rather than from traditional religious communities. It is well suited to the secular stance of public institutions, particularly educational and medical institutions. It furnishes a vague and non-offensive vocabulary that cloaks the materialism of secular assumptions, while allowing the listener or reader to supply whatever construction he or she chooses to give it. In medicine it provides a sense of reverence that offers comfort and a feeling of mystery when confronting issues of life and death. Candy Gunther Brown argues that it can be equally well adapted to the right and left ends of the social and political spectrum, to atheism as well as religious belief. But more surprising has been its appeal to conservative American religious groups, including evangelicals (Brown, 2013, pp. 227–229).

HOLISTIC HEALING AND SPIRITUAL INFLUENCES

While there is much discussion of holistic healing today, and an increasing call for more personal and more compassionate medicine, the complaints of patients are often heard sympathetically, while the financial means to meet their concerns—by adding personnel or increasing resources—are often lacking. But increased staffing and resources do not necessarily produce compassion. Compassion is a quality that is fully compatible with bio-medicine and with progress in medical technology, but it is not one that grows organically out of either. It is deeply personal and in many (though by no means all) caregivers it is rooted in spiritual values. The removal or minimizing of those values as a result of the secularization of medical care has made it more difficult than in previous generations for compassion to flourish in the care of the sick. Holistic medicine requires care of the spirit as well as the body. The best that medicine offers today grows out of the values that a non-religious worldview encourages: medical positivism and the research that has provided us with our understanding of disease and its cure; and egalitarian health care, which strives to ensure that the finest medical attention is available to all without regard to gender, ethnicity, or social or economic distinction. But the unintentional, if perhaps inevitable, result of the removal of religious values from health care has been to cut compassion off from the very source from which it springs. In many health care facilities today, especially in Europe and North America, care-givers have been prohibited from expressing any personal religious values. Anecdotal examples abound. A nurse in the United Kingdom who had been caring for a patient asked the patient if she would like the nurse to pray for her. The patient complained to the nurse's supervisors, who suspended her "for promoting causes that are not related to health." A nurse who had worn a crucifix as a necklace in the workplace for more than 30 years while on duty was hailed before a hospital tribunal, though on appeal the charge was dropped on a technicality (McSherry and Ross, 2012, p. 215). Such prohibitions in health care facilities deny free-speech privileges that are everywhere taken for granted in matters other than religion. But more disturbing, they prevent caregivers from offering spiritual help based on their deepest personal beliefs. If one's own spiritual values grow out of the personal experience of the caregiver, those values deserve to have a place in caregiving. It is in those values that faith-based compassion is rooted, and it is that very compassion that lessens the distance that patients often perceive as the result of being cared for in large, complex, and sometimes patronizing health care systems. By denying those values space in professional relationships in medicine they become choked off and replaced with vague phrases that are the only ones allowed in those medical cultures that have become unnecessarily sensitive. And while improvements in technology bring about continued progress in medicine, at the most basic level much of the healing process still depends on individuals, especially on the doctor and the nurse, who remain the primary caregivers. Where the personal relations of doctor or nurse and patient exist, there will always be space for compassionate care, spiritual as well as physical (for a fine example see Sweet, 2012).

SPIRITUALITY AND THE HUMAN CONDITION

Finally, in the complex web of health care today, many problems arise that are not susceptible of easy solutions. Some of the most intractable are those that defy medical rationality and economic metrics. They are matters that call not for more or better institutional and economic solutions but for more human contact on a personal level. Two factors in particular are operative here. Religious caregivers often cultivate sensitivity to humane over institutional factors in dealing with issues that arise in personal care; and individuals in the ward often find solutions that escape the notice of those who administer complex systems. I mention, by way of example, two groups—the mentally ill and the dying—for which a personal religious perspective historically has provided the motivation for the creation of compassionate institutional care.

Probably no other kind of illness has suffered from so much misconception as mental illness, from theories of demonic possession to the view that those who suffered from the disease were criminals who had to be confined in chains. The earliest attempts to provide humanitarian treatment of the insane in England were made by two English Quaker philanthropists, William Tuke and Dr. Edward Long Fox, whose Christian convictions led them to pioneer the role of noncoercive treatment of the mentally ill in the early nineteenth century in founding asylums (Tuke founded York Retreat and Fox an asylum in Brislington, near Bristol) that cared for patients in a supportive family setting. Both asylums became model institutions for their treatment of the insane, who at the time were often crowded into horrendous asylums, of which London's Bedlam had long been the most notorious (Digby, 1985).

In the 1960s the medicalization of dying attracted a good deal of critical attention from researchers and the public. Elizabeth Kübler-Ross, among others, argued that death and dying had become a social problem and that the dying were too often dehumanized, isolated, and mistreated by the medical system that claimed to care for them. One study found that in Berlin in 1978 more than three-quarters of the terminally ill in geriatric care were placed, often to die alone, in special rooms for the dying (Imhof, 1992, p. 365). Many attempts were made to overcome the modern loneliness that often surrounds the end of life, but the most successful was the Hospice movement, which began with the vision of Cicely Saunders (1918–2005), an English registered nurse who conceived of the idea of helping the dying as the result of her conversion to Christianity. The idea came to her, she wrote, during a Bible study. She subsequently studied nursing, took a B.A. from Oxford, and qualified as a medical social worker, later working in several hospices. In 1951 she began her medical studies and obtained her medical degree in 1957. She planned the founding of a hospice for some eleven years before she was able to establish a hospice-care institution, St. Christopher's, which she said was inspired by her reading of Psalm 37 in her personal devotions: "Commit thy way unto the Lord; trust also in him and he shall bring it to pass." She sought to emphasize concern for the spiritual, social, and psychological well-being, as well as for the physical pain, of patients who were facing death. Saunders traveled internationally to spread her vision and in 1963 influenced Florence Wald—Dean of the Yale School of Nursing, who worked with Saunders in England—to found the Hospice movement in America in 1971 (Siebold, 1992, pp. 1–27; du Boulay, 1984, pp. 85–102). Since then the movement has spread to nearly every country in the world. In 2009 it was estimated that 10,000 programs had been created with the purpose of providing palliative care to the dying.

Is spiritual concern for patients an antiquated idea that no longer has a role to play in patient care? It is unlikely to find a place in the public sphere today, where religious values have largely been eliminated from health care institutions. But it can and should find a place in professional caregiving at the personal level, where those who hold religious or spiritual convictions can be encouraged to bring their vocational callings to patient care in a manner that allows them to meet the needs of those they seek to help. That indeed is true holistic medicine.

ACKNOWLEDGMENTS

In this essay I draw on several themes that I have touched on in earlier publications. I gratefully acknowledge the kind permission of Johns Hopkins University Press to incorporate certain short passages from my *Medicine and Religion: A Historical Introduction* (2014); and of Oxford University Press to incorporate brief portions of my chapter, "Medicine and Religion: A Historical Perspective" from the *Oxford Textbook of Spirituality in Healthcare*, edited by Mark Cobb, Christina Puchalski, and Bruce Rumbold (2012).

I owe special thanks to Dr. Simon Chaplin of the Wellcome Trust, whose lectures in Sidney, Australia, June 30 to July 4, 2015, provided several ideas for this chapter, particularly for my treatment of William and John Hunter. I am also grateful for the information regarding the religious options furnished to those admitted to state public hospitals in Queensland, Australia, which I owe to my friend Dr. John Pearn, OA, Emeritus Professor, School of Medicine, University of Queensland, Australia.

REFERENCES

al-Khalili, Jim. 2010. *The House of Wisdom*. New York: Penguin.

Amundsen, Darrel W. 1996. *Medicine, Society, and Faith in the Ancient and Medieval Worlds*. Baltimore and London: Johns Hopkins University Press.

Baruman, E., A. I. Brint, L. Piper, and P. A. Wright, eds. 1981. *The Holistic Health Handbook: A Tool for Attaining Wholeness of Body, Mind, and Spirit*. Berkeley, CA: And/Or Press.

Bivins, Roberta. 2007. *Alternative Medicine? A History*. Oxford: Oxford University Press.

Brown, Candy Gunther. 2013. *The Healing Gods: Complementary and Alternative Medicine in Christian America*. New York: Oxford University Press.

Digby, Anne. 1985. *Madness, Morality and Medicine: A Study of the York Retreat, 1796–1914*. Cambridge U.K. and New York: Cambridge University Press.

du Boulay, Shirley. 1984. *Cicely Saunders: Founder of the Modern Hospice Movement*. London: Hodder and Stoughton.

Ebrahimnejad, Hormoz. 2011. "Medicine in Islam and Islamic Medicine." In *The Oxford Handbook of the History of Medicine*. Oxford and New York: Oxford University Press.

Eusebius. 1965. *The History of the Church*. Trans. G. A. Williamson. Harmondsworth, Middlesex: Penguin.

Ferngren, Gary. 2009. *Medicine and Health Care in Early Christianity*. Baltimore: Johns Hopkins University Press.

Fessenden, Tracy. 2007. *Culture and Redemption: Religion, the Secular, and American Literature*. Princeton, NJ: Princeton University Press.

Garland, Robert. 1995. *The Eye of the Beholder: Deformity and Disability in the Graeco-Roman World*. Ithaca, NY: Cornell University Press.

Green, Monica, ed. and trans. 2001. *The* Trotula: *A Medieval Compendium of Women's Medicine*. Philadelphia: University of Pennsylvania Press.

Harrison, Peter, Ronald L. Numbers, and Michael H. Shank, eds. 2011. *Wrestling with Nature: from Omens to Science*. Chicago: University of Chicago Press.

Henderson, John. 2001. "Healing the Body and Saving the Soul: Hospitals in Renaissance Florence." *Renaissance Studies* 15: 188–216.

Horden, Peregrine. 2006. "How Medicalised Were Byzantine Hospitals?" *Medicina e Storia* 10: 45–74.

Horden, Peregrine. 2007. "A Non-natural Environment: Medicine without Doctors and the Medieval European Hospital." In *The Medieval Hospital and Medical Practice*, ed. Barbara S. Bowers. Burlington, VT and Aldershot, UK: Ashgate, 133–145.

Houlbrooke, Ralph. 1989. *Death, Ritual, and Bereavement*. London and New York: Routledge.

Imhof, Arthur E. 1992. "The Implications of Increased Life Expectancy for Family and Social Life." In *Medicine in Society: Historical Essays*, ed. Andrew Wear, trans. Elizabeth Rushden. Cambridge, UK: Cambridge University Press, 347–376.

Inglis, Brian. 1979. *Natural Medicine*. Glasgow: Fontana/Collins.

Jackson, Mark, ed. 2011. *The Oxford Handbook of the History of Medicine*. New York: Oxford University Press.

Jones, W. H. S. 1923–31. *Hippocrates*. 4 vols. Loeb Classical Library. Cambridge, MA: Harvard University Press.

Jones, W. H. S. 1924. *The Doctor's Oath: An Essay in the History of Medicine*. Cambridge, UK: Cambridge University Press.

Jonsen, Albert R. 2000. *A Short History of Medical Ethics*. New York: Oxford University Press.

Jouanna, Jacques. 1999. *Hippocrates*. Trans by M. B. DeBevoise. Baltimore: Johns Hopkins University Press.

Judt, Tony. 2010. *The Memory Chalet*. New York: Penguin.

Ludmerer, Kenneth M. 1999. *Time to Heal: American Medical Education from the Turn of the Century to the Era of Managed Care*. New York: Oxford University Press.

McSherry, Wilfred, and Linda Ross. 2012. "Nursing." In *Oxford Textbook of Spirituality in Healthcare*, ed. Mark Cobb, Christina M. Puchalski, and Bruce Rumbold. New York: Oxford University Press, 211–217.

Numbers, Ronald L. 1998. *Darwinism Comes to America*. Cambridge, MA and London: Harvard University Press.

Numbers, Ronald L. 2007. *Science and Christianity in Pulpit and Pew*. New York: Oxford University Press.

Numbers, Ronald L., and Darrel W. Amundsen. 1986. *Caring and Curing: Health and Medicine in the Western Religious Traditions*. New York: McMillan.

Nutton, Vivian. 1993. "Roman Medicine: Tradition, Confrontation, Assimilation." In *ANRW* II. 37, (1): 49–78.

Nutton, Vivian. 2004. *Ancient Medicine*. London and New York: Routledge.

Porter, Roy. 1989. "Death and the Doctors in Georgian England." In *Death, Ritual, and Bereavement*, ed. Ralph Houlbrooke. London and New York: Routledge, 77–94.

Richardson, Ruth. 2000. "A Necessary Inhumanity." *Journal of Medical Ethics: Medical Humanities* 26:104–106.

Siebold, Cathy. 1992. *The Hospice Movement: Easing Death's Pains*. New York: Twayne Publishers.

Sigerist, Henry E. 1943. *Civilization and Disease*. Chicago: University of Chicago Press.

Sigerist, Henry E. 1977. "The Special Position of the Sick." In *Culture, Disease, and Healing*, ed. David Landy. New York: Macmillan, 388–394.

Siraisi, Nancy G. 1990. *Medieval and Early Renaissance Medicine: An Introduction to Knowledge and Practice*. Chicago and London: University of Chicago Press.

Smuts, Jan Christiaan. 1926. *Holism and Evolution*. London: Gestalt Journal Press.

Spaeth, Donald A. 2000. *The Church in the Age of Danger: Parsons and Parishioners, 1660–1740*. Cambridge, UK and New York: Cambridge University Press.

Starr, Paul. 1982. *The Social Transformation of American Medicine*. New York: Basic Books.

Sutcliffe, S. J. 2003. *Children of the New Age: A History of Spiritual Practices*. London: Routledge.

Sweet, Victoria. 2012. *God's Hotel: A Doctor, a Hospital, and a Pilgrimage to the Heart of Medicine*. New York: Riverhead Books.

Thucydides. 1974. *History of the Peloponnesian War*. Trans. Rex Warner with an Introduction and Notes by M. I. Finley. Harmondsworth, UK: Penguin.

Turner, Frank M. 1993. "The Victorian Conflict Between Science and Religion: A Professional Dimension." In *Contesting Cultural Authority: Essays in Victorian Intellectual Life*. Cambridge, UK: Cambridge University Press, 171–200.

van der Eijk, Philip J. 2005. "The Theology of the Hippocratic Treatise, *On the Sacred Disease*." In Phillip J. van der Eijk, *Medicine and Philosophy in Classical Antiquity: Doctors and Philosophers on Nature, Soul, Health and Disease*. New York and Cambridge, UK: Cambridge University Press, 45–73.

von Staden, Heinrich. 1996. "In a Pure and Holy Way: Personal and Professional Conduct in the Hippocratic Oath." *Journal of the History of Medicine* 51: 404–437.

Watson, Patricia Ann. 1991. *The Angelical Conjunction: The Preacher-Physicians of Colonial New England*. Knoxville: University of Tennessee Press.

CHAPTER 20

PHILOSOPHICAL PERSPECTIVES ON MEDICINE AND RELIGION

James A. Marcum

Within the past several decades, the fortunes of spirituality and religion with respect to their possible role(s) in medicine have shifted from irrelevance to constituting a major factor in clinical practice and outcomes (Ferngren, 2104; Koenig et al., 2012; Lucchetti and Lucchetti, 2014). The demise of spirituality and religion vis-à-vis medical practice is traditionally located, especially in the United States, with the publication of the 1910 Flexner report (Puchalski et al., 2014a). As such, the demise was tethered to scientification of medicine, much to the chagrin of clinicians like Francis Peabody (1927). Peabody envisioned the patient as an "impressionistic painting," composed not only of narrow brush-stokes such as pathophysiology but also of broad brush-strokes such as family, employment, and even religion.

During most of the nineteenth and twentieth centuries, the focus of medicine was almost exclusively on the patient's diseased body part, accompanied with the reduction of human life and health to their material components. By mid-twentieth century, however, the impact of this myopia on the quality of health care was devastating, especially in terms of patient dissatisfaction with health care delivery and with respect to ethical issues surrounding the beginning and end of human life. Theologians in particular inaugurated a movement to correct this myopia by humanizing modern medicine (Barron and Marcum, 2013). By the end of the century, various disciplines emerged including biomedical ethics, medical humanities, and the intersection of spirituality and religion with medicine.

In this chapter, select metaphysical, epistemological, and ethical issues surrounding the intersection of spirituality and religion with medicine are explored and analyzed. The metaphysical issues involve the nature of spirituality and religion, as well as the causal mechanisms underlying their impact on health and clinical outcomes and the presuppositions informing clinical research on their intersection with medicine. A clear understanding or definition of what spirituality and religion, as well as the presuppositions animating clinical studies, is necessary to determine whether they have a causal impact on health and clinical outcomes. The epistemological issues, which are intimately related to the metaphysical issues, pertain to whether empirical evidence from clinical trials investigating the impact of spirituality and religion on clinical outcomes can justify that impact. The ethical issues pertain to how best to integrate spirituality and religion with clinical practice, if they should be integrated at all. The chapter concludes by addressing the main philosophical issue of whether the intersection of spirituality and religion with medicine leads to a humanized medicine that achieves medicine's chief goal of relieving or reducing human suffering caused by illness (Cassell, 2004).

METAPHYSICAL ISSUES

Although scientification of medicine succeeded by mid twentieth century, its success came at a cost—the dehumanization of patients, especially in terms of reducing them to machines (Haque and Waytz, 2012). In a popular analogy, patients are often compared to automobiles in disrepair and physicians to auto mechanics who repair them. To reclaim the patient's humanity, as well as the art of medicine but still maintain its science, efforts were undertaken to re-humanize modern medicine, especially through the introduction of humanities courses into the medical curriculum (Marcum, 2008). For example, the Yale philosopher Theodore Greene advocated the inclusion of such courses in order to sensitize medical students to the patient simply not as a diseased body part but "as a complete human being, with his socially conditioned, yet individual, hopes and fears, beliefs and aspirations, living in a complex society whose forces impinge upon him in many conflicting ways" (1947, p. 370). The result was the development of bioethical and medical humanities programs within medical schools.

Although the inclusion of spirituality and religion within the past several decades represents an important component in the re-humanization of modern medicine, it has been controversial—with some advocating their inclusion and others decrying it. Proponents of inclusion claim that spirituality and religion are intimately connected to improved health and clinical outcomes (King, 2000; Koenig, 2001; Levin, 2002; Peteet and D'Ambra, 2011; Puchalski, 2006). Harold Koenig, for instance, who has spent a career investigating the intersection of spirituality and religion with medicine, champions their benefits for healthier and longer lives. Opponents of inclusion argue that spirituality and religion are not the proper domains of clinical practice for physicians (Sloan, 2006). Raymond Lawrence (2002), for example, claims that spirituality and religion are the domain of chaplains; and, Neil Scheurich (2003) calls for a "separation of church and medicine."

One of the more problematic issues concerning the inclusion of spirituality and religion into clinical practice is ontological and involves how best to define them. Without an adequate consensus over what constitutes spirituality and religion, their impact on clinical outcomes becomes difficult to justify, especially through clinical trials. John Hiatt (1986) identified seven attributes of spirituality that could be used to expand George Engel's biopsychosocial model of health care to include it. The first pertains to a person's concern with the "ultimate reality of things," particularly in terms of the meaning or purpose of something. And, ultimate reality consists not only of the tangible but also of the intangible, the next attribute of spirituality. Moreover, spirituality fluctuates dynamically and evolves towards a particular goal or end-point, two other of its attributes. Another attribute refers to how spirituality or ultimate reality is known, which is experientially and intuitively rather than conceptually. This then has an impact on how a person conceives the world and behaves in it. The final attribute pertains to an "integrative function" that provides unity and wholeness for a person's life. Hiatt then defines spirituality as "that aspect of the person concerned with meaning and the search for the absolute reality that underlies the world of the sense and the mind" (1986, p. 737).

Although Hiatt provides a comprehensive definition of spirituality and recognizes that it differs from most definitions of religion, he does not specifically demarcate it from religion or even religious faith in general. Denise McKee and John Chappel, utilizing a definition of spirituality based on a life's meaning and purpose, do demarcate it from religion. According to McKee and Chappel, religion pertains to "doctrine, dogma, metaphors, myths, and a way of perceiving the world" (1992, p. 201). It represents a socially sanctioned way of expressing spirituality. Daniel Sulmasy also demarcates spirituality from religion on similar grounds, as McKee and Chappel. Specifically, Sulmasy defines spirituality as "the characteristics and qualities of one's relationship with the transcendent" (1999, p. 1002). Religion, on the other hand, pertains to "a specific set of beliefs about the transcendent" (1999, p. 1002). Spirituality is a comprehensive term and pertains to almost everyone, including atheists, while religion less so. Although Sulmasy distinguishes between spirituality and religion on their respective scope, he does acknowledge that spirituality can be "ultimately personal" based on personal preferences.

Recently, Christina Puchalski and colleagues have proposed a consensus definition of spirituality, which was the product of a 2013 international conference on the role of spirituality in "whole person care."

> Spirituality is a dynamic and intrinsic aspect of humanity through which persons seek ultimate meaning, purpose, and transcendence, and experience relationship to self, family, others, community, society, nature, and the significant or sacred. Spirituality is expressed through beliefs, values, traditions, and practices (Puchalski et al., 2014b, p. 646).

The definition is meant to be broad enough to include religion, although the authors do not demarcate between spirituality and religion. The goal of proposing a consensus definition for spirituality is to afford a conceptual means for integrating spirituality and medicine (Brémault-Phillips et al., 2015). Additionally, the definition provides a means for standardizing the role of spirituality in both medical practice and clinical research.

Although apparent consensus in defining spirituality vis-à-vis medicine is available, problems with defining it, as well as its relationship to religion, remain controversial. Scheurich calls the conjunction of religion and spirituality as represented by "R/T" an "odd amalgam" (2003, p. 357). It is such an odd amalgam that Lawrence (2002) calls it a "witches' brew," which in the end simply trivializes religion. In a very important way, both Scheurich and Lawrence are correct; and although spirituality and religion share certain features, they are very different and the differences between them may have important implications for integrating spirituality and religion with medicine and then incorporating them into clinical practice. Lawrence (2002) in particular points out that most physicians and health care professionals are simply not equipped to address the spiritual dimension of illness, as clinically trained chaplains are. For him, the patient's soul is best served by chaplains while the patient's body by physicians.

A major problem with defining spirituality broadly is that the term itself becomes meaningless. For example, Scheurich claims, "'Spirituality' is fundamentally ambiguous and flawed term that can be made to mean anything" (2003, p. 357). For him, the term's meaning is so permissive that even atheists can be considered spiritual (Scheurich, 2003, p. 357). Pär Salander and Katarina Hamberg also criticize the definition of spirituality as too broad, with respect to medical practice. Citing the definition of Puchalski and colleagues (Puchalski et al., 2014a), Salander and Hamberg query, "What is left outside of spirituality?" (2014, p. 1430). Instead of donning the label of spirituality, they advocate simply the "humanistic side of medicine." In response, Puchalski and colleagues admit that their definition of spirituality is broad but not in terms of being meaningless but with respect to being inclusive. Moreover, they note that even the term humanism is often broadly defined but generally limited to the patient's biopsychosocial dimensions. By broadening spirituality's scope, their intent is to include the patient's spirituality to provide "compassionate, whole-person care" (Puchalski et al. 2014c, p. 1431). This raises the issue of the relationship between humanism, spirituality, and medicine, especially in terms of extending the biopsychosocial model to a biopsychosocial-spiritual model, which is addressed later in the chapter's concluding section.

Another pressing metaphysical issue is the causal relationship between spirituality and health, especially in terms of mechanistic pathways. In other words, is spirituality, however defined, an efficient cause for promoting health and treating patients? And if so, what is the mechanism responsible for this causal relationship? Jeffrey Levin addresses the issue of causation using Bradford Hill's nine aspects for determining causality in epidemiological studies. He concludes from an analysis of the literature that there "maybe" is a causal relationship between spirituality and health but "examining the evidence in light of Hill's guidelines or aspects is inconclusive" (1994, p. 1480). Specifically, Levin argues that Hill's guidelines of consistency, plausibility, and analogy support a causal relationship, while those of temporality and biological gradient, as well as strength and experimental studies are "insufficient" for supporting a causal relationship. Use of Hill's nine aspects of causality is at best problematic for establishing a causal relationship between spirituality and health, since a biological or causal mechanism has yet to be determined for the relationship—the next subject.

Several different mechanisms are proposed for explaining the impact of spirituality and religion on health and clinical outcomes (Hussain, 2011; Thoresen and Harris, 2002). For example, Levin (2009) identifies five mechanisms to account for the impact. The first is a behavioral/conative mechanism in which religious faith motivates conduct that avoids risky behavior, such as smoking and alcohol abuse, and promotes healthful behavior, such as diet and exercise. This mechanism may operate through the endocrine and immune systems. The next is an interpersonal mechanism in which a religious community provides social and emotional support. This mechanism is thought to operate by reducing stress and anxiety, which can have deleterious health consequences. The third is a cognitive mechanism in which faith provides a mental framework for confronting and coping with illness. The mechanism may involve affirmation of innate healing capabilities. The fourth is an affective mechanism in which religious faith elicits emotions that mitigate the impact of illness. The mechanism is thought to involve positive psychological states. The final is a psychophysiological mechanism in which faith enhances mental states that influence physical states. The mechanism includes a close correlation between the mind and body. Levin concludes that regardless of the existence of the supernatural, "we can make sense of a faith-healing connection through explanations firmly situated within naturalistic bounds" (2009, p. 90).

Doug Oman and Carl Thoresen (2002) also broach the question, "Does religion cause health?" Oman and Thoresen identify four mechanisms to account for the causal relationship between religion and health. The first three are similar to mechanisms discussed by Levin (2009) and include health behaviors, psychological states, and social support. They also discuss a fourth mechanism that Levin only briefly mentions, a superempirical or psi mechanism. According to this mechanism, "subtle energies" exist that obey as-yet unknown physical laws and that can have an impact on physical events at a distance.[1] The best-known example is intercessory prayer in which a collective or nonlocal consciousness of those praying for others can influence the health of others (Olver, 2012). Although Oman and Thoresen answer the question concerning the impact of religion on health affirmatively, they recognize ambiguity associated with the evidence supporting an impact but are optimistic that further research may reduce it.[2]

A final metaphysical issue pertains to the presuppositions informing clinical research investigating the impact of spirituality and religion on health and clinical outcomes. Traditionally, the biomedical model assumes that disease can be understood by reducing it to component parts. According to the presupposition of reductionism, the properties of a phenomenon, like disease, can be understood through the summation of the properties of the individual parts composing the phenomenon (Sachse, 2007). Recently, however, medicine is shifting from a reductionistic presupposition to a holistic one vis-à-vis systems medicine (Federoff and Gostin, 2009). Holism is generally defined as the whole is greater than the sum of its parts because of the emergence of properties within the whole that are not reducible to the properties of any individual part that constitutes the whole (Freeman, 2005; Marcum, 2009). In other words, phenomena involve the appearance of properties that are not accountable by or reducible to the summation of the properties of its individual parts. Rather, a synergy exists in the interaction of the parts that leads to novel properties.[3] Moreover, a reciprocal relationship exists between parts and whole with respect to causation (Figure 20.1). There is an upward causal relationship between them, where the parts are causally necessary but insufficient for accounting for the whole's emergent properties. And, there is a downward causal relationship in which the whole can bring about change in the parts and thereby have an impact on its emergent properties.[4]

Recently, Christian Smith (2011) analyzed the nature of personhood from a "critical realist personalism" framework. Smith defines personhood as

> a conscious, reflexive, embodied, self-transcending center of subjective experience, durable identity, moral commitment, and social communication who—as the efficient cause of his or her own responsible actions and intentions—exercises complex capacities for agency

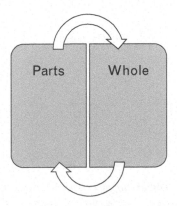

FIGURE 20.1: Relationship of parts to whole in holism. The arrows represent causal relationships.

Philosophical Perspectives on Medicine and Religion • 329

and intersubjectivity in order to develop and sustain his or her own incommunicable self in loving relationships with other personal selves and with the nonpersonal world (2011, pp. 74–75).

For him, a person is a "center with purpose" that emerges from the interactions of capacities, ranging from lower level capacities, such as subconscious embodiment and consciousness awareness of self and surroundings, to upper level capacities, such as creativity, inter-subjective understanding, identity formation, self-reflexivity, self-transcendence, and aesthetic and moral judgment, which can then have a causal impact on lower level capacities.

According to Smith, interpersonal communion and love are the two most defining capacities of a person. Interpersonal communion involves mutual giving of one another in terms of fellowship for the good of each person. The good with respect to human personhood is to flourish and to realize fully a person's potential not only individually but also collectively as a functional community. For Smith, love is not simply a feeling of attraction, especially in terms of self-gratification, but involves

> relating to other persons and things beyond the self in a way that involves the purposive action of extending and expending oneself for the genuine good of others—whether in friendships, families, communities, among strangers, or otherwise (2001, p. 73).

Humans as persons, then, care not just for themselves but also for others and the world itself, through gifting themselves for the good of every person and thing.

If holism is presumed, then spirituality and religion may be conceptualized as complex and multifaceted phenomena that cannot be reduced to the physical, psychological, and social

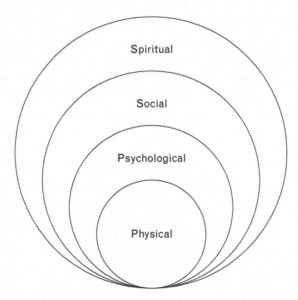

FIGURE 20.2: Dimensions of personhood assuming holism. The properties of included circles are embedded in properties of larger circles, which contain emerget properties not reducible to the included circles.

dimensions, which constitute a person. As shown in Figure 20.2, the core dimension of a person consists of the physical from which the psychological dimension emerges, due to synergistic interactions associated with the structure of the components constituting the physical dimension. In other words, a person's psychological dimension transcends the physical dimension, i.e. the properties of the psychological dimension are not reducible to the individual properties of the physical collectively. In like manner, a person's social dimension emerges from the physical and psychological dimensions. And, finally, a person's spiritual or religious dimension emerges from the physical, psychological, and social dimensions.

Presupposing holism, as illustrated in Figure 20.2, can influence the design of clinical studies on the intersection of spirituality and religion with medicine and the interpretation of evidence obtained from them. For example, methodological design must control as many variables within a person's non-spiritual dimensions as possible in order to isolate the causal element responsible for the impact of the spiritual on physical and mental health. Unfortunately, the problem with presuming holism is that quantifying the parts of the spiritual dimension can be problematic at best (see next section). Moreover, the methodological design and the technology to investigate the spiritual dimension are simply unavailable presently. The challenge for researchers is to develop both new conceptual and technological tools to test the impact of spirituality on health.[5]

If reductionism is presumed, then spirituality and religion may still be conceptualized as complex and multifaceted phenomena but are reducible to the physical, psychological, and social dimensions that constitute a person. As shown in Figure 20.3, the all-encompassing dimension of a person consists of the physical in which the psychological, social, and spiritual dimensions are embedded. In other words, a person's psychological, social, and spiritual dimensions can be explained sufficiently by the physical dimension. Consequently, a person's spiritual or religious dimension is an epiphenomenon, i.e. the result of the physical, psychological, and social dimensions.

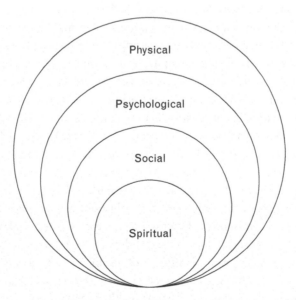

FIGURE 20.3: Dimensions of personhood assuming reductionism. The properties of included circles are embedded in properties of larger circles and explained by them.

Presupposing reductionism, as illustrated in Figure 20.3, can influence the design of clinical studies on the intersection of spirituality and religion with medicine and the interpretation of evidence obtained from them. For example, the mechanisms proposed to account for the impact of spirituality and religion on health and clinical outcomes bear out this influence. Specifically, the interpersonal mechanism reduces spirituality and religion to the social dimension so that their impact on health is explained through social support. The affective, behavioral/conative, cognitive, and psychophysiological mechanisms reduce spirituality and religion to the physical and psychological dimensions so that their impact on health and clinical outcomes can be accounted for through mental states and physiological states, such as the endocrine and immune systems. Even the superempirical or psi mechanism is reducible to the physical dimension in terms of "subtle energies" that are assumed to be subject to physical laws.

EPISTEMOLOGICAL ISSUES

The debate over the definition of spirituality and religion is not trivial philosophically, but it has important consequences for how best to incorporate either into clinical practice or whether they should even be incorporated. Besides the ontological issues of the nature of spirituality and religion and their causal relationship to health and clinical outcomes, there are also epistemological issues, especially with respect to justifying the impact of religion and spirituality on health through clinical trials. In other words, can justified true beliefs be made concerning the intersection of spirituality and religion with medicine? In this section, epistemological and methodological issues surrounding clinical trials designed to investigate the impact of spirituality and religion on health and clinical outcomes are discussed, after first entertaining a brief warning about empirical evidence.

Although evidence-based medicine is the standard for defining best clinical practices, the notion of evidence is problematic. Briefly, scientific evidence and observations are not independent of a particular theoretical construct or background but rather they are theory laden (Hanson, 1958; Harari, 2001). Consequently, scientific theories and the assumptions underlying them can have an impact not only on the design of empirical studies and experiments, but also on the interpretation of the data obtained from them. Care concerning theory ladenness of empirical observation should be exercised when analyzing claims based on empirical evidence. However, this does not mean that claims cannot be made, only that the limits or constraints concerning the robustness of the evidence must be acknowledged (Brown, 1993; Franklin et al., 1989). But it must be emphasized, caution needs to be exercised with respect to the limitations of evidence in justifying scientific theories.

The above warning over the theory ladenness of empirical observation has important implications for clinical research into the impact of spirituality and religion on health and clinical outcomes. Failing to heed this warning can lead to misrepresentation of the robustness of evidence in terms of justifying claims about spirituality and medicine. In other words, empirical evidence can be uncritically claimed to justify a positive impact of spirituality and religion on health and clinical outcomes. For example, as one commentator exclaimed, the fact that "faith can heal" is experimentally justified since "the empirical data speak for themselves" (Levin, 2009, p. 78). Although this commentator realizes that presuppositions, biases, and prejudices can influence how data are interpreted, still the claim that empirical data from clinical trials investigating the impact of religion and spirituality on health and clinical outcomes "speak for themselves" belies naiveté concerning not only the nature of scientific evidence but also its role in justifying scientific claims and theories.[6]

Besides the epistemological problem of evidence's theory ladenness, critics also point out methodological problems with the clinical studies investigating the impact of spirituality and religion on clinical outcomes (Flannelly et al., 2004; Hussain, 2011; Lee and Newberg, 2005; Powell et al., 2003). Among the chief and most vocal critics are Richard Sloan and colleagues, who have identified several methodological problems with such studies (Sloan et al., 1999; Sloan and Bagiella, 2002; Sloan and Ramakrishnan, 2006; Sloan, 2006). Generally, Sloan and colleagues focus on the complexity of spiritual and religious phenomena and the problems such complexity poses in designing clinical trials, especially in terms of controlling the numerous variables associated with them. Specifically, confounding variables such as age, education, gender, race, and socioeconomic factors, if not adequately controlled within a trial, can adversely bias or influence interpretation of empirical results. In addition, they claim that many clinical trials fail to control for multiple comparisons, particularly in terms of outcome variables. Lastly, they note a lack of consistency among the studies on the impact of spirituality and religion on health and clinical outcomes. Interestingly, they point out that lack of precise definitions for spirituality and religion might be responsible for inconsistency among these studies.

Finally, imprecise definitions of spirituality and religion, as well as the notions of health and illness, can hamper interpretation of evidence obtained from clinical trials. If definitions are too ambiguous or imprecise, then what is really being measured becomes problematic along with whether spirituality and religion causally influence health. The issue is how best to operationalize definitions in order to measure spirituality and religion accurately or meaningfully, as well as to quantify their impact on health and illness (Hussain, 2011; Miller and Thoresen, 2003; Monod et al., 2011). For example, Kevin Flannelly and colleagues discuss both simple and complex operational definitions of religion and health in terms of clinical research (Flannelly et al., 2014). Simple definitions of either religion or health generally focus on a single dimension of either, such as religious service attendance and longevity, whereas complex operational definitions expand the number of dimensions involved in the putative relationship between religion and health. The problem with simple operational definitions is that they may fail to account for other confounding variables. The problem with complex operational definitions is that with the expanded definitions—especially with the shift, as the authors note, from religion to spirituality—some other confounding variable not related to spirituality and religion, such as a psychological state of positive emotions, might be responsible for the empirical results.

ETHICAL ISSUES

In this section, several ethical issues surrounding the incorporation of spirituality and religion into medicine are examined and discussed. The first and probably chief ethical issue pertains to whether physicians should be involved in incorporating spirituality and religion into their clinical practice. For advocates, the answer is a resounding yes in the sense of providing comprehensive medical care. For example, Christina Puchalski (2001) insists that assessing and attending to the patient's spirituality is an important element in delivering compassionate care to relieve the patient's suffering and in assisting the patient to find meaning in the illness experience.

> By recognizing that all dimensions of care (physical, emotional, social, and spiritual) are important and by creating care environments where all these dimensions can be addressed, we will reclaim the most honorable of our profession's values: to serve others and to help them heal (2001, p. 18).

Indeed, Koenig (2013) identifies nine reasons why physicians and other health care professionals should include the patient's spiritual history, along with the standard medical history, into treating patients. The reasons range from reducing health care costs to its impact on health care decisions.

Critics, however, are less than sanguine about incorporating spirituality and religion into the clinic. Again, Sloan and colleagues led the charge initially in addressing the ethical issues (Sloan et al., 1999). First, they are concerned that physicians are not prepared to address adequately a patient's spirituality or religion vis-à-vis the illness experience. The fear here is that physicians might abuse their status in terms of proselyting patients.[7] The next ethical issue pertains to the limits of counseling patients in terms of clinical studies investigating the impact of spirituality or religion on health. In other words, if evidence demonstrates that people participating in a particular religion enjoy better health, should a physician accordingly inform the patient?[8] The final ethical issue is the possibility of harming the patient existentially. In other words, the patient might be laboring under the impression that the illness is a result of moral failure and thereby add to the patient's suffering.

Since Sloan and colleagues voiced their criticisms, changes to medical curriculum and practice have been made in terms of integrating spirituality and religion into patient care. For example, medical schools offer courses in how to incorporate spirituality and religion into clinical practice (Fortin and Barnett, 2004; Lucchetti et al., 2012). Also, several instruments are available for taking the patient's spiritual history, including FAITH, FICA, HOPE, and SPIRITual History (Lucchetti et al., 2013; Sulmasy, 2009). Finally, several models have been proposed for integrating spirituality and religion into patient care (Brémault-Phillips et al., 2015; Balboni et al., 2014). Koenig (2012), for instance, proposes the following integrative model.[9] Initially, the physician should take the patient's spiritual history using an appropriate instrument. The physician should respect the patient's beliefs; and, if the physician feels apprehensive in advising the patient, then referral to a chaplain is recommended. If a referral is made, the physician should follow-up with the patient. If the physician feels confident, and the patient agrees, the physician may proceed with caution and sensitivity to the patient's beliefs. At no time should the physician's own beliefs compromise those of the patient. Importantly, the physician should be knowledgeable about the patient's spiritual or religious beliefs.

The ethical issues surrounding the incorporation of spirituality and religion into health care seem intractable, especially with some insisting on including them to provide comprehensive health care while others denounce their inclusion for fear of possible proselytization. There is probably no simple solution to these ethical issues. But one guiding ethical principle that is certainly relevant to the inclusion of spirituality and religion into health care practice is respect for patients' autonomy based on the dignity of their personhood. In the end, what is most important for the inclusion or exclusion of spirituality and religion during the clinical encounter is what is best or good for the patient, as well as for the health care system. The question is not so much whether the physician should conduct a spiritual history, along with the medical history, but rather under what clinical conditions should the history be taken. Only after the health care team determines that taking the spiritual history would provide the patient with the best possible health care and after permission of the patient to take the history, should the history be taken and then by someone qualified to take and interpret it vis-à-vis the patient's illness experience.

CONCLUSION

Has the intersection of spirituality and religion with medicine led to a humanized medicine that achieves the primary goal of relieving or reducing human suffering associated with illness? The answer to this question strikes at the very heart of medicine itself. As Sulmasy (1999) frames the question, "Is medicine a spiritual practice?" His answer is affirmative. For Sulmasy,

> To heal a person, one must first *be* a person. We are all spiritual beings. Medicine is a spiritual discipline (1999, p. 1004).

In other words, patients are certainly interested in having their diseases cured. Why?—because they want to be whole again. But medicine can only cure a handful of diseases. At best, it offers only management for the many chronic illnesses plaguing humanity. In the end, every person must grapple with the existential questions surrounding death and not in the abstract, as Vivian Bearing remarks in *Wit* (Edson, 1999).

Currently, two metaphysics dominate approaches to human personhood—especially as it relates to the intersection of spirituality and religion with medicine. The first is the reduction of the human person to the physical, as illustrated in Figure 20.3. Although this metaphysics provides a powerful means for explicating and controlling the person, its limitations prevent it from providing a comprehensive and effective account of human phenomena—particularly in treating illness and the suffering associated with it. Spirituality and its impact on health and disease, then, are accounted for in terms of physical mechanisms. Interestingly, the humanism associated with this metaphysics eliminates the traditional approach to spirituality as transcending the physical dimension, i.e. the supernatural (Koenig, 2008). Consequently, this approach to humanism results in mechanization of what it means to be a person and it is at root in the delivery of health care that compromises the patient's integrity, as well as dignity, and the quality of care crisis facing contemporary medicine (Institute of Medicine, 2001).

The second type of metaphysics is holism in which the person emerges from the complex network of interactions within the various dimensions comprising a human being (Smith, 2011). As illustrated in Figure 20.2, although a person's psychological, social, and spiritual dimensions are rooted in the physical dimension, they are not reducible to it since novel properties emerge that transcend and expand what it means to be a person vis-à-vis the physical dimension. Indeed, the spiritual dimension subsumes a person's other dimensions, including the physical, psychological, and social. It is not something tacked onto the biopsychosocial model that expands its scope. Rather, it is the foundation for what constitutes humanity in general. In other words, it provides the foundation for a robust and comprehensive humanism. Theoretically, this is why spirituality is so hard to define and operationalize precisely for clinical trials.

In conclusion, spirituality and religion are important dimensions of a person's constitution and thereby important to medicine and its practice, if its goal is to reduce a patient's suffering associated with illness. Medicine then is not simply a science, whether natural, behavioral, or social, but it is also spiritual and thereby humanistic in the fullest sense. If medicine is going to treat patients and relieve suffering, spirituality and religion must be an integral part of it. This is not to say that every clinical encounter is going to include a patient's spiritual history. Obviously, treating a minor wound would most likely not raise existential questions, but treating a patient with terminal cancer might. And so physicians, as well as other health care professionals, must be open to including the spiritual and religious dimension in order to fulfill medicine's chief goal of relieving or reducing human suffering associated with illness (Cassell, 2004).

NOTES

1. See Drew Leder (2005) for discussion of four possible models to account for psi forces vis-à-vis distant healing and health.
2. See also Koenig (2012) for theoretical models to account for the causal relationship between monotheistic religions and physical and mental health. He, too, evokes many of the causal mechanisms prevalent in other models, such as positive psychological states, health behaviors, and social support.
3. An example of holism in terms of disease mechanisms is carcinogenesis. A tumor represents an emergent property of tissue disorganization in which synergistic cooperation among the various genomic, cellular, and tissue parts, along with the extracellular matrix, leads to tumor formation (Marcum 2009).
4. Reductionism is an important assumption for investigating a complex phenomenon, especially for identifying the upward causal pathway involved in its emergence. But it is limited in terms of providing guidance for investigating and explicating a complex phenomenon comprehensively. To that end, holism provides the additional guidance required.
5. A possible vexing problem is that terms like spirituality and religion cannot be defined precisely to design appropriate methodology to test the impact of spirituality and religion on health. Another associated problem is that a spiritual element identified from clinical studies is simply a residual effect of those studies. As Levin and Preston Schiller note, "if it were possible to control for every confounding, intervening, and effect-modifying variable ostensibly related to religion, and a 'religious factor' still remained, what would be the nature of this factor?" (1987, p. 23)—a question for which there is possibly no answer, given the nature of the spiritual dimension.
6. For example, the commentator does acknowledge that theory influences all aspects of scientific investigation.

> A particular theory or theoretical perspective, then, is a lens or psychic grid through which the world is viewed and understood. It is theory, more than anything else, that enables us both to make sense of our existing observations and to craft expectations as to what we will find in subsequent investigations (Levin et al. 2011, p. 403).

He also acknowledged that theories are not so easily "proven" in the natural sciences. If this is so for the natural sciences, as well as for the behavioral and social sciences, then what about a phenomenon like spirituality or religion?
7. But the issue here, as Daniel Hall and Farr Curlin (2004) point out, is whether physicians can remain neutral with respect to the spiritual or religious dimension of health care, especially since the majority of

patients are concerned about it. Hall and Curlin propose that physicians use prudence to navigate spiritual or religious dimensions of treating patients.

8. The issue here is the distinction between intrinsic and extrinsic spiritual or religious motivation (Allport and Ross, 1967; Koenig et al., 2012). In other words, if the patient is motivated extrinsically to join a particular religion for the health benefits then clinical studies must be conducted to demonstrate that such motivation yields the expected benefit.

9. Koenig's model incorporates the elements of the three models discussed by Michael Balboni and colleagues (Balboni et al., 2014).

REFERENCES

Allport, G. W., and Ross, J. M. (1967). Personal religious orientation and prejudice. *Journal of Personality and Social Psychology* 5(4): 432–443.

Balboni, M. J., Puchalski, C. M., and Peteet, J. R. (2014). The relationship between medicine, spirituality and religion: Three models for integration. *Journal of Religion and Health* 53(5): 1586–1598.

Barron, L. A., and Marcum, J. A. (2013). Undergraduate premedical humanities: Relationship to medical school education and graduate medical humanities. In A. P. Giardino and E. R. Giardino (eds.), *Medical Education: Global Perspectives, Challenges and Future Directions*. Hauppauge, NY: Nova Science Publishers, 61–74.

Brémault-Phillips, S., Olson, J., Brett-MacLean, P., Oneschuk, D., Sinclair, S., Magnus, R., . . . Puchalski, C. M. (2015). Integrating spirituality as a key component of patient care. *Religions* 6(2): 476–498.

Brown, H. I. (1993). A theory-laden observation can test the theory. *British Journal for the Philosophy of Science* 44: 555–559.

Cassell, E. J. (2004). *The Nature of Suffering and the Goals of Medicine*, 2nd ed. New York, NY: Oxford University Press.

Edson, M. (1999). *Wit*. New York, NY: Farber and Farber.

Federoff, H. J., and Gostin, L. O. (2009). Evolving from reductionism to holism: Is there a future for systems medicine? *Journal of American Medical Association* 302(9): 994-996.

Ferngren, G. B. (2014). *Medicine and Religion: A Historical Introduction*. Baltimore, MD: The Johns Hopkins University Press.

Flannelly, K. J., Ellison, C. G., and Strock, A. L. (2004). Methodologic issues in research on religion and health. *Southern Medical Journal* 97(12): 1231–1241.

Flannelly, K. J., Jankowski, K. R., and Flannelly, L. T. (2014). Operational definitions in research on religion and health. *Journal of Health Care Chaplaincy* 20(2): 83–91.

Fortin, A. H. VI, and Barnett, K. G. (2004). Medical school curricula in spirituality and medicine. *Journal of the American Medical Association* 291(23): 2883.

Franklin, A., Anderson, M., Brock, D., Coleman, S., Downing, J., Gruvander, A., Lilly, J., . . . Toering, D. (1989). Can a theory-laden observation test the theory? *British Journal for the Philosophy of Science* 40(2): 229–231.

Freeman, J. (2005). Towards a definition of holism. *British Journal of General Practice* 55(511): 145–155.

Greene, T. M. (1947). The education of the doctor in social and moral responsibility. *Journal of Association of American Medical Colleges* 22(6): 370–372.

Hall, D. E., and Curlin, F. (2004). Can physicians' care be neutral regarding religion? *Academic Medicine* 79(7): 677–679.

Hanson, N. R. (1958). *Patterns of discovery: An inquiry into the conceptual foundations of science*. Cambridge, England: Cambridge University Press.

Haque, O. S., and Waytz, A. (2012). Dehumanization in medicine causes, solutions, and functions. *Perspectives on Psychological Science* 7(2): 176–186.

Harari, E. (2001). Whose evidence? Lessons from the philosophy of science and the epistemology of medicine. *Australian and New Zealand Journal of Psychiatry* 35(6): 724–730.

Hiatt, J. F. (1986). Spirituality, medicine, and healing. *Southern Medical Journal* 79(6): 736–743.

Hussain, D. (2011). Spirituality, religion, and health: Reflections and issues. *Europe's Journal of Psychology* 7(1): 187–197.

Institute of Medicine (US). Committee on Quality of Health Care in America. (2001). *Crossing the Quality Chasm: A New Health System for the 21st Century.* Washington, DC: National Academy Press.

King, D. E. (2000). *Faith, Spirituality, and Medicine: Toward the Making of the Healing Practitioner.* Binghamton, NY: Haworth Pastoral Press.

Koenig, H. G., (2001). *The Healing Power of Faith: How Belief and Prayer Can Help You Triumph over Disease.* New York: Simon & Schuster.

Koenig, H. G. (2008). *Medicine, Religion, and Health: Where Science and Spirituality Meet.* West Conshohocken, PA: Templeton Foundation Press.

Koenig, H. G. (2012). Religion, spirituality, and health: The research and clinical implications. *ISRN Psychiatry,* doi: 10.5402/2012/278730.

Koenig, H. G. (2013). *Spirituality in Patient Care: Why, How, When, and What.* West Conshohocken, PA: Templeton Press.

Koenig, H. G., King, D. E., and Carson, V. B. (2012). *Handbook of Religion and Health,* 2nd ed. New York, NY: Oxford University Press.

Lawrence, R. J. (2002). The witches' brew of spirituality and medicine. *Annals of Behavioral Medicine* 24(1): 74–76.

Leder, D. (2005). "Spooky actions at a distance": Physics, psi, and distant healing. *Journal of Alternative & Complementary Medicine* 11(5): 923–930.

Lee, B. Y., and Newberg, A. B. (2005). Religion and health: A review and critical analysis. *Zygon* 40(2): 443–468.

Levin, J. (2002). *God, Faith, and Health: Exploring the Spirituality-Healing Connection.* New York, NY: John Wiley & Sons.

Levin, J. (2009). How faith heals: A theoretical model. *EXPLORE: Journal of Science and Healing* 5(2), 77–96.

Levin, J., Chatters, L. M., and Taylor, R. J. (2011). Theory in religion, aging, and health: An overview. *Journal of Religion and Health* 50(2): 389–406.

Levin, J. S., and Schiller, P. L. (1987). Is there a religious factor in health? *Journal of Religion and Health* 26(1): 9–36.

Levin, J. S. (1994). Religion and health: Is there an association, is it valid, and is it causal? *Social Science & Medicine* 38(11): 1475–1482.

Lucchetti, G., Lucchetti, A. L. G., and Puchalski, C. M. (2012). Spirituality in medical education: Global reality? *Journal of Religion and Health* 51(1): 3–19.

Lucchetti, G., Bassi, R. M., and Lucchetti, A. L. G. (2013). Taking spiritual history in clinical practice: A systematic review of instruments. *Explore: The Journal of Science and Healing* 9(3): 159–170.

Lucchetti, G., and Lucchetti, A. L. G. (2014). Spirituality, religion, and health: Over the last 15 years of field research (1999–2013). *International Journal of Psychiatry in Medicine* 48(3): 199–215.

Marcum, J. A. (2008). *An Introductory Philosophy of Medicine: Humanizing Modern Medicine.* New York, NY: Springer.

Marcum, J. A. (2009). *The Conceptual Foundations of Systems Biology: An Introduction.* New York, NY: Nova Scientific Publishers.

McKee, D. D., and Chappel, J. N. (1992). Spirituality and medical practice. *Journal of Family Practice* 35(2): 201–205.

Miller, W. R., and Thoresen, C. E. (2003). Spirituality, religion, and health: An emerging research field. *American Psychologist* 58(1): 24–35.

Monod, S., Brennan, M., Rochat, E., Martin, E., Rochat, S., and Büla, C. J. (2011). Instruments measuring spirituality in clinical research: a systematic review. *Journal of General Internal Medicine* 26(11): 1345–1357.

Olver, I. (2012). *Investigating Prayer: Impact on Health and Quality of Life*. New York: Springer.

Oman, D., and Thoresen, C. E. (2002). 'Does religion cause health?' Differing interpretations and diverse meanings. *Journal of Health Psychology* 7(4): 365–380.

Peabody, F. W. (1927). The care of the patient. *Journal of the American Medical Association* 88(12): 877–882.

Peteet, J. R., and D'Ambra, M. N., eds. (2011). *The Soul of Medicine: Spiritual Perspectives and Clinical Practice*. Baltimore, MD: The Johns Hopkins University Press.

Powell, L. H., Shahabi, L., and Thoresen, C. E. (2003). Religion and spirituality: Linkages to physical health. *American Psychologist* 58(1): 36–52.

Puchalski, C. M. (2001). The critical need for spirituality in our healthcare system. *New Theology Review* 14(4): 9–21.

Puchalski, C. M., ed. (2006). *A Time for Listening and Caring: Spirituality and the Care of the Chronically Ill and Dying*. New York, NY: Oxford University Press.

Puchalski, C. M., Blatt, B., Kogan, M., and Butler, A. (2014a). Spirituality and health: The development of a field. *Academic Medicine* 89(1): 10–16.

Puchalski, C. M., Vitillo, R., Hull, S. K., and Reller, N. (2014b). Improving the spiritual dimension of whole person care: Reaching national and international consensus. *Journal of Palliative Medicine* 17(6), 642–656.

Puchalski, C. M., Blatt, B., and Handzo, G. (2014c). In reply to Salander and Hamberg. *Academic Medicine* 89(11), 1430–1431.

Sachse, C. (2007). *Reductionism in the Philosophy of Science*. Piscataway, NY: Transaction Books.

Salander, P., and Hamberg, K. (2014). Why "spirituality" instead of "the humanistic side of medicine"? *Academic Medicine* 89(11), 1430.

Scheurich, N. (2003). Reconsidering spirituality and medicine. *Academic Medicine* 78(4): 356–360.

Sloan, R. P. (2006). *Blind Faith: The Unholy Alliance of Religion and Medicine*. New York, NY: St. Martin's Press.

Sloan, R. P., Bagiella, E., and Powell, T. (1999). Religion, spirituality, and medicine. *Lancet* 353(9153): 664–667.

Sloan, R. P., and Bagiella, E. (2002). Claims about religious involvement and health outcomes. *Annals of Behavioral Medicine* 24(1): 14–21.

Sloan, R. P., and Ramakrishnan, R. (2006). Science, medicine, and intercessory prayer. *Perspectives in Biology and Medicine* 49(4): 504–514.

Smith, C. (2011). *What Is a Person? Rethinking Humanity, Social Life, and the Moral Good from the Person Up*. Chicago, IL: University of Chicago Press.

Sulmasy, D. P. (1999). Is medicine a spiritual practice? *Academic Medicine* 74(9), 1002–1005.

Sulmasy, D. P. (2009). Spirituality, religion, and clinical care. *CHEST Journal* 135(6): 1634–1642.

Thoresen, C. E., and Harris, A. H. (2002). Spirituality and health: What's the evidence and what's needed? *Annals of Behavioral Medicine* 24(1): 3–13.

CHAPTER 21

MEDICINE, RELIGION, AND SPIRITUALITY IN THEOLOGICAL CONTEXT

Brett McCarty and Warren Kinghorn

W hat is theology, and what does it mean to consider medicine in a theological context? The term "theology" is broad, and is used to describe a wide array of practices and ways of speaking. Sometimes theology emerges within the practices and language of religious communities as they relate to God or to what they understand to be divine or transcendent. This mode of theology may be called "primary theology (Kelsey, 2009, pp. 12–31)." When Jews affirm that "Hear, O Israel: the LORD our God, the LORD is one," Christians affirm that "Jesus is Lord," or Muslims affirm that "there is no god but God and Muhammad is the messenger of God," they are giving voice to primary theology. Primary theology is not limited to specialized scholarly discourse or even to language, but rather emerges within the context of religious community life and can emerge within unexpected forms of worship, new practices of relating to each other in community, innovations in institutional life, and so on.

Growing out of primary theology, however, is what theologian David Kelsey calls "secondary theology," an "analytically descriptive, critical, and revisionary practice" that seeks to clarify the work of primary theology in changing cultural, historical, and religious contexts (Kelsey, 2009, p. 21). Secondary theology is speech that reflects upon God's (or the gods') nature, the way that God is present in the world and to humans, and the implications of God's presence and activity in the world for all forms of human presence and activity before God. It is discourse about God (or gods; Griffiths, 2016), and is generally what people do who consider themselves "theologians." But secondary theology takes a wide range of disciplinary and methodological forms. Scholars interested in the practices of religious communities, for example, may describe their work as practical theology, though their methods may be very similar to sociology or anthropology. Scholars interested in the development of religious doctrines over time may describe their work as historical theology, though their methods may resemble those of intellectual and cultural history. Similarly, moral theology may draw upon ethics; philosophical theology may draw upon philosophy and metaphysics; biblical theology may draw heavily on particular models of scriptural interpretation. At other times, theology is associated with a particular moral aim or purpose, as in liberation theology. At still others, theology is denoted insofar as it originates within and reflects the interests of particular communities, as in Black, feminist, womanist, *mujerista*, deaf, and queer theologies. In yet others, theology is denoted insofar as it meets a particular functional role in religious life, as in liturgical, sacramental, or pastoral theology. Furthermore, scholars who are speaking or writing from any discipline can participate in the work of secondary theology insofar as they specifically and meaningfully reflect on the difference that God makes (or gods make) for the discipline's work.

In this chapter we argue that theology—especially "primary theology" that emerges within the practices of religious communities in particular historical and cultural contexts—has been influential, and continues to be influential, in the development of medical and health-related practices and institutions. As communities of faith have grappled over time with how best to serve the needs of those who are sick, they have altered the contexts within which health care is understood and practiced, sometimes in innovative and transformative ways. Though this work of "primary theology" has often preceded the discursive activity of "secondary theology"— that is, over time the work of Jewish, Christian, and Muslim healers and communities has preceded that of theologians reflecting on the precise meanings of health and healing—we nonetheless argue that "secondary theology" has also been important both for narrating the work of primary theology and also for informing future practices.

Our argument in this chapter is threefold. First, after briefly considering two common but insufficient ways that theology is used within contemporary religion-and-medicine conversations, we argue that in the past theology has informed the contexts within which influential medical institutions and practices, including the hospital itself, have developed. Second, we will argue that theology continues to inform contexts of health care in the present, most obviously in the case of "faith-based" institutions and programs but also, more subtly, in nonsectarian, "secular" medicine. Finally, turning to prescription and recommendation, we will discuss several ways that clinicians, patients, and scholars of medicine and health care might draw more deeply on theological context to inform future moral commitments, practices, and institutions in health care.

Before we begin, it is important to note that theology—both primary and secondary theology—is never done in the abstract, but rather in particular cultural, historical, and religious contexts. Every theologian, including each of us, writes within a particular context. The authors interpret our own Christian context to mean that when we say "God," we speak of a three-in-one unity of Father, Son, and Holy Spirit who (among many other things) creates all that is and calls it good, who unites Godself to human nature in the person of Jesus Christ, and who in Christ has defeated sin and death and beckons all creation into God's peace. Someone performing Jewish or Islamic theology would interpret God's nature and God's action in creation in differing ways, though also with some shared monotheistic similarities. In this essay we do not seek to adjudicate among different religious traditions, nor to set forth a detailed account of Christian theology. But we do acknowledge that although we will discuss Jewish and Muslim as well as Christian examples in this chapter, our own Christian context shapes our interpretation of how theology might inform practices of medicine and health care.

TWO INSUFFICIENT USES OF THEOLOGY IN HEALTH CARE

In order to clarify how theology has provided and can continue to provide meaningful contexts for health care practices and institutions, we first will describe and then set aside two common modern uses of theology with respect to medicine that we take to be important but insufficient.

First, theology often is thought to contribute to medicine insofar as it provides positive content for the "spirituality" of patients and clinicians, where spirituality is understood as a content-neutral, individual human capacity, as in the often-cited Association of American Medical Colleges formulation that spirituality is "expressed in an individual's search for ultimate meaning through participation in religion and/or belief in God, family, naturalism, rationalism, humanism and the arts" (Medical School Objectives Project, 1999). This articulation treats "spirituality" as somehow prior to theology or religion, as if theology (or "religion or belief in God") were simply colorful frosting applied to an already-baked "spirituality" cake (Hall et al., 2004). But this is inadequate. Theology does not simply provide content for an individual's "spirituality." Rather, the very idea that "spirituality" could be "expressed in an individual's search for ultimate meaning" *already* displays theological commitments, common within liberal protestant Christian theology since the 19th century, that human life can be meaningful, that "ultimate meaning" is a worthwhile object of pursuit, and that human subjectivity is a valid locus for such a search (Lindbeck, 1984). In our view, then, theology does more than contribute to the content of spirituality; it rather shapes the meaningfulness of "spirituality" as a concept.

Second, theology often shows up in health care and medicine in the context of contentious disputes about the proper allocation of health care resources and about the appropriate limits of medical technology. Political debates about research on stem cells, abortion, physician-assisted suicide, end-of-life care, and reproductive technology have long been influenced by theological claims. Often, in these cases, theology seems to play a negative or cautionary role, a roadblock to medical "progress." And indeed theology does play an important role in these debates, and others. Particularly for people formed in religious communities and shaped by religious traditions, theology plays an important role in the formation of conscience. It would be a mistake, however, to assume that theology informs medicine and health care only in these contentious limit-situations, or that theological postures to medicine and medical technology are primarily cautionary or obstructionist. Indeed, we will show that just the opposite has often been the case.

HOW THEOLOGY HAS SHAPED THE CONTEXTS OF HEALTH CARE

In order to understand the ways in which theology has shaped both the vision and the practice of health care, we begin with fundamental theological claims that, in their interpretation, have proven deeply influential in the history of Western medicine (a history informed largely, but not exclusively, within predominantly Christian cultures). The proclamation "Hear, O Israel: the LORD our God, the LORD is one" (Deut. 6:4) is the opening line of what is known within

Judaism as the Shema, a prayer that begins and ends each day for the faithful. An injunction immediately follows: "You shall love the LORD your God with all your heart, and with all your soul, and with all your might" (Deut. 6:5). Famously, Jesus is recorded as having paired this command in Deuteronomy with the admonition, "You shall love your neighbor as yourself" (Lev. 19:18). "On these two commandments," Jesus said, "hang all the law and the prophets" (Matt. 22:40). The evangelist Luke (himself, by tradition, a physician) reports that when a lawyer pressed Jesus to clarify his claim by asking, "And who is my neighbor?" (Luke 10:29), Jesus answered with a story that resonates within the history of Western medicine down to the present day:

> Jesus replied, "A man was going down from Jerusalem to Jericho, and fell into the hands of robbers, who stripped him, beat him, and went away, leaving him half dead. Now by chance a priest was going down that road; and when he saw him, he passed by on the other side. So likewise a Levite, when he came to the place and saw him, passed by on the other side. But a Samaritan while travelling came near him; and when he saw him, he was moved with pity. He went to him and bandaged his wounds, having poured oil and wine on them. Then he put him on his own animal, brought him to an inn, and took care of him. The next day he took out two denarii, gave them to the innkeeper, and said, 'Take care of him; and when I come back, I will repay you whatever more you spend.' Which of these three, do you think, was a neighbor to the man who fell into the hands of the robbers?" He said, "The one who showed him mercy." Jesus said to him, "Go and do likewise" (Luke 10:30–37, NRSV).

Characteristic of Jesus' teaching, this "parable of the Good Samaritan" challenged established religious, political, and ethnic hierarchies of his time, and proclaimed that radical hospitality—including medical care for those who are sick and ostracized—is inseparable from loving God fully and loving one's neighbor as oneself. Jesus intensifies this connection even further when he proclaims that taking care of "the least of these," which includes the sick, is actually caring for Jesus himself (Matthew 25:31–46).

Between the fragmentary nature of the ancient historical record and the rootedness of primary theology in practices rather than texts, we do not know exactly how early Christians (many of them Jews, and all drawing on Jewish moral and prophetic teaching) reflected on Jesus' teaching as they developed new practices of care for those who were sick. But it is well-documented that Christians distinguished themselves within the late Roman Empire by the way that they cared for victims of various plagues who were left to die by Roman elites fleeing the contagion. As historian Gary Ferngren has argued, early Christians risked their own health and safety to care for victims of plagues, serving "the least of these" as if they served Jesus himself. Indeed, as Ferngren contends, in their care for those who were marginalized, Christians pioneered a new concept of philanthropy that was devoted not to the glory of cities and their populations (and, reflexively, of the philanthropist) but rather to the well-being of "the poor" and "the sick" (Ferngren, 2009). In fact, historian Peter Brown goes so far as to say that Christians "invented the poor" in their practices of care for the destitute, who had previously been invisible in the Greco-Roman world (Brown, 2002, p. 8).

As noted earlier, this radical hospitality has deeply Jewish roots, and these Jewish and Christian practices of care did not go unnoticed by the emperor Julian, who sought in the fourth century to reestablish worship of the Roman pantheon of gods in an empire that was becoming predominantly Christian. Julian recognized the witness of Jewish and Christian care as a threat to

Greco-Roman religious practices, saying, "For it is disgraceful that, when no Jew ever has to beg, and the impious Galileans [the Christians] support not only their own poor but ours as well, all men see that our people lack aid from us [that is, from the pagan priesthood]" (Brown, 2002, p. 2). Julian sought to combat this charity by funding pagan temples to care for the poor, but in so doing he became one of the first examples of how the witness of theological commitments can transform a wider society's moral vision and vocabulary of care. Because of the theological trajectory begun in the Jewish law and the prophets and intensified with Jesus' admonition to "go and do likewise," Roman emperors now thought in terms of categories and institutions with distinctly theological origins.

The emperor Julian was acting in response to the rise of institutions known as *xenodocheia* and *ptôchotropheia* ("houses for strangers" and places for "nourishing the poor"), institutions set up to care for poor travelers in need of shelter and care (Brown, 2002). These Christian institutions were a loose network of hostels established to provide the kind of care offered by the Good Samaritan and the innkeeper in Jesus' parable. Shortly after Julian wrote about the care offered by these "impious Galileans," a Christian bishop, Basil of Caesarea, provided a further institutional innovation that has proved decisive for the history and practice of medicine. Basil, who had received a classical education alongside Julian in Athens, founded what many consider to be the first hospital, a space marked by the combination of professional medical care, inpatient facilities, and charitable care (Crislip, 2005, pp. 100–142). In bringing these three aspects together, Basil was both institutionally innovative and theologically creative. By combining professional medical care with the institutional models of the *xenodocheia* and *ptôchotropheia*, Basil united Jesus' admonition to care for the sick, as seen in Matthew 25, with the emphasis on hospitality found in the parable of the Good Samaritan.

In Western Europe, this theological innovation in medical care was carried forward in monasteries governed by the *Rule of St. Benedict*, written by Benedict of Nursia in the middle of the 6th century CE. This short but influential document has animated Western monasticism for nearly 1,500 years, and in it we see an explicit identification of the sick and the stranger with the person of Christ. "Care of the sick," Benedict says, "must rank above and before all else, so they may be served truly as Christ, for he said, 'I was sick and you visited me' (Matt. 25:36), and, 'What you did for one of these least brothers you did for me' (Matt. 25:40)" (Benedict, 1981, ch. 36). Similarly, "All guests who present themselves are to be welcomed as Christ, for he himself will say, 'I was a stranger and you welcomed me' (Matt. 25:35)" (Benedict, 1981, ch. 53). Throughout the centuries, seeing service to the sick and stranger as service to Christ has provided a crucial theological vision of and influence on the practice of medicine.

Theologically informed health care innovation has not been confined to Christianity. Examples within Islam display important similarities as well as differences. By the end of his life, the Prophet Muhammad had organized his community in such a way that submission to Allah was working itself out in all aspects of life, including political life. Because of this, political leaders were expected to attend to the bodily health of those whom they governed. We can see this theopolitical trajectory on display in the development of the Islamic hospital, known by the Persian name *bīmāristān* ("place for the sick"). These hospitals were generally larger and more organized than their Christian counterparts, and they were often founded by an endowment (*waqf*) set aside by the ruling elite. In a typical *bīmāristān*, medical care was provided by well-trained medical experts in an institution with less overt religious practices than in an analogous Christian hospital. Both

Christian and Islamic medical institutions display the way that practices were formed within particular theological contexts: Christian medical practices developed in a theological context that marked a tension between current society and the in-breaking kingdom of God, whereas Islamic (especially Sunni) thought fostered medical practices with less overtly theological underpinnings because they originated in a society that understood itself as integrated in its submission to Allah. The Islamic hospital was inspired in part by Christian precursors, and the *bīmāristān* also influenced later Byzantine Christian hospitals in both scope and organization (Dols, 1987; Pormann and Savage-Smith, 2007; Risse, 1999, pp. 125–130).

The fact that theological commitments inspired new health care practices and institutions in the early centuries of Christianity and Islam, however, does not mean that all such practices and institutions were good or healthy. Indeed, some of the characteristics of modern health care that are considered harmful also find historical roots in the early centuries of Christian medical care. While Basil of Caesarea's hospital did indeed offer an innovative expression of theological concerns for radical hospitality and care for the sick, it also was remembered for the ways it removed from public sight "the terrible and piteous spectacle of men who are living corpses" (Crislip, 2005, p. 115). This mixed legacy was not limited to the earliest Christian hospitals. The Priory of St. Mary of Bethlehem in London was founded in 1247 by a Christian monastic order as a site of hospitality and by 1403 had become one of the first institutions in Europe providing residential care to persons with mental illness—but it was founded within the dubious social context of the Crusades and even in the 1400s was beginning to develop confinement practices that would in later centuries contribute to its notoriety as "Bedlam" (Porter, 1997). Guenter Risse explores this legacy by devoting an entire chapter of his history of the hospital to examining "Hospitals as Segregation and Confinement Tools," as Christian religious institutions were mobilized for hundreds of years as sites of containing bodies suffering from leprosy or the plague (Risse, 1999, pp. 167–229).

Institutional and social developments like these did not develop *in spite of* theological commitments but rather, in many cases, *in the context of* them. Indeed, historians and theorists of culture have argued that deep-seated theological commitments can be traced within cultural practices and assumptions that do not seem to be explicitly theological at all. Philosopher Charles Taylor, for example, argues that in the religious and political milieu known as the Protestant Reformation in the 1500s, northern Europeans increasingly expected individuals to display ordered, holy lives not only within monastic orders, but rather throughout all of society. Taylor argues that this reformist zeal resulted in "the rise of the disciplinary society" (Taylor, 2007, pp. 90–145). Drawing from the work of Michel Foucault and others, Taylor describes how active state intervention, drawing on the theological roots of the Reformation, worked to mold populations into subjects fit for the ambitions of emerging nation states. These governmental efforts combined with a Protestant emphasis on the sacred importance of ordinary life to create an ideal "rationalized, disciplined, and professionalized mode of life" (Taylor, 2007, p. 119). One important result was that views of poverty radically shifted. No longer was a poor person regarded primarily as a potential bearer of Christ; instead, he or she became the object of scrutiny, deserving charity only if he or she was somehow unable to work. Similarly, sick patients were now categorized based upon their disease, and hospitals were spatially redesigned to group patients by their diagnoses (Foucault, 1994). These two shifts resulted in a practice of medicine no longer centered around hospitable care for the poor and sick; instead, health care was an important part of a disciplined society looking to eliminate inefficiencies like disease and poverty. For Taylor, this modern western social order has distinctive Protestant roots.

Similarly, scholars including theologian Gerald McKenny have argued that Protestant theological commitments about the use of nature and the relief of human suffering were deeply influential in the thought of early modern thinker Francis Bacon. These theological commitments helped shape a moral drive to overcome the limitations of the human body and "to relieve the human condition" (McKenny, 1997). Dissatisfied with the diseases afflicting the human body and the suffering that seems to naturally accompany finite embodied existence, the "Baconian project" in medicine has sought to overcome the body and its limitations. "As a result," claims McKenny, "medicine is [now] based on practices and techniques of control over the body rather than on traditions of wisdom about the body" (McKenny, 1997, p. 20). This kind of medicine is marked by a relentless drive to mobilize technology for the relief of suffering. Genetic therapies, pharmacological remedies, surgical technologies, and a host of other interventions are all seen as potential means of saving people from the problems of their bodies. But these also, for McKenny, display distinctively Protestant theological roots.

THEOLOGICAL CONTOURS WITHIN CONTEMPORARY HEALTH CARE

So far we have touched briefly on various ways that theology—especially the "primary theology" of embodied communities of faith—has made a difference for the contexts of health care. Specifically, we have traced the theological contours of specific institutions (like Basil's hospital), of innovative practices of health care (such as caring for strangers and the poor) and, more subtly, in health-related motivations and assumptions that bear theological roots, even if they are not self-consciously religious or theological. But how does theology shape the contexts of health care today? As in the past, we can point to specific institutions, to innovative models of care, and to ongoing cultural motivations and assumptions.

Specific faith-related health care institutions are perhaps easiest to recognize as theological, because they often cultivate active relationships with religious believers and congregations, incorporate theological approaches to care into their programming, and make their faith commitments clear in their foundational statements. The Church Health Center in Memphis, Tennessee, for example, which is a thriving Christian clinic and community center serving a diverse and socioeconomically marginalized community, names as its mission the desire "to reclaim the Church's biblical commitment to care for our bodies and our spirits" (http://www.churchhealthcenter.org/mission). Founded in 1987 by a physician with theological training, the Church Health Center has grown from a small medical clinic for the uninsured into a multispecialty health center that also offers wellness programs, child life programs, a fitness center, and nutrition education, framing all of this work within the biblical narrative of sin and redemption (Hotz & Mathews, 2012). In many other faith-based health care institutions, explicit theological grounding is less obvious, but nonetheless, many of these institutions would not have existed apart from theological convictions enacted in particular historical and cultural contexts.

Second, theology informs the contexts of modern health care by contributing to the innovation of new practices and models of care. The modern hospice and palliative care movement, for example, emerged from the work of Cicely Saunders, a British nurse, social worker, and physician whose broad medical training and deep Christian faith converged in the foundation of St. Christopher's Hospice in London in 1967 (du Boulay, 1984). Though more recent critics have lamented the increasing instrumentality and medicalization of palliative care (Bishop, 2011, pp. 253–278), the attentiveness of most hospice clinicians to spiritual concerns and the structural Medicare requirement that chaplains serve on hospice teams reflect this theologically-informed foundation.

More broadly, with Taylor and McKenny we affirm that many of the taken-for-granted moral assumptions informing health care have traceable theological roots, even if they do not make this explicit. The Protestant "affirmation of ordinary life" identified by Taylor, which placed a moral obligation on every person (and not just those consecrated to religious or monastic life) to live holy and disciplined lifestyles, continues to inform the assumption that every individual has a responsibility to engage in healthy behavior and to seek his or her own health (and that those who do not do so should be stigmatized). The Baconian focus on the use of science to relieve human suffering described by McKenny continues to inform the common assumption that technologies capable of reducing mortality or relieving identified human suffering are *prima facie* goods.

HOW MIGHT THEOLOGY BENEFIT MEDICINE AND HEALTH CARE GOING FORWARD?

We have discussed so far specific ways that theology has informed the contexts of health care in the past, and ways that theology continues to inform the contexts of health care in the present. In a modern culture that is increasingly pluralistic and non-religious, it may seem that theology has little constructive role to play moving forward, both in society at large and in health care in particular. To many proponents of a secular culture, true progress entails the unleashing of health care from the hindrance of religious commitments and contexts. For this vision of the future of health care, theology is at best irrelevant if not downright harmful. In response, many religious actors and organizations have assumed a combative posture towards what they regard as corrosive forces of secularism. For them, the future of health care depends upon the victory of like-minded religious voices united in their commitment to traditional theological values.

Our argument in this chapter points toward the possibility of a third way forward for theology's constructive role within the practices of health care. In contrast to the proponents of a thoroughly secular vision of health care, we have shown several examples of how core commitments, practices, and institutions in modern medicine have deeply theological roots. Even if overt theological discourse were to be completely eradicated from health care, these theological influences would remain, though perhaps they would become less coherent and so less sustainable. Moreover, a growing number of scholars have begun criticizing the very premises that undergird the secularization thesis, and are instead calling for a postsecular politics, one that seeks to promote the ability of individuals and institutions to navigate the public sphere without giving up their basic commitments, religious or otherwise (Bretherton, 2010, pp. 10–16). At the same time, those religious voices decrying secularism seem to ignore these postsecular possibilities for faithful action. They also seem to forget the ways in which certain theological influences have not been wholly laudable, from the "Baconian project" and its sacralization of technological progress to the use of religious justifications for the work of medical institutions to segregate and contain those who are poor or marginalized.

Given the presence of this complex theological legacy in modern health care, what then is a constructive role for theology moving forward? Rather than accepting an inevitable secularism or seeking its inverse, religious triumphalism, we propose that theology can serve to help enable faithful witness within the moral commitments, practices, and institutions of modern health care. For us, witness is *the* crucial category for theology's role in health care's postsecular future. By thinking in terms of witness, religious agents can avoid both the constraints of secularism and the pretensions of religious triumphalism, while at the same time being reminded of the necessity for judgment between helpful and unhelpful forms of religious witness. As Christian theologian Stanley Hauerwas claims:

> Calling attention to the necessity of witness suggests to many people, particularly those of the philosophical bent, the end of argument. For Christians, however, "witness" names the condition necessary to begin argument. To be a witness does not mean that Christians are in the business of calling attention to ourselves but that we witness to the One who has made our lives possible. Witness, at least the witness to which Christians are called, is, after all, about God and God's relation to all that is (Hauerwas, 2001, p. 207).

If we are to continue debating the role of theology in health care, religious witnesses are necessary for such an argument to even be made possible. To that end, we conclude by examining particular instances of how theology might matter for the moral commitments, practices, and institutions of health care moving forward. In creative ways, these religious individuals and organizations selectively retrieve and embody core theological insights from their religious traditions and so display the postsecular possibilities contained within health care.

First, we suggest that theology can continue to shape the moral commitments that patients and clinicians express through health care practices. In a medical culture increasingly marked by both competition for scarce resources and the language of service provision (the two are not unrelated), ingrained theological commitments—for example, the Jewish commitment to work toward *tikkun olam*, the repair of the world, or the Christian commitment to treat each sick person as if Jesus himself were present—can be both constructive and deeply important. The commitments to care found within these theological traditions can help provide the frameworks sufficient to sustain the professional virtues of medical practitioners. Rather than artificially excluding these theological commitments from its discourse, postsecular medicine could be marked by an "open pluralism: a commitment to explore, understand, and hear the voices of the particular moral communities that constitute our culture" (Kinghorn et al., 2007). Such postsecular open pluralism in medicine helps make possible the witness of medical practitioners whose moral commitments are explicitly theological.

But what might it look like in practice for medical practitioners to be these kinds of virtuous witnesses, shaped by their particular theological traditions and communities? For one such example, we turn to the Physician's Vocation Program at Loyola University Chicago Stritch School of Medicine. This voluntary program runs alongside their standard medical training, and in it students combine coursework and the practices of Ignatian spirituality in order to discern religious contours in their medical practice and calling. By integrating their medical formation with their religious identity and practices, the students are able to see and be shaped in new and surprising ways, and so become witnesses to alternate ways of inhabiting modern medicine. John Hardt, who directs the program, tells of one particular practitioner who displayed one such alternate way clearly as he began reimagining his routine practice of sanitizing his hands before entering patients' rooms. Instead of mindlessly applying the sanitizer, he instead pictured his Catholic priests washing their hands in preparation for handling the Eucharist, the body and blood of Christ. Through this theological vision, he prepared to meet Christ in the body of a sick patient, and to attend to the patient with patience and care. In an innovative way, therefore, this student has allowed the theological trajectory begun in Matthew 25 to animate his current medical practice (McCarty, 2016).

Through the example of the Physician's Vocation Program and this student's story, we can see an instance of how Christian theology can encourage both patients and clinicians to develop the much-needed virtue of *patience.* For Christians, we suggest, the radical hospitality of Jesus requires recognizing time as a gift to be received and not controlled, for the very practice of welcoming the sick, the poor, and the stranger requires patience. Crucially, the theological legacy of the Good Samaritan parable and Matthew 25 demands that medicine makes space for the sick guest to become the host as they are recognized as Christ himself, as seen in Basil's hospital and *The Rule of St. Benedict* (Swinton, 2015). This patience is not quietism, for welcoming the sick as guests and working to allow them to become hosts demands all the wisdom of the body medicine can provide. At the same time, this vision of patience in medicine resists the overreaching effort at control expressed in the modern disciplinary society and the Baconian project (Hauerwas and Pinches, 1997, p. 176). Health care that can patiently bear with the sufferings of the sick while working to enable them to do the same is a witness in a world ever-increasingly marked by its impatience.

Second, as it has done in the past, theology can continue to inform the development of health-related practices and models of care that promote flourishing. Though theology is often thought to exert primarily a restraining influence on the development of new technologies (e.g., embryonic stem cell research), the history of Christian theology's relationship with medicine shows that the bounds of this "no" actually exist to make clear Christian theology's more fundamental "yes" to health. For example, the refusal of early Christians to allow plague victims to suffer unattended demonstrated a "yes" to health that by its witness provoked the Emperor Julian to change the health care practices of the Roman Empire.

Witnesses to such a theological "yes" to health continue today in innovative health-related practices. Within the last century, for example, Alcoholics Anonymous—a religious movement with roots in Protestant Christianity and a nonsectarian but recognizably Christian structure of personal transformation—has deeply informed clinical and societal approaches to addiction. Christian commitments to social justice and to the dignity of meaningful work birthed the development of progressive institutions like Hull House in Chicago, and, from there, whole clinical disciplines like social work and occupational therapy. Eastern meditative traditions like Zen have strongly influenced the development of particular forms of psychotherapy (e.g., dialectical behavior therapy) and mindfulness interventions. There is no reason to believe that the twenty-first century will not give rise to equally transformative theologically informed practices and models of care.

It is possible that theology's most important influences in modern health care will be reflected not in cutting-edge medical technologies but rather by undergirding the mundane, everyday practices of care for the sick and vulnerable without which any medical system would fail. For example, increased life expectancy and a rapidly aging population in the United States make for particularly acute difficulties when coupled with weakening intergenerational family support networks, rising costs of assisted-living care, and an elderly population that is increasingly isolated and unappreciated. While these challenges certainly extend beyond the bounds of health care, modern medicine's current fixation on acute care renders medicine poorly situated to help with the health of the elderly. It is here that the witness of theologically informed practices and models of care becomes especially compelling.

One such witness is the elder care offered through Sant'Egidio, an international association of approximately sixty thousand lay Christians dedicated to serving the poor and marginalized in a variety of ways. Sant'Egidio began as a Roman Catholic lay movement in 1968 and has since spread to become international and ecumenical in its scope. Through care for immigrants, prisoners, the homeless, those with HIV/AIDS, abused and abandoned children, and the elderly, Sant'Egidio seeks to promote friendship through solidarity. In the United States, care for the elderly has been a particular focus of Sant'Egidio. By focusing on building relationships, lay volunteers spend time with the elderly at home and in institutions, seeking to increase their sense of belonging and agency while also learning from their wisdom and experience. Sant'Egidio members have basic medical care training, and they also raise funds to coordinate more advanced paid care services. They work to collaborate with family and nonprofit governmental care programs, all the while seeking to integrate the elderly more fully in the local community (Moses, 2015). Rather than pursuing new medical techniques, Sant'Egidio instead reclaims the theological commitment to hospitality and friendship found in the parable of the Good Samaritan and the earliest Christian hospitals. This care for the elderly represents a theological "yes" to the health of all, and in this way Sant'Egidio's refusal to disregard those who are marginalized is an important witness in a culture that is increasingly incapable of valuing aging lives.

Finally, theology can continue to inform the contexts of health care by giving rise to specific institutions capable of bearing witness in an increasingly pluralistic and postsecular context. One already-mentioned example is that of St. Christopher's Hospice in London, founded by Dame Cicely Saunders, that birthed the hospice movement which in turn profoundly altered medical approaches to death and dying. Yet another is L'Arche, a network of supportive homes for people with intellectual disabilities. In 1964, Jean Vanier founded the first L'Arche community in Trosly-Breuil, France when he invited two men with intellectual disabilities to share life together in a small home that he named L'Arche ("The Ark"), in reference to Noah's ark. Vanier was reacting against what he perceived as abuse and neglect of people with disabilities. His actions are rooted in a deep Roman Catholic spirituality that seeks to respond to a wounded and divided world in love and community. Rather than treating disabled persons as clients, L'Arche communities work hard to foster friendships marked by mutuality and joy. Such friendships do involve basic and often difficult acts of bodily care and service, but these medical practices are transfigured within the institutional context of L'Arche.

Although Vanier claims that he never meant to create an "institution," he admits that the communities of L'Arche have had to navigate the institutional complexities of governmental regulation. Moreover, L'Arche has worked hard to be intentionally interreligious, with Catholic houses welcoming residents from other religious traditions while remaining Catholic. The same is true of houses that are primarily Protestant, Hindu, and Muslim. Through patience and joy, Vanier and L'Arche have become witnesses to ways in which theological commitments can take surprising and important form in our modern context. Vanier beautifully summarizes the importance of this kind of theological and institutional witness when he says,

> I have been trying to point out that our deep need is to meet those on the other side of the wall, to discover their gifts, to appreciate them. We must not get caught up in the need for power over the poor. We need to be with the poor. . . . Maybe the world will be transformed when we learn to have fun together. I don't mean to suggest that we don't talk about serious things. But maybe what our world needs more than anything is communities where we celebrate life together and become a sign of hope for our world. Maybe we need signs that it is possible to love each other (Vanier, 2008, 75).

The Physician's Vocation Program, Sant'Egidio, and L'Arche witness to theology's constructive role in contemporary medicine and health care. They are living examples of the work of primary theology, as religious communities seek to discern what it means to respond faithfully to God in changing contexts. As an exercise in secondary theology, this essay has sought to narrate the work of primary theology and, in so doing, provide conceptual resources capable of discerning the challenges and opportunities of our present context in hopes of informing future practices. We write secondary theology out of our own Christian context, and so have focused largely on Christian examples throughout, but precisely as Christians we have also learned from the witness of Jewish and Muslim moral commitments, models of care, and institutions of health care. For all those seeking a theological context for medicine and health care, we have implicitly argued throughout that such a context is not provided in the abstract, but in the lived realities of religious communities and practitioners. Christian theologian John Swinton makes just this point when he writes about L'Arche, saying,

> Its presence reminds us that Christianity is not a theory but a practice. To believe in Christianity we need not only to know about God; we need to see God, to feel God and to love God in all things and at all times. That is our peace, our shalom. Peace follows the shape of the gospel; it needs to be seen to be believed. L'Arche helps us to begin to see what peace looks like (Swinton, 2008, pp. 104–105).

What Swinton writes of Christianity and L'Arche is true of theology and health care as a whole. The embodied witness of primary theology is necessary for us to understand what it means to set medicine and health care in theological context. Indeed, now more than ever, theology needs to be seen to be believed.

REFERENCES

Benedict of Nursia (1981). *The Rule of St. Benedict: In Latin and English with Notes*, ed. Timothy Fry. Collegeville, MN: The Liturgical Press.

Bishop, Jeffrey (2011). *The Anticipatory Corpse: Medicine, Power, and the Care of the Dying*. Notre Dame, IN: University of Notre Dame Press.

Bretherton, Luke (2010). *Christianity and Contemporary Politics: The Conditions and Possibilities of Faithful Witness*. Chichester, West Sussex, England: Wiley-Blackwell.

Brown, Peter (2002). *Poverty and Leadership in the Later Roman Empire*. Hanover, NH: University Press of New England.

Crislip, Andrew (2005). *From Monastery to Hospital: Christian Monasticism and the Transformation of Health Care in Late Antiquity*. Ann Arbor, MI: The University of Michigan Press.

Dols, Michael W. (1987). The origins of the Islamic hospital: myth and reality. *Bulletin of the History of Medicine* 61(3): 367–390.

du Boulay, Shirley (1984). *Cicely Saunders: Founder of the Modern Hospice Movement*. London: Hodder and Stoughton.

Ferngren, Gary B. (2009). *Medicine & Health Care in Early Christianity*. Baltimore, MD: The Johns Hopkins University Press.

Foucault, Michel (1994; 1963). *The Birth of the Clinic: An Archaeology of Medical Perception*, trans. A. M. Sheridan Smith. New York: Vintage Books.

Griffiths, Paul J. (2016). *The Practice of Catholic Theology: A Modest Proposal*. Washington, D.C.: Catholic University of America Press.

Hall, Daniel E., Koenig, Harold G., and Meador, Keith G. (2004). Conceptualizing "religion": How language shapes and constrains the study of religion and health. *Perspectives on Biology and Medicine* 47:386–401.

Hauerwas, Stanley (2001). *With the Grain of the Universe: The Church's Witness and Natural Theology*. Grand Rapids, MI: Brazos Press.

Hauerwas, Stanley, and Pinches, Charles (1997). *Christians among the Virtues: Theological Conversations with Ancient and Modern Ethics*. Notre Dame, IN: University of Notre Dame Press.

Hotz, Kendra, and Mathews, Matthew T. (2012). *Dust and Breath: Faith, Health, and Why the Church Should Care About Both*. Grand Rapids, MI: Eerdmans.

Kelsey, David (2009). *Eccentric Existence: A Theological Anthropology*. Louisville, KY: Westminster John Knox Press.

Kinghorn, Warren A., McEvoy, Matthew D., Michel, Andrew, and Balboni, Michael (2007). Professionalism in modern medicine: Does the emperor have any clothes? *Academic Medicine* 82(1): 40–45.

Lindbeck, George (1984). *The Nature of Doctrine: Religion and Theology in a Postliberal Age*. Louisville, KY: Westminster John Knox Press.

McCarty, Brett (2016). Diagnosis and therapy in *The Anticipatory Corpse*: A second opinion. *Journal of Medicine and Philosophy* 41(6): 621-641.

McKenny, Gerald (1997). *To Relieve the Human Condition: Bioethics, Technology, and the Body*. Albany, NY: State University of New York Press.

Medical School Objectives Project (1999), *Report III: Contemporary Issues in Medicine: Communication in Medicine*. Washington, DC: Association of American Medical Colleges.

Moses, Sarah M. (2015). *Ethics and the Elderly: The Challenge of Long-Term Care*. Maryknoll, NY: Orbis Books.

Pormann, Peter E., and Emilie Savage-Smith (2007). *Medieval Islamic Medicine*. Washington, D.C.: Georgetown University Press.

Porter, Roy (1997). Bethlem/Bedlam: Methods of madness? *History Today* 47:41–47.

Risse, Guenter B. (1999). *Mending bodies, saving souls: A history of hospitals*. Oxford: Oxford University Press.

Swinton, John (2008). Conclusion: L'Arche as a peace movement. In *Living Gently in a Violent World: The Prophetic Witness of Weakness*, by Stanley Hauerwas and Jean Vanier. Downers Grove, IL: InterVarsity Press.

Swinton, John (2015). Ordinary things with extraordinary love: Mental health and congregational care. *ABC Religion and Ethics Newsweekly*, Oct 7, 2015. Available at: http://www.abc.net.au/religion/articles/2015/10/07/4326417.htm.

Taylor, Charles (2007). *A Secular Age*. Cambridge, MA: The Belknap Press of Harvard University Press.

Vanier, Jean (2008). The vision of Jesus: Living peaceably in a wounded world. In *Living Gently in a Violent World: The Prophetic Witness of Weakness*, by Stanley Hauerwas and Jean Vanier. Downers Grove, IL: InterVarsity Press.

PART 3

SYNTHESIS AND INTEGRATION

CHAPTER 22

RELIGION AND HEALTH: A SYNTHESIS

Tyler J. VanderWeele

This review is concerned with the relationships between religion and health. Its principle purpose is to provide an overview of the empirical research literature on this relationship, relating different forms of religious participation, especially religious service attendance, to various health outcomes. However, it also briefly considers theological and religious traditions and themes concerning health, healing, and wholeness. It further reviews interventions related to religious communities that promote health, considers relations between the empirical literature on religion and health and the theological and religious traditions, and discusses where there is convergence, where there is tension, and where various open questions for further reflection and research remain. It concludes with a number of summary propositions attempting to capture the major themes of the present survey.

EMPIRICAL RESEARCH ON RELIGION AND HEALTH

Religious beliefs and participation are ubiquitous within and across populations. Approximately 84% of the world's population report a religious affiliation: 31.5% Christianity, 23.2% Islam, 15% Hinduism, 7.1% Buddhism, 5.9% Folk religions, 0.2% Judaism, and 0.8% Other. Only 16.3% report being religiously unaffiliated (Pew Forum, 2012). Within the United States, 89% believe in God or a universal spirit, 78% consider religion a very important or fairly important part of life, 79% identify with a particular religious group, and 36% report having attended a religious service in the last week (Gallup Poll, 2015–2016). Not only is participation substantial, but as will be described in this review, the associations between religious participation and health are likewise considerable in magnitude. Public health relevance is often described as a function of the prevalence of the exposure and the size of the effect. On these grounds, religious participation, as will be argued in this review, is a powerful social determinant of health. Here we will review the empirical research on religion that makes clear the important implications for health of this very common and powerful human phenomenon.

BRIEF HISTORICAL OVERVIEW

Modern accounts of religion and health research sometimes begin with Emile Durkheim's work *Suicide*. Durkheim (1897) noted that suicide rates were higher in Protestant areas within Europe than in Catholic areas, and argued that this was due to greater social cohesion and control within the Catholic religion. The study used ecologic (or group-averaged) data and has been criticized on that account subsequently, but the work exerted a powerful influence within sociology. Another substantial influence on research on religion and health was the writing of Sigmund Freud who viewed religion, for the most part, as an irrational neurotic phenomenon. His writing shaped views on religion and health for decades. Early empirical studies on religion and health with individual level data began to appear during the period of 1950–1980, and increased more substantially during the 1980's. As the field continued to gain momentum, substantial critique and skepticism concerning the work emerged during the 1990s, as many of the early studies were methodologically quite weak (cf. Sloan et al., 1999; Chatters, 2000). The research continued to rapidly expand throughout the first decade and a half of the 21st century, with thousands of studies having now been published (Koenig et al., 2012). Many of these studies are methodologically still quite weak, but an increasing number of rigorous studies, in this area, have been published. These too, like the previous literature, suggest evidence for a protective effect of religious participation, especially religious service attendance, on health, for outcomes as diverse as all-cause mortality, depression, suicide, cancer survival, and subjective well-being. Our focus in this chapter will be on quantitative, rather than qualitative, empirical research on religion and health with an eye towards the strongest studies methodologically that help establish the knowledge-base in this field.

RELIGION AND ALL-CAUSE MORTALITY

While religion and spirituality have been defined variously within the religion and health literature (Koenig, 2008; Hill and Pargament, 2003; Chatters, 2000; see Oman, 2013, for a review of various definitions of each term used within psychology), in most of the empirical research relating religion and health, fairly specific measures have been employed. Such measures have included self-assessed measures of religiosity and spirituality, service attendance, private practices such as prayer, Scripture reading and mediation, religious coping, spiritual experience, and specific beliefs (Hill and Hood, 1999; Fetzer, 1999; Pargament et al., 2000; Underwood and Teresi, 2002; Idler et al., 2003; Koenig and Bussing, 2010). We will begin our discussion of the empirical literature on religion and health by reviewing the existing literature on religious participation and all-cause mortality. It is for this health outcome that the evidence concerning the empirical research on the effects of religious participation is arguably the strongest. Within the present literature, the measure that seems most strongly associated with health is service attendance. This holds true both with research on all-cause mortality and, as will be seen later, with research on many other health outcomes. This may be partially because service attendance is the measure most often available, but also perhaps because of the powerful effect of communal participation on health, issues we will return to later in this review.

Studies using individual level data examining associations between religion and mortality with relatively large sample sizes began to appear in the 1970s, 1980s, and 1990s. Religious participation of course does not protect against "death" itself in the end. However, the research suggests that religious participation might increase longevity, that is, decrease the odds of death within a 5-year or 10-year follow-up. Most early studies had small sample sizes and often inconclusive results. One early study with a much larger sample size was conducted by Comstock and Tonascia (1977; cf. Comstock and Patridge, 1972) who examined 38,839 adults in Washington County, Maryland. Attending religious services once or more per week was associated with 39% lower mortality in follow-up than those not attending at all. Rates were adjusted for demographic factors but not for baseline health. As we will discuss further in this chapter, if baseline health status is not controlled for, the direction of causality is difficult to assess because it may be that those with poorer health are less able to attend services and more likely to die.

If we turn to some of the stronger studies—ones that were able to control for baseline health— a study by Hummer et al. (1999) is sometimes pointed to as an important turning point in the rigor of the research on service attendance and all-cause mortality. Their study, using data from the National Health Interview Survey, that surveyed 21,204 adults, was nationally representative. Control was made for age, sex, race, and region, and, importantly, baseline health (activity limitations, self-reported, health-related bed days) was also controlled for, along with socioeconomic status. Those never attending compared to those attending more than once per week had a hazard of dying that was 1.72 ($p < 0.01$)[1] times higher during follow-up. The analyses also suggested a clear "dose-response" relationship with increasingly greater service attendance associated with increasing lower mortality. Compared to those attending more than once per week, those attending only weekly had a hazard ratio (HR) of 1.23, those attending less than weekly of 1.34, and those not attending of 1.72, with all of these being statistically significant. Hummer et al. reported that those attending services more than weekly had a roughly 7 year greater life expectancy at age 20 than did those not attending at all. Although the effect estimates are fairly substantial in this study, Hummer et al. (1999) report that, without control for baseline health, the estimates were even larger. This again emphasizes the importance of controlling for baseline health and other confounders in these analyses of religion and health. Hummer et al. (1999) further controlled for social ties and various health behaviors, such as smoking, and this reduced the hazard ratio estimate comparing never attenders to those attending more than once per week to 1.5 ($P < 0.01$). Social ties and health behaviors may be on the pathway, or mediators, from service attendance to mortality, and this further analysis suggests some evidence for such mediation, a point to which we will later return.

Although the Hummer et al. (1999) study is often pointed to as an important step forward in the literature, there were certainly prior studies that also contributed strong evidence. For

---

1. We will, throughout this review, make reference to various measures of statistical uncertainty such as p-values and confidence intervals. The p-value is a measure of how likely the outcome obtained, or one more extreme, would be if there were in fact no true association and the result was simply due to chance. More formally, it is the probability of obtaining a result as extreme or more extreme than the one actually obtained if there were in fact no true association. It is a measure between 0 and 1; the value $p = 0.05$ is sometimes used as a cut-off below which the evidence is considered reasonably strong (sometimes also referred to as "statistically significant"); however, the p-value is a continuous measure and the lower the p-value, the stronger the evidence that the result is not simply due to chance variation. A 95% confidence interval is a range of plausible values for an estimate given the statistical uncertainty. More formally, it is constructed so that, under repeating sampling of the same underlying population, the true value of the estimate will lie within the constructed interval at least 95% of the time. Two numbers in brackets that follow estimates will indicate the 95% confidence interval.

example, the same sample was used somewhat earlier by Rogers (1996) who looked at associations with "service attendance in previous two weeks." That paper looked at various associations and did not specifically focus on religion. Fairly strong evidence was also reported by Strawbridge at al. (1997) using data from Alameda county (cf. Oman et al., 2002 for additional analyses) with a somewhat smaller sample size of 5,286. Although this study, unlike the Hummer et al. study, was not a nationally representative sample, there was good confounding control and the evidence, once again, suggested an effect of service attendance on all-cause mortality.

In 2000, McCullough et al. (2000) conducted a meta-analysis of 42 studies in the literature that included 125,826 participants. Their meta-analysis included studies with various measures of religious participation, mostly service attendance, but others as well. All measures were dichotomized for the purpose of this study. In their meta-analysis, they found that being less religious was associated with a 1.29 (95% CI: 1.20, 1.39) higher odds of death during follow-up. There was stronger evidence for an effect for women than men, and there was some evidence that private religious measures were less strongly associated with mortality during follow-up than institutional measures, such as service attendance. The quality of studies in this meta-analysis and the adequacy of control for confounding varied considerably across studies. Not all of the studies were equally rigorous. However, as the literature has developed, an increasing number of rigorous studies, with large sample sizes and with control for baseline health and other confounding variables, have become available. In addition to the Hummer et al. (1999) and Strawbridge et al. (1997) studies mentioned, other prominent studies have included, for example, Gillum et al. (2008) and Musick et al. (2004), which both controlled for baseline health and suggested a 20–35% reduction in mortality for those regularly attending services. The analyses of Musick et al. (2004) suggested also that private religious practices, volunteering, and subjective religiosity were not associated with mortality once control was made for service attendance. Service attendance seemed the more powerful predictor. Further studies on religious participation and mortality are summarized in Idler (2011).

An updated meta-analysis by Chida et al. (2009) of the research on religion and mortality, with somewhat stricter inclusion criteria than the McCullough et al. (2000) study, included results from 44 studies and about 121,000 participants. Those with higher levels of religious participation had 0.82 (95% CI: 0.76, 0.87) lower hazard of death during follow-up. The effect size was more substantial for women, HR = 0.70 (0.55, 0.89) than men HR = 0.87 (0.81, 1.02), and also larger for organizational involvement, HR = 0.77 (0.71, 0.83), than for non-organizational religious activity, HR = 0.95 (0.80, 1.13). Those attending services at least once per week had a 0.73 (0.63, 0.84) lower hazard of death during follow-up.

Similar protective associations between service attendance and all-cause mortality have been found in Denmark (la Cour et al., 2006) and Finland (Teinomen, 2005), in Taiwan (Yeager et al., 2006) with a predominantly Taoist and Buddhist population, and in Israel (Litwin, 2007) with a predominantly Jewish population. Further research is still needed for other religious groups. The effect sizes seems larger for women than for men (Chida et al., 2009; Teinonen et al., 2005; la Cour et al., 2005); they appear larger for African Americans than for the white population (Hummer et al., 1999; Chatters, 2000; Dupre et al., 2006) and there is perhaps some evidence that the effect of attendance is larger earlier in life (Dupre et al., 2006), but this has arguably not yet firmly been established. The effect sizes on all-cause mortality are similar to or only slightly less substantial than those for many other important health exposures such as physical activity, tobacco smoking cessation, the use of beta-blockers for congestive heart failure, screening for mammography, and fruit and vegetable consumption (Lucchetti et al., 2011).[2]

RELIGION AND DEPRESSION

Sigmund Freud believed that religion contributed to neuroses. He wrote that religion works "by distorting the picture of the real world in delusional manner. . . by forcibly fixing [adherents] in a state of psychical infantilism and by drawing them into a mass delusion" (Freud, 1930, pp. 31–32, "Civilization and Its Discontents"). It has been argued that, in part due to Freud, for almost an entire century, religious participation was thought to be associated with poor mental health (Koenig, 2009). A review written by Sanua in 1969 concluded: "The contention that religion as an institution has been instrumental in fostering general well-being. . . is not supported by empirical data. . . there are no scientific studies which show that religion is capable of serving mental health" (Sanua, 1969). The literature on religious participation and mental health over the past couple of decades has shown this contention to be wrong.

In 1992, Larson and co-authors assessed measures of religious commitment in two psychiatric research journals from 1978–1989 and found 35 studies (Larson et al., 1992). Of those 72% reported a positive association between religion and mental health, 16% reported a negative association, and 12% found no association. Since then, there have been over a thousand studies examining religion and mental health. Like much of the research on mortality, many of these studies are methodologically weak. Here we will focus on the literature that examines depression, and we will again see that weak methodology and design is especially problematic, again due to the possibility of reverse causation. We will focus on those studies that, methodologically, are the strongest. See also Blazer (2017) for discussion of research on religious participation and mental health and some of the methodological challenges.

Koenig et al. (2012) summarize the literature on religious participation and depression for research published through 2010. The majority of these suggest that religious participation of various forms is associated with lower rates of depression. Koenig et al. note that of 272 cross-sectional studies published since 2000, 63% suggested a protective effect; only 6% a detrimental effect; and of 45 cohort studies since 2000, 47% suggested a protective effect and only 11% a detrimental effect. Of these studies, then, the vast majority are cross-sectional (i.e., all data are collected at a single point in time) and they thus examine associations between religious participation and depression measured at the same time. There has been meta-analysis of the religion and depression literature (e.g., Smith et al., 2003) that has likewise suggested a protective association but these in general include studies that are cross-sectional or that do not control for baseline depression and so can contribute almost no evidence towards whether the relationships are causal. The problem arises because depression might itself affect service attendance. Without data on service attendance and depression over time, it is impossible to assess the direction of causality. And in fact, there is evidence for an effect in the reverse direction. Maselko et al. (2012),

---

2. Lucchetti et al. (2011) report mortality odds ratios: Physical activity OR = 0.67; Tobacco smoking cessation OR = 0.71; Beta-blocker-congestive heart failure OR = 0.72; Screening for mammography OR = 0.74; Fruit and vegetable consumption OR = 0.74; Service attendance OR = 0.75

using longitudinal data, assessed evidence for an effect of depression on service attendance. They showed that, among women, depression at age 18 predicted lower service attendance subsequently, controlling for baseline service attendance. Because of this effect in the reverse direction, cross-sectional studies evaluating the relationship between service attendance and depression are useless for establishing causality. Even if there were no effect of service attendance on depression, one would find a "protective association" simply because those who became depressed would stop attending (Maselko et al., 2012; VanderWeele, 2013). In order to assess evidence for a causal relationship, one needs to assess service attendance and depression over time, and to control for baseline levels of depression to address issues of reverse causation.

In fact, several studies, though comparatively few in relation to the whole of the literature, have done precisely that; that is, they have used longitudinal data with relatively large sample sizes to assess associations between service attendance and depression with control for depression at baseline (Strawbridge et al., 2001; Van Vorhees et al. 2008; Norton et al., 2008; Balbuena et al., 2013; Li et al., 2016a). These studies too suggest a protective effect of service attendance on depression. Strawbridge et al. (2001) in a study of 2,676 persons in the Alameda Country Study followed from 1965 to 1994, found evidence that service attendance at least once per week for those depressed increased odds of depression recovery by 2.3 (1.23, 4.35) fold; and some evidence that attendance at least weekly was associated with 0.76 (0.55, 1.05) lower odds of becoming depressed. Van Voorhees et al. (2008) using a nationally representative sample of 4,791 adolescents in the AddHealth study, followed for one year, and controlled for race, family income, age, gender, and baseline depressive symptoms. They found those with religious identity had 0.57 (0.34, 0.96) lower odds of depression onset; those praying at least once per week had 0.52 (0.29, 0.94) times lower odds; and those attending services at least once per month had 0.37 (0.15, 0.88) times lower odds. Norton et al. (2008) report analyses in a sample of 2,989 persons that, after controlling for sociodemographic variables, health, and baseline depression, found that those attending more than once per week had 0.51 (0.28, 0.92) lower odds of a depressive episode in 3-year follow-up compared to those not attending services. Balbuena et al. (2013) using a sample of 12,583 persons from the Canadian National Population Health Survey who were not depressed at baseline, and followed for 14 years found that, after controlling for age, household income, family and personal history of depression, marital status, education, and perceived social support, those attending at least monthly had 0.78 (0.63, 0.95) lower rate of depression compared with non-attenders; neither self-reported importance of spiritual values nor identification as a spiritual person was related to major depressive episodes. There thus seems to be evidence for an effect of service attendance on depression. There may in fact be an effect in both directions: service attendance protects against depression, but depression itself also leads to lower levels of service attendance.

The strongest evidence to date for these relationships between service attendance and depression comes from a longitudinal analysis of the Nurses' Health Study data. Li et al. (2016a) used data on 48,984 U.S. nurses followed for 12 years, using statistical models that handle feedback and reverse causation (Robins et al., 2000), controlling for confounding by baseline depression and an extensive demographic, socioeconomic, behavioral, and health variables. The results suggest both that (1) women who attended services more than once per week had a lower risk of becoming depressed (RR = 0.71, 95% CI: 0.62, 0.82) compared with women who did not attend; but also that (2) women with depression were less likely to subsequently attend religious services once or more per week (RR = 0.74, 95% CI: 0.68, 0.80) compared with women who were not depressed.

Once again, the effects seemed to be present in both directions even with the study designs using repeated measures on both service attendance and depression, with a very large sample size, with methods to address feedback, and with extensive confounding control.

While it is again the case that service attendance seems to contribute to health by lessening depression, the results on the effects of depression on service attendance also arguably have important implications for religious communities. Those who become depressed are more likely to stop attending services, which may of course exacerbate depression further. The research perhaps suggests a role for clergy and other members of religious communities to more actively be aware of, or even screen for (Hankerson et al., 2015), those who might be depressed, and to offer help, support, and possible referral, before depression becomes worse. The empirical research helps inform religious communities and clergy that those who may be most in need may be the least likely to be present to receive it; they may need to be sought out.

The results reported here for a protective effect of service attendance on depression also depend at least in part on the context. The effect of attendance on depression seems larger for women than for men (Strawbridge et al., 2001). And in certain contexts, it seems participation can have detrimental effects on depression. There is some evidence that religious participation may be associated with higher depression rates for unwed mothers (Sorenson et al., 1995; Koenig, 2009), and negative interactions at church can lead to higher levels of psychological distress (Krause et al., 1998; Ellison et al., 2009). Such research may also have important implications for religious communities and pastoral practice.

One important lesson for research that emerges from this discussion of the literature on service attendance and depression is that although hundreds of studies have been published on the topic, only a very small number contribute substantially to the evidence base for a causal relationship. We do not need more studies on religion and depression; what we need are more *rigorous* studies. The *associations* between religion and health are clearly established; what is needed is to continue to accumulate evidence for *causation* concerning specific aspects of religious participation and specific health outcomes. There are some strong studies available that provide reasonably good evidence. Additional studies concerning certain aspects of the religion and health relationship might be helpful, but if further studies are to be conducted, they should be such that they contribute to questions that are still open, not merely reiterate a well-documented association that contributes little to the existing knowledge base or our understanding of the actual causal relationships.

RELIGION AND SUICIDE

The major world religions have strong traditions that prohibit suicide. In the major monotheistic religions—Islam, Judaism, and Christianity—this prohibition has, traditionally, been especially strong. Theological and ethical reasons sometimes given for prohibiting suicide include that life is a sacred gift from God, that it injures the community, that it is contrary to love of self and of others, that it might encourage others to follow, and that death itself is a great evil and should not be brought about. As noted in the introduction, one of the very early empirical studies on religion and health was Durkheim's study of suicide comparing Catholics and Protestants. Suicide rates were lower in Catholic countries and geographic regions, which Durkheim attributed to greater social control and social cohesion among Catholics (Durkheim, 1897). There have been over a hundred empirical studies of religion and suicide since. Koenig et al. (2012) report that in 106 of 141 of studies surveyed (75%), religious participation was associated with fewer suicides and suicide attempts, or less suicide ideation, or more negative attitudes towards suicide. As with depression, many of these studies, especially with attitudes and ideation are cross-sectional; a number of them, including Durkheim's, make use of ecologic (i.e., group-averaged) data and cannot make control for individual level confounding. Some of these use survey data for suicide attempts, but these obviously cannot capture successful suicides. Further methodological challenges arise because suicide, as an outcome, is relatively rare and therefore requires extremely large sample sizes and long follow-up for longitudinal designs to be feasible. There are however a few relatively large longitudinal studies; sometimes case-control designs have also been used to study suicide. We will review a few of the stronger studies here.

Nisbet et al. (2000) analyzed data from the National Followback Study, a case-control study comparing 584 completed suicides and with 4,279 natural deaths as controls. Those who did not attend religious services had 4.34 (2.52, 7.49) higher odds of having died by suicide than those who attended regularly. Thompson et al. (2007) used Add Health data, consisting of a sample of 15,034 adolescents ages 12–17, with 1-year and 7-year follow-up. After controlling for gender, race, problem drinking, self-esteem, impulsivity, depression, and delinquency, adolescents who indicated that religion was very or fairly important at baseline had odds of suicide attempt requiring medical attention 0.54 (0.26, 1.13) times lower than others at 1-year follow-up; and 0.43 (0.19, 0.93) times lower at 7-year follow-up. Rasic et al. (2009) used data from Waves 3 and 4 of the Baltimore Epidemiologic Catchment Area Study with a sample size of 1,091. After control for age, gender, race, education, income, and marital status, as well as baseline suicidal ideation/attempts, comorbid mental disorders, social support, and chronic physical conditions, respondents who attended religious services at least once per year had 0.33, (0.13, 0.84) times lower odds of subsequent suicide attempts compared with those who did not attend religious services.

Spoerri et al. (2010) conducted a longitudinal study linking Switzerland census data in year 2000 to mortality through 2005. The study consisted of about 3.6 million persons (46% Catholic, 42% Protestant, and 12% with no religious affiliation). After adjustment for age, marital status, education, type of household, language and degree of urbanization, the rate of suicide was lower for Catholics than Protestants: Age 35–64 Men: HR = 0.80 (0.73, 0.88); Age 65–94 Men: 0.60 (0.53, 0.67); Age 35–64 Women: 0.90 (0.80, 1.03); Age 65–94 Women: 0.67 (0.59, 0.77). Suicide rates were higher for those with no religious affiliation than for Protestants: Age 35–64 Men 1.09 (0.98, 1.22); Age 65–94 Men 1.96 (1.69, 2.27); Age 35–64 Women 1.46 (1.25, 1.72); Age 65–94 Women 2.63 (2.22, 3.12). The study suggests that Durkheim's observation persists, at least in Switzerland, even with individual level analyses.

Using NHAANES III cohort data involving 20,014 persons and controlling for a number of demographic characteristics and behavioral variables, Kleinman and Liu (2014) report that those attending services at least 24 times per year were about one third as likely to commit suicide (HR = 0.33, $p < 0.05$) than those who attended less frequently. Unfortunately, however, they were not able to control for depression, which is related both to suicide, and as discussed, to service attendance. A similar large cohort analysis was carried out with the Nurses' health data described above, in an analysis using 89,708 women and controlling for numerous demographic, health, and behavioral variables, including depression, and found that attending services at least weekly was associated with an approximately five-fold lower rate of suicide, compared with never attending services

(HR = 0.18, 95% CI: 0.06-0.51; VanderWeele et al., 2016). The results also appeared to differ by religious affiliation. Service attendance once or more per week, versus less often, was associated with a suicide hazard ratio of HR = 0.05 (0.006–0.46) for Catholics, but only HR = 0.37 (0.11–1.19) for Protestants (p-value for heterogeneity = 0.05).

As was the case with depression, here also with suicide, the strongest evidence comes from only a few studies. Even though there have been over one hundred studies on religion and suicide published in the literature, most are weak. The studies suggest that the effects of religious participation on suicide are quite strong, likely larger than mortality, with effects sizes as large as 2- to 5-fold. Affiliation also appears to have an effect, and as of 2010, Durkheim's study had received additional support using individual level data. Proposed mechanisms for a protective effect have included the hypotheses that religious participation reduces depression, is associated with better physical health, increases social support, and reduces drug and alcohol use. Of course, the belief that suicide is wrong likely also affects suicide attempts, and there is some evidence suggesting that this may indeed be an important factor (Oquendo et al., 2005). However, the existing empirical studies that directly assess the mechanisms for the relationship between religious participation and suicide are limited.

OTHER RELIGION-SPIRITUALITY MEASURES AND HEALTH

We have seen then that there is evidence for service attendance being strongly associated with lower mortality, less depression, and lower likelihood of suicide. Religious service attendance is of course only one form of religion and spirituality. The literature on the associations between other form of religious participation and spirituality with all-cause mortality is more limited and mixed. Some of the gap in the literature is likely due to the fact that in most large cohort studies, in which these associations could be examined rigorously with longitudinal data, questions on religion and spirituality, if asked at all, focus almost exclusively on religious service attendance, often as a measure of social integration (Berkman and Syme, 1979). The studies that do have other religion and spirituality measures often tend to be of smaller sample size.

Of the literature that does exist, the results from longitudinal studies for other measures of religion and spirituality are somewhat more mixed. In general, service attendance appears to be the strongest predictor. The Musick et al. (2004) study discussed suggested that private religious practices, such as prayer and Scripture reading, had little association with mortality. Using longitudinal cohort data from the Black Women's Health Study, with mortality as the outcome, VanderWeele et al. (2016b) found no association with religious coping, religious or spirituality identity, or prayer, after multivariate control for demographic and health variables, but strong association with service attendance. Similar weak or null associations between mortality and private religious practices and also with intrinsic religiosity is suggested in systematic review (Chida et al., 2009; Koenig et al., 2012). Some studies of other religion or spirituality measures have suggested a protective association with mortality. Ironson and Kremer (2009) report lower mortality among HIV patients who experience religious transformation. There is some literature on the use of religious coping in the face of illness. In clinical populations, there is some evidence that positive coping is associated with lower all-cause mortality in follow-up (Oxman et al., 1995) but other studies find weaker results (Pargament et al., 2001). There is also evidence from longitudinal analyses that negative religious coping is related to higher mortality (Pargament et al., 2001). There may also be a difference in the effects of various forms of religion and spirituality for ill clinical populations versus the general population. Schnall et al. (2010), in a large longitudinal study of 92,395 women, report an association between service attendance and all-cause mortality, but much weaker, and in many cases null, associations between strength and comfort from religion and all-cause mortality. It is also possible that with non-clinical populations, high levels of religious coping and prayer in fact also serve as markers for health problems or threats already present, thus partially confounding the association.

With depression, the Balbuena et al. (2013) study mentioned found reduced depression incidence for those attending religious services but neither self-reported importance of spiritual values nor identification as a spiritual person was related to major depressive episodes. Likewise, in a study of 8,318 medical patients in several European countries, Leurent (2013) found either no association or mild causative association between self-assessed religiosity/spirituality and depression. A longitudinal study by Koenig et al. (1998) found that, for a clinical population, measures of intrinsic religiosity were associated with a quicker time to depression remission. More research is needed on the relationships with other measures of religious participation and spirituality with mortality, depression, suicide and other health outcomes. While there is some suggestive evidence from cross-sectional studies for some other measures—for example, belief in life after death appears to be cross-sectionally associated with better mental health outcomes (Flannelly et al., 2006)—it is also the case, as has already been discussed, that such cross-sectional data contributes little to evidence for causality. Future work could also examine whether specific religious beliefs, intrinsic religiosity, practices of forgiveness (Fetzer, 1999), and also religious/spiritual experiences (Underwood and Teresi, 2002; Underwood, 2011), are predictors of mortality. It would also be of interest to see whether such associations persist after controlling for service attendance, since religion and spirituality measures will be associated with each other and service attendance is clearly a strong predictor for many health outcomes. Incorporating such measures into existing cohort studies could be a very powerful way to examine these associations with large sample sizes and adequate confounding control.

OTHER HEALTH OUTCOMES

There is a large literature on other health outcomes as well. Koenig et al. (2012) summarize evidence that suggests that religious participation is, in over half of published studies, for each outcome, related to lower blood pressure, better cardiovascular function, less coronary artery disease, better immune function, better endocrine function, better social support, greater marital stability, greater purpose in life, and overall higher levels happiness and subjective well-being. Other outcomes that have been examined with some evidence of a protective effect of service attendance include lower usage rates of cigarettes or marijuana or alcohol among pregnant and postpartum women, and lower rates of low infant birth weight (Page et al. 2009; Burdette et al. 2012); lower rates of smoking and drug use among adolescents attending services (Koenig et al., 2012; Idler, 2014a); lower rates of disability among the elderly for those who attend services, even after adjustment for baseline disability (Idler and Kasl, 1997), and slower decline for those with Alzheimer's among those attending (Koenig et al., 2012; Coin et al., 2010; Idler, 2014a).

Of course, many of these studies summarized are again cross-sectional and methodologically weak. Some of the outcomes, such as disability or Alzheimer's disease or cardiovascular health, may themselves affect service attendance. Longitudinal studies, and careful control for confounding, including control for baseline outcome, are thus needed. For some outcomes, the relationship may not stand up against more rigorous scrutiny. For example, in what is arguably the strongest and largest study of cardiovascular health, Schnall et al. (2010), using Women's Health Initiative data, with a sample of 92,395 women, find that although service attendance is associated with lower all-cause mortality, there is essentially no effect (if anything a slightly detrimental effect) of service attendance on the incidence of coronary heart disease. Similar results of a near-null association between religious service attendance and incidence of cardiovascular disease were also obtained with the Nurses Health Study data (Li et al., 2016b; VanderWeele et al., 2016c). In this case, at least with two rigorous studies, the results from the weaker studies did not seem robust to more careful analysis. In other cases, such as with the effect of attendance on disability, the evidence from longitudinal studies, even when controlling for baseline disability outcome, may be more robust (Idler and Kasl, 1997), but each of these outcomes needs careful assessment as to the strength of the available evidence from rigorous longitudinal studies. The evidence for mortality, depression, and suicide is relatively strong, but other outcomes may still need more careful examination. An important step forward in religion and health research would be a series of meta-analyses for different health outcomes in which restriction was made to longitudinal studies, with good confounding control, including control for baseline outcome (e.g., controlling for initial immune function when examining subsequent immune function outcomes).

For most health outcomes, the evidence suggests a protective effect of religious participation on health, but such protective associations are not universal and do depend on context. There is some evidence that the effect of attendance is less pronounced and even detrimental in countries which restrict freedoms, or in countries in which religious participation is less common (Hayward and Elliott, 2014). One study suggested that students in schools where their own religious affiliation was in the minority were 2 to 4 times more likely to attempt suicide or self-harm (Young et al. 2011). We noted earlier that another study presented some evidence that religious participation was associated with higher depression rates for unwed mothers (Sorenson et al., 1995; Koenig, 2009). Spiritual struggles have also been shown to be associated longitudinally with worse health (Pargament et al., 2001, 2004; Winkelman et al., 2011), and negative congregational interactions are associated with lower measures of well-being (Krause et al., 1998; Ellison et al., 2009). While much of the evidence thus points to a beneficial effect of religious participation on health, it is clear that there are contexts and settings for which this is not so. Such research can also be of importance to religious communities in informing communal and pastoral practices.

OTHER OUTCOMES RELATED TO WELL-BEING

Service attendance is also associated with a number of other important outcomes that are not generally considered to fall under "health," a point to which we will return later, but do concern well-being more broadly. Numerous studies have examined service attendance and life satisfaction or subjective well-being. Unfortunately, almost all of these studies are cross-sectional (Koenig et al., 2012) and contribute little evidence towards causality. The associations, at least with service attendance, appear to hold up under much better longitudinal designs as well. For example, Lim and Putnam (2010) report that religious service attendance is strongly associated longitudinally with higher life satisfaction, after control for baseline life satisfaction and other confounders, and they provide some evidence that the development of within-congregation friendships constitutes an important mechanism for this effect.

Another important outcome for which religious service attendance appears to have a protective effect is divorce. Numerous studies have examined associations between attendance and divorce, but, as with other outcomes, many of those studies are cross-sectional or weak methodologically (Koenig et al., 2012; Mahoney et al., 2008). A few, however, use strong longitudinal designs and supply compelling evidence (Call and Heaton, 1997; Amato and Rogers, 1997; Strawbridge et al., 1997, 2001). Call and Heaton (1997) provide some evidence that the wife's attendance has a stronger influence on the likelihood of divorce than the husband's, but that any difference between the attendance patterns of the two also has a detrimental effect. The Nurses Health Study data described likewise gives evidence for an effect of attendance on reducing divorce. After extensive covariate control, service attendance once per week was associated with a 0.57 (0.45, 0.71) times lower risk of divorce during follow-up and service attendance more than once per week with a 0.51 (0.38, 0.69) times lower risk of divorce during follow-up. Other studies have examined social support. Again, most of these are cross-sectional but some good longitudinal studies can be found in the literature (Strawbridge et al., 1997; Lim and Putnam, 2010). For example, the Strawbridge et al. (1997) study mentioned found that the service attendance was longitudinally associated with a greater number of close friends, non-religious community membership, and likelihood of staying married (Strawbridge et al., 1997).

Yet other studies have examined meaning and purpose. The vast majority of these have suggested that various forms of religious participation and service attendance are associated with a greater sense of meaning or purpose in life, but, once again, the vast majority of these studies are cross-sectional (Koenig et al., 2012). However, there is at least some evidence, using stronger longitudinal designs (Krause and Hayward, 2012), examining service attendance and meaning in life which likewise provide evidence that service attendance is associated over time with greater meaning in life, even after control for social and demographic covariates and baseline meaning in life.

Other studies have examined virtue and character as outcomes. This literature is somewhat more complex than in the other areas above which relied entirely on observational studies. With questions of virtue and character, there have been numerous randomized priming experiments suggesting at least short term effects of religious prompts on pro-social behavior (Shariff et al., 2016), possibly with "affiliation" primes having an effect only on in-group behavior but "God" primes on both in-group and out-group pro-social behavior (Preston et al., 2010; Preston and Ritter, 2013), but also evidence that religious primes may increase aggression (Bushman et al., 2007). There is longitudinal evidence that those who attend services are subsequently more generous and more civically involved (Putnam and Campbell, 2012). There is also some experimental evidence that encouragement to prayer increases forgiveness, gratitude, and trust (Lambert et al., 2009, 2010, 2012).

In the research on these other outcomes such as life satisfaction, divorce, social support, and meaning and purpose, although there are a few strong longitudinal studies that suggest attending religious services may lead to better outcomes in these dimensions, the current evidence base, at present, comes from a very small number of studies and so the results are at best tentative. More research using good designs and rigorous analytic methodology is needed on the relationships between service attendance, and other forms of religious participation, and these various outcomes related to well-being. See also VanderWeele et al. (2016c) for further discussion of rigorous methodology for causal inference using longitudinal data in religion and health research.

CRITIQUE AND RESPONSE

As noted, many of the early studies on religion and health were methodologically fairly weak and thus subject to criticism. In 1999, Sloan et al. (1999) published a critique in which it was argued that in the empirical studies on religion and health it was often the case that confounding control was inadequate, that often when control for confounding was adequate the associations would disappear, that there was typically failure to control for multiple comparisons, that results were inconsistent across studies and measures of religion, that the studies raised ethical concerns regarding whether physicians might start "prescribing religion," and that physicians overstep boundaries in addressing religion. The paper further objected to the suggestion that physicians should ask how they can support patients' faith, proposing that religion should not be "intervened upon" (as would be the case also, say, with marriage, which has been linked to health), and that the religion and health links might inappropriately suggest that illness is due to religious or moral failure; the critique granted that some discussion may be more appropriate when it is clear that the physician and patient share a common faith.

Many of the methodological critiques were, at the time, reasonable concerning the literature taken as a whole. However, the field was rapidly advancing, and has advanced since. The relatively strong Hummer et al. (1999) study had been published just that year. The Strawbridge et al. (1997) study discussed, had been published a couple of years earlier. Even at that earlier stage in the development of the literature, Koenig et al. (1999) offered a rebuttal of some of the points. Koenig et al. agreed with Sloan et al. that control needed to be made for confounding, that adjustment needed to be made for multiple comparisons, and that the ethical questions are complicated, but further argued that Sloan et al. had presented a very selective review and had omitted evidence from some of the strongest studies, that they had inaccurately reported some results, that they had failed to distinguish between confounding variables and mediating variables (i.e., those that may be on the pathway) in "explaining away" associations, that the claim of inconsistent results in the literature had failed to distinguish between different populations and different measures and aspects of religion and spirituality, and that, taken as a whole, the strongest evidence suggested that certain forms of religious participation had a beneficial effect on health. They briefly addressed Sloan et al.'s ethical concerns, arguing that health care providers deal with other private practices, and other settings where moral failure is seen as an issue, as is perhaps sometimes may be viewed as being the case with inability to quit smoking. We will return to some of these ethical concerns later in this review.

The timing of this debate and critique is important to keep in mind. It essentially took place at the first appearance of the strongest evidence for a relationship between religious participation and health beginning to appear. The first edition of Koenig et al.'s *Handbook on Religion and Health* was in press at the time. The McCullough et al. (2000) meta-analysis came out the following year. However, many of Sloan's critique were reasonable with respect to the vast majority of the literature, and many of these same critiques are still applicable to much of the literature today. However, as discussed, the strongest studies do seem to suggest a relatively strong protective relationship between forms of religious participations, especially religious service attendance and health.

IS IT CAUSAL?

One of Sloan et al.'s critiques was that confounding control in many of the studies on religion and health was weak. For many studies, this critique was reasonable. However, we have also noted that there are now numerous longitudinal studies examining service attendance and mortality, depression, and suicide, with very good control for potential confounders; and in these studies, the associations still persist. Nevertheless, these studies still make use of observational data, and it is always possible that unmeasured or residual confounding may explain some of these associations. It is, however, possible to use sensitivity analysis to examine how strong such unmeasured confounding would have to be to explain away the associations. For example, in using the Nurses' Health Study data to examine associations between service attendance and mortality, after extensive confounding control, Li et al. (2016b) reported that those attending services more than weekly had 0.67 (0.62, 0.71) lower rate of mortality in follow-up than those not attending. Using sensitivity analysis, they further noted that for an unmeasured confounder to explain away the association, the unmeasured confounder would have to both increase the likelihood of service attendance and decrease the likelihood of mortality by 2.35-fold, above and beyond the measured confounders. Such substantial confounding by unmeasured factors seems unlikely, given adjustment already made for an extensive set of covariates. While causality cannot be definitely established, the evidence that some of the association is causal seems fairly strong.

Likewise, for depression, Li et al (2016a) reported that for an unmeasured confounder to explain away the estimate that those attending services multiple times per week were 0.71 (0.62, 0.82) less likely to become depressed, an unmeasured confounder would have to both increase the likelihood of service attendance and decrease the likelihood of depression by 2.1-fold, above and beyond the measured confounders. Similarly, for suicide, VanderWeele et al. (2016a) reported that for an unmeasured confounder to explain away the estimate that those attending services at least weekly were 0.18 (95% CI: 0.06, 0.51) times less likely to commit suicide, an unmeasured confounder would have to both increase the likelihood of service attendance and decrease the likelihood of suicide by 10.5-fold, above and beyond the measured confounders. In this case, extremely strong unmeasured confounding would be required. With observational data, one can never be certain about causality, but the results of sensitivity analysis, after extensive control for measured covariates, suggest that the evidence that some of the association is causal is quite strong.

Another form of evidence that some of the associations between religion and health are causal is that there are a number of plausible mechanisms by which religious participation may affect health and it is to these that we now turn.

POTENTIAL MECHANISMS

Numerous mechanisms have been suggested for what might be responsible for the associations between religious participation and health (George et al., 2002; Koenig et al., 2012). For example, for mortality and service attendance, it has been suggested that social support, less smoking, lower depression, greater self-regulation, hope and optimism, and meaning and purpose may be potential mechanisms. There is some empirical evidence that some of these might indeed explain some of the relationship. For example, in a number of studies examining service attendance and mortality (Strawbridge et al., 1997; Hummer et al., 1999; Musick et al., 2004; la Cour et al., 2006), after control is made for social support, the magnitude of the associations decreases by about 20–30%, which is sometimes interpreted as social support mediating about 20–30% of the effect. There are some difficulties with analyses of this type. First, to interpret such analyses as evidence of mediation require confounding control not only for service attendance, but also for factors that might be confounding the relationship between the mediator and the outcome; for example, with social support as a mediator one would want to control for common causes of social support and mortality (VanderWeele, 2015). Second, while it is the case that service attendance probably does increase social support, it is also possible that social support might increase the likelihood of attendance. There may be effects in both directions. Said another way, social support may be both a confounder and a mediator of the relationship. Social support may mediate the effect of prior service attendance but confound the effect of subsequent service attendance. Assessing the extent of mediation and quantifying the importance of a mechanism in the presence of such two-way effects, can be done, but is much more challenging (VanderWeele, 2015). With repeated measures one can make progress but additional analytic methods are needed.

It is nonetheless somewhat easier to qualitatively establish mechanisms than it is to precisely quantify their exact contributions. For example, we discussed how there is fairly strong evidence, from longitudinal studies with good confounding control, that service attendance is related to lower smoking, less depression, more social support, and a greater sense of meaning and purpose. It is also known from other studies that these variables are related to mortality, thereby establishing fairly strong evidence that smoking, depression, social support, and meaning and purpose, are mechanisms that relate service attendance to mortality. However, more work using newer, more sophisticated methods (VanderWeele, 2015) that assess mediation with time-varying exposures and mediators with time-varying confounding will be needed to adequately *quantify* the relative contributions of these different mechanisms.

Likewise, a number of mechanisms have been suggested relating religious participation to better mental health including higher social support, better physical health, comfort from religion, systems of meaning, and relaxation of nervous system through prayer/meditation (Koenig et al., 2012). Several mechanisms have likewise been suggested governing associations between service attendance and suicide including social support, less alcohol, less depression, less drug use, and the moral belief that suicide is wrong (Dervic et al., 2004; Oquendo et al., 2005; Koenig et al., 2012). Qualitatively many of these mechanisms can be established by similar arguments to those we have given for mortality. However, once again, further research will be needed to quantify the relative contributions of these various potential mechanisms. That these plausible mechanisms are present does, however, contribute some further evidence that some of the association between service attendance and health is in fact causal, and helps elucidate further how this is so.

FORGIVENESS AND HEALTH

A final topic on the empirical research on religion and health that we will cover in this review and that has received considerable attention in past years is the relationship between forgiveness and health. Many religious traditions encourage some form of forgiveness. As we will see, the empirical research literature has suggested that forgiveness itself is closely tied to health.

There are difficult conceptual issues regarding what forgiveness itself is, and how it is defined. It is sometimes seen as a victim's replacing resentment towards the wrongdoer with compassion, or the reduction of negative thoughts, emotions, and behaviors and replacing these with positive thoughts, emotions, and behaviors towards the offender (cf. Worthington, 2005; Worthington et al., 2013). Distinctions are sometimes drawn between "trait forgiveness," the degree to which a person tends to forgive across time and situations, and "state forgiveness" a person's forgiveness of a specific offense. Distinctions are likewise sometimes drawn between "decisional forgiveness," the behavioral intention to forgo revenge and to treat the offender as a person of value, and "emotional forgiveness," the replacement of negative unforgiving emotions with positive other-centered emotions (Worthington, 2006). Decisional forgiveness will often precede emotional forgiveness; one can decide to forgive even with unforgiving emotions like resentment, bitterness, hostility, hatred, anger, fear, and desire for vengeance. Forgiveness takes place in time and there may be both general trends in the temporal process of forgiveness but also daily fluctuations (McCullough et al., 2003). Repeated offenses may also alter dynamics (Worthington et al., 2013). Forgiveness itself is sometimes distinguished from communicating forgiveness which may occur at a different occasion. Forgiveness is likewise often distinguished from condoning, reconciling, forgetting, forbearing, justifying, not demanding justice, and excusing, points we will return to later. Most of the empirical literature on forgiveness is focused on forgiveness of another for an offense committed. Other forms of forgiveness include self-forgiveness—that is, the forgiving of oneself for doing wrong to another or falling short of one's own standards—though some argue this would be better formulated as self-acceptance (Vitz and Meade, 2011; cf. Kim and Enright, 2014); and divine forgiveness, a person's sense of being forgiven by the deity that they consider to be sacred. Some discussion has been given to settings in which forgiveness might be seen as problematic such as contexts in which forgiveness and restoration of relationships may facilitate dynamics of prolonged intimate partner violence (Gordon et al., 2004). Various empirical measures have been developed to assess forgiveness (McCullough et al., 2006; Thompson et al., 2005; Brown, 2003). Sample items from these scales include "Even though his/her action hurt me, I have goodwill for him/her" or "I'll make him/her pay" or "I have released my anger so I can work on restoring our relationship to health."

Numerous analyses, and also meta-analysis, suggest that religiousness and spirituality measures are associated with greater levels of forgiveness (Davis et al., 2013). There is some evidence that religiousness is more consistently associated with forgiveness than is spirituality (DeShea et al., 2006), and also some evidence that spirituality is more strongly associated with self-forgiveness than is religiosity (Davis et al., 2013). There is some evidence that forgiveness varies across religious groups (Cohen et al., 2006). However, these studies are cross-sectional and so the direction of causality is difficult to determine and it is hard to rule out a potential common cause. For example, empathy may incline people towards forgiveness and towards religion. Religious participation may likely have some effect on forgiveness, as most religions instruct forgiveness, but more research is needed to establish this empirically.

Forgiveness is itself associated with better health. In a recent review, McCullough et al. (2009) note that forgiveness is associated with lower measures of depression, anxiety, and hostility; reduced risk for nicotine dependence and substance abuse; higher positive emotion; higher satisfaction with life; higher social support; and fewer self-reported health symptoms. The mechanisms are generally thought to be beneficial emotion regulation and forgiveness being an alternative to maladaptive psychological responses like rumination and suppression. There is some evidence that forgiveness of self or others may be associated with better physical health as well, but the associations are less consistent (Toussaint et al., 2015). Once again, however, most of the research is cross-sectional and from such studies it is difficult to determine the direction of causality.

However, in the case of the potential effects of forgiveness on health, various forgiveness interventions have been developed, and in fact even evaluated in randomized trials. Two prominent intervention classes are based on specific models of forgiveness including Enright's Process model and Worthington's REACH model. Most interventions require a trained professional to implement but workbook interventions have also been developed (Harper et al., 2014; Greer et al., 2014). In Enright's Process model, treatment takes place over twenty steps (Enright and Fitzgibbons, 2000) organized into four phases: uncovering negative feelings about the offense, deciding to pursue forgiveness for a specific instance, working towards understanding the offending person, and discovery of unanticipated positive outcomes and empathy for the forgiven person. Interventions using this model have been shown to be effective with groups as diverse as adult incest survivors (Freedman and Enright, 1996), parents who have adopted special needs children (Baskin et al., 2011), and inpatients struggling with alcohol and drug addiction (Lin et al., 2004). In Worthington's REACH model, each letter of "REACH" represents a component of the process (Worthington, 2001): Recall the hurt one has experienced and the emotions associated with it; Empathize with the offender and take the other's perspective in considering reasons for action (without condoning the action or invalidating one's feelings); Altruistic gesture of recalling one's own shortcomings and realizing others have offered forgiveness Commitment to forgive publicly; and Hold onto or maintain the forgiveness through times of uncertainty or through the returning of anger and bitterness.

Numerous randomized trials and intervention studies have made use of these forgiveness models. A recent meta-analysis of 54 studies suggested a fairly sizable average effect on forgiveness among the studies (Wade et al., 2014). The size of the effect depended on length of the intervention; the interventions based on the Enright model were generally of longer duration than those of the Worthington model and thus had larger effects. The same meta-analysis examined the average effects across studies for other outcomes and also found evidence for an effect of the forgiveness interventions on depression, anxiety, and hope. Some smaller individual randomized studies have found effects of forgiveness interventions on aspects of physical health (Waltman et al., 2009; Ingersoll et al., 2009). Although most of these forgiveness interventions require a trained professional, there is some preliminary evidence that even workbook forgiveness interventions, that can be done on one's own, are effective in bringing about forgiveness and perhaps alleviating depression (Harper et at., 2014; Greer et al., 2014). Workbooks have been developed both for the forgiveness of others (Harper et al., 2014; Greer et al., 2014) and for the forgiveness of self (Griffin et al., 2015). Such workbooks are freely available online (http://www. evworthington-forgiveness.com/diy-workbooks). More research is needed, but if these workbook resources prove to be effective, the potential for outreach and promotion of both forgiveness and mental health, may be substantial and could have profound public health implications.

INTERVENTIONS CONCERNING RELIGION AND HEALTH

Our focus thus far in this review has been ways in which religious institutions, and participation in them, contribute to a variety of health outcomes. However there is also a literature on health-focused interventions within religious institutions, and also on religious institutions providing resources for health promotion, such as the work of many faith-based organizations delivering health care. In this second part of the review we will thus describe potential interventions related to religion and health that have been developed, and also partnerships between religious and public health institutions, to promote health. We will summarize the research literature on religiously oriented interventions that may promote health.

HEALTH PROMOTION INTERVENTIONS IN RELIGIOUS SETTINGS

Various health promotion interventions have been developed for use within specific religious contexts or institutions. In this literature, a distinction is sometimes also drawn between "faith-based" versus "faith-placed" interventions, the former involving some sort of spiritual or religious approach and the latter simply indicating that the intervention is merely taking place at a religious institution (DeHaven et al., 2004; cf. Lasater et al., 1997). Much of the literature on interventions is descriptive in nature. There is a much smaller literature on empirically assessing the effectiveness of interventions. Campbell et al. (2007) review about 60 studies on church-based health promotion and find that most are descriptive with only 13 involving some formal evaluation. Most that do have an evaluative component are within African-American Churches. They report evidence from randomized trials that interventions can increase fruit and vegetable consumption lead to smoking cessation, and perhaps promote weight-loss, and increase cancer screening (cf. Chatters, 2000; Allen et al., 2014).

In reviewing the literature, Campbell et al. (2007) also discuss five important elements of design of such interventions including: true partnerships and trust, adequately constructing membership lists, understanding the social and environmental context of the religious community in designing the intervention, incorporating appropriate spiritual/religious content and involving the community members in delivery, and leaving something behind; for example, providing training, leaving materials behind, or assisting churches is finding funding to continue the program. There are also important questions concerning evaluation in such religious community-based settings for interventions. In evaluating the impact of an intervention, it is not only of interest to discern whether the intervention itself is more effective than a control condition, but also whether the intervention itself is more effective than other religious non-health related meetings, and possibly whether a religiously based intervention is more effective than a secular alternative, a point to which we will return later. See Campbell et al. (2007) for further discussion and review.

HEALTH CARE PROVISION BY RELIGIOUS AND FAITH-BASED INSTITUTIONS

Religious institutions also often provide important resources that make partnerships with public health institutions possible. Such resources include spaces to meet, often with kitchens, regular gatherings with large numbers, a community with relationships of trust, and a shared spiritual and moral message. Idler (2014b) discusses in detail a number of such partnerships. See also Levin (2014, 2016) for further discussion. Examples of partnerships in which the resources or space have been important include soup kitchens and food pantries; Alcoholics Anonymous programs;

H1N1 vaccination and education programs (Kiser and Santibanez, 2014); La Leche (cf. Idler, 2014b) in the promotion of breastfeeding; and breast cancer screening programs (Allen et al., 2014); and church-based health promotion/prevention programs for diabetes, maternal and child health, and hypertension (Chatters, 2000).

Moreover, religious groups and faith-based organizations often have as their mission some health related goal. Religious groups have also often provided material resources and infrastructure for hospitals, clinics, and medical missions. Most 19th-century homes for the aged in the United States were started by Christian and Jewish groups; even in mid-20th century most remained religious (Maves, 1960). L'Arche communities for the disabled had religious origins (cf. Idler, 2014). A recent report (Brown, 2014) indicated that the Catholic Church, as one of the largest global health care providers, operated 5,246 hospitals, 17,530 dispensaries, 577 leprosy clinics, and 15,208 houses for the chronically ill and handicapped worldwide. In a number of African countries, it is estimated that faith-based organizations provide between 30% and 50% of health-related facilities (Mwenda, 2011).

Religious groups have also provided a powerful moral message and advocacy. Important examples include the role of religious institutions in civil rights advocacy in the United States (Morris, 1986) and in the Truth and Reconciliation Commission in South Africa (Tutu, 2000). Yet another example of such efforts include the role religious institutions played in community advocacy concerning the link between environmental pollution and leukemia in Woburn, Massachusetts (Van Ness, 1999; Harr, 1996).

Although there have been a number of very effective partnerships between religious groups and public health institutions, there have also been tensions. A prominent example of tension is the role of religious organizations in providing care for HIV/AIDs patients. Within the United States, some Christian commentary suggested that AIDS was a divine punishment for sins of homosexuality, adultery, or premarital or extramarital sex. It has been argued that this may have affected government funding and policy (Dalmida and Thurman, 2014). However, faith-based hospitals also provided much of the care early in the epidemic and considerable institutional support. In 1986, the Episcopal Church sponsored a national AIDS-related faith gathering. In 1989, Catholic programs united as the Catholic AIDS network. In the 1990's an AIDS National Interfaith Network was formed. Globally, early faith-based efforts focused on care and support for those with HIV/AIDS, but later programs have focused more on education and prevention (Derose et al., 2011). There is some evidence that faith-based organizations may have first contributed to increasing discrimination and stigmatization in Uganda, but later made important contributions to decreasing discrimination and stigmatization (Otolok-Tanga et al., 2007). Religious groups have focused more on providing care, raising awareness, and testing. Partnerships between religious and public health institutions, such as between the Catholic Church and Brazil's National AIDS program (Murray et al., 2011), were also formed. One of the most important controversies in this regard has been the use of condoms, with public health groups advocating for their use in preventing the spread of HIV, and religious groups sometimes advocating against condom use as either encouraging more promiscuous sexual activity, or as wrong in and of itself. See Murray et al. (2011) for discussion of how these tensions were handled, but not eliminated, in partnerships between Brazil's National AIDS Program (NAP) and the Catholic Church, with some willingness on each side to tolerate different ideological perspectives. In a number of instances, partnerships between religious organizations and public health institutions have been powerful and effective, but they have not been without various tensions. See Trinitapoli and Weinreb (2012) for further discussion.

FORGIVENESS INTERVENTIONS

We discussed in the first section of this review that forgiveness interventions have been developed, and that there is evidence from randomized trials that these interventions not only effectively promote forgiveness but also alter depression, anxiety, and hope, and perhaps even promote physical health. There is some evidence that such forgiveness interventions can be effective in even very difficult contexts such as among adult incest survivors (Freedman and Enright, 1996), in reconciliation after the 1994 Rwandan genocide (Staub et al., 2005), and in trials of restorative justice meetings between convicted criminals and their victims (Sherman et al., 2005). While most of the interventions that have been developed require a trained counselor or professional to implement, there have recently been developed "do-it-yourself" workbook interventions to promote forgiveness. These too have been tested in randomized trials with some preliminary evidence that they also are effective (Harper et al., 2014; Greer et al., 2014; Griffin et al., 2015). Further research is needed, as the sample sizes in the randomized workbook trials were quite small, but if these do prove to be effective, they could constitute powerful forgiveness and public health promotion resources. Further research on intervention development might incorporate perspectives from the philosophical literature (e.g., North, 1987; Holmgren, 1993) on the moral conditions for forgiveness, and help ensure that practical interventions sufficiently distinguish forgiveness from condoning, reconciling, forgetting, forbearing, justifying, not demanding justice, and excusing so as to ensure more effective interventions and to appropriately handle contexts that may be problematic (Gordon et al., 2014).

SPIRITUALLY INTEGRATED MEDICAL CARE AND PSYCHOTHERAPY

A number of religiously based or spiritually integrated psychotherapy interventions have also been developed, and some of these have been assessed in randomized trials. Such interventions are intended to draw upon the spiritual resources, motivations, and coping strategies that may be available to those with religious beliefs. Reasons sometimes given for employing spiritually integrated psychotherapy include the broad participation in religion within America and worldwide and its embeddedness within culture, spirituality itself being a resource to many people, an acknowledgement that spirituality can also be the source of problems and difficulties, and the fact that, when surveyed, patients often state that they would prefer spiritually integrated interventions. See Pargament (2011) for a fuller overview of such spiritually integrated interventions.

In some cases, these spiritually integrated or tailored interventions have been shown to have larger effects, among specific religious samples, than secular alternatives. For example, there is some evidence that, with Christian patients, certain forms of Christian cognitive behavioral therapy may yield higher recovery rates than is achieved with regular cognitive behavioral therapy (Koenig et al., 2009). Likewise, in the forgiveness workbook interventions described, although different samples were used, there was some preliminary evidence that the effect size for the workbook tailored to Christian participants was larger than the more generic forgiveness workbook intervention (Harper et al., 2014; Greer et al., 2014). However, in other cases, these larger effect sizes for religiously tailored interventions are not observed (Rye et al., 2005; Koenig et al., 2015). Koenig et al. (2015) do, however, report evidence for an interaction between religiously integrated therapy and the religiosity of patients, in which the religiously integrated therapy is somewhat more effective for more religious patients. Even in cases in which effects do not differ, however, it may be preferable to use a spiritually integrated or religiously-based psychotherapy intervention if it is likely to have broader outreach among certain religious populations who might otherwise be skeptical of, and hesitant to participate in, more secular types of psychotherapy.

Considerable research has been devoted to providing spiritual care in end-of-life health care settings. Spiritual care is included in many national and international palliative care guidelines (World Health Organization, 2004; National Consensus Project, 2009; Joint Commission 2013). Spiritual care can take many forms, including taking a spiritual history, referrals to hospital chaplaincy, and inviting conversation regarding religious and spiritual issues, among others (Hanson et al., 2008). The provision of spiritual care by medical teams has been shown to be associated with better quality of life at the end of life, less aggressive treatment, and lower costs (Astrow et al., 2007; Balboni et al., 2010, 2011), and is desired by patients (Steinhauer et al., 2000). However, it continues to be given infrequently (Phelps et al., 2012; M. J. Balboni et al., 2013). Training is an important predictor of the provision of spiritual care, but training itself is received by health care providers infrequently (M. J. Balboni et al., 2013). Interventions have been developed to provide training in the provision of spiritual care and have been assessed observationally (Zollfrank et al., 2015), but randomized trials are needed to adequately assess the effectiveness of these interventions on increasing the provision of care and on patient outcomes.

Research on spiritual care provided by a patient's religious community in the end-of-life context with terminal illness somewhat surprisingly indicates that the provision of such care is associated with seeking more aggressive treatment (T. A. Balboni et al., 2013), perhaps indicating that when spiritual care and medical care are not integrated, and the prognosis is not taken into account in spiritual care, patients may be more likely to believe a miracle is possible and that all aggressive treatment options ought to be sought out. Further research on integrating spiritual care and medical care would be of importance, along with the development of training interventions for clergy providing end-of-life care, to be assessed in randomized trials.

The development of training interventions for the provision of spiritual care is relevant also outside of the end-of-life context. The majority of patients in the United States would like to receive some form of such care (King& Bushwick, 1994; Astrow et al., 2007). Guidelines on and tools for taking a spiritual history in a medical context are available (Koenig, 2000b; Puchalski, 2014) and now some form of spiritual care training is available in over 80% of U.S. Medical School curricula (Koenig et al., 2010; Puchalski et al., 2012). Guidelines for competencies in spirituality and health for medical education have been developed (Puchalski et al., 2014). However, the majority of the courses available in medical curricula are electives, and most physicians report not having received any training (M. J. Balboni et al., 2013). Curricular and training interventions have been developed but their efficacy remains, for the most part, unclear (Fortin and Barnett, 2004). It may be necessary to incorporate spiritual care training and competencies throughout medical school and residency, rather than only as a single module (Puchalski et al., 2014; Sulmasy, 2009). Future research could consider the development of more effective training interventions for the provision of spiritual care, potentially integrating these with training on having "difficult conversations" with patients, and assessing the effects of these interventions on provision of spiritual care and also patient outcomes in randomized trials.

In the first part of this review, we summarized some of the strongest evidence from observational studies concerning the associations between religious service attendance and health outcomes such as mortality, depression, and suicide. It is often pointed out in the literature that it is not possible to randomize service attendance or other forms of religious involvement; it would be both unethical and infeasible; and thus that one must rely on observational data to explore the relationships between religious participation and health. We saw that, based on numerous large studies, with reasonably good methodology and study design, the evidence for the relationships between service attendance and mortality, depression, and suicide being causal was, if not conclusive, at least fairly strong. The sensitivity analysis for unmeasured confounding supported this conclusion. The evidence for other health outcomes was often less definitive.

While it is true that it is not possible to randomize service attendance directly, the impossibility of direct intervention is sometimes dealt with in the intervention literature by what is called an encouragement trial. In such encouragement trials, rather than attempting to intervene directly on the actual behavior or activity of interest, the intervention instead consists of some form of encouragement for the activity under study. With careful design and selection of study population, it would seem that such a design might in fact be possible also for religious service attendance, partially circumventing the issue that service attendance is not possible to randomize directly. Careful thought would need to be given to a number of practical and ethical issues. However, a study could potentially be designed to be conducted among those who already self-identify with a particular religious affiliation, but who may not regularly attend services. Each participant could be randomized to receive either written encouragement to attend religious services (e.g., mailings summarizing the empirical research on service attendance and health, perhaps accompanied also by more religiously oriented reasons for participating, prepared say by the religious group under study, along with a listing of the names and addresses of relevant religious groups nearby) or alternatively randomized to receive some neutral reading material (e.g., a summary of the most recent sporting event). The design might involve multiple such mailings. Follow-up could examine whether the mailings did in fact alter religious service attendance participation and also various health outcomes. An alternative design, in the setting of therapy for depression, but again for a study population who already self-identifies as religious, might be to randomize individuals to either receive standard cognitive behavioral therapy or to receive the same cognitive behavioral therapy but supplemented with discussion of participation in faith communities. In designs such as this, a relatively large sample size would likely be needed for such a trial to have adequate power to detect relevant effects, in part because many who self-identify with a particular religious affiliation would likely already be attending, and in part because the effectiveness of a mailing may be limited in changing longer term participation. The former difficulty could potentially be partly addressed by only including, within the study, those who did not attend or were only occasionally attending. Even with a large sample, the effects would have to be carefully interpreted as the effects of encouraging attendance rather than attendance itself, and would be specific to the religious group or groups under study. Some of the ethical issues regarding such a trial would be at least partially addressed by limiting the study population to those who already self-identify with the particular religious tradition being studied.

The ethical issues related to encouraging religious service attendance have also been raised within the medical literature on religion and health. In 2000, Sloan and colleagues published a

New England Journal of Medicine Sounding Board piece entitled "Should physicians prescribe religious activities?" (Sloan et al., 2000). In it, the authors argue that prescription of religious service attendance is unethical since the content of religious services varies considerably, religion can also often cause tensions and antagonism, religious views often differ across patients and physicians, physicians are not trained in such matters, and that the empirical literature on religion and health is a veiled attempt to validate religion by associations with health and that this literature moreover trivializes religion itself. The piece, which raised many important issues, elicited also numerous letters to the editors. Koenig (2000a) argued that Sloan et al. approach the question by setting up and attacking an extreme position, that physicians should prescribe religious activities, and that this is very different from a recognition that such activities may be important in the patient's life and understanding of illness. He notes that this is again different from current recommendations (Koenig, 2000b) for physicians to take a short four-question spiritual history and that for those who are not religious, the discussion can quickly move on. Other responses were of a more personal nature. Nicklin (2000), a family physician, responded that in 16 years of practice none of his inquiries about patients' religious or spiritual lives in the face of progressive, incurable or fatal illness led to a negative response, and that often they had been helpful.

The issue of addressing religious concerns within the medical and public health context has been, as can be seen, somewhat controversial. A detailed review of the literature on the topic is beyond the scope of this review. Encouraging religious community participation for those who already hold the specific beliefs of the religious community may be somewhat more appropriate as a source of community involvement, social support, and shared framework of meaning and understanding. However, careful thought would certainly have to be given to these ethical issues if the effects of service attendance itself were to be studied in a randomized encouragement trials as described.

RANDOMIZED TRIALS OF PRAYER

We will conclude our description of religion and health interventions with a brief discussion of what is perhaps an even more controversial topic: randomized trials of prayer. The standard design of these trials is that patients are randomized to receive intercessory prayer from someone else; patients themselves, however, are often "blinded" in the sense that they don't know whether or not they are being prayed for. Some of these randomized trials have suggested an effect of prayer; other studies have suggested no effect; and the research remains controversial. Two reviews have attempted to synthesize all available evidence but they themselves are divided. Astin et al. (2000) conducted a systematic review with fairly broad inclusion criteria and include 23 randomized trials. Astin et al.'s review concluded that there was some evidence for an effect: 57% (13 studies) reported an effect; 39% (9 studies) no effect; 4% (1 study) a negative effect. Meta-analysis has also been done by the Cochran Collaboration and has been repeated a number of times (Roberts et al., 2000, 2007, 2009). Using stricter inclusion criteria than the Astin et al. (2000) study, the Cochran meta-analysis in 2000 was inconclusive; the meta-analysis in 2007 suggested an effect on mortality with summary odds ratio OR = 0.88 (95% CI: 0.80, 0.97) but no effect on clinical state or complications. The meta-analysis in 2009 still had a protective odds ratio, OR = 0.77 (95% CI: 0.51, 1.16), but one for which the confidence interval included the null of no effect. The conclusion seemed to depend somewhat on what studies were included. Moreover, much commentary on the studies themselves and the meta-analyses questions the objectivity of those conducting these randomized trials of prayer.

Reactions to such research range from dismissal to intrigue to outrage. Objections to this research on prayer come from those both with and without religious commitments. Some object to this research on the grounds that it is the wasting money and valuable research resources that could be redirected to questions which have true benefit to health. Yet others claim that such research is nearly impossible to carry out rigorously, that the investigators conducting such studies almost always have an agenda—for or against—and that the research will thus rarely be credible. Those who do believe in prayer have also leveled objections against this research. Some object to the research on the grounds that such research is "putting God to the test"; such research, using these randomized trials, seems to assume that God, if he exists, is somehow outside of the trial; that he does not know it is happening; that he wouldn't be able to determine the outcome but is somehow constrained by what "usually happens." Yet others object to these trials on the grounds that they seem to implicitly assume that those in the control arm are not being prayed for by anyone (e.g., family and friends outside of the trial), which may not be a reasonable assumption. Another objection to these trials is that the forms of prayer examined in these "double blinded" trials do not correspond to the forms of prayer that are actually practiced within religious communities. Prayer for healing within religious communities often occurs within the context of a relationship and often involves the laying on of hands, which is very different it is claimed from what is being studied in the randomized trials. Clearly objections exist to such research from very different perspectives. The research employing randomized trials to examine the effects of intercessory prayer seem to bring us to the boundary of what questions can actually be studied empirically concerning religion and health. Whether the methodology is appropriate and whether the subject matter lends itself to empirical study is likely to remain controversial. See Brown (2012) for further discussion of various aspects of the study of prayer.

THEOLOGICAL THEMES CONCERNING RELIGION AND HEALTH

In this section we will provide a brief overview of various religious and theological themes concerning religion and health. We will describe some important common elements concerning views of health shared by many of the world religions, we will briefly summarize certain Biblical themes on religion and health from the Christian tradition, we will give an overview of some work within philosophy on forgiveness, and finally discuss religious objections that have been put forward concerning the empirical research on religion and health. The focus of this brief summary will be the themes most relevant to the empirical research literature on religion and health surveyed, in order to, in the final section of this review, consider points of convergence and tension, and where the empirical and theological and philosophical literatures might inform each other.

RELIGION AND HEALTH IN THE WORLD RELIGIONS

The topic of the conceptions of health within the various world religions is very broad, and it is far beyond the scope of this review to even attempt to adequately represent each religious tradition. Here we will only proceed with a summary of some common elements that emerge from the various conceptions of health encountered in many of the world religions. We will summarize some of the various conclusions suggested in other work.

Ketchell et al. (2011), summarizing various literatures and also a prior book-length survey on world religions and health (Sullivan, 1989), consider perspectives on physical, mental, social and spiritual health from Buddhist, Confucian, Hindu, Islamic, Judaic, and Shamanic traditions and summarize three major themes across traditions. First, that disharmony between the individual, community, and Ultimate Reality is the principal source of suffering and illness. Second, the various world religions offer a variety of remedies or pathways to healing for this disharmony including prayer, meditation, good deeds, rituals and ceremonies, and practical institutions of health and social support. And third, that community health is integrally related to individual health. It is noted that in many ancient societies, priests both met religious needs and also provided healing, again tying together religion and health. We have already seen, to a certain extent, some of these themes in our survey of the empirical literature on religion and health and in the final section of this review we will consider in more detail the relation between the various religious themes and the empirical research.

Fuller consideration of major distinct themes concerning religion and health in each of the world's religions is again beyond the scope of this review. The interested reader is referred to Desai (1989) for a review of themes and ideas on religion and health from within the Hindu tradition, Rahman (1987) from an Islamic tradition, Fledman (1986) from a Jewish tradition, Birnbaum (1989) from a Buddhist tradition, and the collected volume by Sullivan (1989) for summaries of these and many other individual religious traditions. See also McCarty and Kinghorn (2017) for discussion of how Islamic, Jewish and Christian theology has shaped and continues to shape medical institutions and practice.

BIBLICAL TRADITIONS CONCERNING RELIGION, HEALTH, AND HEALING

As most of the empirical literature on religion and health has been conducted within the United States, and thus pertains to predominantly Christian populations, we will briefly survey, in somewhat more detail, some of the themes concerning religion and health within Christianity, focusing here on Biblical traditions. Specifically, we will consider eight themes which have some prominence in the Hebrew Bible or Old Testament, and within the New Testament. These themes will include broad conceptual relations such (1) health as wholeness, (2) sin as the cause of ill health and brokenness, (3) God as the source of healing, and (4) relations between health and salvation; along with pathways to healing and health including (5) healing as response to prayer, (6) healing and forgiveness, (7) healing and community, and (8) healing and caregiving. See Kee (1992), Kelsey (1995), Avalos (1999), Wilkinson (1998), and Pilch (2000) for fuller treatments of this topic, upon which the summary that follows is based. The aim of this section will be, once again, to eventually relate some of the theological themes on religion and health to the empirical literature on religion and health, and to explore where these literatures converge, where there are tensions, and how one might inform the other.

With regard to the concept of health found in the Biblical texts, there is a close connection between health and wholeness. The Hebrew word *rapha* is often translated "heal," and connotes a "restoring to normal." The Hebrew word perhaps closest to "health" is *marpe*, but it is used relatively infrequently. Instead the Hebrew word *shalom*, often translated as "peace," is frequently employed and conveys a sense of general well-being or right relation to self, others, and God. Three Greek words are predominantly used in the New Testament for "heal": *therapevo, iaomai,* and *sozo. Therapevo* is associated with care or attention; *iaomai* is associated with cure or restoration; and *sozo* more literally means "save." The Greek word for "to be in health," *hygiano,* is somewhat similar to the concept in English, "to be whole, sound and well." Both the Hebrew and Greek concepts of health thus relate closely to well-being generally or wholeness. As will be discussed further, healing in the Biblical accounts often concerned the whole person and included both physical and spiritual healing.

The Biblical narrative suggests that sin, wrongdoing, and rejection of God is ultimately the root cause of brokenness, illness, and death. While certainly not every instance of ill health is attributed to wrongdoing, the connection between the two is portrayed in various ways. Ill health is pictured as the consequence of sin sometimes directly by someone's actions harming another. At other times, the relationship is depicted as disordered behaviors and actions bringing about ill health for oneself or, as in the Proverbs, through a deficiency in character and virtue. Sometimes the relationship between sin and ill-health is pictured as divine punishment. Perhaps more profoundly, the relationship is sometimes pictured as the general all-pervasive fallenness and brokenness of the created order being the consequence of sin and the rejection of God.

Healing in the Bible is often seen as the work of God and of those whom he empowers. In many of the Biblical stories, God heals after intercessory prayer is made by another. The prophetic books speak of the renewal, restoration, and healing of the entire people of Israel. Many of the Gospel accounts are occupied with accounts of Jesus' healing by God's power. Jesus' death on the cross and his resurrection is pictured as being for the healing and salvation of the world with, once again, God pictured as agent. The Spirit of God is also spoken of as accomplishing transformation of one's character and person, bringing about a restoration to wholeness.

Closely related to this point, healing is often also tied to salvation in the Biblical accounts. The prophetic books speak of the "healing" of apostasy and faithlessness; healing and restoration or salvation are also often spoken of in parallel in the prophetic books. In the healing accounts of the Gospels, in several instances when Jesus uses the words "your faith has healed you," it is the Greek word sozo that is used and the more direct translation would thus be "your faith has saved you." Jesus' care for the physical ailments of those he heals highlights the importance of the body, but the healings themselves often symbolically point towards, or are accompanied by speech concerning, spiritual healing and salvation. The New Testament Epistles also suggest a link between salvation and healing with faith leading to conversion and transformation of character, by following the example of Jesus, and by the work of the Spirit. While healing is never completely accomplished in this life, ultimate healing and restoration is pictured as coming fully and finally in the resurrection of the dead.

Our discussion thus far has focused on broad conceptual relations between religion and health: health and wholeness, sin as the root cause of brokenness and ill-health, God as the agent of healing, and healing coming from salvation. The Biblical account, however, also suggests a number of more concrete pathways to healing including prayer, forgiveness, caregiving, and community.

As already noted, prayer is pictured as a pathway to healing in many of the Biblical stories. In some of the healing accounts, such prayer is accompanied by the laying on of hands; it is often tied to faith in God. The book of James suggests that this prayer for healing may be in a congregational context and accompanied by anointing with oil. Prayer does not always result in healing in the Biblical accounts, but it is clearly one pathway to it.

Forgiveness is pictured as another pathway to healing. Healing and forgiveness are spoken of in parallel in the prophetic books. The New Testament pictures Jesus' life and death as being for the forgiveness of sins and restoration of the person to wholeness and communion with God. Emphasis is also placed in the New Testament on forgiving others, which is to be done irrespective of the number of offenses, and is important for community and religious life. Forgiveness of others is to follow from God's forgiveness, a connection explicitly made in Jesus' parables and in the Lord's Prayer. In some of the Gospel healing accounts, Jesus likewise ties healing to the forgiveness of sins. Illness itself can become the path to conversion, forgiveness, and true healing. In the book of James, healing is tied to confession and the forgiveness of sins in the context of congregational life. The various writings thus suggest that forgiveness from God brings healing, wholeness and salvation; one's forgiveness of others brings healing to oneself, to the offender, and to the community; and confession of sins to God and to the community, and accompanying forgiveness, can likewise bring healing.

In the Biblical accounts, care and healing are also to take place in ways that are more physical and direct, through care-giving. The prophets command care for the sick and crippled and rebuke the people when they do not do so. Jesus expected that his followers would be involved in healing, and in the care for the sick. In Paul's letters, healing is spoken of as one of the gifts of the Spirit, and it is suggested that even one's own suffering and illness can be for the consolation of others. The giving of care to those in need is thus also pictured as an important pathway for healing.

Relatedly, throughout the Biblical account, the community itself was understood as the context within which salvation, forgiveness, and healing would come. The community was to provide for the needs of each other, to issue rebuke for wrong action when necessary, to participate together in religious life and ritual, and to love, support and encourage one another. The community was thus itself an important part of salvation and healing. Spiritual healing would bring one into this community and the community itself was a source of healing. In Jesus' healings of those with leprosy or hemorrhaging, the healing was not only physical, but also constituted a full restoration to community and religious life which illness had prevented. Jesus' life, death, and resurrection, with the healing and salvation which this brought, was to be remembered within the community by a common meal following the model of the last supper of Jesus with his disciples. Love was to be the central defining feature of this community, following Jesus' life and example, with Jesus himself having also summarized the whole of the law as love of God and love of one's neighbor. In Paul's writing, love was described as the greatest end of communal and religious life.

Subsequent developments of many of these Biblical themes concerning health and healing, as it relates to wholeness, sin, God, salvation, prayer, forgiveness, caregiving, and community have taken place within theology. For example, later theology ties the sacraments quite closely to healing and the aforementioned modes of healing. The Catechism of the Catholic Church (2000) connects the sacrament of the Eucharist to community, forgiveness, and healing and restoration; it relates the sacrament of the anointing of the sick to prayer, forgiveness, caregiving, and healing; and it relates the sacrament of penance and reconciliation to forgiveness, prayer, community, and conversion and healing. Due to space limitations and the focus of this review, we will not, however, further survey the subsequent theological development of these various themes. See McCormick (1984) for further discussion of health and medicine from the Catholic tradition; Smith (1986) from an Anglican tradition; Vaux (1984) from a Reformed tradition; Sweet (1994) from an evangelical tradition; Marty (1983) from a Lutheran tradition; Fledman (1986) from a Jewish tradition; and also shorter summaries in Numbers and Amundsen (1985) for these and various other Western religious traditions. We will return to some of these themes in the final section of this review, and we will consider their relation to the empirical research on religion and health that we surveyed.

PHILOSOPHICAL LITERATURE ON FORGIVENESS

In the first two sections of this review (Empirical Research on Religion and Health; and Critique and Response) we discussed some of the empirical research on forgiveness and forgiveness interventions. Here we will summarize some of the philosophical literature, focused primarily on the nature of forgiveness and the conditions under which forgiveness is to be considered morally appropriate. We will examine two fairly prominent philosophical articles on forgiveness in the work of North (1987) and Holmgren (1993).

In our summary of the empirical research on forgiveness, we noted that forgiveness itself is often distinguished from condoning, reconciling, forgetting, forbearing, justifying, the foregoing of justice, and excusing. North (1987) provides some justification for these distinctions and argues that punishment is not in fact inconsistent with forgiveness. Forgiveness, she argues, is the overcoming of resentment by endeavoring to view the wrongdoer with compassion, benevolence and love, while recognizing that the wrongdoer has, in some sense, willfully abandoned his right to them. Forgiveness thus does not necessarily logically exclude punishment. She notes that forgiveness recognizes a wrong has been done and thus is different from excusing someone. While punishment is not inconsistent with forgiveness, she also argues that neither punishment nor repentance is necessary for forgiveness, though they might sometimes help facilitate it. North further notes that forgiveness recognizes that a wrong has been done and thus requires effort; it is not given lightly. Someone might have a forgiving disposition but this is only established through considerable development of character. She concludes by noting that forgiveness has moral worth in that it (1) recognizes a wrong has been done; (2) is a step towards reconciliation; and (3) helps promote mutual affection, trust, and sympathy that are fundamental human values at the root of our relations with one another.

Holmgren (1993) is concerned principally with the morality of forgiveness, under what circumstances it is to be considered morally appropriate, and what morality requires in terms of forgiveness. She argues that forgiveness itself involves several interrelated components: someone injured, wrong-doing on the part of the offender, an overcoming of negative feelings with the intent of reaching an appropriate attitude, and an internal acceptance of the wrongdoer. Genuine forgiveness, it is argued, involves numerous steps including the recovering of self-esteem, a recognition that a wrong has been done, an acknowledgement of one's feelings, possibly an opportunity to express beliefs and feelings to the wrongdoer, assessing the situation and the future relationship with respect to the offender, and determining whether or not to seek restitution. Holmgren argues that essentially all of this ought to happen prior to forgiveness in order for forgiveness to be genuine. After these steps are complete, genuine forgiveness, the replacement of negative feelings by compassion and good will for the offender, can take place. She moreover argues that, provided these conditions are met, unconditional forgiveness is *always* appropriate and does not depend on the action or beliefs of the wrongdoer.

She further argues that such genuine forgiveness is beneficial to the one forgiving, that it retains self-respect, that it respects morality, that it respects the wrong-doer as a moral agent, and that it builds character and virtue. Genuine forgiveness is beneficial to the one forgiving because it frees the victim from the past, does not make the victim dependent on the wrongdoer, and further promotes love compassion, acceptance, and harmony in human relations. Such genuine forgiveness furthermore retains self-respect because esteem is established, needs are addressed, the wrong is acknowledged, and the victim is no longer dependent on the wrongdoer; moreover, the perpetrator's perspective, even if confused, is acknowledged without the victim necessarily having responsibility for changing it. Such genuine forgiveness, it is argued, also respects morality because it acknowledges a wrong, it separates the sin and the sinner, and it gives the wrongdoer space to change.

Genuine forgiveness, Holmgren argues, further respects the wrongdoer as a moral agent. As sentient and morally free, human persons ought to be respected as persons, and forgiveness does this by creating an attitude of empathy and understanding while acknowledging the other's freedom. Because of these things, forgiveness, it is argued, is thus not only compatible with respect for oneself, morality, and the wrongdoer as a moral agent, but it is, in fact, *required* by these things. The pursuit of these things and of forgiveness thus builds virtue and character. In attempting to synthesize some of the empirical and theological and philosophical literature, we will return to some of these arguments and positions again.

RELIGIOUS OBJECTIONS TO EMPIRICAL RESEARCH ON RELIGION AND HEALTH

We considered some of the methodological critiques of the empirical religion and health literature earlier in this review, and mentioned some of the ethical questions that were raised by such research and we will return to these again later. Some objections to this type of research, however, have also been raised by those from religious communities concerning the entire enterprise of empirical research on religion and health. For example, Bishop (2009) argues that the empirical research on religion and health tends to strip religion of its distinctive content, and that the measures used are often too generic. He notes that religion itself is generally concerned with questions of salvation, the nature of God, and worship. However, the empirical research generally does not address such questions and instead replaces them with much more generic and functional notions of religion. Bishop argues that, in doing so, such research poses the danger of taking a utilitarian or functional view of religion. It risks making use religion for health while in fact neglecting religion's own goals and internal goods. Related arguments are put forward by Shuman and Meador (2002) who argue that the religion and health research likewise risks replacing the true meaning of faith with a self-interested individualism which enlists faith to simply get what we want.

From the perspective of a religious community, Bishop's and Shuman and Meador's concerns arguably are reasonable. Often relatively generic measures of religion and spirituality have been used in such research, and the research often is not focused on the primary goals and ends of religious communities. However, these concerns can also be, at least partially, addressed by more appropriately shaping this research area. More specific religious measures could be introduced and used concerning particular beliefs, or measures of particular relevance to specific denominations or religious traditions. Questions concerning notions of salvation, or beliefs such as that in life-after-death or the nature of right and wrong, could be developed and incorporated into research studies. Future empirical research studies, perhaps with the involvement of religious communities, could focus more on the particular goals and ends of religious communities, taking religious variables not simply as "exposures" but also as "outcomes," viewed as ends in their own right. Such research could arguably be of use to religious communities, and not simply serving generic functional or utilitarian ends.

Moreover, it is arguably the case that some of the empirical research on religion and health is potentially already of use to religious communities. The empirical research on service attendance and health gives religious communities a powerful message that it is not simply solitary spirituality that matters, but that the communal religious experience has important and powerful effects. The empirical research on service attendance and health thus may provide a message to help religious communities call people back to communal life. As a second example, the research on service attendance and depression, suggested that not only did service attendance decrease the likelihood of depression but also that those who were depressed were more likely to stop attending services. Such knowledge suggests that religious communities might take steps to seek out those struggling with depression, before the depression gets so severe that they cease attending, perhaps thereby exacerbating depression further. Such research may have important implications for pastoral practice; screening programs for depression within churches have also begun to be developed (Hankerson et al., 2015). As a third example, the research on forgiveness, not only highlights the importance of the practice of forgiveness, but also provides powerful and effective tools and interventions to promote forgiveness, tools and interventions that can be used by religious communities. With further engagement from religious communities, more of the empirical research could be made useful, not simply to academics and health care providers, but to religious communities themselves. Greater engagement from religious communities may be necessary to counter functionalist views of religion and to make clear the ultimate ends which religious traditions pursue.

SYNTHESIS

In this final section of the review we will consider the relations between the empirical research on religion and health and some of the theological and philosophical themes on this topic, and various aspects of convergence and tension across the different literatures. We will also consider how the empirical research on religion and health can inform theological perspectives, as well as how the theological and philosophical ideas might shape subsequent empirical research. We will conclude with a few summary propositions emerging from this review of the literature.

We saw in our discussion of the relations between religion and health across the world religions, as well as specifically in the more detailed consideration of the Christian and Jewish Biblical texts, that community emerged as a prominent theme tying religious participation to health. There was clear indication in these literatures that individual health is closely tied to the health of the community, that community participation is itself an aspect of health or wholeness, and that community is often the means through which caregiving and healing come. The empirical research on religion and health likewise appeared to indicate that it was communal forms of religious participation that appeared to matter most for health. Many of the substantial and well-established associations with health in the empirical literature concerned religious service attendance. Religious service attendance seemed to be a stronger protective predictor of subsequent mortality, depression, suicide, and other outcomes, than was individual spiritual or religious practice or identity. The associations with many of these other religious or spiritual variables were generally weak and often diminished further when control was made for religious service attendance. The literature highlights the powerful effects of communal aspects of religious participation. The importance of religious community in health is thus one area in which there is fairly clear convergence between the empirical and theological literatures on religion and health. Communal religious life contributes to health.

We have described how the empirical research indicated that forgiveness itself was strongly related to mental health outcomes such as depression, anxiety, and hope, and possibly related to physical health as well. The empirical research literature in psychology has not only established these associations, but has developed interventions to help promote forgiveness that have been rigorously tested in randomized trials, concerning both forgiveness of others (Harper et al., 2014; Greer et al., 2014), and forgiveness of self (Griffin et al., 2015). Forgiveness was likewise an important theological theme in the Biblical literature surveyed. In that literature, forgiveness from God constituted a central part of healing and restoration to wholeness; it was a central aspect of the very notion of salvation. Forgiveness of others was strongly emphasized as well, following from forgiveness granted by God. Forgiveness of others was tied both to the health of the individual and to the health of the community. The relationship between forgiveness and health might thus also be seen as another area in which there is strong convergence between the empirical and theological literatures. Forgiveness is important for health.

Our survey of the theological literature also emphasized caregiving from religious communities as an important pathway to health and wholeness. The very notion of love as seeking the good of another entails caring for those in need; caring for those who are ill and seeking their health and healing was a prominent theme in its own right. We saw also, in our survey of partnerships between public health institutions and religious institutions, that such caregiving by religious groups plays an important role in the overall public health and medical landscape, both historically and today. In parts of Africa such efforts include as much as half of all health care services. The theme of religious persons and institutions caring for the ill is thus very clearly manifest in actual current health care and caregiving practices, and constitutes a third area of convergence of the empirical and theological literatures. Religious institutions support, and provide, caregiving which contributes to health.

In addition to these areas in which the empirical and theological literatures appear to converge there were also areas in which tensions were in one way or another manifest. We have discussed tensions between the Catholic Church and Brazil's National AIDS Program over condom use in the prevention of HIV/AIDs. Similar tensions are manifest in other partnerships or potential partnerships between religious and public health institutions in harm reductions programs such as needle exchange programs or safer sex condom distribution programs, which, to religious groups, may appear also to implicitly condone risky actions that they would judge immoral. In these settings, the values and ends in view differ between public health institutions and religious institutions, with public health institutions focused principally on what are perceived to be as better health outcomes, while religious institutions often place equal or greater weight on moral belief and religious teachings. See Van Ness (2013) for discussion of how utilitarian versus deontological views of ethics are likely manifest within the tensions present in such partnerships. Such tensions are, in some cases at least, unlikely to be able to be resolved entirely and partnerships will often require both parties tolerating some level of difference in ideological perspective. Research on how to facilitate partnerships, in the face of irreconcilable tensions, may prove to be important. These tensions may also be present in religion and health research in less politically and ideologically charged forms. For example, Pargament et al. (2004) notes that those experiencing spiritual struggles have higher mortality in follow-up, but the same study reports that these individuals also experience more spiritual and character growth. While, from a perspective focused on physical health, rapid elimination of these spiritual struggles may seem desirable, the individual facing these struggles may consider them an important part of their religious experience and development, fostering character and spiritual growth and transformation. There are prominent spiritual traditions concerning the "dark night of the soul" (Saint John of the Cross, 1585; May, 2004). Clearly here the health goals, at least with health viewed in a narrow sense, may well be in tension with broader religious values. While many religious groups emphasize and seek to promote health, physical health is typically not taken as the highest or most important value; other considerations and ends are given more importance. Here, health, viewed narrowly, and religion may be in tension.

Other types of tensions, concerning the very possibility of empirical study, are also manifest. We discussed empirical attempts to assess the efficacy of intercessory prayer. We noted that even though such research had been subjected to numerous randomized trials, investigator biases and agendas arguably make this research difficult to carry out objectively. Religious objections included that the trials arguably assess a form of prayer very different from what is in fact practiced by many religious communities. In contrast to what is often done in a blinded trial, in which the patients do not know whether or not they are being prayed for, prayer in many religious communities takes place in the context of long-term well-established relationships and may involve the laying on of hands. Other religious, even epistemological, objections to the research include noting that God, if he exists, would not be "unaware" of what was taking place or bound by acting in any specific manner. Prayer thus appears to be an area in which, while there is emphasis on prayer and healing in many religious traditions, empirical research on the topic may be challenging to adequately carry out.

We also saw that there are objections, from religious communities and persons, not simply to the research on prayer, but to the entire broader enterprise of empirical research on the relationships between religion and health. Religious objections that are sometimes put forward concerning this research are that it is too utilitarian in purpose, seeking to use religion for more secular ends, rather than focusing on the ends that religions and religious groups deem important, and that, moreover, the existing empirical research often uses very generic measures of religion and spirituality, stripping religions of their distinctive and, often, most central content. While the objections carry some weight, it may be possible to partially address these objections by involving religious communities in the empirical religion and health research itself, from study design, to planning, to research agendas, so as to use more specific and distinctive religious measures, and to focus more on the goals and ends of religious communities. Nevertheless, it is clear that the study questions involved, the measures used, and the uses to which empirical religion and health research is put, are potential areas of tension.

In addition to areas of convergence and tensions, we have also, in the review, highlighted at least some areas in which the empirical literature and the theological literature may benefit from perspectives and themes of the other. A prominent theme across world religions, and in the more specific Biblical material surveyed, was the notion of health as wholeness. Indeed, the notion of health as wholeness appears elsewhere as well, including the World Health Organization (WHO) definition of health as: "Health is a state of complete physical, mental and social well-being and not merely the absence of disease or infirmity," (World Health Association, 1948), a definition which manifests similar concern with health taken holistically and may well have been influenced by broader perspectives on health from religious communities. See Larson (1996) for discussion of possible expansion of the World Health Organization definition to include a spiritual dimension to health. Religious understandings of health and wholeness are, arguably yet broader still than the WHO definition, focusing also on right relationship to, or communion with, the divine, and notions of salvation. While such understandings of health may not be universally shared, they do point to, and emphasize, the potential breadth of the notion of health, and emphasize further how values and ends of individuals and communities may extend well beyond physical health. In seeking to develop effective interventions for health, it may be important to consider the whole range of a person's or community's goals and ends. We noted how, in some cases, other values and ends may be considered more important than, and in tension with, physical health. The theological literatures on health emphasizes and reminds the research community of the potential need for a broad conception of health and well-being.

The theological and philosophical literatures are, have been, and likely will continue to be, helpful for the conduct of empirical research in other ways as well. We discussed how philosophical perspectives on forgiveness, and the conditions under which forgiveness is morally grounded, might be integrated into existing forgiveness interventions and how theological themes likewise can be included in such interventions. Indeed the adaptation of the forgiveness workbook interventions to specifically Christian communities is one such example of this (Greer et al., 2014). Spiritually integrated psychotherapy (Pargament, 2011) is likewise an example of theological ideas finding an important place in the development of interventions that are to be tested empirically. Religious communities and theological ideas may also, as discussed, be important in developing better, and more specific and distinctive measures of religious participation, beliefs, understanding, and identity, and in helping direct the empirical research to consider not only health-related ends but also other ends and outcomes relevant to religious communities themselves.

While the theological and philosophical literature can, and has, helped shape and inform empirical research efforts, it is also the case that empirical research itself may be of use and can help inform religious communities. The empirical research on religion and health such as relating religious service attendance to lower all-cause mortality, lower depression, less suicide, and better health outcomes generally provides a powerful message for religious communities to convey concerning the importance of the communal aspects of religious participation. In an era in which an increasingly large number of persons, at least in the West, self-identify as spiritual but not religious, religious communities can point to empirical data that suggest that it is not just belief that matters but attendance and community participation as well. Community matters, not just theologically, but empirically for physical health also. The empirical research on service attendance and depression likewise suggests a protective effect of attendance but, in this relationship, there was also an important effect in the reverse direction: those who become depressed are more likely to cease attending services. This empirical research likewise is important to religious communities in that it suggests that efforts might be made to reach out to members who become depressed before they potentially leave their community, perhaps exacerbating depression further. We also saw that the empirical research literature had developed effective forms of forgiveness interventions that have been tested in randomized trials. Forgiveness itself is an important emphasis for many religious communities, and the interventions that have been developed may be effective tools for promoting forgiveness within these communities. Workbook forms of these interventions have been developed to allow for easy and more widespread use, and the workbooks have been tailored also to address specifically religious contexts, currently in the form of Christian workbook interventions, but others could also potentially be developed. Here too the empirical research contributes to and helps inform the life of religious communities.

There are thus areas in which the empirical and theological literatures converge, there are areas of tensions, and also areas in which one literature can inform, and help shape, the other. However, for certain aspects of the religion and health connection, the relation between the empirical research and the theological themes is less clear. In our survey of theological themes, sin and fallenness are the sources of ill-health and brokenness was important in the Biblical conception of health. Likewise, health and healing were itself tied to the notion of salvation, with God ultimately being the source of both healing and salvation. Such ideas provide a powerful interpretative framework for religious communities, and help make sense systematically of the Biblical material and narratives. However, the relation of these interpretative ideas to empirical research is much less clear. To assess the potential truth claims of these interpretative frameworks, there is no empirical study that can directly provide evidence. At best, the interpretative frameworks themselves have to be assessed through other modes of inquiry such as inference to the best explanation, generally within the context of the entire religious system of meaning and understanding (Pannenberg, 1976). The interpretative ideas are powerful but not subject to direct empirical inquiry.

In summary, we have seen a number of areas in which the empirical and theological literature on religion and health suggest convergence including community and health, forgiveness and health, and caregiving and health. We have seen other areas in which there are various forms of tensions including empirically evaluating intercessory prayer, different goals and values of public health and religious institutions in partnerships, as well as potentially different agendas and goals in carrying out the research. The tensions sometimes concern the limits of the very possibility of studying empirically various religious practices, and sometimes concern different goals, ends, and values of research of public health and religious communities. We have also seen areas in which theological or philosophical perspectives might enhance religion and health research including broadening the very notion of health; using theological and philosophical perspectives on forgiveness to help improve forgiveness interventions; and potentially working with religious communities to use more specific and distinctive measures of religious participation and to address questions, goals, and values of religious communities themselves. We have also seen areas in which the empirical literature can contribute to the life of religious communities including providing a powerful message, corroborated by empirical evidence, for the importance of communal aspects of religious participation; empirical demonstration of the need to reach out to members of religious communities who are suffering from depression before they leave their communities, perhaps exacerbating depression yet further; and further the potential power of forgiveness interventions to facilitate forgiveness in settings in which this might otherwise be difficult. We have further noted some areas in which there seems to be relatively little potential overlap between the empirical and theological literatures, such as the notion of sin as the ultimate source of ill-health, and the relationship between healing and salvation. Here, the theological literature offers more of an interpretative perspective that is difficult to assess directly empirically. Finally, as discussed in the second part of this review, it is clear that there are concrete, religiously based, interventions that can contribute to well-being including, for example, church-based health promotion interventions, religious and faith-based organizations providing health care and public health services, spiritual care in end-of-life and medical settings, forgiveness interventions, and possibly also encouragement to attend services and participate in community life.

Having surveyed the literature on religion and health, we will close with a series of summary propositions, encapsulating much of the discussion of the present review, but offered so as to be subject to further discussion, refinement and potential empirical inquiry:

1. Religion is concerned with health in its broadest sense, that of wholeness or well-being.
2. Religious participation contributes to physical and mental health, and subjective well-being, through shaping behavior, creating systems of meaning, altering one's outlook on life, building community and social support, supporting moral beliefs, and through an experience of the transcendent.
3. It is communal forms of religious participation, rather than merely private practices, that most powerfully affect health.
4. Religious communities and persons can promote health through caregiving, health-promotion interventions, spiritual care in medical and end-of-life settings, forgiveness interventions, and by simply offering a form of meaningful communal participation.
5. A religious understanding of health, illness, and well-being, and of the actions needed to promote health, will often make appeal to theological concepts such as sin, salvation, character, love, divine action, and forgiveness.

From the perspective of faith, religion itself may be seen as essential in complete wholeness and well-being, in coming to a communion with God. From a more strictly empirical perspective, the literature surveyed in this review suggests that religious participation is an important determinant of health: it is strongly associated, over time, with a variety of health outcomes. Religious participation, on these grounds, thus ought to be included in discussions of, and analyses of, health, as is already common practice for other social determinants of health such as race, gender, or income. Religion affects individual behavior, shifts cognition and emotion, shapes communities and public life, and offers justification for values and moral discourse. In these and other ways, it has a profound effect on health. While much of the past empirical research was weak, there is now, for outcomes such as mortality, depression, and suicide, a reasonably strong knowledge base, built upon good study designs and rigorous analyses. Further research, using longitudinal designs, is still needed for other health outcomes, and for measures of religious participation other than service attendance. However, it is clear that certain forms of religious participation do affect health, that religious institutions play an important role in the provision of health care and public health services, and that religious groups have formed broad, and sometimes profound, conceptions of health itself. Religious participation affects health, it should be considered in discussions of and approaches to health, and it is ultimately concerned with health in its very broadest sense.

ACKNOWLEDGMENTS

The author thanks Harold Koenig, Michael Balboni, and John Peteet for insightful comments on an earlier version of this chapter.

REFERENCES

Allen JD, Pérez JE, Tom L, Leyva B, Diaz D, Torres MI. (2014). A Pilot Test of a church-based intervention to promote multiple cancer-screening behaviors among Latinas. Journal of Cancer Education; 29(1): 136–143.

Amato PR, Rogers SJ. (1997). A longitudinal study of marital problems and subsequent divorce. Journal of Marriage and Family, 59:612–624.

Astin JA, Harkness E, Ernst E. (2000). The efficacy of "distant healing": A systematic review of randomized trials. Annals of Internal Med. 2000;132:903–910.

Astrow AB, Wexler A, Texeira K, He MK, Sulmasy DP. (2007). Is failure to meet spiritual needs associated with cancer patients' perceptions of quality of care and their satisfaction with care? Journal of Clinical Oncology 25(36):5753–5757.

Avalos H. (1999). Health Care and the Rise of Christianity. Peabody, MA: Hendrickson Publishers.

Balboni MJ, Sullivan A, Amobi A, Phelps AC, Gorman D, Zollfrank A, . . . Balboni TA. (2013). Why is spiritual care infrequent at the end of life? Spiritual care perceptions among patients, nurses, and physicians and the role of training. Journal of Clinical Oncology, 30:2538–2544.

Balboni TA, Paulk ME, Balboni MJ, et al. (2010) Provision of spiritual care to patients with advanced cancer: associations with medical care and quality of life near death. Journal of Clinical Oncology, 28: 445–452.

Balboni, TA, Balboni, MJ, Phelps, AC, Wright, AA, Peteet, JR, Block, SD, Lathan C, VanderWeele TJ, Prigerson HG. (2011). Support of terminal cancer patient spiritual needs and associations with medical care costs at the end of life. Cancer, 117:5383–5391.

Balboni TA, Balboni MJ, Enzinger AC, Gallivan K, Paulk ME, Wright A, . . . Prigerson HG. (2013). Provision of spiritual support to advanced cancer patients by religious communities and associations with medical care at the end of life. JAMA Internal Medicine, 73:1109–1117.

Balbuena L, Baetz M, Bowen R. (2013). Religious attendance, spirituality, and major depression in Canada: a 14-year follow-up study. Canadian Journal of Psychiatry 58:225–232.

Baskin TW, Rhody M, Schoolmeesters S, Ellingson C. (2011). Supporting special-needs adoptive couples assessing an intervention to enhance forgiveness, increase marital satisfaction, and prevent depression. The Counseling Psychologist 39:933–955.

Berkman LF, Syme SL. (1979), Social networks, host resistance, and mortality: A nine-year follow-up study of Alameda County residents. American Journal of Epidemiology 109(2):186–204.

Birnbaum R. (1989). Chinese Buddhist traditions of healing and the life cycle. In L. Sullivan (ed.), Healing and Restoring: Health and Medicine in the World's Religious Traditions (pp. 33–58). New York: Macmillan.

Bishop JP. (2009). Biopsychosociospiritual medicine and other political schemes. Christian Bioethics, 15: 254–276.

Blazer DG. (2017). The empirical study of religion/spirituality and psychiatric disorders: Implications for clinical practice. In Balboni MJ, Peteet J (eds.), Spirituality and Religion within the Culture of Medicine: From Evidence to Practice. Oxford University Press.

Brown C G. (2012). Testing Prayer. Boston: Harvard University Press.

Brown PJ. (2014). Religion and global health. In Idler E, (ed.), Religion as a Social Determinant of Public Health. New York: Oxford University Press.

Brown RP. (2003). Measuring individual differences in the tendency to forgive: Construct validity and links with depression. Personality and Social Psychology Bulletin, 29:759–771.

Burdette AM, Weeks J, Hill TD, Eberstein IW (2012). Maternal religious attendance and low birth weight. Social Science & Medicine, 74: 1961–1967.

Bushman BJ, Ridge RD, Das E, Key CW, Busath GM. (2007). When God sanctions killing: Effect of scriptural violence on aggression. Psychological Science 18(3):204–207.

Call VRA, Heaton TB. (1997). Religious Influence on Marital Stability. Journal for the Scientific Study of Religion, 36:382–392.

Campbell MK, Hudson MA, Resnicow K, et al. (2007). Church-based health promotion interventions: Evidence and lessons learned. Annual Review of Public Health 28:213–234.

Catholic Church. Catechism of the Catholic Church. 2nd ed. Libreria Editrice Vaticana, 2000.

Chatters LM (2000). Religion and health: Public health research and practice. Annual Review of Public Health 21:335–367.

Chida Y, Steptoe A, Powell LH. (2009). Religiosity/spirituality and mortality. A systematic quantitative review. Psychotherapy and Psychosomatics 78(2):81–90.

Cohen AB, Malka A, Rozin P, Cherfas L (2006). Religion and unforgiveable offenses. Journal of Personality and Social Psychology 74:85–117.

Coin A, Perissinotto E, Najjar M, Girardi A, Inelmen EM, Enzi G. . . .Sergi G. (2010). Does religiosity protect against cognitive and behavioral decline in Alzheimer's dementia? Current Alzheimer Research, 7:445–452.

Comstock GW, Partridge KB. (1972). Church attendance and health. Journal of Chronic Disease 25: 665–672.

Comstock GW, Tonascia JA. (1977). Education and mortality in Washington County, Maryland. Journal of Health and Social Behavior, 18(1):54–61.

Dalmida SG, Thurman S. (2014). HIV/AIDS. In E. Idler (ed.), Religion as a Social Determinant of Health. New York: Oxford University Press, 369–381.

Davis DE, Worthington EL Jr., Hook JN, Hill PC. (2013). Research on religion/spirituality and forgiveness: A meta-analytic review. Psychology of Religion and Spirituality, 5(4), 233–241.

DeHaven MJ, Hunter IB, Wilder L, Walton JW, Berry J. (2004). Health programs in faith-based organizations: Are they effective? American Journal of Public Health 94(6):1030–36.

Derose KP, Mendel, PJ, Palar K, Kanouse DE, et al. (2011). Religious congregations' involvement in HIV: A case study approach. AIDS and Behavior, 15:1220–1232.

Dervic K, Oquendo MA, Grunebaum MF, Eliis S, Burke AK, Mann JJ. (2004). Religious affiliation and suicide attempt. American Journal of Psychiatry 161:2303–2308.

Desai PN. (1989). Health and Medicine in the Hindu Tradition: Continuity and Cohesion. New York: Crossroad Publishers.

DeShea L, Tzou J, Kang S, Matsuyuki M (2006). Trait forgiveness II: Spiritual vs. religious college students and the five-factor model of personality. Poster presented at the annual conference of the Society for Personality and Social Psychology, Palm Springs, CA.

Dupre ME, Franzese AT, Parrado EA. (2006). Religious attendance and mortality: Implications for the black-white mortality crossover. Demography 43(1): 141–164.

Durkheim E. (1897/1951). Suicide: A Study in Sociology. New York: Free Press.

Ellison CG, Zhang W, Krause N, Marcum JP (2009). Does negative interaction in the church increase psychological distress? Longitudinal findings from the Presbyterian Panel Survey. Sociology of Religion 70 (4): 409–431.

Enright RD, Fitzgibbons RP. (2000). Helping Clients Forgive: An Empirical Guide for Resolving Anger and Restoring Hope. Washington, DC: American Psychological Association.

Fetzer Institute. (1999). Multidimensional measurement of religiousness/spirituality for use in health research: A report of the Fetzer Institute/National Institute on Aging Working Group. Kalamazoo, MI: Author.

Flannelly KJ, Koenig HG, Ellison CG, Galek K, Krause N. (2006). Belief in life after death and mental health: Findings from a national survey. Journal of Nervous and Mental Disease 194(7): 524–529.

Fledman DM. (1986). Health and Medicine in the Jewish Tradition: L'Hayyim—To Life. New York: Crossroad Publishers.

Fortin AH, Barnett KG. (2004). Medical school curricula in spirituality and medicine. Journal of the American Medical Association 291 (23): 2883.

Freedman SR, Enright RD. (1996). Forgiveness as an intervention goal with incest survivors. Journal of Consulting and Clinical Psychology, 64:983–992.

Freud S. (1930/1962). Civilization and Its Discontents. In Standard Edition of the Complete Psychological Works of Sigmund Freud, ed. and trans. by J. Strachey. London: Hogarth Press, 25, 36.

Gallup Poll. (2015–2016). http://www.gallup.com/poll/1690/religion.aspx. Accessed July 28, 2016.

George LK, Ellison CG, CG Larson CG. (2002). Explaining the relationships between religious involvement and health. Psychological Inquiry, 13:190–200.

Gillum RF, King DE, Obisesan TO, Koenig HG (2008). Frequency of attendance at religious services and mortality in a U.S. national cohort. Annals of Epidemiology, 18(2):124–129.

Gordon KC, Burton S, Porter L. (2004). Predicting the intentions of women in domestic violence shelters to return to partners: Does forgiveness play a role? Journal of Family Psychology, 18: 331–338.

Greer CL, Worthington EL Jr, Lin Y, Lavelock CR, BJ Griffin BJ. (2014). Efficacy of a self-directed forgiveness workbook for Christian victims of within-congregation offenders. Spirituality in Clinical Practice, 1(3):218–230.

Griffin BJ, Worthington EL Jr, Lavelock CR, Greer CL, Lin Y, Davis DE, Hook JN. (2015). Efficacy of a self-forgiveness workbook: A randomized controlled trial with interpersonal offenders. Journal of Counseling and Psychology, 62(2):124–136.

Hankerson SH, Lee YA, Brawley DK, Braswell K, Wickramaratne PJ, Weissman MM. (2015). Screening for Depression in African-American Churches. American Journal of Preventive Medicine, 49: 526–533.

Hanson LC, Dobbs D, Usher BM, Williams S, Rawlings J, Daaleman TP. (2008). Providers and types of spiritual care during serious illness. Journal of Palliative Medicine, 11(6):907–914.

Harper Q, Worthington EL, Griffin BJ, Lavelock CR, Hook JN, Vrana SR, Greer CL (2014). Efficacy of a workbook to promote forgiveness: A randomized controlled trial with university students. Journal of Clinical Psychology 70:1158–1169.

Harr J (1996). A Civil Action. New York: Random House.

Hayward RD, Elliott M. (2014). Cross-national analysis of the influence of cultural norms and government restrictions on the relationship between religion and well-being. Review of Religious Research, 56:23–43.

Hill PC, and Hood RW. (1999). Measures of Religiosity. Birmingham, AL: Religious Education Press.

Hill PC, Pargament K I. (2003). Advances in the conceptualization and measurement of religion and spirituality: Implications for physical and mental health research. American Psychologist 58(1): 64–74.

Holmgren MR. (1993). Forgiveness and the intrinsic value of persons. American Philosophical Quarterly, 30: 341–352.

Hummer RA, Rogers RG, Nam CB, Ellison CG. (1999). Religious involvement and US adult mortality. Demography, 36(2):273–285.

Idler EL. (2011). Religion and adult mortality: Group-and individual-level perspectives. In R Rogers, E Crimmins, eds., International Handbook of Adult Mortality. New York, Berlin: Springer, pp.345–377.

Idler EL. (2014a). Religion and physical health from childhood to old age. In EL Idler, ed., Religion as a Social Determinant of Public Health. New York: Oxford University Press.

Idler EL. (2014b). Ingenious institutions: religious origins of health and development organization. In EL Idler, ed., Religion as a Social Determinant of Public Health. New York: Oxford University Press.

Idler EL, Kasl SV. (1997). Religion among disabled and nondisabled elderly persons II: Attendance at religious services as a predictor of the course of disability. Journal of Gerontology: Social Sciences 52B:S306–S316.

Idler EL, Musick MA, Ellison CG, George LK, Krause N, Ory MG, et al. (2003). Measuring multiple dimensions of religion and spirituality for health research: Conceptual background and findings from the 1998 General Social Survey. Research on Aging 25(4): 327–365.

Ingersoll-Dayton B, Campbell R, Ha J (2009). Enhancing forgiveness: A group intervention for the elderly. Journal of Gerontological Social Work 52:2–16.

Ironson G, Kremer H. (2009). Spiritual transformation, psychological well-being, health, and survival in people with HIV. International Journal of Psychiatry in Medicine 39: 263–281.

Joint Commission. (2013). Spirituality, Religion, Beliefs and Cultural Diversity to JCAHO's Standards/Elements of Performance. Manual for Hospitals.

Kee HC. (1992). Medicine and healing. In DN Freedman (ed.), Anchor Bible Dictionary. New York: Doubleday.

Kelsey MT (1995). Healing and Christianity. Minneapolis, MN: Ausburg.

Ketchell A, Pyles L, Canda E. (2011). World Religious Views of Health and Healing. http://spiritualdiversity.ku.edu/sites/spiritualitydiversity.drupal.ku.edu/files/docs/Health/World%20Religious%20Views%20of%20Health%20and%20Healing.pdf

Kim J, Enright RD (2014). A theological and psychological defense of self-forgiveness: Implications for counseling. Journal of Psychology and Theology, 42:260–268.

King DE, Bushwick B. (1994). Beliefs and attitudes of hospital inpatients about faith healing and prayer. Journal of Family Practice 39 (4): 349–352, 1994.

Kiser M, Santibanez S. (2014). Influenza pandemic. In Idler EL, ed, Religion as a Social Determinant of Public Health. New York: Oxford University Press.

Kleinman EM, Liu RT. (2114). Prospective prediction of suicide in a nationally representative sample: Religious service attendance as a protective factor. British Journal of Psychiatry, 204:262–266.

Koenig HG. (2000a). Medicine and religion, Letter to the editor. New England Journal of Medicine, 343:1339.

Koenig, H.G. (2000b). Religion, spirituality, and medicine: Application to clinical practice. JAMA, 284(13):1708.

Koenig, HG. (2008). Medicine, religion, and health: Where science and spirituality meet. West Conshohocken, PA: Templeton Foundation Press.

Koenig, HG. (2009). Research on religion, spirituality and mental health: A review. Canadian Journal of Psychiatry 54(5): 283–291.

Koenig HG, Büssing A. (2010). The Duke University Religion Index (DUREL): A five-item measure for use in epidemiological studies. Religions, 1:78–85.

Koenig HG, George LK, Peterson, BL. (1998). Religiosity and remission of depression in medically ill older patients. American Journal of Psychiatry, 155:536–542.

Koenig HG, Hooten EG, Lindsay-Calksin E, Meador KG. (2010). Spirituality in medical school curricula: Findings from a national survey. International Journal of Psychiatry in Medicine 40(4): 391–398.

Koenig HG, Idler E, Kasl S, Hays JC, George LK, Musick MA. (1999). Religion, spirituality, and medicine: A rebuttal to skeptics. International Journal of Psychiatry in Medicine, 29:123–131.

Koenig HG, King DE, Carson VB. (2012). Handbook of Religion and Health. 2nd ed. Oxford, New York: Oxford University Press.

Koenig HG, Pearce MJ, Nelson B, Shaw SF, Robins CJ, Daher NS, . . . King MB. (2015). Religious vs. conventional cognitive behavioral therapy for major depression in persons with chronic medical illness: A pilot randomized trial. Journal of Nervous and Mental Diseases, 203(4):243–251.

Krause N, Ellison CG, Wulff KM (1998). Church-based emotional support, negative interaction, and psychological well-being: Findings from a national sample of Presbyterian. Journal for the Scientific Study of Religion 37:725–741.

Krause N, Hayward RD. (2012). Religion, meaning in life, and change in physical functioning during late adulthood. Journal of Adult Development, 19: 158–169.

la Cour P, Avlund K, Schultz-Larsen K. (2006). Religion and survival in a secular region. A twenty year follow-up of 734 Danish adults born in 1914. Social Science and Medicine, 62(1):157–164.

Lambert NM, Fincham F, Braithwaite SR, Graham S, Beach S. (2009). Can prayer increase gratitude? Psychology of Religion and Spirituality, 1, 39–49.

Lambert NM, Fincham FD, LaVallee DC, Brantley CW. (2012). Praying together and staying together: Couple prayer and trust. Psychology of Religion and Spirituality. 4:1–9.

Lambert NM, Fincham F, Stillman T, Graham S, Beach S. (2010). Motivating change in relationships: Can prayer increase forgiveness? Psychological Science, 21, 126–132.

Larson DB, Sherrill KA, Lyons JS, Craige FC, Thielman SB, Greenwold MA, Larson SS (1992). "Dimensions and valences of measures of religious commitment found in the American Journal of Psychiatry and the Archives of General Psychiatry, 1978–1989." American Journal of Psychiatry, 149: 557–559.

Larson JS (1996). The World Health Organization's definition of health: Social versus spiritual health. Social Indicators Research 38:181–192.

Lasater TM, Becker DM, Hill MN, Gans KM. (1997). Synthesis of findings and issues from religious-based cardiovascular disease prevention trials. Annals of Epidemiology, 7(57):S47–53.

Levin J. (2014). Faith-based initiatives in health promotion: History, challenges, and current partnerships. American Journal of Health Promotion, 28:139–141.

Levin J. (2016). Partnerships between the faith-based and medical sectors: Implications for preventive medicine and public health. Preventive Medicine Reports, 4:344–350.

Li S, Okereke OI, Chang SC, Kawachi I, VanderWeele TJ (2016a). Religious service attendance and lower depression among women: A prospective cohort study. Annals of Behavioral Medicine. 50:876-884.

Li S, Stamfer M, Williams DR, VanderWeele TJ. (2016b). Association between religious service attendance and mortality among women. JAMA Internal Medicine, 176(6):777–785.

Lim C, Putnam RD. (2010). Religion, social networks, and life satisfaction. American Sociological Review, 75:914–933.

Lin WF, Mack D, Enright RD, Krahn D, Baskin TW. (2004). Effects of forgiveness therapy on anger, mood, and vulnerability to substance use among inpatient substance-dependent clients. Journal of Consulting and Clinical Psychology, 72:1114–1121.

Litwin H. (2007). What really matters in the social network-mortality association? A multivariate examination among older Jewish-Israelis. European Journal of Ageing 4(2): 71–82.

Lucchetti G, Lucchetti ALG, Koenig HG (2011). Impact of spirituality/religiosity on mortality: Comparison with other health interventions. Explore, 7:234–238.

Mahoney A, Pargament KI, Tarakeshwar N, Swank AB. (2008). Religion in the home in the 1980s and 1990s: A meta-analytic review and conceptual analysis of links between religion, marriage, and parenting. Psychology of Religion and Spirituality, S(1), 63–101.

Marty ME (1983). Health and Medicine in Lutheran Tradition: Being Well. New York: Crossroad Publishing.

Maselko J, Hayward RD, Hanlon A, Buka S, Meador K. (2012). Religious service attendance and major depression: A case of reverse causality? American Journal of Epidemiology 175(6):576–83.

Maves PB (1960). Aging, Religion, and the Church. Handbook of Social Gerontology. Chicago, IL: University of Chicago Press.

May GG. (2004). The Dark Night of the Soul. A Psychiatrist Explores the Connection Between Darkness and Spiritual Growth. New York City: HarperCollins.

McCarty B, Kinghorn W. (2017). Medicine, religion, and spirituality in theological context. In MJ Balboni, J Peteet J, eds., Spirituality and Religion within the Culture of Medicine: From Evidence to Practice. Oxford University Press.

McCormick, RA. (1984). Health and Medicine in the Catholic Tradition: Tradition in Transition. New York: Crossroad Publishing.

McCullough ME, Hoyt WT, Larson DB, Koenig HG, Thoresen C. (2000). Religious involvement and mortality: A meta-analytic review. Health Psychology. 19(3):211.

McCullough ME, Fincham FD, Tsang J. (2003). Forgiveness, forbearance, and time: The temporal unfolding of transgression-related interpersonal motivations. Journal of Personality and Social Psychology, 84, 540–557.

McCullough ME, Root LM, Cohen AD. (2006). Writing about the benefits of an interpersonal transgression facilitates forgiveness. Journal of Consulting and Clinical Psychology, 74(5):887–897.

McCullough ME, Root LM, Tabak B, Witvliet CVO. (2009). Forgiveness. In SJ Lopez, CR Snyder, eds., Handbook of Positive Psychology, 2nd ed., (pp. 427–435). New York: Oxford.

Morris, AD (1986). Origins of the Civil Rights Movements. New York: Free Press.

Murray LR, Garcia J, Munoz-Laboy M, Parker RG. (2011). Strange bedfellows: The Catholic Church and Brazilian National AIDS Program in the Response to HIV/AIDS in Brazil. Social Science and Medicine 72:945–952.

Musick MA, House JS, Williams DR. (2004). Attendance at religious services and mortality in a national sample. Journal of Health and Social Behavior, 45(2):198–213.

Mwenda S. (2011). The African Christian Health Association Platform: Showcasing the Contributions of CHAs. Contact 190:2.

National Consensus Project (2009). NCP Clinical Practice Guidelines for Quality Palliative Care. http://www.nationalconsensusproject.org/guideline.pdf. Accessed March 15, 2014.

Nicklin DE (2000). Medicine and religion, letter to the editor. New England Journal of Medicine, 343:1340.

Nisbet PA, Duberstein PR, Conwell Y, Seidlitz L. (2000). The effect of participation in religious activities on suicide versus natural death in adults 50 and older. Journal of Nervous and Mental Disorders, 188(8): 543–546.

North J (1987). Wrongdoing and forgiveness. Philosophy 62: 499–508.

Norton MC, Singh A, Skoog I, et al. Church attendance and new episodes of major depression in a community study of older adults: The Cache County study. Journal of Gerontology B: Psychological Science and Social Science 63(3):P129–P137.

Numbers RL Amundsen DW (1985). Caring and Curing: Health and Medicine in the Western Religious Traditions. London: Macmillan Publishing.

Oman D (2013). Defining religion and spirituality. In RF Paloutzian, CL Park eds., Foundations of the Psychology of Religion. New York: Guilford Press.

Oman D, Kurata JH, Strawbridge WJ, Cohen, RD. 2002. Religious attendance and cause of death over 31 years. International Journal of Psychiatry in Medicine 32(1):69–89.

Oquendo MA, Dragatsi D, Harkavy-Friedman J, et al. (2005). Protective factors against suicidal behavior in Latinos. Journal of Nervous and Mental Diseases 193:438–443.

Otolok-Tanga E, Atuyambe L, Murphey CK, Ringheim KE, Woldehanna S. (2007). Examining the actions of faith-based organizations and their influence on HIV/AIDS-related stigma: a case study of Uganda. African Health Sciences 7(1): 55–60.

Oxman TE, Freeman DH Jr., Manheimer ED. (1995). Lack of social participation or religious strength and comfort as risk factors for death after cardiac surgery in the elderly. Psychosomatic Medicine, 57(1):5–15.

Page RL, Ellison CG, Lee J. (2009). Does religiosity affect health risk behaviors in pregnant and postpartum women? Maternal Child Health Journal 13: 621–632.

Pannenberg W (1976). Theology and the Philosophy of Science. St. Louis, MO: Westminster Press.

Pargament KI (2011). Spiritually Integrated Psychotherapy: Understanding and Addressing the Sacred. New York: Guilford Press.

Pargament KI, Koenig HG, Perez LM. (2000). The many methods of religious coping: Development and initial validation of the RCOPE. Journal of Clinical Psychology, 56(4):519–543.

Pargament KI, Koenig HG, Tarakeshwar N, Hahn J. (2001). Religious struggle as a predictor of mortality among medically ill elderly patients: A two-year longitudinal study. Archives of Internal Medicine, 161: 1881–1885.

Pargament KI, Koenig HG, Tarakeshwar N, Hahn J. (2004). Religious coping methods as predictors of psychological, physical and spiritual outcomes among medically ill elderly patients: A two-year longitudinal study. Journal of Health Psychology, 9:713–730.

Pew Forum. (2012). The Global Religious Landscape. http://www.pewforum.org/files/2014/01/global-religion-full.pdf

Phelps AC, Lauderdale KE, Alcorn S, Dillinger J, Balboni MT, Van Wert M, . . . Balboni TA (2012). Addressing spirituality within the care of patients at the end of life: Perspectives of advanced cancer patients, oncologists, and oncology nurses. Journal of Clinical Oncology, 30:2538–2544.

Pilch JJ (2000). Healing in the New Testament. Minneapolis, MN: Fortress Press.

Preston JL, Ritter RS, Hernandez JI. (2010). Principles of religious prosociality: A review and reformulation. Social and Personality Psychology Compass 4(8):574–590.

Preston JL, Ritter RS. (2013). Different effects of religion and God on prosociality with the ingroup and outgroup. Personality and Social Psychology Bulletin, 39:1471–1483.

Puchalski CM, Rumbold B, Cobb M, Zollfrank A, Garlid CF. (2012). Curriculum development, courses, and CPE. In CM Puchalski, M Cobb, B Rumbold B, eds., Oxford Textbook of Spirituality in Healthcare, New York, London: Oxford University Press,.

Puchalski CM. (2004). The FICA spiritual history tool. Journal of Palliative Medicine, 17(1):105–106.

Puchalski CM, Blatt B, Kogan M, Butler A. (2014). Spirituality and health: The development of a field. Academic Medicine, 89(1):10–16.

Putnam RD, Campbell DE. (2012). American Grace. New York: Simon & Schuster.

Rahman F. (1987). Health and Medicine in the Islamic Tradition: Change and Identity. New York: Crossroad Publishers.

Rasic DT, Belik SL, Elias B, Katz LY, Enns M, Sareen J. (2009). Spirituality, religion and suicidal behavior in a nationally representative sample. Journal of Affective Disorders, 114:32–40.

Roberts L, Ahmed I, Hall S. (2000). Intercessory prayer for the alleviation of ill health. Cochrane Database of Systematic Reviews 2000, Issue 2.

Roberts L, Ahmed I, Hall S. (2007). Intercessory prayer for the alleviation of ill health. Cochrane Database of Systematic Reviews 2007, Issue 1.

Roberts L, Ahmed I, Hall S, Davison A. (2009). Intercessory prayer for the alleviation of ill health. The Cochrane Library 2009, Issue 3.

Robins JM, Hernán M, Brumback B. (2000). Marginal structural models and causal inference in epidemiology. Epidemiology, 11(5);550–560.

Rogers RG. (1996). The effects of family composition, health, and social support linkages on mortality. Journal of Health and Social Behavior, 37(4);326–338.

Rye MS, Pargament KI, Pan W, Yingling DW, Shogren KA, Ito M. (2005). Can group interventions facilitate forgiveness of an ex-spouse? A randomized clinical trial. Journal of Consulting and Clinical Psychology, Oct;73(5):880–892.

Saint John of the Cross. (1585). The Dark Night of the Soul.

Sanua VD. (1969). Religion, mental health, and personality: A review of empirical studies. American Journal of Psychiatry, 125:1203–1213.

Schnall E, Wassertheil-Smoller S, Swencionis C, et al. (2010). The relationship between religion and cardiovascular outcomes and all-cause mortality in the Women's Health Initiative Observational Study. Psychology and Health, 25(2):249–263.

Shariff AF, Willard, AK, Andersen T, Norenzayan A. (2016). Religious priming: A meta-analysis with a focus on prosociality. Personality and Social Psychology Review 20(1):27–48.

Sherman LW, Strang H, Angel C, Woods D, Barnes GC, Bennett S, Inkpen N. (2005). Effects of face-to-face restorative justice on victims of crime in four randomized, controlled trials. Journal of Experimental Criminology 1:367–395.

Shuman JJ, Meador KG. (2003). Heal Thyself: Spirituality, Medicine, and the Distortion of Christianity. New York: Oxford University Press.

Sloan RP, Bagiella E, Powell T. (1999). Religion, spirituality, and medicine. Lancet, 353(9153):664–667.

Sloan RP, Bagiella E, VandeCreek L, et al. (2000). Should physicians prescribe religious activities? New England Journal of Medicine, 342:1913–1916.

Smith D. (1986). Health and Medicine in the Anglican Tradition: Conscience, Community, and Compromise. New York: Crossroad Publishing.

Smith TB, ME McCullough ME, and Poll J. (2003). Religiousness and depression: Evidence fora main effect and the moderating influence of stressful life events. Psychological Bulletin 129(4): 614–636.

Sorenson AM, Grindstaff CF, Turner RJ. (1995). Religious involvement among unmarried adolescent mothers: A source of emotional support? Sociology of Religion, 56:71–81.

Spoerri A, Zwahlen M, Bopp M, Gutzwiller F, Egger M.; Swiss National Cohort Study. (2010). Religion and assisted and non-assisted suicide in Switzerland: National Cohort Study. International Journal of Epidemiology, 39(6):1486–1494.

Staub E, Pearlman LA, Gubin A, Hagengimana A. (2005). Healing, reconciliation, forgiving and the prevention of violence after genocide or mass killing: An intervention and its experimental evaluation in Rwanda. Journal of Social and Clinical Psychology, 24:297–334.

Steinhauer KE, Christakis EC, Clipp EC, et al. (2000). Factors considered important at the end of life by patients, family, physicians, and other care providers. Journal of the American Medical Association, 284:2476–2482.

Strawbridge WJ, Cohen RD, Shema SJ, Kaplan GA. (1997). Frequent attendance at religious services and mortality over 28 years. American Journal of Public Health, 87(6):957–961.

Strawbridge W J, Shema SJ, Cohen RD, Kaplan GA. (2001). Religious attendance increases survival by improving and maintaining good health behaviors, mental health, and social relationships. Annals of Behavioral Medicine 23(1): 68–74.

Sullivan LE (1989). Healing and Restoring: Health and Medicine in the World's Religious Traditions. New York: Macmillan.

Sulmasy DP. (2009). The Rebirth of the Clinic: An Introduction to Spirituality in Health Care. Washington, DC. Georgetown University Press, 2009.

Sweet L. (1994). Health and Medicine in the Evangelical Tradition: "Not by Might Nor Power." Philadelphia, PA: Trinity Press International.

Teinonen T, Vahlberg T, Isoaho R, Kivela SL. (2005). Religious attendance and 12-year survival in older persons. Age and Ageing 34(4): 406–409.

Thompson, LY, Snyder CR, Hoffman L, Michael ST, Rasmussen HN, Billings LS, . . .Roberts DE. (2005). Dispositional forgiveness of self, others, and situations. Journal of Personality 73: 313–359.

Thompson MP, Ho CH, Kingree JB. (2007). Prospective associations between delinquency and suicidal behaviors in a nationally representative sample. Journal of Adolescent Health, 40(3):232–237.

Toussaint LL, Worthington EL, Williams DR. (2015). Forgiveness and Health. New York: Springer.

Trinitapoli J, Weinreb A. (2012). Religion and AIDS in Africa. New York: Oxford University Press.

Tutu, D. (2000). No Future Without Forgiveness. New York: Image.

Underwood LG (2011). The daily spiritual experience scale: Overview and results. Religions, 2:29–50.

Underwood LG, Teresi JA. (2002). The daily spiritual experience scale: Development, theoretical description, reliability, exploratory factor analysis, and preliminary construct validity using health-related data. Annals of Behavioral Medicine 24(1): 22–33.

VanderWeele TJ. (2013). Re: "Religious service attendance and major depression: a case of reverse causality?" American Journal of Epidemiology, 177(3):275–276.

VanderWeele TJ (2015). Explanation in Causal Inference: Methods for Mediation and Interaction. New York: Oxford University Press.

VanderWeele TJ, Li S, Tsai A, Kawachi I. (2016a). Association between religious service attendance and lower suicide rates among US women. JAMA Psychiatry, 73:845-851.

VanderWeele TJ, Yu J, Cozier YC, Wise L, Rosenberg L, Shields AE, Palmer JR. (2016b). Religious service attendance, prayer, religious coping, and religious-spiritual identity as predictors of all-cause mortality in the Black Women's Health Study. American Journal of Epidemiology, 03 March 2017; DOI: https://doi.org/10.1093/aje/kww179.

VanderWeele TJ, Jackson JW, Li S. (2016c). Causal inference and time-varying exposures: A case study of religion and mental health. Social Psychiatry and Psychiatric Epidemiology, 51:1457–1466.

Van Ness PH. (1999). Religion and public health. Journal of Religion and Health, 38:15–26.

Van Ness PH. (2013). Religion, public health, and the revaluation of risk. HSPH Lecture Series on Religion and Health March 29, 2013. http://webapps.sph.harvard.edu/accordentG3/episeminar-20130329/main.htm?layout=default&type=ms&archived=visible&bandwidth=high&audioonly=no

Van Voorhees BW, Paunesku D, Kuwabara SA, et al. (2008). Protective and vulnerability factors predicting new-onset depressive episode in a representative of U.S. adolescents. Journal of Adolescent Health, 42(6):605–616.

Vaux KL. (1984). Health and Medicine in the Reformed Tradition: Promise, Providence, and Care. New York: Crossroad Publishing.

Vitz PC, Meade JM. (2011). Self-forgiveness in psychology and psychotherapy: A critique. Journal of Religion and Health, 50:248–263.

Wade NG, Hoyt WT, Kidwell JE, Worthington EL. (2014). Efficacy of psychotherapeutic interventions to promote forgiveness: A meta-analysis. Journal of Consulting and Clinical Psychology, 82:154–170.

Waltman MA, Russell DC, Coyle CT, Enright RD, Holter AC, Swoboda CM. (2009). The effects of a forgiveness intervention on patients with coronary artery disease. Psychology and Health, 24:11–27.

Wilkinson J. (1998). The Bible and Healing. Grand Rapid, MI: WM. B. Eerdmans Publishing.

Winkelman WD, Lauderdale K, Balboni MJ, Phelps AC, Block SD, VanderWeele TJ, Balboni TA (2011). The relationship of spiritual concerns to the quality of life of advanced cancer patients. Journal of Palliative Medicine, 14:1022–1028.

World Health Association. (1948). Preamble to the constitution of the World Health Organization. In International Health Conference (Official records of the World Health Organization, no. 2, p. 100). New York, NY: World Health Association.

World Health Organization. (2004). Palliative care: Symptom management and end of life care. Integrated management of adolescent and adult illness. Available from http://www.who.int/hiv/pub/imai/generic-palliativecare02004.pdf. Accessed March 15, 2014.

Worthington E.L Jr. (2001). How can I ever forgive? Catholic Digest, 65 (7), 34–43.

Worthington EL. (2005). Handbook of Forgiveness. New York: Brunner-Routledge.

Worthington EL. (2006). Forgiveness and Reconciliation: Theory and Application. New York: Routledge.

Worthington EL, Davis DE, Hook JN, Van Tongeren DR, Gartner AL, Jennings II DJ, Greer CL, Lin Y. Religion and spirituality and forgiveness. (2013). In R Paloutzian, C Park, eds., Handbook of Religion and Spirituality, 2nd ed. New York: Guilford Press, pp. 476–497.

Yeager D, Glei DA, Au M, Lin H-S, Sloan RP, and Weinstein M. (2006). "Religious involvement and health outcomes among older persons in Taiwan. Social Science and Medicine 63(8):2228–2241.

Young R, Sweeting H, Ellaway A. (2011). Do schools differ in suicide risk? The influence of school and neighbourhood on attempted suicide, suicidal ideation and self-harm among secondary school. BMC Public Health, 11:874.

Zollfrank AA, Trevino KM, Cadge W, Balboni MJ, Thiel MM, Fitchett G., . . . Balboni TA. (2015). Teaching healthcare providers to provide spiritual care: A pilot study. Journal of Palliative Medicine, 18:408–414.

INDEX

Grossoehme, D. H., 39, 45
GTRR. *See* GWish-Templeton Reflection Rounds
guidelines, 152, 200–204, 202*t*–203*t*
Gustafson, James, 269, 269n1
Gutenberg, Johannes, 313
GWish. *See* George Washington Institute for
    Spirituality and Health
GWish-Templeton Reflection Rounds (GTRR),
    201, 208
gynecology. *See* obstetrics and gynecology

Halakhah, 188–89
Hall, Daniel E., 85, 283, 285, 337n7
Hamberg, Katarina, 328
Hammonds, Clare, 271
Handbook of Religion and Health (Koenig et al.),
    110, 369
*Handbook (of) Patients' Spiritual and Cultural Values
    for Health Care Professionals* (Healthcare
    Chaplaincy Network), 93
Hardt, John, 350
Hart, D., 42
*Harvard Initiative on Health, Religion, and
    Spirituality*, 2
Harvard Medical School, 206, 210
Hauerwas, Stanley, 349
healing
    biblical traditions with religion, health
        and, 381–84
    energy, 154
    holistic, 319
    miracles, 93
health, 110, 196, 211, 240, 362, 368, 369, 370.
        See also George Washington Institute for
        Spirituality and Health; mental health;
        physical health; religion, health and;
        reproductive health
    of African American women with spirituality, 81
    behaviors with gerontology, 115
    biblical traditions with healing, religion,
        and, 381–84
    defined, 389
    family medicine with evidence base of, 52–53
    forgiveness and, 371–73
    medical education with national competency
        behaviors in spirituality and, 202*t*–203*t*
    NIH, 266
    outcomes with research on religion and, 366–67
    religion and benefits for, 216–17
    religious objections to research on religion
        and, 385–86
    R/S measures and, 365–66
    world religions and, 381

health care, 16, 201, 206. *See also* reproductive health
    by religious and faith-based institutions, 374–75
    sexual and reproductive, 182–84
    spirituality of practice within, 60–61
    theology and, 343–52
Healthcare Chaplaincy Network, 93
health care providers
    best practices for family physicians, 59–60
    pediatrics, 37–38, 41–45
health care providers, OBG
    best practices for, 24–29
    reflections for non-religious, 27
    reflections for religious, 25–27
    research, religion of, 22–23
health services frameworks, 54, 56
Heaton, T. B., 368
Hellenistic period (323–30 B.C.), 307
Henderson, Lawrence J., 264
herbal remedies, 318
The Hero with a Thousand Faces (Campbell,
    J.), 270–71
Hexem, K. R., 45
Hiatt, John, 326–27
Hight, E., 85–86
Hill, Bradford, 328
Hinduism, 16, 23, 117, 247, 357
Hippocrates (c. 460–380 B.C.), 306, 310, 312
Hippocratic Corpus, 306–7, 310
Hippocratic Oath, 209, 307, 310–11
HIV/AIDS, 97, 248, 351, 365, 375, 388
Hmong people, 25, 287
Hobby Lobby, 233, 296, 298
holism
    carcinogenesis and, 336n3
    defined, 329
    dimensions of personhood assuming, 330*f*
    parts to whole relationship and, 329*f*
    role of, 336n4
holistic healing, spiritual influences and, 319
Holmgren, M. R., 384–85
Homer, 306
HOPE spiritual assessment tool, 85–86, 174,
    207, 334
Horden, Peregrine, 309
Hospice Conditions of Participation Final Report
    (CMS), 56
hospices, 52, 56, 320, 348, 351
hospital chaplains, 6, 25
"hospitalists," 79
hospitalization, isolation with, 36
hospitals, 2, 98, 345
    Arabic medicine and, 311, 346
    Christianity and, 310, 313–15, 346

founding of first, 309
in Middle Ages, 310, 313
reorganization, 316–17
role of, 314–15
"houses for strangers" (*xenodocheia*), 309, 345
Houskamp, B. M., 42
Hull House, 350
human anatomy cadaver donors, memorial services
for, 209
human condition, spirituality and, 320–21
human experience, immaterial dimension of, 4–5
Hummer, R. A., 359, 360, 369
humoral theory, 307
Hunter, John, 314
Hunter, William, 314
hypertension, 111
Ibn Sina, 312

ICUs. *See* intensive care units
Idler, Ellen L., 268, 271
Iliad (Homer), 306
illness, 131, 134, 189, 211
children with drawings of, 44*f*
disease, 110–11, 120, 148–49, 276, 307
disorientation of, 219–20, 223
medicine and spirituality with meaning of, 305–6
as narrative, 217–18, 270
narratives, case studies, 222–28
reclaiming and framing, 51–52
reorientation, 218–19, 224
Ultimate Reality of, 381
Illness Narratives (Kleinman), 277
immaterial dimension, of human experience, 4–5
Immigration and Nationality Act of 1965, 275
"incompatibility thesis," 294
"indirect" referrals, 28
infertility, reproductive health, 22
Institute for Spirituality and Health, Texas Medical
Center, 2
Institute for the Study of Health & Illness
(ISHI), 211
Institute of Medicine (IOM), 52–53, 101–2
"institutionalized spirituality," 281
intensive care units (ICUs)
best practices, 173–75
challenges to therapeutic alliance, 167
chaplains in, 98, 171, 175
clinicians with R/S in, 171–72
culture of, 165–68
family stresses and surrogate decision
making, 167–68
with mortality, high, 165–66
PICU, 37

with prognostic uncertainty and unaligned
expectations, 166–67
R/S, miracle language, 169–71
R/S, visible and invisible, 167–68
intercessory prayer (IP)
dying and, 52
role of, 55
"subtle energies" of, 329
surgery and, 94
internal medicine
arguments, conceptual, 85–87
best practices for, 87–89
evidence, empirical, 80–85
patient perspective, 80–82
physician perspective, 82–85
physicians, practicing, 83–85
research, future, 89
R/S and patient-clinician relationship, 89–90
scenarios, common, 79–80
trainees in, 82–83
interventions
evaluations with medical education and teaching
methods, 204–6
forgiveness, 376
palliative care, 53
psychiatry, 68, 71–72
psycho-spiritual, 245–48
with religion and health, 373–80
religious settings and health promotion, 374
service attendance, 378–79
interviews, after-death, 55
IOM. *See* Institute of Medicine
IP. *See* intercessory prayer
Ironson, G., 365
ISHI. *See* Institute for the Study
of Health & Illness
Islam, 345. *See also* Arabic medicine; Muslims
isolation, with hospitalization, 36
Israel, 21, 360

Jehovah's Witness, 80, 88, 96, 280
Jews, 16, 188–89, 192n3, 341, 357
abortion and Israeli, 21
EOL and, 185
sexuality and, 17
Shema prayer and, 343–44
suicide and, 73
Johnson, Diane, 142
John Templeton Foundation, 2
Joint Commission, 1, 52, 59, 102–3, 149
Judaism, 16, 357
Julian (Roman Emperor), 344–45, 350
Jung, Carl, 280

theory, science and, 336n6

Thompson, M. P., 364

Thoresen, Carl, 328–29

Thucydides, 308

Tibetan medicine, 280, 318

Tilburt, J. C., 188

Tillich, Paul, 3–4, 5

Title VII. *See* Civil Rights Act of 1964, Title VII of

Tonascia, J. A., 359

touch, pediatrics health care providers with, 43

traditional Chinese medicine (TCM), 318

trainees, in internal medicine, 82–83

training

    for Arabic medicine, 312

    in ICUs, best practices, 174, 175

    medical professionals with spiritual
        care, 152–53

    science in pediatrics and need for, 38–39

    spiritual care, need for, 244–45

"trait forgiveness," 372

"transfer of care," 28

trauma, surgery, 94–95

treatment

    mental health and interactions with, 119

    of patients, spiritual influences on, 155–56

    physical health and interactions
        with, 121–222

    religion and life-sustaining, 96

Treloar, L. L., 80

Truth and Reconciliation Commission, South
    Africa, 375

Tuke, William, 320

Turner, Victor, 279

Uganda, 375

ultimate concern, religion and, 3–4, 5

Ultimate Reality, 381

United Kingdom, 79, 200, 205, 319

University of Chicago, 2, 211

University of North Carolina at Chapel Hill, 54

University of Pennsylvania, 51

University of South Carolina Psychiatry
    Residency, 208

USA Weekend, 56

U.S. Supreme Court, 298

Vaillant, G., 66

VanderWeele, T. J., 365, 368, 370

Vanier, Jean, 351–52

Van Ness, P. H., 4, 388

Van Voorhees, B. W., 362

Vaux, K. L., 384

Vesalius, Andreas, 313

Walco, G. A., 39–40

Wald, Florence, 320

Walker, Matthew, 94

Wehtje-Winslow, B. J., 86

Weldon Amendment, 299

well-being, 131, 134

    mental health and, 110

    R/S and, 367–68

Wesley, John, 276

White, Katherine, 296

White Coat Ceremony, 209

Wicclair, Mark, 294–95

Wilkinson, J., 381

Winkelman, W. D., 150

Winslow, G. R., 86

Wisconsin Longitudinal Study, 115

Wisconsin v. Yoder (1972), 298

women, 21, 81, 365. *See also* obstetrics and
    gynecology

    medical profession and role of, 1–2

    R/S and, 16–17

Women's Health Initiative data, 366–67

World Health Organization, 149, 389

world religions, religion and health in, 381

Worthington, E. L., 373

Wuthnow, Robert, 60

xenodocheia ("houses for strangers," first hospitals),
    309, 345

Yale University, 2

Yates, F. D., 43, 45

Yi, M. S., 82–83

yoga, 245, 276

Zen, 350

Zilboorg, Gregory, 66